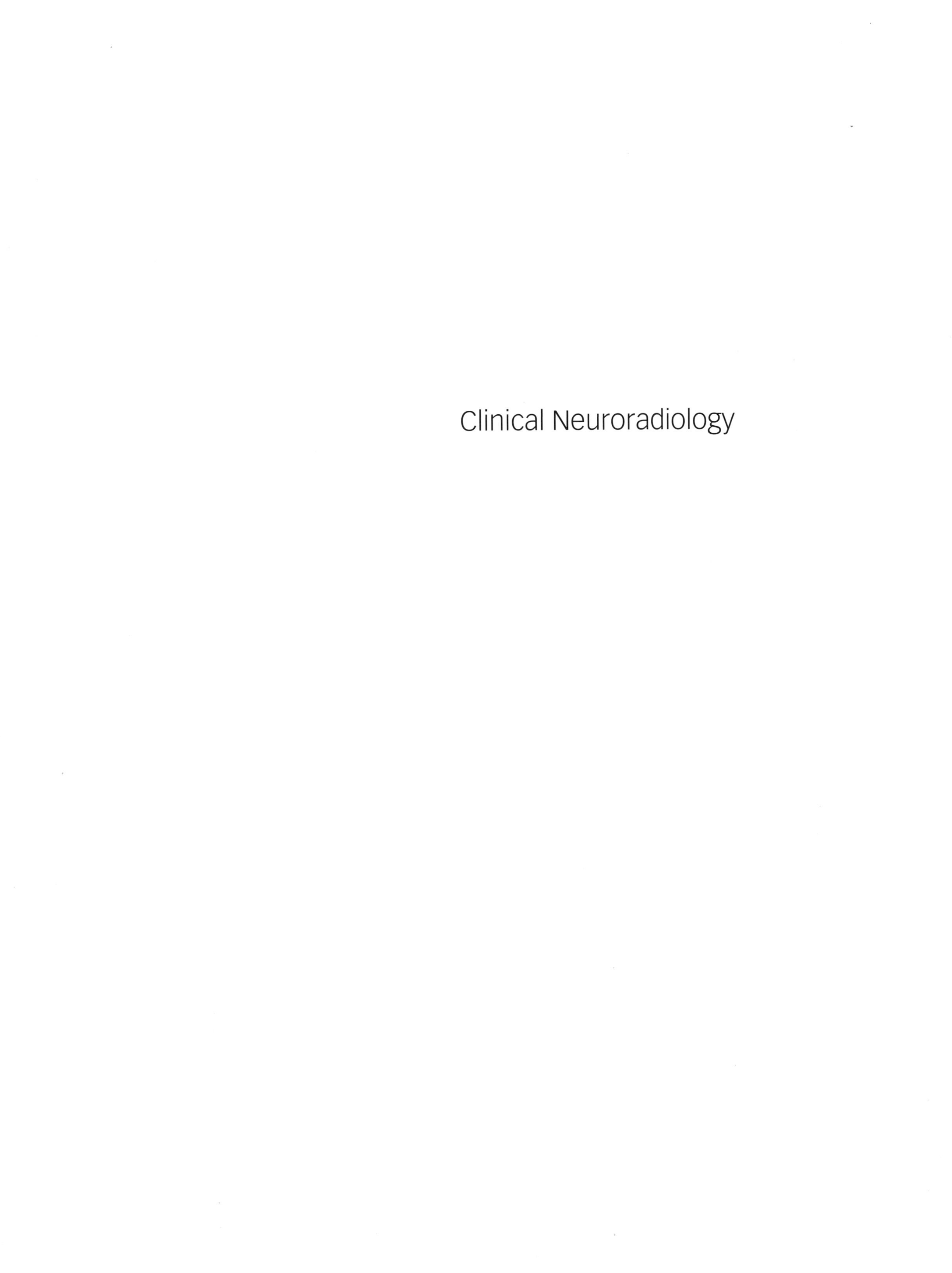

Clinical Neuroradiology

Clinical Neuroradiology

A Case Based Approach

By

GASSER M. HATHOUT

Illustrated by

TANYA FERGUSON

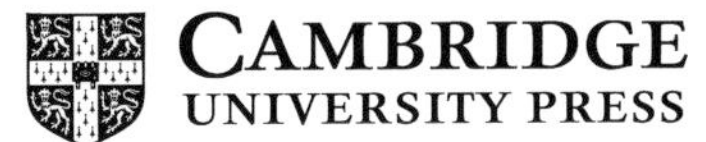

CAMBRIDGE
UNIVERSITY PRESS

CAMBRIDGE UNIVERSITY PRESS
Cambridge, New York, Melbourne, Madrid, Cape Town, Singapore,
São Paulo, Delhi

Cambridge University Press
The Edinburgh Building, Cambridge CB2 8RU, UK

Published in the United States of America by Cambridge University
Press, New York

www.cambridge.org
Information on this title: www.cambridge.org/9780521600545

First published 2009

Printed in the United Kingdom at the University Press, Cambridge

A catalog record for this publication is available from the British Library

Library of Congress Cataloging in Publication data
Hathout, Gasser M., 1963–
Clinical neuroradiology : a case based approach / by Gasser M.
Hathout; illustrated by Tanya Ferguson.
     p.   ;   cm.
Includes bibliographical references and index.
ISBN 978-0-521-60054-5
1. Brain – Radiography – Case studies.   2. Brain – Imaging – Case
studies.   I. Title.
[DNLM: 1. Brain Diseases – diagnosis.
2. Brain – anatomy & histology.   3. Diagnostic Imaging.   WL 141
H364c 2008]
RC386.6.R3H38   2008
616.8′047572–dc22

                                                        2008025553

ISBN 978-0-521-60054-5 hardback

To my parents, with boundless love and limitless gratitude. I owe you a debt I can never repay.

Contents

Color plates will be found between p. xii and p. 1.

Preface

One of my early mentors in radiology told me the following aphorism: "You see what you look for, and you look for what you know." In the past two decades, the increasing spatial and contrast resolution of modern imaging techniques has vastly expanded the scope of what we can see, and hence, of what we must know. The past dozen years of teaching radiology residents, neurology residents, and neuroradiology fellows has convinced me that this is particularly true in neuroimaging, and applies both to the depth and the scope of our requisite knowledge base. The ability of MRI to show precise neuroanatomical details has made the practices of neurology and neuroradiology more intertwined than ever before. This, in turn, makes it necessary for neuroradiologists to learn more neurology and for neurologists to learn more neuroradiology than practitioners of a generation ago.

This book seeks to fulfill that aim. Focusing on the intersection between these two closely related specialties, it attempts to bridge a gap sometimes found in the many excellent standard textbooks in both fields – an insufficient stress on the overlap between them. To give a rudimentary example, when a neurologist comes down to radiology stating that he has a patient with internuclear ophthalmoplegia (INO), the neuroradiologist needs to recognize the syndrome, understand its underlying neuroanatomic substratum, and look carefully in the brainstem tegmentum for the small lesion involving the medial longitudinal fasciculus which might otherwise be missed. Conversely, when a neuroradiologist proclaims to his neurology colleagues that a parkinsonian patient's MRI scan shows the stigmata of multiple system atrophy (MSA), they would like to be familiar enough with the particulars of MRI to recognize those stigmata. Thus, this book attempts to provide imaging correlates for typical cases seen in neurology and clinical correlates for the findings made with neuroimaging.

The book is divided into individual chapters, from the cerebellum through the brainstem, diencephalon, basal ganglia, and cortex. Each chapter provides a discussion of the clinically relevant neuroanatomy of that part of the brain. Following this introductory discussion, structure–function correlations in the CNS are illustrated through consideration of actual clinical cases. The cases are presented in an interactive question–answer "noon conference" format, leading from the clinical history to a presentation of imaging findings and a discussion of the relationship between those findings and the patient's clinical deficits. This format allows neuroanatomical details to take on an immediate clinical relevance, thus making them easier to remember, and also allows the clinician to appreciate the elegance and specificity of modern neuroimaging. By its very nature – i.e., a case-based approach – this is not meant to be a comprehensive text. However, it attempts to present many of the common entities seen in a hospital-based neurology practice in some detail, and to enhance these presentations with discussions of the relevant neuronal circuitry, pertinent neurochemistry and sometimes the basic therapeutic approaches to particular syndromes of the CNS. Since many of the structure–function correlations we discuss are best displayed with stroke cases, the book ends with a detailed chapter on imaging in stroke and the role of imaging in stroke therapy.

As you read through the book, you will notice that I have tried to keep it light-hearted and informal in style, with sporadic attempts at humor which I hope will be neither feeble nor offensive. If they are either, or both, please accept my apologies in advance.

I need to credit several individuals for their help, and to thank others for their support. For the most part, I will do that in the Acknowledgments section, as is customary. Here, however, I must both thank and credit Dr. Tanya Ferguson for her invaluable help. She not only provided the many excellent neuroanatomical illustrations, which are the crux of the structure–function correlations, but also edited the midbrain chapter and helped edit the neuroanatomy sections throughout the book, keeping me honest with her exquisite knowledge of neuroanatomy. The manuscript is better for her participation.

Acknowledgments

I would like to credit my friend and colleague Dr. Michael Waters for writing a wonderful midbrain chapter, thus helping me when time was short. I must also credit Dr. Roongroj Bhidayasiri for his assistance in the early stages of this project, both in helping to conceptualize it and in helping to get it off the ground. Of course, I must also credit my absolutely wonderful publishers and editors at Cambridge University Press, Deborah Russell and Katie James, Mary Sanders, and most especially, Dawn Preston. It was truly a pleasure working with them, and their indulgence throughout this process is sincerely appreciated.

In terms of thanks, I owe a debt of gratitude to many. Especially deserving of my thanks is my friend and colleague Dr. Suzie El-Saden. She has been very generous in always trying to provide me opportunities to work on this book, and equally generous in providing me with some excellent cases. My sincerest thanks also go to Dr. Noriko Salamon and Dr. Whitney Pope of the UCLA Division of Neuroradiology for generously providing me with several excellent cases, and for their enthusiasm and friendship. The same goes for Dr. Ashok Panigrahy of the Los Angeles Children's Hospital. Additionally, I thank Dr. Suzie Bash for her enthusiastic support and positive feedback at the inception of this project. I also wish to thank all of the residents and fellows at UCLA who have allowed me the privilege of teaching them, and learning with them, over these many years. Finally, I must thank my loving (and beautiful) wife Mona and my lovely children for their support, encouragement, and forbearance during all the evenings and weekends which this project took.

References

At the end of many case discussions, I have provided one or several references, which serve both as footnotes for some of the cited facts and as sources for further reading on particular topics. At this juncture, though, I would like to credit several excellent sources which I have heavily relied on throughout the writing of this book. This makes more sense than referencing them again and again at the end of each case. Those sources are:

Afifi, A. K. and Bergman, R. A. *Functional Neuroanatomy: Text and Atlas.* 1998, McGraw-Hill Companies, Inc.

Baehr, M., and Frotscher, M. *Duus' Topical Diagnosis in Neurology.* 2005, Thième Publishers.

Blumenfeld, H. *Neuroanatomy Through Clinical Cases.* 2002, Sinauer Associates, Inc.

Nolte, J. *The Human Brain: An Introduction to Its Functional Neuroanatomy*, 5th edn. 2002, Mosby, Inc.

Victor, M. and Ropper, A. *Adams and Victor's Principles of Neurology*, 7th edn. 2001, McGraw-Hill Inc.

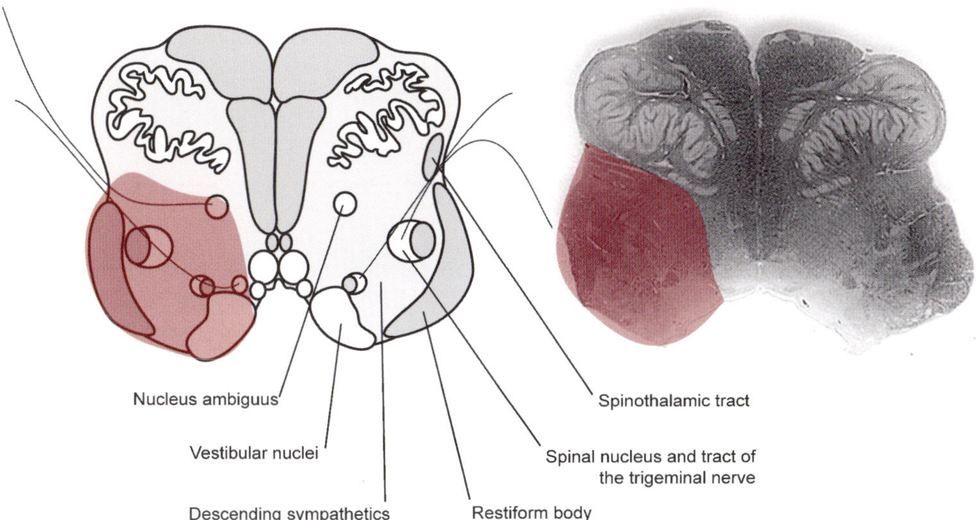

Fig. 2.16. **Schematic diagram of brainstem structures involved in Wallenberg's syndrome.**

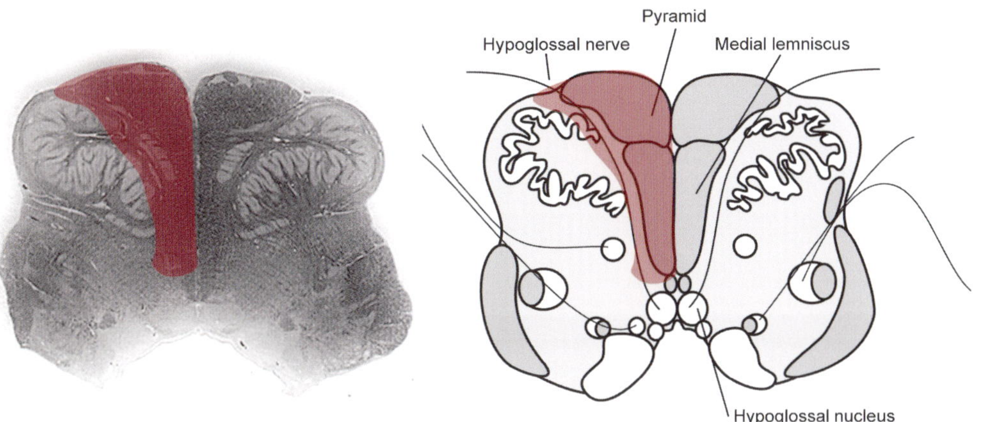

Fig. 2.19. **Schematic diagram of the structures involved in Dejerine's syndrome.**

Fig. 3.44. **Schematic diagram showing the blood supply of the pons.**

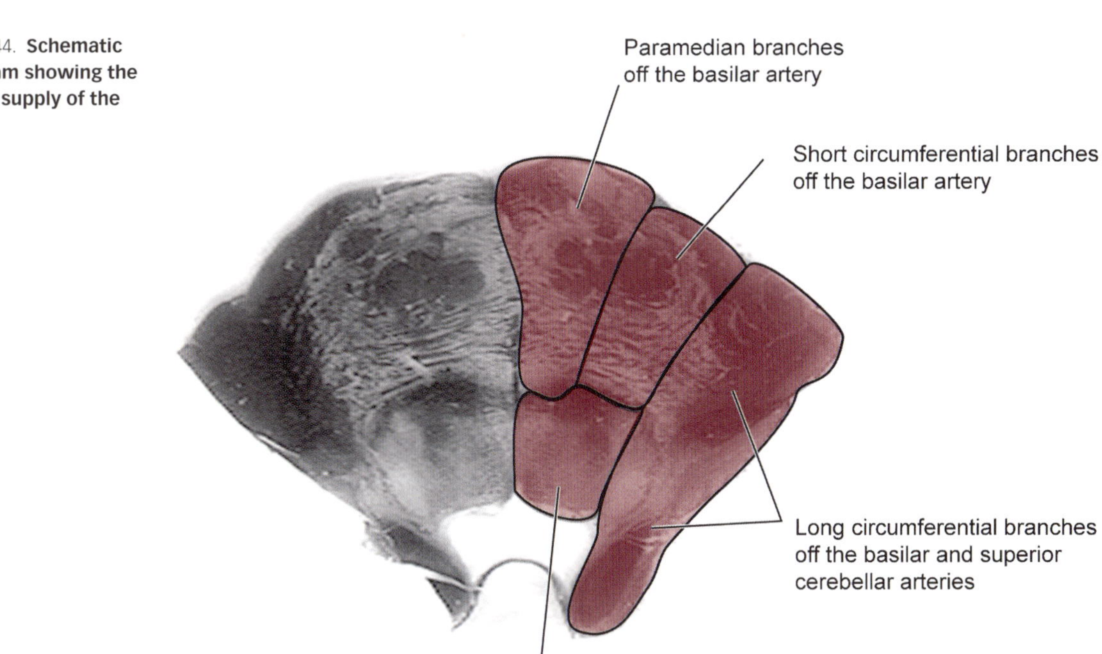

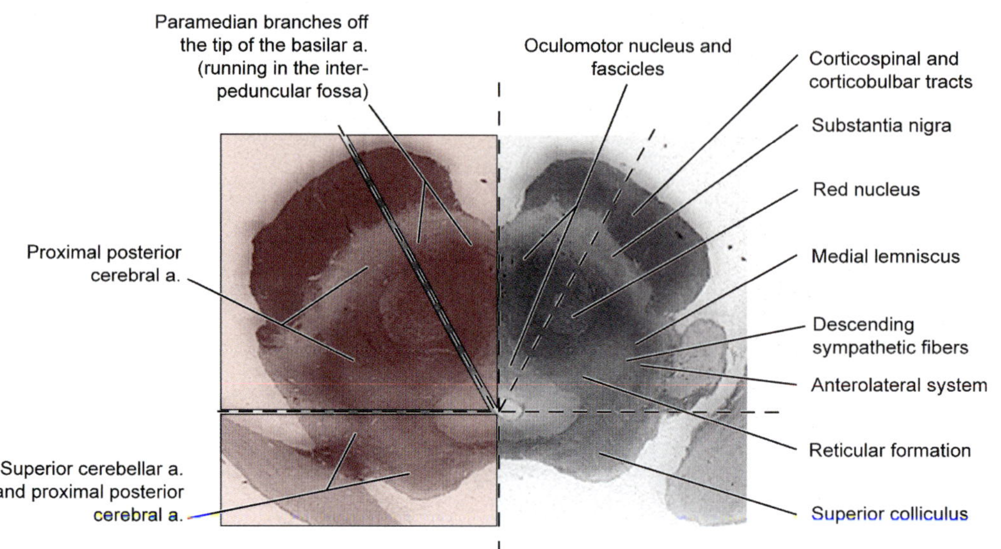

Fig. 4.10. **Vascular distribution of the midbrain.**

Fig. 5.23a. **Fluorodeoxyglucose PET scans at the level of the striatum our patient.**

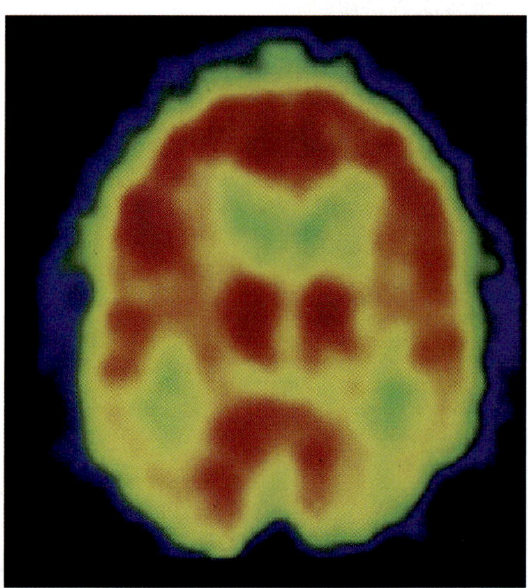

Fig. 5.23b. **Fluorodeoxyglucose PET scans at the level of the striatum with normal control.**

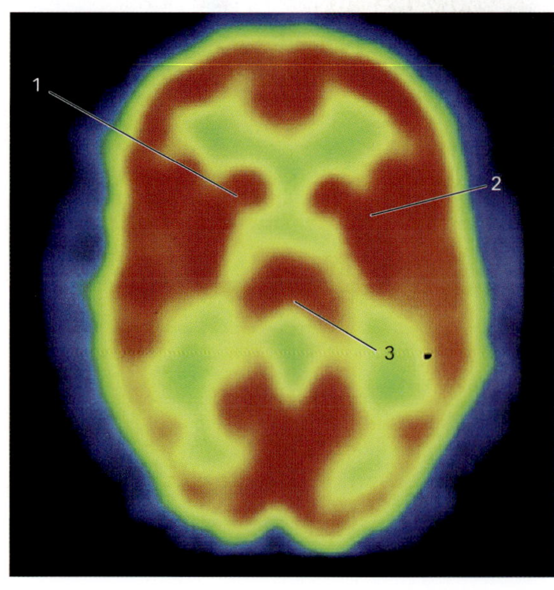

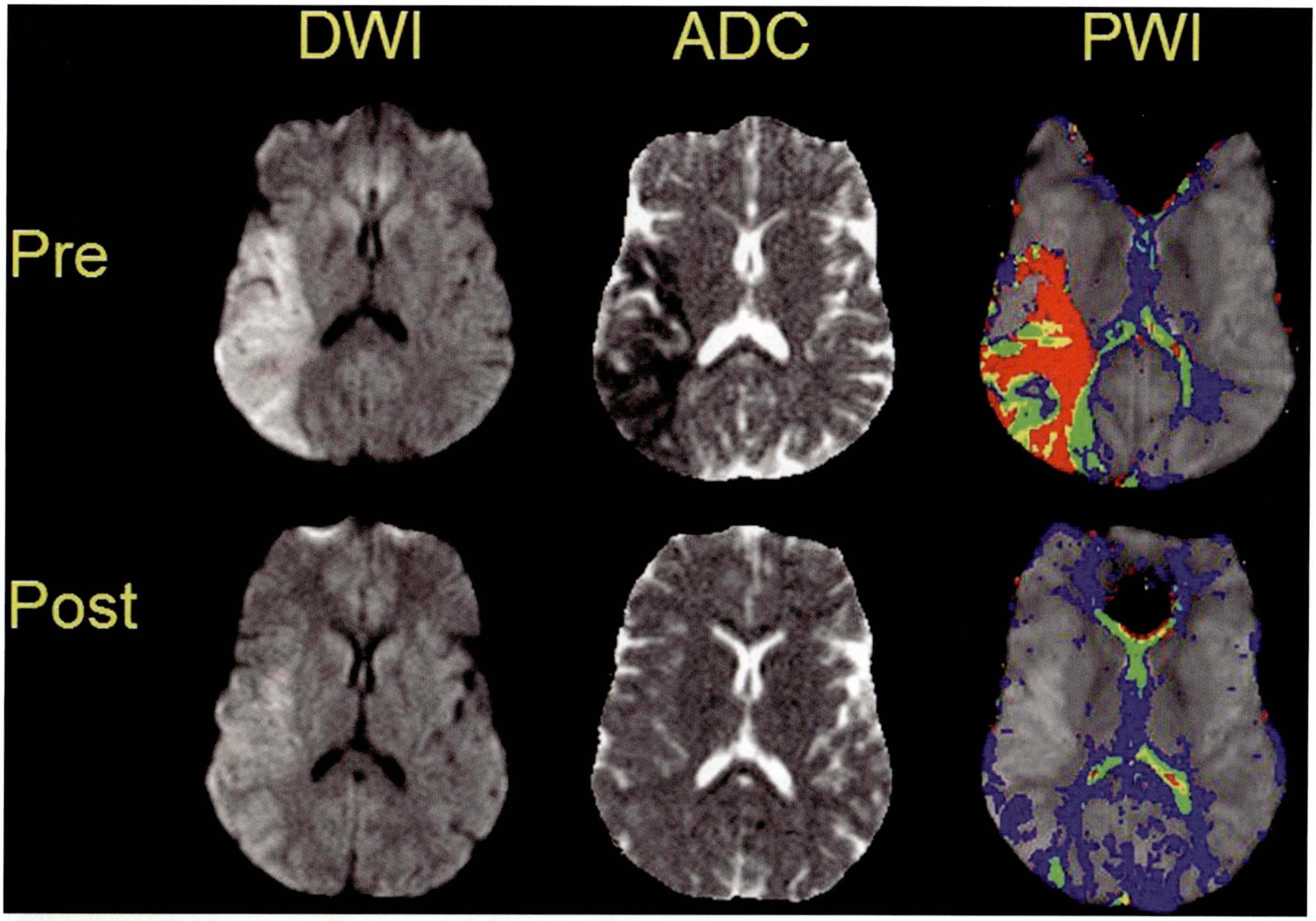

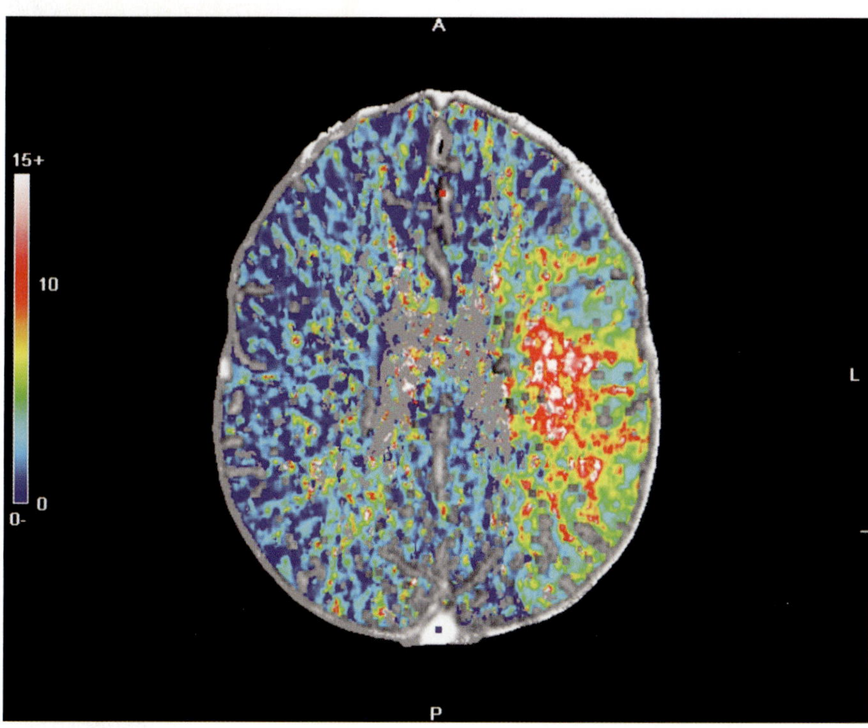

Fig. 8.33. **Pre- and post-thrombolysis images of a patient with right MCA infarct. The pre-treatment images show a matched DWI–PWI defect. Post-treatment, both the PWI and the DWI abnormalities have resolved. (Image courtesy of Dr. Michael Waters, Director of the Stroke Progam, Cedars-Sinai Medical Center, Los Angeles, CA.)**

Fig. 8.38c. **CT perfusion study in a patient with recurrent TIAs, but without acute infarct. MTT image shows a clearly prolonged MTT in the left MCA territory consistent with hypoperfusion. CT can also provide direct quantitation for specified regions of interest.**

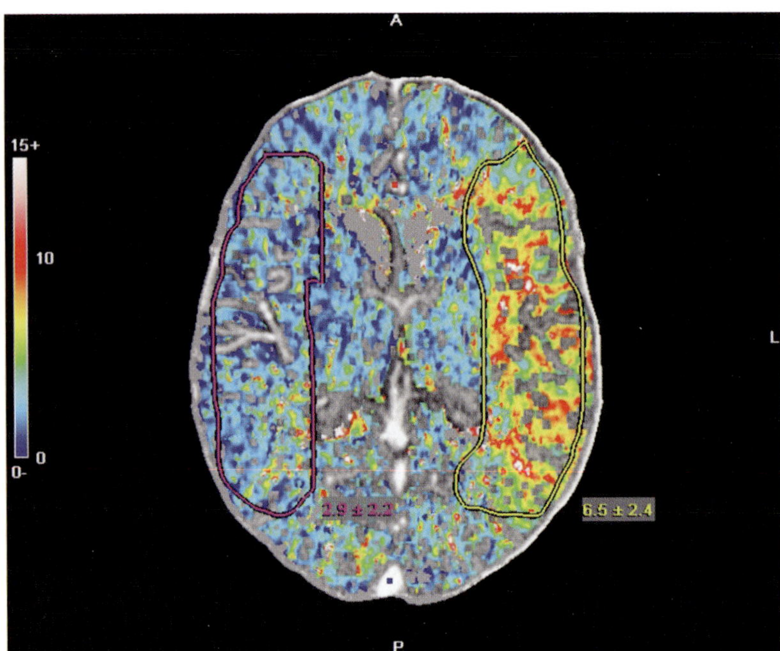

Fig. 8.38d. **CT perfusion study in a patient with recurrent TIAs, but without acute infarct.** Quantitative MTT estimates show an MTT of 2.9 seconds on the right, and a markedly prolonged MTT of 6.5 seconds on the left.

Fig. 8.38e. **CT perfusion study in a patient with recurrent TIAs, but without acute infarct.** Quantitative CBF mapping shows a normal CBF of 64 ml/100 g per min on the right, and a significant reduction to 29 ml/100 g per min on the left.

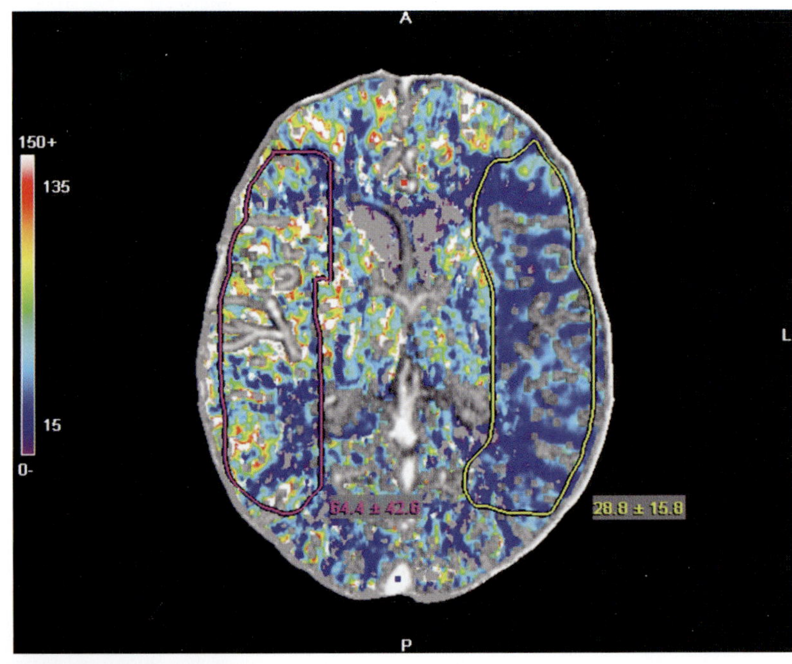

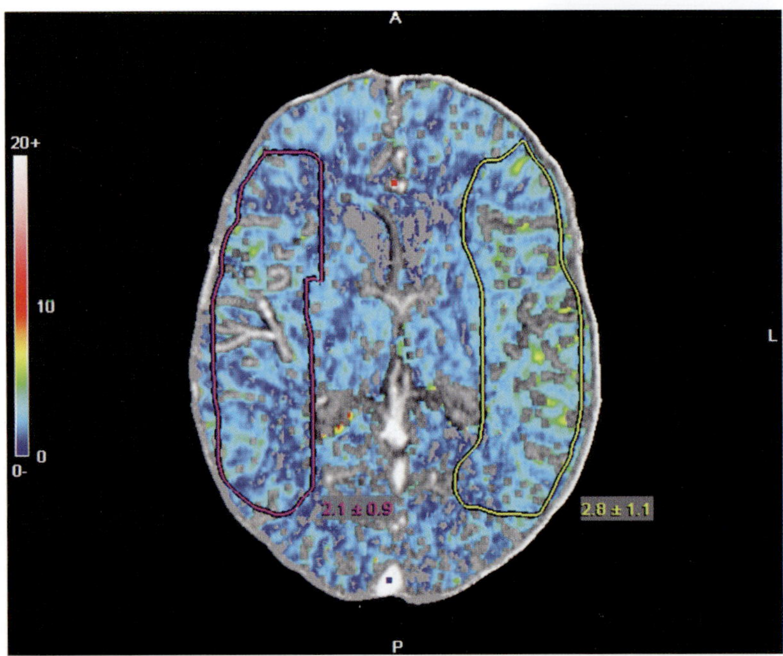

Fig. 8.38f. **CT perfusion study in a patient with recurrent TIAs, but without acute infarct.** The quantitative CBV map shows a value of 2.1 ml/100 g on the right and 2.8 ml/100 g on the left, reflecting the known compensatory increase in CBV in the face of hypoperfusion.

1 | The cerebellum

Introduction

It may come as a surprise to know that the cerebellum (literally "little brain") has nearly as many neurons as the entire cerebrum. While the cerebellum has, at various epochs, been postulated to be the seat of love or of sexual desire in the CNS, we now know that its main function is to assist the primary motor system in the control of motion. This includes helping to control equilibrium, posture, eye movements, and the control of voluntary movements through careful monitoring of their strength, velocity, and trajectory. Recent research is also revealing that the cerebellum may have significant non-motor functions, including some input in cognition.

While neuroanatomists often describe the cerebellum as "simple" in structure, "uniform" may be a better word. Detailed descriptions of the different cell types, neuronal connections, feedback loops between different cell populations, which cells are inhibitory and which are excitatory, etc., is at this time of little clinical significance. This is because, although the cytoarchitecture has been well described, the link between this and how the cerebellum actually performs its functions remains unclear. Therefore, we will give only a brief and necessarily incomplete description of microscopic anatomy, followed by a discussion of cerebellar functional zones, which is clinically more relevant.

Anatomic overview

The cerebellum can be thought of as a white matter core covered by convolutions of gray matter cortex called folia. Imbedded within the white matter core are four pairs of deep cerebellar nuclei, all adjacent to the fourth ventricle (Fig. 1.1). Moving lateral to medial, they are the dentate, emboliform, globose, and fastigial nuclei. The emboliform and globose nuclei are a single functional unit and are therefore often referred to as the interposed nucleus.

The motor and premotor cortex of the cerebrum communicate with the cerebellar cortex regarding planned movements, while essentially all sensory modalities also input into the cerebellar cortex to apprise it regarding the status of movements in progress. The cerebellar cortex processes this very complex information and sends its output to the deep cerebellar nuclei, which communicate back to the cerebral cortex.

Therefore, at heart, the organizational schema seems straightforward: motor cortex to cerebellar cortex to deep cerebellar nuclei back to motor cortex (Fig. 1.2).

We have found, though, that medical students and junior residents are sometimes confused about this basic schema. When asked, "How does the cerebellum help modulate the motion of my finger to touch my nose? Is it by communicating with the anterior motor horn cells of my cervical spinal cord to control my arm muscles or by communicating with my cerebral cortex?", well over half of those asked believe that the cerebellum modulates a finger-to-nose movement by communicating with the spinal cord. However, it actually does so mainly by communicating with the cerebral cortex. There are some indirect communications with the spinal cord through the red nucleus, as well as through the vestibular and reticular nuclei of the brainstem through the vestibulospinal and reticulospinal tracts respectively. These pathways are especially important for automatic functions such as posture, and for programmed movements such as walking.

Cytoarchitecture

So what then is this cerebellar cortex which does all of this processing? It is composed of three cellular layers (Fig. 1.3). The most superficial of these is the molecular layer, a region filled primarily with axons and dendrites and only a few cells. Next is a single layer of large distinctive neurons known as the Purkinje cells. The third and deepest layer is the granule cell layer composed mostly of neurons called "granule" cells. Both the molecular layer and the granular layer contain some specific types of intrinsic cerebellar neurons such as Golgi cells, stellate cells, and basket cells, but we won't be concerned with that level of detail.

With a modicum of inaccuracy, we can consider the Purkinje cells as the key players in the cerebellar cortex. All

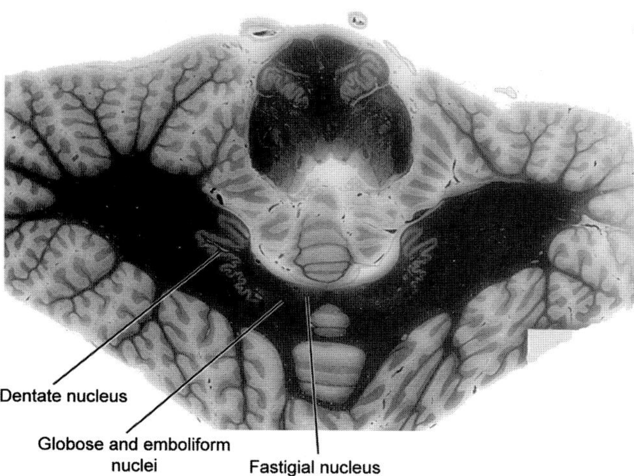

Fig. 1.1. **Anatomic diagram showing the deep cerebellar nuclei.**

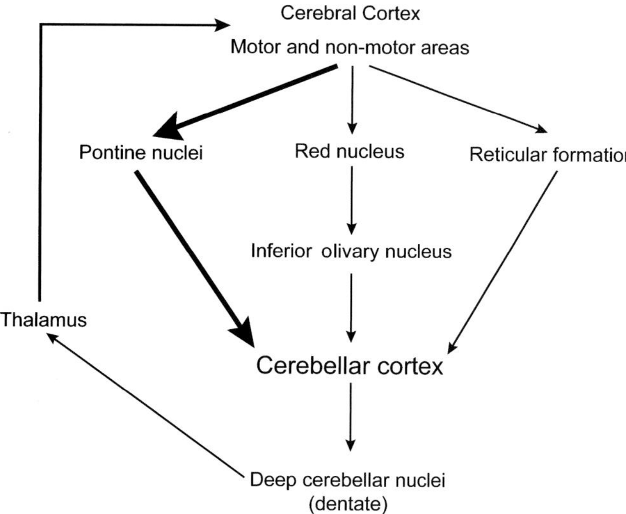

Fig. 1.2. **Schematic diagram showing the basic organizational schema of cerebellar communication. The cerebral cortex communicates with the cerebellar cortex through a main pathway which relays in the pons and through accessory pathways that involve the red nucleus and the reticular formation. These pathways constitute afferent or input information to the cerebellar cortex. After processing these inputs, output (efferent) information from the cerebellar cortex is relayed to the deep cerebellar nuclei, which then communicate back to the cerebral cortex via thalamic relays.**

inputs eventually come to them, and they are the only cells that are able to project outside the cerebellar cortex. They send their axons to the deep cerebellar nuclei, which then communicate the output of the cerebellum to the remainder of the brain.

There are only two ways for incoming (afferent) information to reach the Purkinje cells: either through *climbing* fibers or *mossy* fibers. The climbing fibers to one cerebellar hemisphere arise predominantly from the contralateral inferior olivary nucleus of the medulla. Each climbing fiber ends on one Purkinje cell. The mossy fibers, on the other hand, deliver their information to the Purkinje cells indirectly. They synapse on granule cells in the granular layer, which in turn send their axons to the molecular layer where they synapse with the dendrites of the Purkinje cells.

The mossy fibers arise from three principal afferent sources:
(1) the cerebral cortex, which sends large numbers of cortico-cerebellar fibers that relay on pontine nuclei and then enter the cerebellum;
(2) the vestibular nuclei;
(3) the spinal cord.

The inferior olivary nuclei, the source of climbing fibers, receive information from multiple sources, such as the contralateral spinal cord and, most prominently, the ipsilateral red nucleus. The red nucleus receives multiple inputs to pass to the inferior olives and then the cerebellum, such as prominent cortical inputs, as well as a significant input from the dentate nucleus of the cerebellum, forming a feedback loop.

All communication (afferent and efferent) between the cerebellum and the rest of the CNS takes place through three fiber tracts, known as the inferior, middle, and superior cerebellar peduncles.

Inferior cerebellar peduncles

These are also known as the restiform and juxtarestiform bodies, and bring inputs (afferents) to the cerebellum. The major afferent tracts in the restiform body are the dorsal spinocerebellar tract, the cuneocerebellar tract, and the olivocerebellar tract, arising in the contralateral inferior olivary nucleus. The juxtarestaform body contains axons from the vestibular system. Efferent information from the cerebellum originates from the fastigial nuclei, and terminates in the brainstem.

Middle cerebellar peduncles

These are also known as the brachium pontis. They are an input tract to the cerebellum, originating from the pontine nuclei. There are no efferent axons in the middle cerebellar peduncle.

Superior cerebellar peduncles

These are also known as the brachium conjunctivum. They have a minor input from the spinal cord, but are primarily a major output pathway of the cerebellum. They contain the important dentatothalamic tracts, from the dentate nucleus to the thalamus, as well as outputs from the interposed nuclei, which terminate in the brainstem.

Thus, in rough terms, we can think of the inferior and middle cerebellar peduncles as the input pathways to the cerebellum, carrying inputs from the spinal cord and the cortex, respectively, and the superior cerebellar peduncles as the major output pathway of the cerebellum. There are some exceptions. For example, the ventral or anterior spinocerebellar tract enters the cerebellum through the superior cerebellar peduncles – but we're thinking BIG PICTURE here!

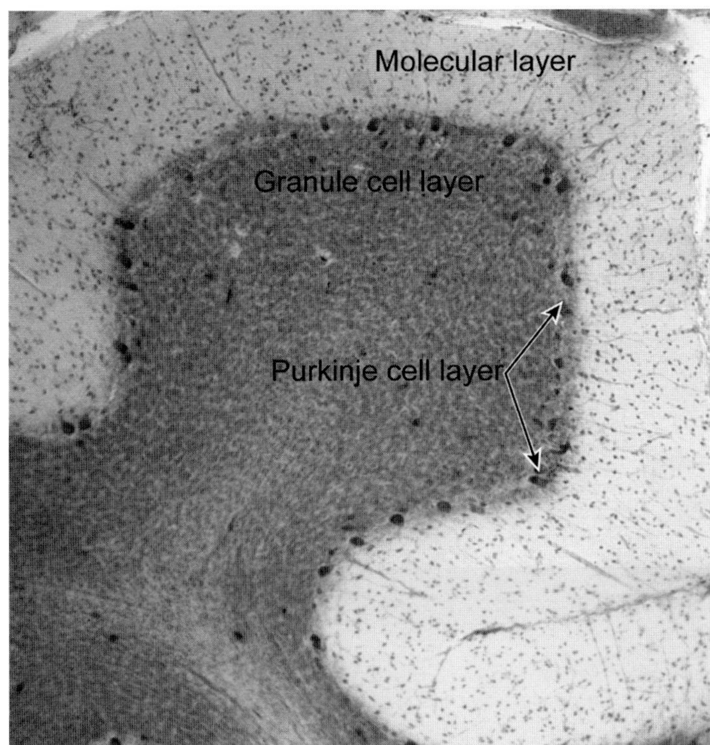

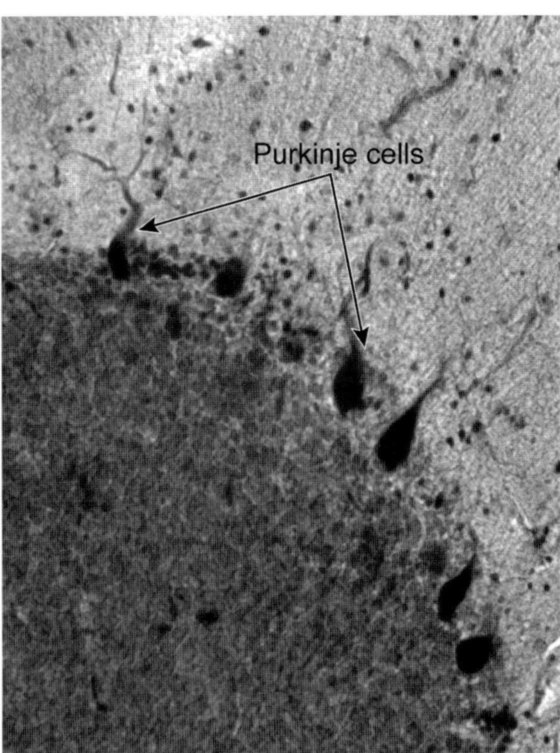

Fig. 1.3. **Cytoarchitecture of the cerebellum. On the left is a photomicrograph of a single folium, showing the loosely packed molecular cell layer adjacent to the pia, and the deep granule cell layer adjacent to the cerebellar white matter. Between these two is a single layer of Purkinje cells. On the right is a magnified view of the Purkinje cells.**

Macroscopic organization

The cerebellum is formed from a midline vermis and two laterally placed cerebellar hemispheres (Fig. 1.4). These can be further subdivided both transversely and longitudinally into clinically meaningful subdivisions. The transverse division of the cerebellum is anatomic, based on the existence of transversely oriented fissures, which divide the cerebellum into three main lobes (each of which contains portions of the vermis and the hemispheres). The primary fissure divides the cerebellum into anterior and posterior lobes. Also, a postero-lateral fissure nearly pinches off the flocculus of the cerebellum from the main body, thus forming the flocculonodular lobe, which includes the flocculi as well as the nodulus (a lobule) of the vermis.

Sensory inputs from the head and body are somatotopically mapped three times in the cerebellum – once in the anterior lobe and twice (on each side of the midline) in the posterior lobe, with the trunk toward the midline and the extremities more laterally.

The cerebellum can also be divided longitudinally based on neuronal connections delineating three different functional zones. These are the midline vermis, the intermediate or para-vermal zones, and the lateral zones on each side of the vermis. There is some overlap with the previously defined transverse divisions, especially the flocculonodular lobe, which acts as its own functional zone (Fig. 1.5(a), (b)).

Each of these functional zones has fairly distinctive inputs and outputs, leading to important clinical correlations which will be discussed below. Here, we note that each zone sends its output to a different deep nucleus. The lateral zones send their output to the dentate nucleus, the paravermal zones to the interposed nucleus, and the vermis to the fastigial nucleus.

Functional zones and clinical correlations

The lateral zones

These form the bulk of the cerebellar hemispheres. Their major neural connections have been briefly discussed already, and are mostly in the form of a neural circuit between the cerebrum and the cerebellum. Therefore, the lateral zones are also called the *cerebrocerebellum* or the *neocerebellum*. To give a concrete example, let us follow information from the left motor and premotor cortex regarding a planned movement of the right hand, such as a finger-to-nose motion. This information passes through the left internal capsule into the left cerebral peduncle and then into the left pons. In the pons, the axons synapse on pontine reticular neurons and decussate across the belly of the pons (from left to right, in this example). That is why the belly of the pons appears to have horizontal striations on photomicrographs. The axons then enter the right cerebellum via the large right middle cerebellar peduncle. As an aside, this corticocerebellar pathway is significantly

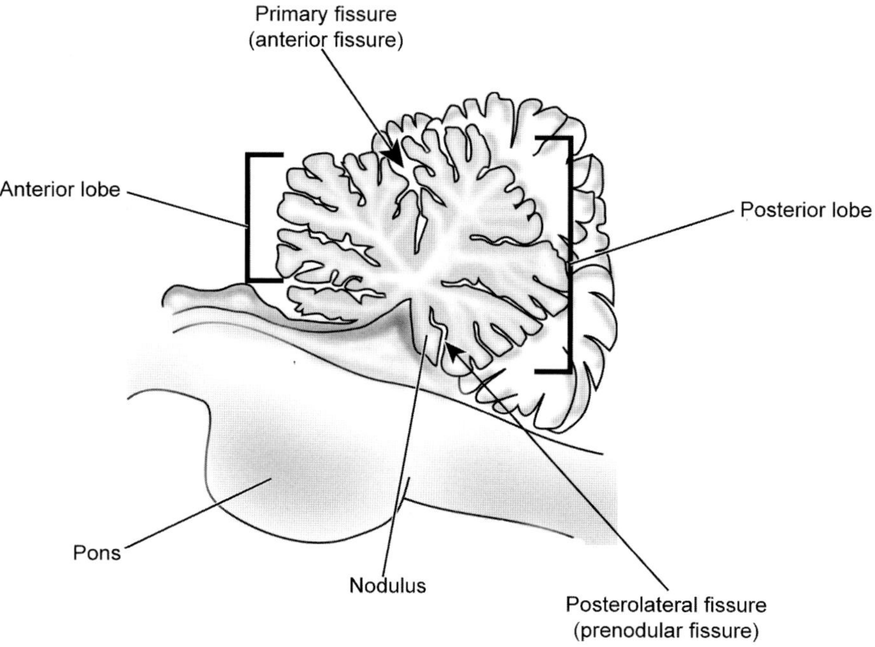

Fig. 1.4. **Schematic diagram of a mid-sagittal slice through the cerebellum and brainstem, outlining the anterior and posterior lobes. The location of the flocculonodular lobe is marked by the nodulus of the vermis, lying just above the posterolateral fissure.**

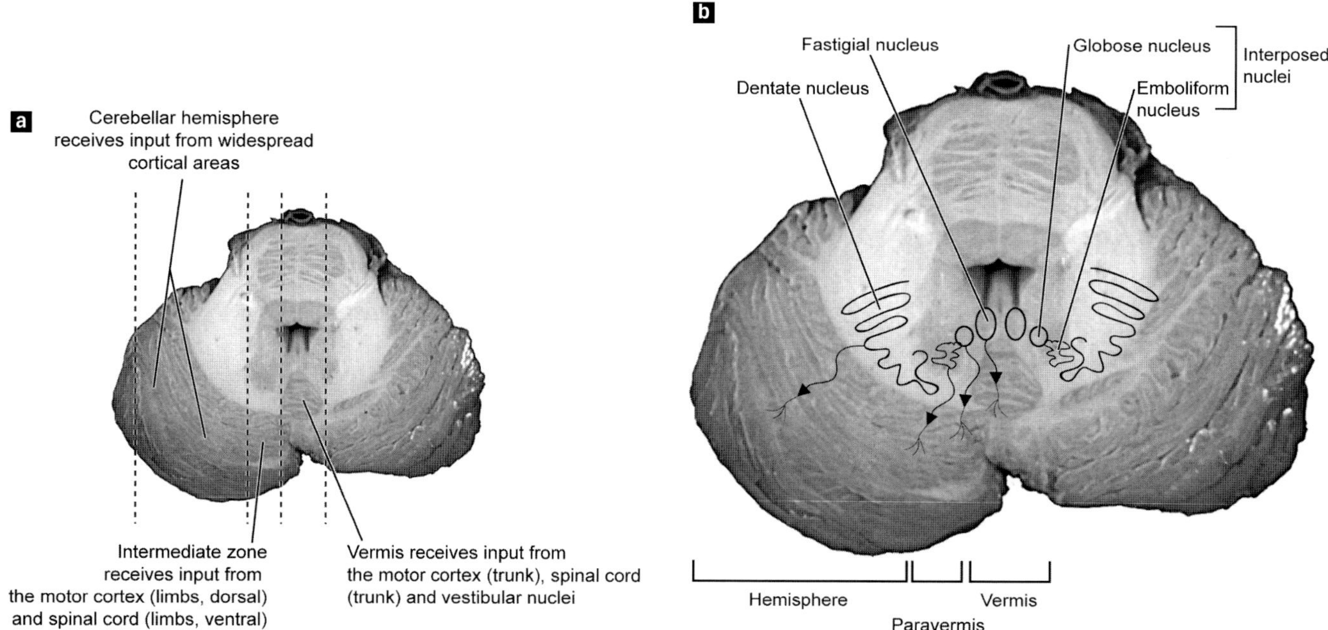

Fig. 1.5 **(a) Schematic showing the different longitudinal functional zones of the cerebellum, and outlining their (a) main inputs and (b) outputs. Note that the lateral zones (hemispheres) output through the dentate nucleus, the paravermal zones output through the interposed (globose and emboliform) nucleus, while the vermis outputs through the fastigial nucleus.**

larger than the corticospinal tracts, perhaps by as much as 20 : 1 in terms of the number of axons.

This afferent information is processed in the cortex of the right cerebellar hemisphere, and the Purkinje cells of the cerebellar cortex send their axons to the right dentate nucleus, which in turn sends its axons out through the right superior cerebellar peduncle. The superior cerebellar peduncles decussate in the caudal midbrain, and the axons pass to the motor nuclei (VA/VL) of the left thalamus (via the dentatothalamic tract). The left thalamus, in turn, projects back to the left

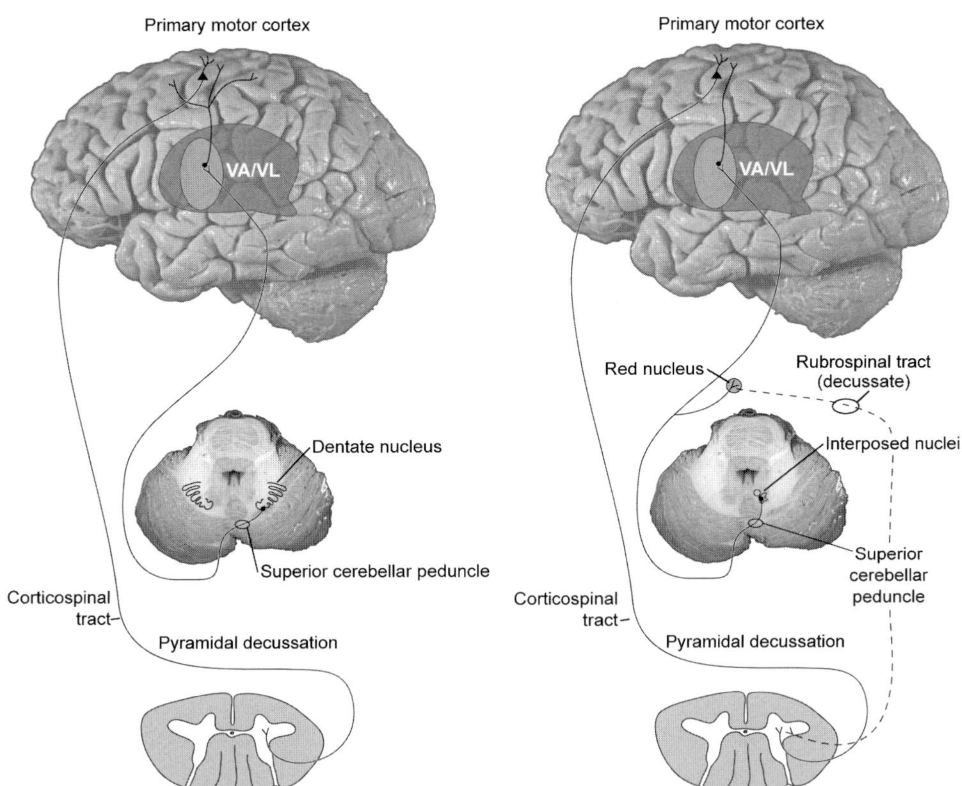

Fig. 1.6. **Schematic diagram of the main output circuits of the lateral (left) and intermediate (right) cerebellar functional zones. Output from the lateral zone goes from the dentate nucleus to the superior cerebellar peduncles, which then decussate to synapse on the contralateral thalamus, which relays to the motor and premotor cortex (e.g., left cerebellum to right thalamus to right motor and premotor cortex). Output from the motor and premotor cortex re-crosses the midline in the pyramidal decussation (e.g., right motor and premotor cortex to left hemicord). The result is that one cerebellar hemisphere influences the ipsilateral side of the body. The intermediate zone output is similarly organized, except that fibers also project to the contralateral red nucleus. The red nucleus projects to the spinal cord via the rubrospinal tract, which also decussates on the way to the cord, upholding the principle that one cerebellar hemisphere influences the ipsilateral cord and body.**

motor and premotor cortex to modulate the motion of the right hand and smoothly guide the right index finger to the nose.

This simplified description highlights a critical clinical fact regarding cerebellar pathology: damage to one side of the cerebellum affects the ipsilateral side of the body. From our example, we see that the left motor cortex "talks to" the right cerebellum, and right cerebellar lesions would, in turn, impact the function of the left motor cortex, which controls the right body. This occurs because of a double decussation of the input–output pathways between the cerebrum and the cerebellum. Information from the cerebrum decussates on the way into the cerebellum in the belly of the pons, and decussates on the way out of the cerebellum in the decussation of the superior cerebellar peduncles.

Similar compensating decussations operate at all levels in the cerebellum to uphold the principle that cerebellar lesions affect the ipsilateral side of the body (Fig. 1.6).

Communication between the cerebellum and the spinal cord is more complex than the cerebrocerebellar circuit described above, but follows similar principles, and a couple of illustrative examples are given (Fig. 1.7). We have already mentioned that climbing fibers (one of the two main inputs to

the Purkinje cells) arise in the contralateral inferior olivary nucleus. The spinal tracts that deliver information to the inferior olivary nucleus, however, arise form the hemicord contralateral to the inferior olivary nucleus in which they synapse. Therefore, left spinal hemicord neurons send axons that cross the cord and synapse with the right inferior olivary nucleus, which sends its axons to the left cerebellar hemisphere (Fig. 1.7). Another example is the ventral spinocerebellar tract. As mentioned parenthetically before, this enters the cerebellum via the superior cerebellar peduncle. For concreteness, we follow neurons from the right hemibody. Axons enter the cord and decussate, then ascend in the left ventral spinocerebellar tract, entering the left superior cerebellar peduncle. The axons then decussate once again to synapse in the right cerebellar hemisphere (Fig. 1.7).

Also, some tracts do not decussate at all, such as the dorsal spinocerebellar tract, which enters the cerebellum through the inferior cerebellar peduncle, and synapses ipsilateral to its side of origin in the cord (Fig. 1.7). We can also look at an example of cerebellar efferents, which send information to the spinal cord. A small part of the output of the paravermal zones goes to the cord. It travels via the

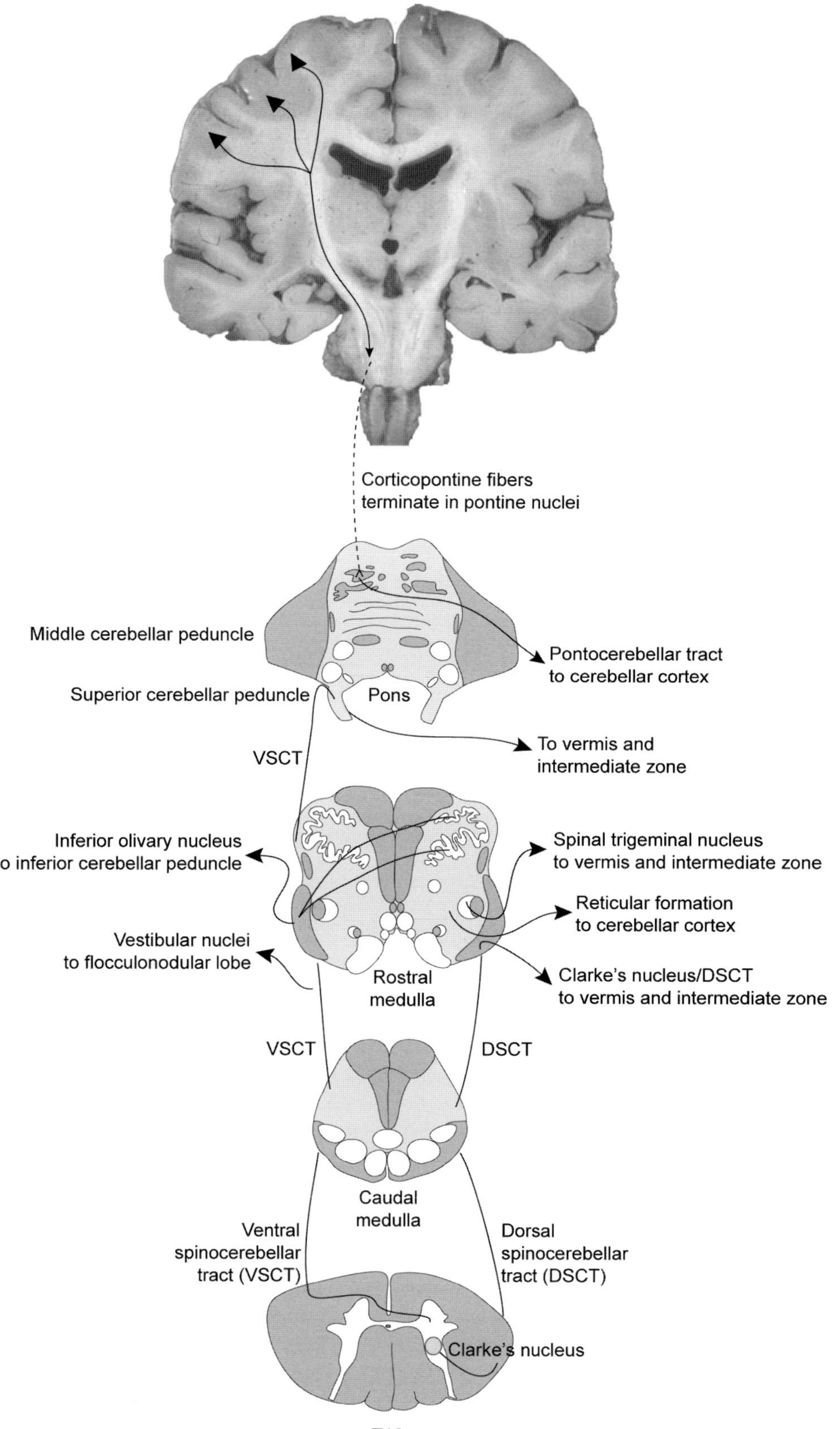

Fig. 1.7. **Schematic of inputs from the cerebral cortex and the spinal cord to the cerebellum. Inputs from the motor and premotor cortex synapse in the pons, and then decussate in the belly of the pons to enter the contralateral cerebellar hemisphere via the middle cerebellar peduncle. Spinal cord inputs are more complex. In the diagram, some fibers from the right hemibody cross the midline in the cord and ascend in the left ventral spinocerebellar tract (VSCT). These fibers enter the left superior cerebellar peduncle, and then decussate to synapse on the right cerebellar hemisphere (right body, left VSCT, right cerebellum). Other fibers, e.g. from the left hemibody, ascend in the ipsilateral cord then decussate to synapse on the contralateral (right) inferior olivary nucleus, which then sends climbing fibers to the contralateral (left) cerebellum (left body, right inferior olivary nucleus, left cerebellar hemisphere). Finally, some fibers, such as the dorsal spinocerebellar tract (DSCT), do not decussate. In the diagram, fibers from the left hemibody ascend in the left DSCT and enter the left cerebellum via the left inferior cerebellar peduncle. In all cases, one cerebellar hemisphere influences the ipsilateral side of the body.**

interposed nucleus and the superior cerebellar peduncle, decussating to synapse on the contralateral red nucleus (Fig. 1.6). The descending rubrospinal (from the red nucleus to the spine) tract decussates again before it enters the cord. Therefore, with regard to communication between the cerebellum and the spinal cord, one side of the cerebellum communicates with the ipsilateral side of the cord, which controls that same side of the body, upholding the principle of cerebellar lesions causing symptoms on the same side of the body.

After this long digression into ipsilaterality, we return to the functional aspects of the lateral zones of the cerebellum. As mentioned previously, the somatotopic maps of the body in the cerebellum have the extremities mapped laterally. Therefore, damage in the lateral zones will cause the so-called neocerebellar syndrome. The most prominent feature here is a peripheral ataxia – an incoordination of voluntary movements characterized by overshooting or undershooting of the target (*dysmetria*), lack of control of the velocity and precise direction of motion (*intention tremor*), difficulty with rapid alternating movements (*dysdiadochokinesia*), and poor timing of different parts of a complex motion (*decomposition of movement*). The complex motor control involved in speaking may be similarly affected, disrupting the normal flow and cadence of speech, causing a cerebellar dysarthria known as *scanning speech*. Other manifestations of the neocerebellar syndrome include hypotonia (part of the function of cerebellar efferents to the motor cortex is to help maintain motor tone) and hyporeflexia. Because of the hypotonia, a limb may continue to swing after a reflex contraction; this is known as a *pendular reflex*.

Vermis and paravermal zones

Both of these zones (except the nodulus of the vermis) receive significant inputs from the spinal cord, and so are together called the *spinocerebellum*. The paravermal zones also receive input from the cerebral cortex. The paravermal zones output through the interposed nucleus and then through the superior cerebellar peduncles. The output decussates and goes predominantly to the contralateral red nucleus, and from there either to the thalamus and then the cortex, or back to the spinal cord through the rubrospinal tract (Fig. 1.8). The paravermal zones work both with the lateral zones in helping to control limb movements and with the vermis.

The vermis receives inputs predominantly from the spinal cord through spinocerebellar tracts. The vermis outputs through the fastigial nuclei, and then to the vestibular nuclei (Fig. 1.9). There are also some direct connections from the vermis to vestibular nuclei bypassing the fastigial nuclei. Since the trunk is primarily represented along the vermis, and since its projections are to the bilateral vestibular nuclei, which function to maintain equilibrium, it is not surprising that damage to the vermis causes central ataxia, manifested by postural instability and gait ataxia. The vermis also functions in concert with the flocculonodular lobe.

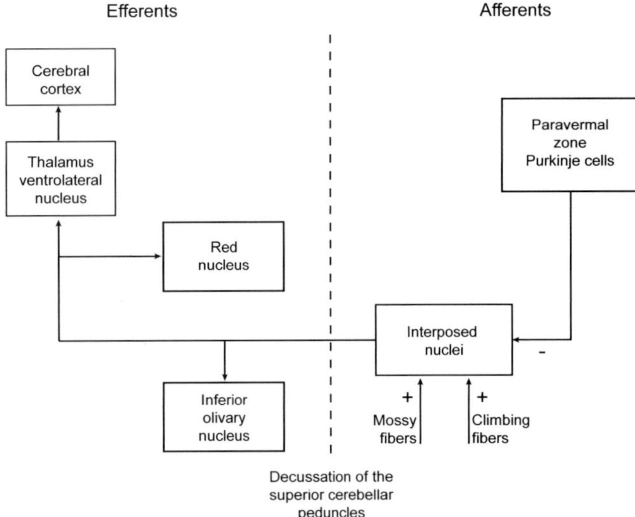

Fig. 1.8. **Schematic diagram showing the inputs (right) and outputs (left) of the paravermal zone of the cerebellum. Outputs of the paravermal zone go through the interposed (globose and emboliform) nucleus. They decussate and go to the contralateral red nucleus, thalamus and cortex, as well as to the inferior olivary nucleus. The red nucleus sends fibers to the spinal cord via the rubrospinal tracts.**

Flocculonodular lobe

This functional zone receives inputs primarily from the vestibular nuclei through the inferior cerebellar peduncles and is therefore known as the *vestibulocerebellum*. Because phylogenetically this zone is the oldest part of the cerebellum, it is sometimes also referred to as the *archicerebellum*. It skips the deep cerebellar nuclei and projects to the vestibular and reticular nuclei (which in turn project to the spinal cord), and to the oculomotor nuclei via the medial longitudinal fasciculus. Damage to the flocculonodular lobe causes the so-called archicerebellar syndrome, characterized by nystagmus and gait and truncal ataxia. Sometimes, there is also a frank sense of disequilibrium, which is noteworthy since sensory manifestations are unusual with cerebellar lesions. The nystagmus is usually horizontal, with the fast component toward the side of the lesion; it is worse when the patient looks toward the side of the lesion.

In an incomplete but pithy summary, then, the lateral zones of the cerebellum (neocerebellum or cerebrocerebellum) receive inputs predominantly from the contralateral cerebral cortex, and output via the dentate nucleus back to that contralateral cerebral cortex via thalamic relays. The intermediate zone (spinocerebellum) is made up of both paravermal cortex and portions of the vermis. The paravermal regions receive inputs from both the spinal cord and the cerebral cortex. They output through the interposed (globose and emboliform) nuclei back to the cerebral cortex via thalamic relays, as well as back to the spinal cord via the red nucleus and the rubrospinal tracts. The vermal portion of the spinocerebellum receives inputs predominantly from the spinal cord, and outputs

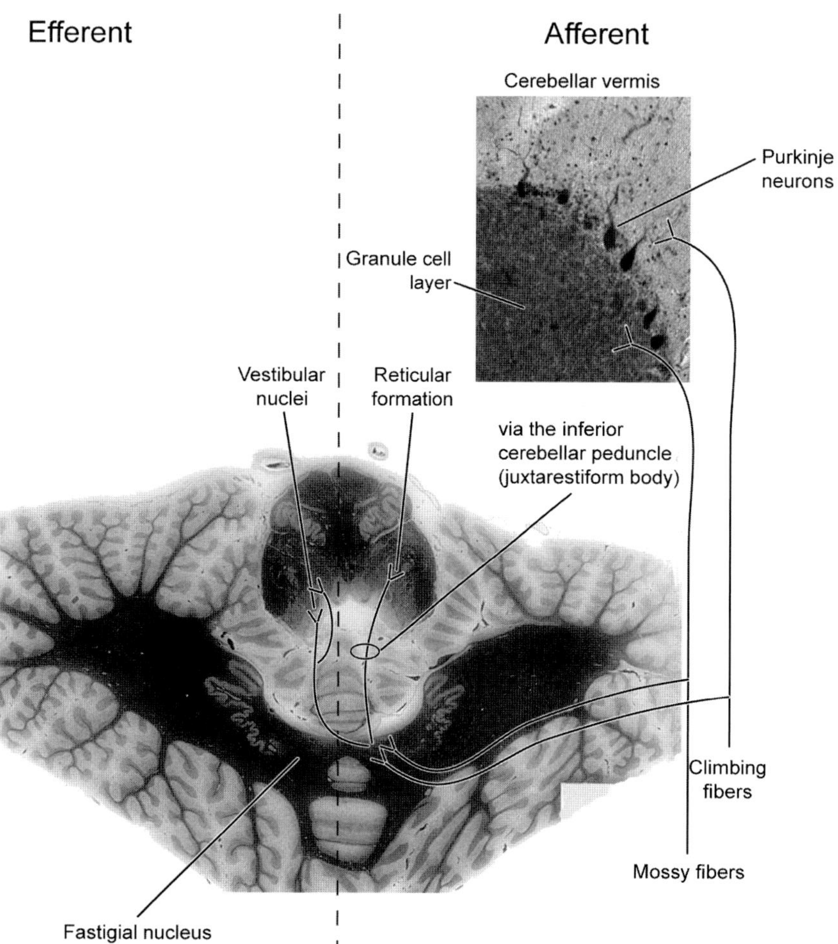

Fig. 1.9. **Inputs and outputs of the cerebellar vermis. Inputs come mainly from the spinal cord through the dorsal and ventral spinocerebellar tracts, as well as by spinoreticular fibers, which synapse on the lateral and paramedian reticular nuclei and then project to the vermis. Outputs of the vermis go predominantly via the fastigial nucleus to the bilateral vestibular nuclei and the reticular formation.**

through the fastigial nucleus to the vestibular nuclei and the reticular formation. The flocculonodular lobe (vestibulocerebellum) receives inputs from the vestibular nuclei predominantly through the inferior cerebellar peduncles. It bypasses the deep cerebellar nuclei and outputs directly to the vestibular and reticular nuclei (which project to the spinal cord) and to the oculomotor nuclei.

Now, let's take some cases!

Case 1.1

56-year-old patient presents with several months of progressive gait ataxia. On examination, the patient walks with a wide-based gait, and has ataxia of the lower extremities on heel-to-shin testing.

A CT examination (Fig. 1.10) is presented below.

What are the findings? What is your differential? What other points of history and physical examination are pertinent?

The patient has marked cerebellar atrophy with prominence of the sulci. There is no gross evidence of brainstem atrophy. The cerebellar atrophy is most pronounced in the anterior–superior vermis and paravermal zones (Fig. 1.10(a)). More inferiorly, there is no significant atrophy of the cerebellar hemispheres (Fig. 1.10(b)). The pattern would be consistent with alcohol-induced cerebellar degeneration.

Diagnosis: alcoholic cerebellar degeneration.

A key point in the patient's history would be the extent of ethanol (ETOH) consumption. Other important aspects of the physical examination would center around whether there is significant involvement of the upper limbs, nystagmus, or speech deficits such as dysarthria. These would be unusual with alcohol-induced cerebellar degeneration. In fact, the presence of cerebellar nystagmus or speech pathology should suggest a search for alternative causes of ataxia (however, sometimes there is a concomitant Wernicke's syndrome which has oculomotor abnormalities).

Discuss the underlying pathophysiology of alcohol-induced cerebellar degeneration.

Cerebellar atrophy secondary to alcohol abuse tends to be most prominent in the anterior–superior vermis and paravermal zones. This region corresponds fairly closely with the anterior

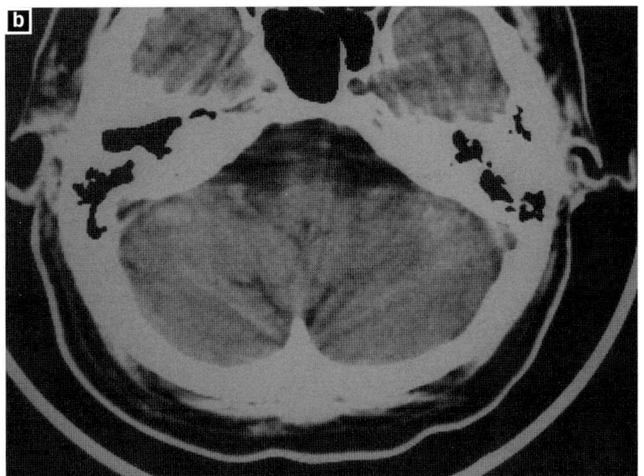

Fig. 1.10. **(a), (b) Axial non-contrast CT images through the cerebellum.**

lobe of the cerebellum. Because the transversely oriented primary fissure occurs so high in the cerebellum, most of the anterior lobe is anterior–superior vermis and paravermal zones. Therefore, as discussed previously, central truncal and gait ataxia would be a prominent feature, with lesser involvement of the upper limbs, and only rarely oculomotor symptoms or cerebellar dysarthria.

The underlying cause of the cerebellar degeneration remains unclear. However, most authorities feel that one of the most likely causes is the thiamine deficiency often associated with alcoholism. This is due to a high degree of correlation, both clinically and pathologically, between alcoholic cerebellar degeneration and cerebellar pathology in Wernicke's syndrome. An interesting clinical aside, however, is that, while there seems to be little sex predilection in Wernicke's when it comes to cerebellar pathology, there is a significant male predilection among alcoholics of alcohol-induced cerebellar degeneration.

Case 1.2

63-year-old male with progressive gait ataxia over several months. Clinical examination reveals a significant truncal, gait and upper extremity ataxia as well as dysarthria.

An MRI is presented (Fig. 1.11).

What are the findings?

There is generalized cerebellar atrophy with prominence of the cerebellar sulci and the fourth ventricle. There is also a suggestion of mild brainstem atrophy involving the basis pontis.

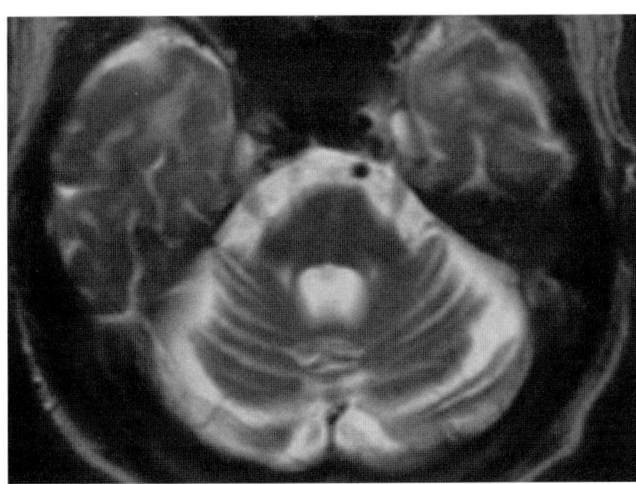

Fig. 1.11. **Axial T2-weighted image of the cerebellum.**

What is your differential diagnosis? What additional clinical history might be useful?

There is a long differential for cerebellar atrophy and ataxia, which will be discussed as part of this case and the subsequent case. Two critical points, however, are worth making now:

(1) The findings, which include dysarthria and upper limb ataxia, would make alcoholic cerebellar degeneration an unlikely diagnosis, despite its ubiquity. However, an ETOH history is always important. Our patient has no history of ETOH abuse, but has an 80-pack/year smoking history.

(2) In patients over the age of 40 with subacute (as opposed to slow or acute) cerebellar syndromes, paraneoplastic cerebellar degeneration probably accounts for 50 percent or more of the cases. It is definitely an under-recognized entity, and you should think about underlying, possibly occult, neoplasia.

Look at the accompanying chest CT (Fig. 1.12). What are the findings and what is your diagnosis?

You are probably thinking that this is highly unfair – even egregious – to be asked to make diagnoses from a chest CT in a neuroradiology book. Sorry. Moving on, the chest CT shows diffuse middle mediastinal and hilar adenopathy with central necrosis. Given the heavy smoking history, this suggests small cell lung carcinoma.

Diagnosis

Paraneoplastic cerebellar degeneration (PCD); small cell lung carcinoma.

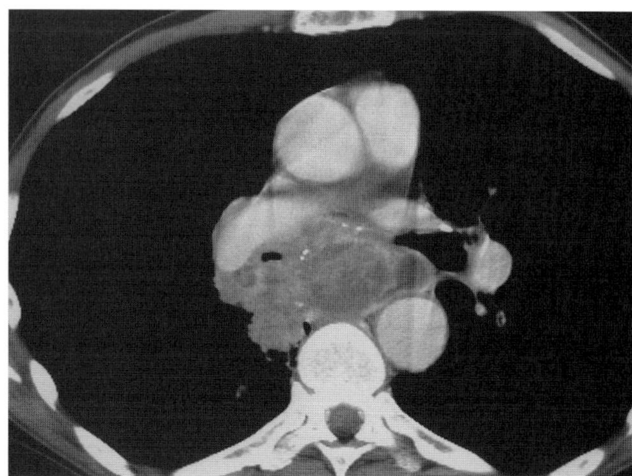

Fig. 1.12. **Contrast CT of the chest.**

Discuss the pathology of paraneoplastic cerebellar degeneration.

When faced with a patient with known cancer and cerebellar ataxia, the leading differential possibility is metastatic disease to the cerebellum. However, paraneoplastic cerebellar degeneration should be considered if there are no metastases visible, and "in the appropriate clinical setting." This phrase is often an irritating hedge, but in this case, it is actually meaningful. There is a definite epidemiology or "appropriate clinical setting" to PCD. Interesting references in this regard are Peterson *et al.* (1992) and Shams'ili *et al.* (2003).

PCD with detectable antibodies

About half of the cases diagnosed as PCD have anti-neuronal antibodies in the serum and cerebrospinal fluid. The antibodies differ based on the underlying malignancy, but they are not seen in other cerebellar disease, so their detection is useful, as it may point to an occult neoplasm, or help confirm the diagnosis of paraneoplastic cerebellar degeneration.

The most common antibody is called anti-Yo. It is directed against the Purkinje cells and can be detected by Western blot testing. It is seen only in women. About half of the cases of anti-Yo associated PCD are due to ovarian carcinoma, while the other half are mainly due to breast carcinoma or other gynecological malignancies.

Other cancers in the PCD with detectable antibody group include Hodgkin's lymphoma, which may be associated with paraneoplastic cerebellar degeneration. In about one-third of the cases of Hodgkin's with associated PCD, there are anti-Purkinje cell antibodies; these are different from anti-Yo. They have a different cytoplasmic staining pattern (diffuse versus granular, as in anti-Yo), and are not detectable on Western blot testing.

Patients with small cell lung cancer sometimes have antibodies against various cells in the central nervous system, known as anti-Hu antibodies. These are not specific to the cerebellum and may be seen in such syndromes as paraneoplastic limbic encephalitis. However, sometimes patients with small cell lung cancer present with isolated PCD.

According to Shams'ili *et al.*, there are nine specific neuronal antibodies associated with PCD, including anti-Yo, anti-Hu, anti-Tr, anti-Ri, and anti-mGluR1.

PCD without detectable antibodies

As already mentioned, this group makes up about one-half of the total cases of PCD. About two-thirds of patients with Hodgkin's lymphoma and associated paraneoplastic cerebellar degeneration are in this group. Other than Hodgkin's disease, the main cancers in this group are lung and breast.

While paraneoplastic cerebellar degeneration is probably under-recognized, its prevalence in lung and ovarian cancer patients is low, probably less than 5 percent. MRI findings may be absent until late in the disease, and the cerebellar symptoms predate the diagnosis of malignancy in a significant proportion of the cases. In fact, in the paper of Peterson *et al.*, cerebellar symptoms preceded the diagnosis of cancer in 34 out of 52 patients, while in the paper of Shams'ili *et al.*, symptoms predated the clinical diagnosis of tumor in 26 out of 42 patients. MRI findings, when present, tend to be diffuse cerebellar atrophy, which may be associated with mild brainstem atrophy as well.

Clearly, a specific diagnosis of PCD simply from a history of cerebellar ataxia and an MRI showing cerebellar atrophy would be difficult, since there is a broad differential for this constellation. An excellent classification of ataxias was introduced by Harding in the early 1980s:

I. Hereditary ataxias

A. Autosomal recessive ataxias

This includes such ataxias as Friedreich's Ataxia, Ataxia Telangiectasia, Congenital Ataxias, and Early-onset Cerebellar Ataxia. It is noted that significant recent progress has been made in uncovering the genetic basis of many of these syndromes, such as the X25 gene on chromosome 19 in Friedreich's ataxia or the phosphatidyl inositol kinase mutation (11q22–23) in Ataxia Telangiectasia.

A quick clinical note regarding Friedreich's ataxia is that it is primarily a spinal degeneration with only occasional involvement of the cerebellum. Therefore, significant cerebellar atrophy is not usually seen on MRI. This is mentioned because residents usually say Friedreich's ataxia first when seeing a case of profound cerebellar atrophy in a young person. Early-onset Cerebellar Ataxia (EOCA) is another autosomal recessive hereditary ataxia. It does show significant cerebellar atrophy. It may be distinguished from Friedreich's ataxia in that patients with Friedreich's ataxia usually lose their tendon reflexes, while patients with EOCA have retained tendon reflexes. Friedreich's ataxia patients also often have other abnormalities, such as cardiomyopathy.

B. Autosomal dominant cerebellar ataxias

This category includes spinocerebellar ataxias types 1 to 6. (SCA1–SCA6) and such entities as the episodic ataxias.

The spinocerebellar ataxias are further subdivided into those without and those with retinal degeneration. The chromosomal disease loci for various SCA syndromes have been determined (SCA1-6p; SCA2-14q; etc.).

The responsible mutation is often a CAG repeat expansion. The various genetic and clinical differences between these syndromes are beyond the scope of this work. However, the degree of cerebellar atrophy on imaging is different among the syndromes, being very profound in SCA2 for example, but quite mild in SCA3, also known as Machado–Joseph syndrome.

II. Non-hereditary ataxias

A. Idiopathic cerebellar ataxias

B. Symptomatic cerebellar ataxias

Discuss the symptomatic cerebellar ataxia category.

This group includes alcoholic and paraneoplastic cerebellar degeneration, which have been discussed. It is basically the group of non-hereditary cerebellar ataxias with a known cause. Several other less common causes are noted:

Hypothyroidism

This is a rare cause of cerebellar syndromes, but it is important because it is potentially treatable. Usually, somatic symptoms of hypothyroidism precede cerebellar signs and symptoms, which are usually a gait ataxia. The cerebellar signs usually resolve completely with thyroid replacement therapy.

Drugs

Most notable here is cerebellar atrophy secondary to prolonged anticonvulsant therapy, especially with phenytoin. Other drugs implicated include 5-FU and cytosine arabinoside, but the cerebellar syndromes here are usually reversible.

Toxins

Such things as toluene, mercury poisoning, and lead poisoning can lead to cerebellar ataxia and possibly degeneration.

Hypoxia and physical insults

Purkinje cells are very sensitive to oxygen deprivation and the cerebellum may be affected with hypoxia; see the CT scan above (Fig. 1.13).

This patient suffered respiratory arrest. There is marked hypodensity of the bilateral globus pallidus and of the cerebellar hemispheres. Both of these zones, along with the hippocampal neurons, are very sensitive to hypoxia. Apparently, the Purkinje cells are very fragile. There may also be significant loss of Purkinje cells after episodes of hyperthermia, such as severe heat stroke, or malignant hyperpyrexia.

Vitamin E deficiency

Vitamin E (alpha tocopherol) is a highly fat-soluble vitamin important for normal neurologic function. There are reports of spinocerebellar syndromes secondary to vitamin E deficiency.

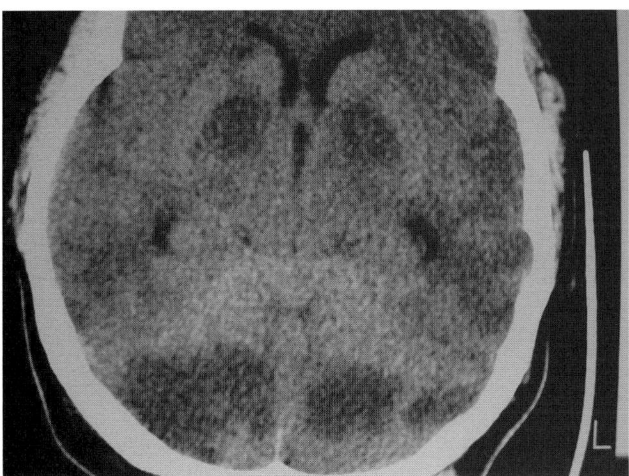

Fig. 1.13. **Axial non-contrast CT images of the cerebellum.**

Some of these disorders are genetic, such as patients with a mutation in the alpha tocopherol transfer gene or patients with abetalipoproteinemia, who lack apoprotein B which carries lipids from the intestine to the plasma. However, acquired vitamin E deficiency from malabsorption, such as after significant intestinal resection surgery from Crohn's disease, represents a potentially treatable cause of cerebellar degeneration. For a case report discussing this rare and fascinating association, see Yokota *et al.* (1987).

References

Peterson, K., Rosenblum, M. K., Kotanides, H. *et al*. Paraneoplastic cerebellar degeneration. I. A clinical analysis of 55 anti-Yo antibody-positive patients. *Neurology* 1992; **42**(10): 1931–1937.

Shams'ili, S., Grefkens, J., de Leeuw, B. *et al*. Paraneoplastic cerebellar degeneration aasociated with anti-neuronal antibodies: analysis of 50 patients. *Brain* 2003; **126**(6): 1409–1418.

Yokota, T., Wada, Y., Furukawa, T. *et al*. Adult-onset spinocerebellar syndrome with idiopathic vitamin E deficiency. *Annals of Neurology* 1987; **22** (1): 84–87.

Case 1.3

55-year-old male patient with a slowly progressive course of gait ataxia. Examination reveals pan-cerebellar findings with truncal, gait, and extremity ataxia.

The patient's MRI examination is provided (Fig. 1.14).

What are the findings, and what is your diagnosis?

There is marked diffuse atrophy of the cerebellum, as well as marked atrophy of the pons, and the middle cerebellar peduncles. There is also some abnormal T2-weighted hyperintensity within the middle cerebellar peduncles.

These findings suggest the diagnosis of olivopontocerebellar atrophy.

Diagnosis

Olivopontocerebellar atrophy (more correctly: Idiopathic Cerebellar Atrophy-Plus, or IDCA-P/MSA, as will be explained below).

Discuss the diagnosis of Olivopontocerebellar Atrophy (OPCA).

Pathologically, OPCA represents neuronal loss in the reticular pontine neurons, inferior olives, and the cerebellum. Until recently, it was considered a specific syndrome, with early-onset familial inherited and late-onset sporadic forms. However, more recently, OPCA has been reclassified as a number of diverse processes, or even as a non-specific pathologic diagnosis which can be seen in a number of different diseases. The familial inherited forms are now in general regarded as part of the spectrum of the autosomal dominant spinocerebellar ataxias discussed previously. The late onset sporadic form is regarded both as part of the spectrum of Multisystem Atrophy (MSA), and part of the spectrum of Idiopathic Cerebellar Atrophy, a subcategory of the non-hereditary ataxias.

Idiopathic Cerebellar Atrophy (IDCA) is a category which comprises late-onset (beginning after 25 years of age) cerebellar

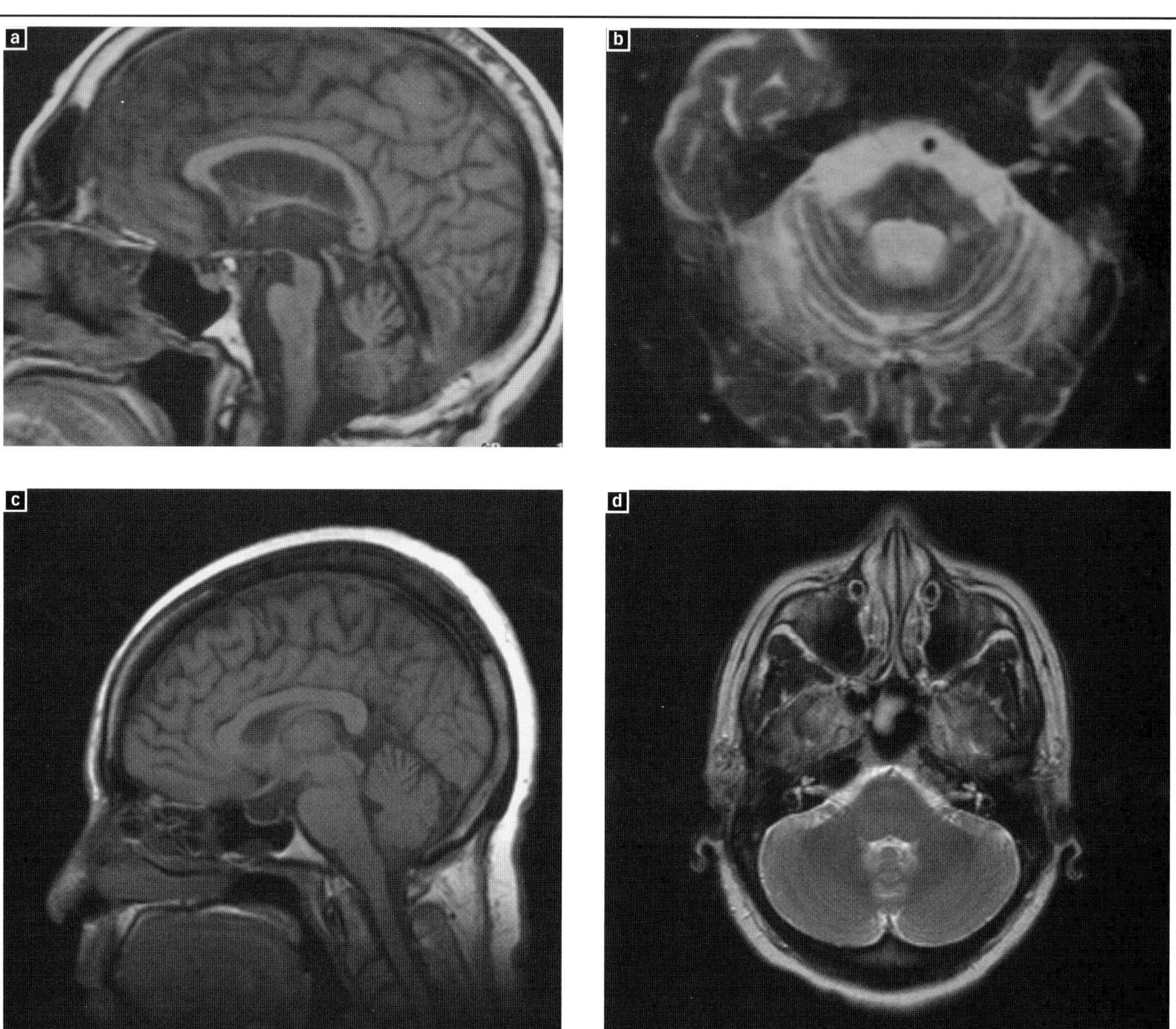

Fig. 1.14. **(a), (b) Sagittal T1- and axial T2-weighted images of our patient. (c), (d) Sagittal T1- and axial T2-weighted images of a normal subject (with an incidental finding of a partially empty sella turcica), provided for comparison.**

ataxia, and degeneration, without a known cause. According to some authors, it is divided into two broad groups: purely cerebellar (IDCA-C), and cerebellar plus (IDCA-P/MSA). The cerebellar-plus group is composed mainly of those cases with extra-cerebellar findings, such as olivopontocerebellar atrophy.

Olivopontocerebellar atrophy is also considered a part of multisystem atrophy (MSA), along with Shy–Drager syndrome, and striatonigral degeneration. All three entities share the presence of characteristic oligodendrocyte glial cytoplasmic inclusions, suggesting that they belong to one large category of disease.

Multisystem atrophy, conversely, is divided into two broad groups: MSA-P, which denotes the parkinsonian form, with prominent striatonigral degeneration, and MSA-C which denotes the cerebellar or OPCA form of MSA. Obviously, there is some overlap between these categories, as well as what was previously called Shy–Drager syndrome. Therefore, both categories may present with variable degrees of autonomic findings.

Our patient, for example, presented not only with cerebellar findings, but with impotence, and urinary urgency. Such symptoms, in the setting of any idiopathic cerebellar degeneration of late onset should suggest IDCA-P/MSA. Thus, to clarify, OPCA is considered the cerebellar form of MSA (i.e., MSA-C) as well as the plus form of IDCA (IDCA-P/MSA). It is estimated that about 15 percent of MSA patients have a cerebellar presentation, and would be classified as MSA-C.

The clinical presentation of IDCA-P/MSA which includes ataxia, dysautonomia and parkinsonism is usually not a difficult clinical diagnosis. However, the categorization scheme is imperfect, in that there are patients who on imaging have an appearance suggestive of OPCA, but never display any dysautonomia or parkinsonian symptoms. It is difficult to know whether they should still be called MSA-C, or whether there is OPCA without MSA. In the opinion of some authors, at least, the latter is true.

Clinical notes:
- Patients with IDCA-C can be very difficult to distinguish from those with symptomatic cerebellar atrophy, and a careful search for one of the etiologies in the symptomatic ataxia group should be undertaken. Imaging in these patients reveals diffuse cerebellar atrophy without brainstem involvement (Fig. 1.15).
- Because patients with OPCA often have degeneration of Onuf's nucleus, EMG of the external sphincter muscles (ouch!) has been suggested as a possible means of distinguishing IDCA-C from incomplete presentations of IDCA-P/MSA. In the latter, EMG of the sphincter muscles would reveal denervation activity.
- Patients with IDCA-P/MSA may have additional findings on MRI, such as increased T2-weighted hypointensity in the putamen (a finding characteristic of striatonigral degeneration, to be discussed later), or abnormal T2-weighted hyperintensity in the middle cerebellar peduncles. Whether or not these findings are present, the OPCA imaging appearance heralds a worse prognosis for the patient than an appearance of isolated cerebellar atrophy.
- Once again, the classification schemes are imperfect, and there are cases of idiopathic cerebellar degeneration that will defy precise categorization.

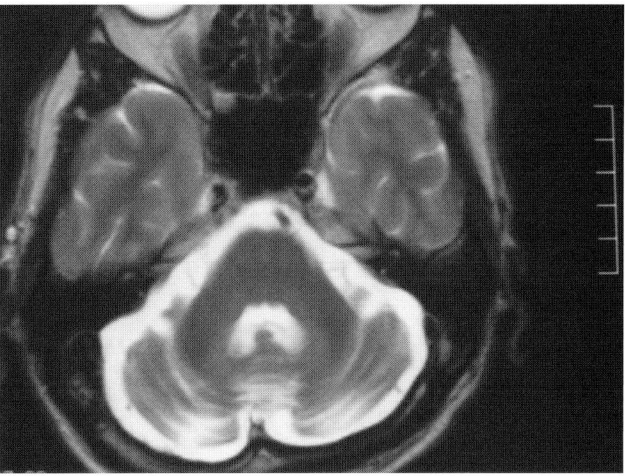

Fig. 1.15. **Axial T2-weighted image of the cerebellum. This 50-year-old male presented with a steadily progressive cerebellar ataxia over one year. No cause could be identified. The MRI shows diffuse cerebellar atrophy. When compared to the patient with OPCA, we see that there is no evidence of atrophy of the pons or the middle cerebellar peduncles.**

Case 1.4

6-year-old male patient who presents with a one-month history of headaches and truncal ataxia. The patient falls when sitting, and has a broad-based ataxic gait. The patient also has difficulty maintaining eccentric gaze, as well as nystagmus. When the trunk is supported, there is no evidence of limb ataxia, with normal heel-to-shin, and normal finger-to-nose testing.

What is your differential?

The patient is showing signs and symptoms typical of a midline cerebellar lesion. As opposed to the anterior lobe syndrome described previousuly, the presence of nystagmus suggests a flocculonodular lobe or archicerebellar syndrome. Because of the patient's young age, a posterior fossa midline tumor would be a likely diagnosis.

Look at the MRI sequences (Fig. 1.16).

What are the findings? What is your differential?

The images show a predominantly solid midline cerebellar tumor filling the fourth ventricle.

Diagnosis: Medulloblastoma (Primitive Neuroectodermal Tumor (PNET) of the cerebellum).

Medulloblastomas are malignant primitive neuroectodermal tumors, which arise predominantly in the vermis along the roof of the fourth ventricle, and hence grow in the midline of the cerebellum, often presenting as an intraventricular mass filling the fourth ventricle. Most tumors present in the first decade of life. They are probably the most common cerebellar tumor in children, just ahead of cerebellar astrocytomas. If cerebellar and brainstem astrocytomas are lumped as one category, though, then they are more common than medulloblastoma. These tumors comprise 15–20 percent of intracranial neoplasms in children and 30–40 percent of posterior fossa tumors.

Medulloblastomas occur in three histologic varieties: classic type (50 percent), desmoplastic type (25 percent) and mixed with neuronal differentiation (25 percent). The desmoplastic variety tends to occur in older age groups, such as adolescents and adults, and may present in the cerebellar hemispheres rather than in the vermis and the fourth ventricle. Because medulloblastomas are composed primarily of densely packed small round cells, they are often hyperdense on non-contrast CT, which is an excellent diagnostic clue. This same feature often causes them to be isointense to cortex on T2, rather than markedly hyperintense as most tumors tend to be. While the typical description is of a solid homogeneously enhancing non-calcified tumor, it is now known that medulloblastomas often have calcifications (up to 20 percent) or cysts and necrotic areas (50 percent). Another

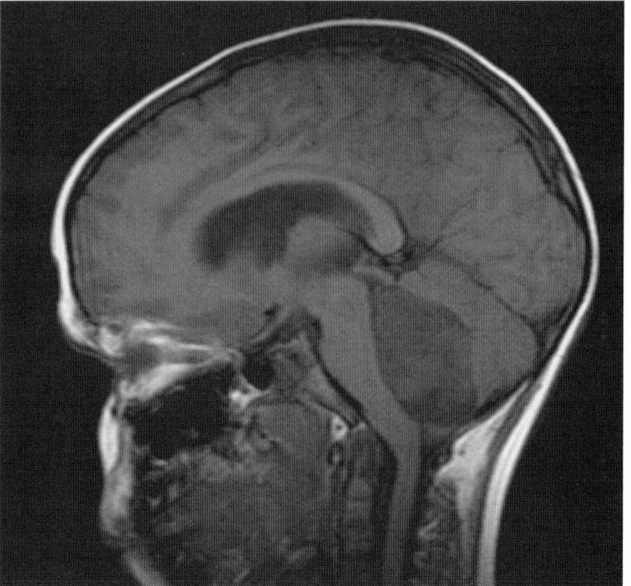

Fig. 1.16. **Sagittal T1-weighted MRI image.**

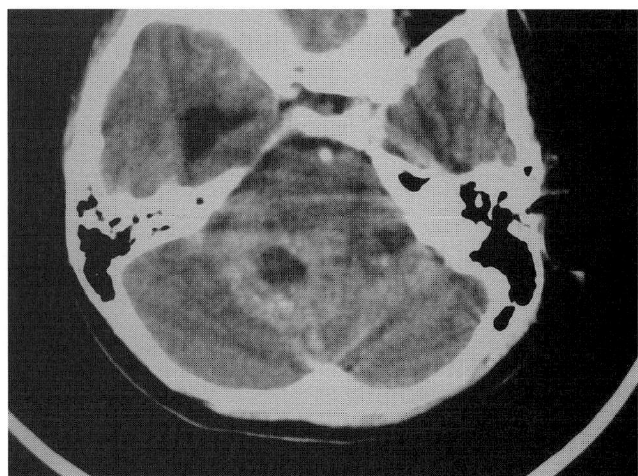

Fig. 1.17. **Axial contrast CT image of the posterior fossa.**

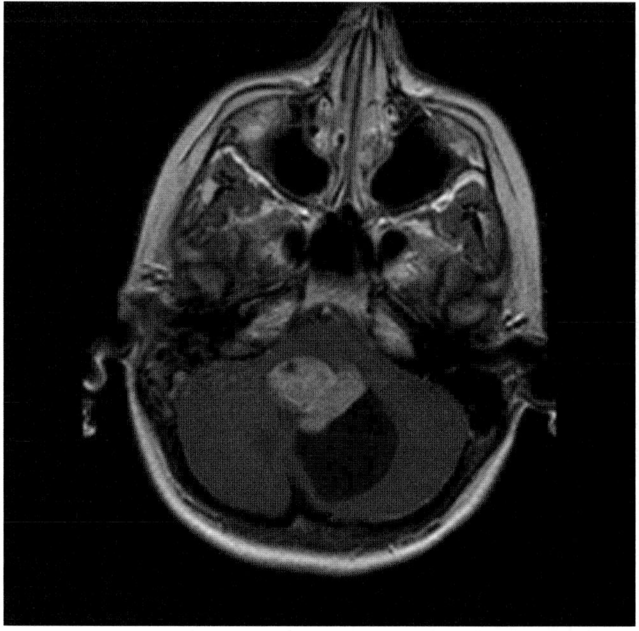

Fig. 1.18. **T1-weighted axial post-contrast image shows a midline mass with an enhancing solid component as well as a non-enhancing cystic portion, characteristic of pilocytic astrocytoma.**

important fact about these tumors is their high predilection for CSF spread. It is noted that medulloblastomas are more common in males than females. While most cases are sporadic, medulloblastomas are also part of some unusual genetic syndromes such as Gorlin's (basal cell nevus) syndrome, blue rubber bleb nevus syndrome, Turcot's syndrome (polyposis and gliomas), and Rubinstein–Taybi syndrome. The genetics of this tumor are being worked out. In perhaps half of the cases there is an abnormality in chromosome 17, possibly involving a regulator of the p53 tumor suppressor gene.

Because of their location, they often present with the flocculonodular cerebellar syndrome of midline ataxia and nystagmus, just as our patient did. In fact, according to Nolte, medulloblastomas are the most common cause of damage to the flocculonodular lobe. Of course, they often also present with hydrocephalus and symptoms of increased intracranial pressure, due to obstruction of the fourth ventricle.

Let us look briefly at a second case of a 5-year-old male with a similar clinical presentation of truncal ataxia and nystagmus (Fig. 1.17).

Once again, there is a midline fourth ventricular mass, heterogeneously enhancing with cystic areas. Certainly, medulloblastoma is on the differential (most likely, in fact). As we ponder the differential, we recall that there are only three common tumors of the pediatric cerebellum: medulloblastoma, astrocytoma, and ependymoma, in that order.

On the CT image, the tumor is noted to extend laterally, along the right foramen of Luschka, a characteristic suggestive of (but not pathognomonic for) an ependymoma, which tends to be a softer tumor, often seeping down the foramen magnum and foramen of Magendie or extending out of the foramen of Luschka. This is a case of an ependymoma, which can also cause a flocculonodular cerebellar syndrome.

Ependymomas tend to be tumors of childhood, with about 70 percent occurring infratentorially, usually in the fourth ventricle. They comprise slightly less than 10 percent of intracranial tumors and about 15 percent of posterior fossa tumors in children. They have more of a tendency to have cysts or calcify than medulloblastomas, but the distinction is difficult. Like medulloblastoma, ependymomas are often associated with hydrocephalus. There is a significant male predilection.

Cerebellar astrocytomas in children tend to be of a histologic subtype called pilocytic astrocytoma (over 75 percent of the time).

These are benign tumors (WHO grade I), with an approximately 95 percent 25-year-survival. They can grow in the midline or more laterally in the cerebellar hemispheres. It is unusual for them to invade the fourth ventricle, which is more commonly effaced by midline tumors. About 50 percent of these tumors are cystic with a solidly enhancing portion, called a mural nodule. The cyst wall is composed of compressed cerebellum, and therefore does not enhance (Fig. 1.18).

About 40 percent of pilocytic astrocytomas are solid tumors with cystic or necrotic centers, while about 10 percent are purely solid.

The remaining 25 percent of cerebellar astrocytomas are usually of the fibrillary subtype, which grows by diffuse infiltration, as opposed to the localized pattern of the benign juvenile pilocytic astrocytoma. Therefore, complete surgical resection is less achievable, and the survival rate decreases to a 40 percent 25-year survival. Fibrillary astrocytomas, when they are grade II, often do not enhance. This is sometimes confusing, since the grade I pilocytic astrocytoma shows exuberant enhancement in its solid portions. This, however, is due to a more leaky blood–brain barrier in pilocytic astrocytomas. A cerebellar astrocytoma which does not enhance at all is extremely unlikely to be a benign juvenile pilocytic astrocytoma, and is probably a grade II fibrillary astrocytoma, actually having a worse prognosis.

It may be worthwhile to also briefly review the most common primary cerebellar tumor in the adult (Fig. 1.19). *What is it?*

The pathology of these lesions, and the answer to our question, is hemangioblastoma. This tumor is bengin (WHO grade I). It comprises about 2 percent of all primary CNS tumors, and about 10 percent of primary posterior fossa tumors. Thus, hemangioblastoma is vastly outnumbered by vestibular schwannoma in the posterior fossa as a whole, and by metastases in the cerebellum. Yet, it is the *most common primary tumor of the cerebellum in the adult.*

About 60 percent of the cases are cystic with a solidly enhancing mural nodule, made up of a fine hypervascular capillary

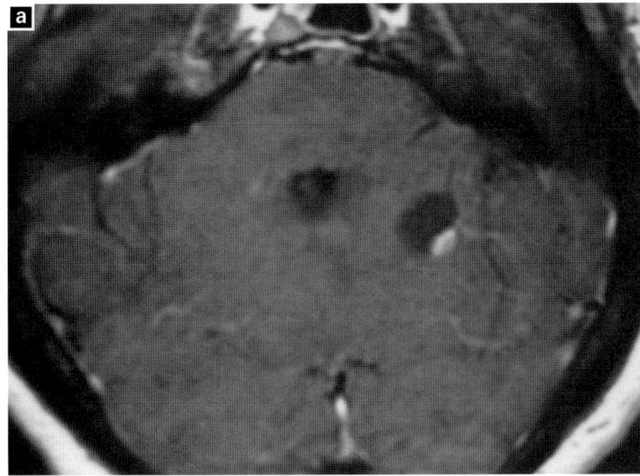
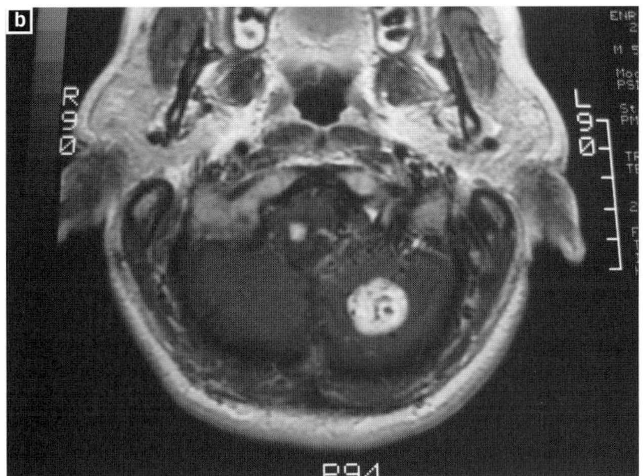

Fig. 1.19. **(a) Axial post-contrast T1-weighted images show a left cerebellar cystic lesion with a solid enhancing mural nodule, as well as (b) a second solidly enhancing lesion with flow voids located more inferiorly. A small solidly enhancing lesion is also noted in the right posterior medulla.**

mesh. The other 40 percent of the cases are solid, often with flow voids. About 85–90 percent of hemangioblastomas occur in the cerebellum, with the rest occurring in the spinal cord and medulla, as well as rarely in the cerebrum. About 20 percent of hemangioblastomas occur in the setting of von Hippel–Lindau (VHL) syndrome, an autosomal dominant disease characterized by CNS and retinal hemangioblastomas, as well as possibly renal cell carcinomas, pheochromocytomas, and liver and pancreatic cysts. About 80 percent of patients with VHL eventually develop cerebellar hemangioblastomas. It is noted that VHL has been mapped to chromosome 3 (p25).

Some clinical notes

- Hemangioblastomas tend to develop in young adults in their 30s–40s. This helps in distinguishing them from pilocytic astrocytomas, which also tend to present as cysts with enhancing solid portions, but at a younger age (5–15 years old). Other helpful factors are that hemangioblastomas tend to have a peripheral location next to a pial surface, and that, on average, the cyst to solid portion of the tumor is bigger in hemangioblastoma. Finally, if need be, an angiogram can be diagnostic. Hemangioblastomas (solid portion) will show an intense blush because they are hypervascular, while pilocytic astrocytomas typically do not show such an intense blush. Yet both have solid portions that enhance with contrast on MRI or CT. This is because they lack a blood–brain barrier. This is a different phenomenon than being hypervascular. Therefore, think of angiography as measuring vessel density, but contrast on CT or MR as measuring vessel leakiness.
- About 40 percent of patients with hemangioblastoma will have some degree of polycythemia, because the tumor secretes erythropoeitin.
- If a patient with VHL has a renal cell carcinoma or a pheochromocytoma, it may be impossible to distinguish whether a cerebellar lesion is a hemangioblastoma or a hypervascular metastasis. This is the case even on pathological examination. A helpful clue may be that the cyst walls of hemangioblastomas do not enhance, while the walls of a cystic metastatic lesion often do.
- Lastly, although fourth ventricular ependymomas tend to be tumors of children, it is noted that adults may sometimes get a tumor in this location with a similar sounding name: subependymoma. This is a rare benign tumor, with a distinctive

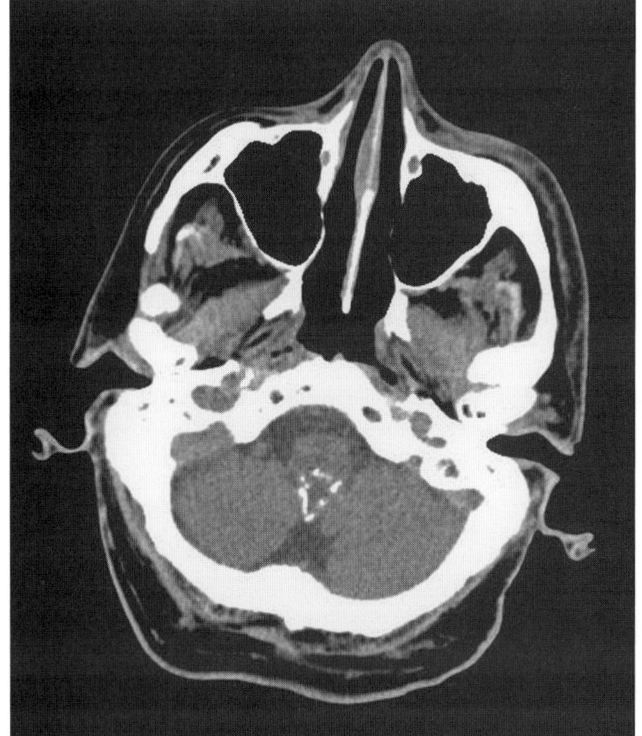

Fig. 1.20. **Axial non-contrast CT. Sixty-year-old male patient who presented with mild truncal ataxia. There is a rim-calcified mass at the inferior aspect of the fourth ventricle. Diagnosis: subependymoma.**

histology and epidemiology. It presents in adults, from middle-aged to elderly. It may be asymptomatic, or cause symptoms secondary to obstruction of CSF flow. Because of its location, it may also conceivably cause a flocculonodular cerebellar syndrome. The tumor may have some calcifications, and only minimally enhances. Such a case is presented above (Fig. 1.20).

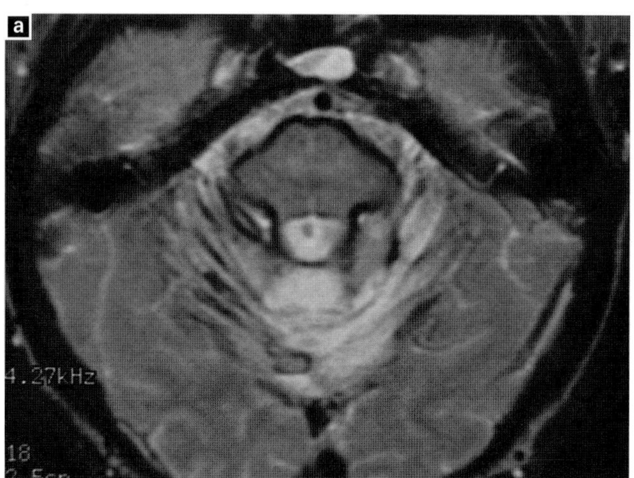
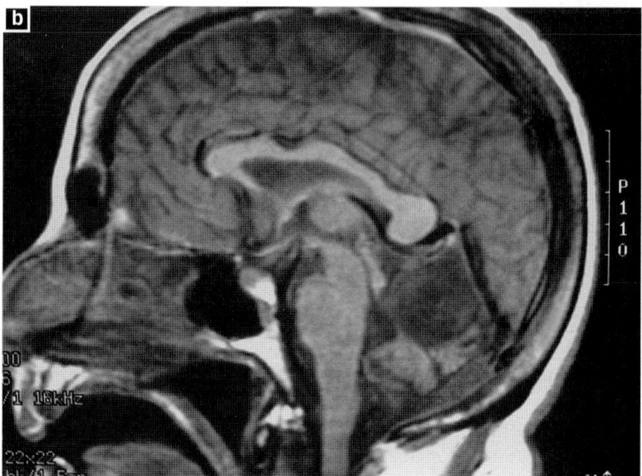

Fig. 1.21. **(a), (b) T2-weighted axial and T1-weighted sagittal images are provided.**

Case 1.5

60-year-old female who presented with a 3-year history of progressive deafness and gait ataxia.

MRI images are provided (Fig. 1.21).

What are the findings? What is your diagnosis?

There is a rim of marked T2-weighted hypointensity surrounding the brainstem (as if someone had drawn around it with a black marker!), and outlining the cerebellar sulci. The sagittal T1 images show marked tissue destruction involving the superior vermis.

The diagnosis here is unusual but pathognomonic. The marked T2 hypointensity outlining the brainstem is consistent with hemosiderin deposition.

Diagnosis

Superficial siderosis of the CNS.

This rare condition is caused by deposition of hemosiderin (an iron-rich blood degradation product) along the leptomeninges due to chronic repeated subarachnoid or intraventricular bleeds. These bleeds are often occult, until the patient presents with the symptoms and signs of superficial siderosis, the most prominent of which are ataxia and progressive deafness.

Pathogenetic studies have suggested that the iron deposited in the leptomeninges is toxic to the microglia. The cerebellar microglia may be especially sensitive. This, coupled with the fact the superior vermis may be more "bathed" in blood than the rest of the cerebellum after subarachnoid bleeds, has been hypothesized as the cause for the marked destruction of the superior vermis seen in these cases. As discussed previously, this would lead to a profound central ataxia.

The significant sensorineural hearing loss is accounted for by marked involvement of the eighth nerves by the superficial

siderosis as well. Experimental and pathologic studies have shown that the siderosis in cranial nerves extends precisely to the transition point between central and peripheral myelin. In most cranial nerves, this occurs very soon after the exit from the brainstem. In the eighth nerves, however, the entire cisternal segment has central myelin until the nerves near the internal acoustic meatus. Therefore, the eighth nerves are especially susceptible.

The majority of reported cases in the literature seem secondary to repeated small bleeds from tumors, especially ependymomas, as well as vascular malformations, or subdural hematomas. Also, the disorder has been described in association with hemispherectomy.

However, about a quarter of the cases are idiopathic, without any source of bleeding identified, even at autopsy. It has been suggested that the bleeds here may be secondary to microsocopic vascular malformations. It is interesting to note, though, that at least a portion of these occult cases, when questioned, will provide a remote history of significant prior trauma.

This diagnosis should be kept in mind in cases of slowly progressive cerebellar ataxia coupled with sensorineural hearing loss. The prognosis for the disorder is unclear, but there have been anecdotal reports of attempted treatment with iron chelating agents.

A nice reference on the imaging of superficial siderosis is Bracchi *et al.* (1993).

Reference

Bracchi, M., Savoiardo, M., Triulzi, F. *et al.* Superficial siderosis of the CNS: MR diagnosis and clinical findings; *American Journal of Neuroradiology* 1993; **14**: 227–236.

Case 1.6

66 year old male patient who presents with right sided ataxia. The patient shows significant dysmetria on finger-to-nose testing, and lower right limb ataxia on heel-to-shin testing and gait ataxia. The patient also complains of vertigo and demonstrates right axial lateropulsion (lateropulsion is the tendency to fall or veer to one side while in motion).

The MRI examination is shown below (Fig. 1.22).

What are the findings?

The images show gray matter edema in the inferior aspect of the right cerebellar hemisphere, manifest as sharply marginated T1-weighted hypointensity. The prominent gray matter edema, sharp margination, and narrow transition zone, as well as confinement of the pathology to a vascular territory are diagnostic.

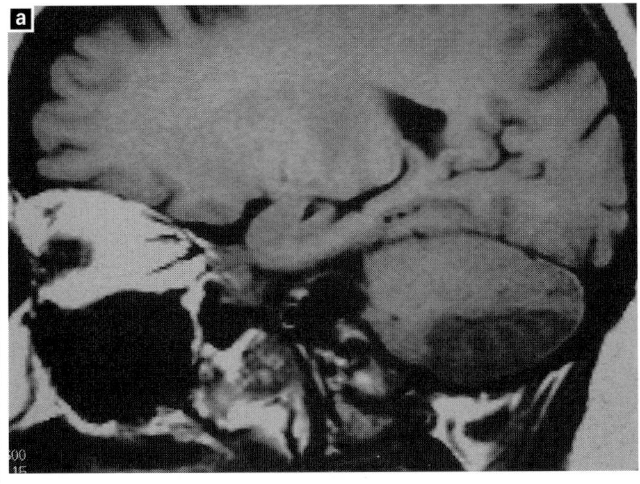
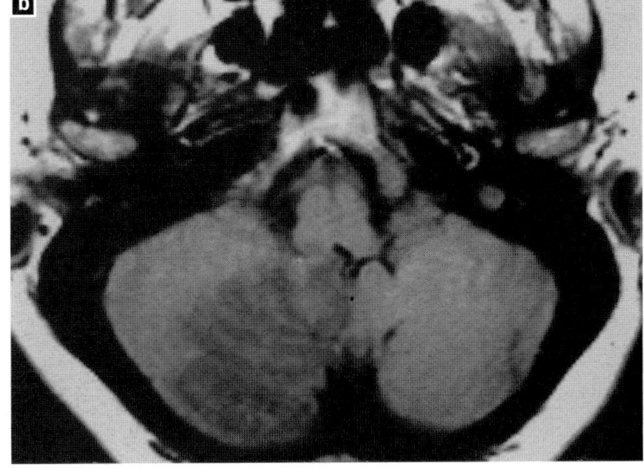

Fig. 1.22. **(a), (b) Sagittal and axial T1 MRI images are provided.**

Diagnosis

Right cerebellar subacute infarct in the posterior inferior cerebellar artery (PICA) territory.

The pathology in this case is consistent with that of both lateral and paramedian cerebellar lesions, with both peripheral and central ataxia, as the infarct involves both zones.

Other interesting clinical correlates may occur if there is an associated posterolateral medullary infarct. This can occur since this portion of the medulla is also supplied by the posterior inferior cerebellar artery and should always be looked for in the setting of PICA infarcts.

In this particular case, there are indeed other interesting yet subtle findings: there is subtle T1-weighted hypointensity in the right posterolateral medulla, indicating that this region is also involved by the infarct. Those ancillary symptoms and signs are discussed in the chapter on the medulla.

Case 1.7

64-year-old male patient, who presents with sudden onset left-sided limb ataxia, as well as dysarthria. The patient does not complain of vertigo.

MRI examinations are presented (Fig. 1.23).

What are the findings? What is your diagnosis?

The T1-weighted sagittal image shows hypointensity in the left superior cerebellum. The diffusion weighted image shows hyperintensity in the left superior cerebellum. Like the previous case,

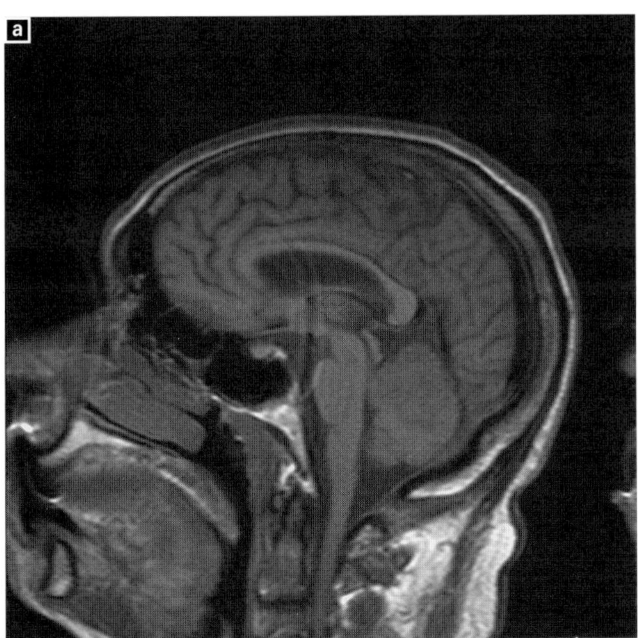
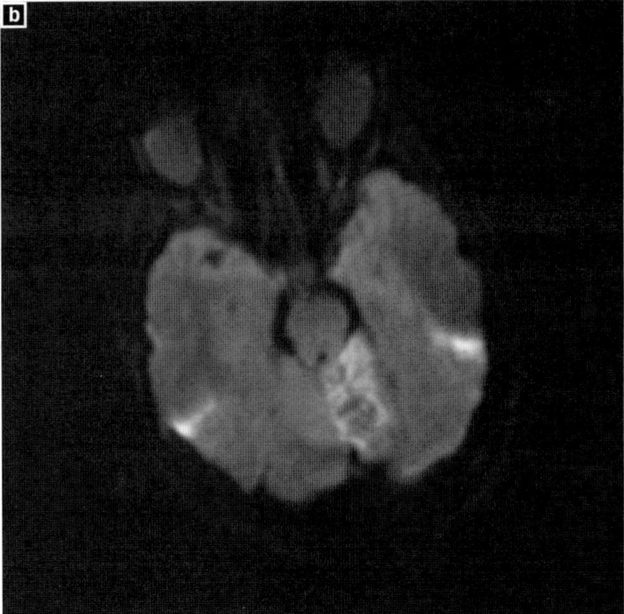

Fig. 1.23. **(a), (b) T1 sagittal and diffusion-weighted axial MRI images are provided.**

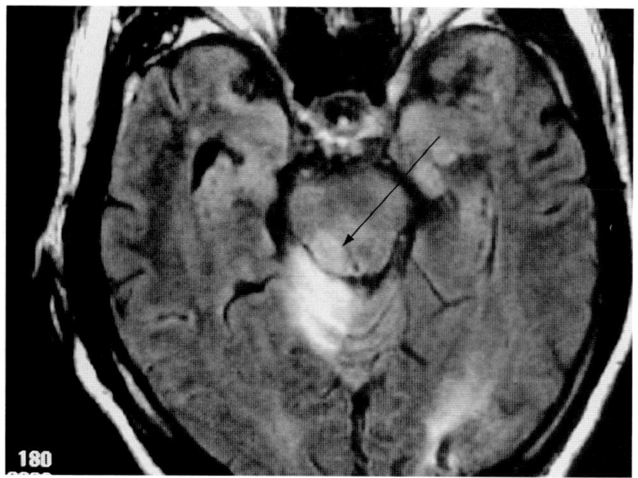

Fig. 1.24. **Axial FLAIR image in a 68-year-old male who presented with right-sided cerebellar ataxia and a right-sided Horner's syndrome, as well as left body pain and temperature sensory loss and a left trochlear nerve palsy (left ocular superior oblique muscle palsy). The infarct extends into the right superior pontine tegmentum (arrow).**

the findings indicate cortical (cytotoxic) edema, and are confined to a vascular territory, sharply respecting the midline on the DWI image.

Diagnosis

Left superior cerebellar artery (SCA) territory infarct.

This patient presents with the typical clinical findings of a superior cerebellar artery infarct. Once again, because the lesion involves the left cerebellar hemisphere, we expect left peripheral ataxia. Unlike posterior inferior cerebellar artery strokes, infarcts in the superior cerebellar artery territory often present with cerebellar dysarthria. In fact, rare cases of isolated dysarthria have been reported with occlusion of the medial branch of the superior cerebellar artery, where the infarct is confined to the paravermal zone. Another difference between PICA and SCA infarcts is that, with SCA infarcts, vertigo is significantly less likely, since this finding is usually seen with flocculonodular lobe pathology in the inferior cerebellum.

Once again, many other interesting clinical correlates may occur if there is concomitant involvement of the pontine tegmentum, and these include an ipsilateral Horner's syndrome, as well as contralateral pain and temperature sensory deficits, and contralateral trochlear nerve palsy. These findings are discussed in more detail in the pons chapter, but the adjacent case provides a nice illustration of such a combined cerebellar–pontine tegmentum syndrome (Fig. 1.24).

The images show a subacute infarct in the right superior cerebellar hemisphere extending into the right pontine tegmentum. The involved structures are the right trochlear nucleus, the right spinothalamic tract, and the right-sided descending sympathetic fibers.

Case 1.8

67-year-old male patient presents with sudden onset of vertigo, falling to the left, and left hand dysmetria.

MRI examination is provided below (Fig. 1.25).

What are the findings? What is your diagnosis?

The images show subtle hyperintensity in the left anterior–inferior cerebellum. This is consistent with infarction in the left anterior inferior cerebellar artery (AICA) territory.

Diagnosis

Left AICA infarct.

Anterior inferior cerebellar artery infarcts are uncommon. They tend to present with ipsilateral dysmetria and vestibular signs. If there is concomitant involvement of the brainstem, there may be ipsilateral facial weakness, an ipsilateral Horner's syndrome, ipsilateral body pain and temperature sensory loss, and contralateral facial pain and temperature sensory loss.

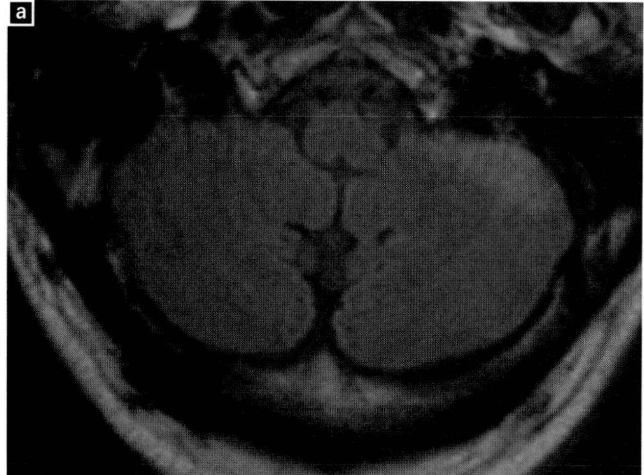
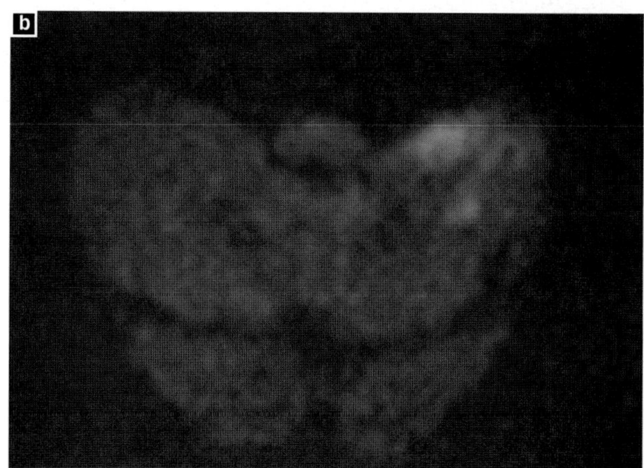

Fig. 1.25. **(a), (b) FLAIR and poor quality diffusion-weighted MRI images.**

Case 1.9

41-year-old alcoholic patient with electrolyte abnormalities. Patient presented with headaches, nausea, vomiting, nystagmus,

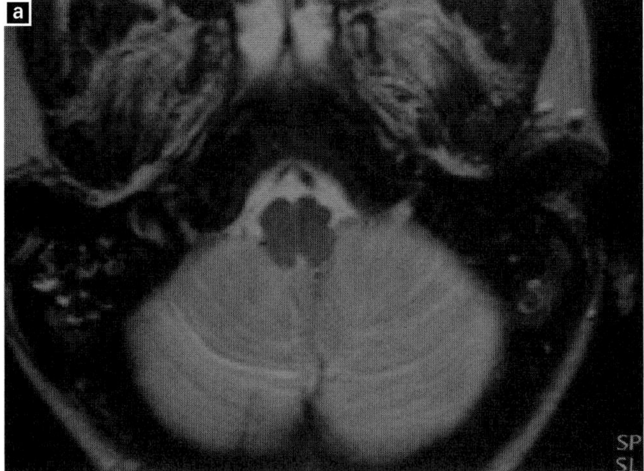

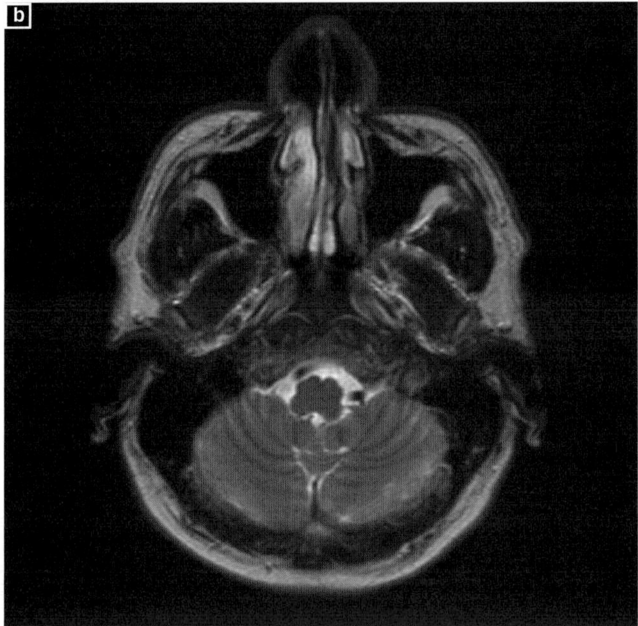

Fig. 1.26. **(a) Axial T2-weighted image (top) from our patient.
(b) Comparison T2-weighted image from a normal control (bottom).**

myoclonic jerks and truncal as well as limb ataxia. The patient progressed to coma.

MR images are presented (Fig. 1.26).
What are the findings? What is your diagnosis?

In comparison to the normal control, we see that there is marked diffuse symmetric abnormal hyperintensity on the T2-weighted images in the cerebellar hemispheres. The appearance is suggestive of demyelination and/or edema. Delving further into the patient's history, we find that he had rapidly corrected hyponatremia.

Diagnosis

Diffuse cerebellar (extrapontine) myelinolysis.

This is part of the spectrum of osmotic myelinolysis usually attributed to over-rapid correction of hyponatremia. Osmotic myelinolysis usually manifests in the pons as central pontine myelinolysis (CPM), but can involve other structures, such as the brainstem, thalami, or cerebellum, in which case it is called extra pontine myelinolysis. Such extensive, isolated cerebellar involvement is unusual, but the appearance suggests only a very limited differential.

Other possible causes of diffuse cerebellar edema/hyperintensity similar to this case would include hypoxia (as we have seen above), lead intoxication, and acute infectious cerebellitis. In children, infectious cerebellitis is often known as "acute ataxia of childhood." It is usually secondary to viral infections, the most common association being with chickenpox. Other infections which may cause a similar picture include Coxsackie virus, EBV, CMV, and Mycoplasma infection, as well as post-vaccine reactions. In adults, the most commonly implicated organisms are probably Mycoplasma and EBV. Infectious cerebellitis usually presents with ataxia, dysarthria and nystagmus of rapid onset. The prognosis is usually benign, with complete recovery. However, permanent deficits, or progression to death may result (sounds like one of those disclaimers for a drug commercial!). Finally, a truly rare cause of symmetric cerebellar hyperintensity is a disease called neuroaxonal dystrophy. This is a progressive disorder seen in children. It involves both the central and the peripheral nervous systems, and the most consistent imaging finding is symmetric cerebellar hyperintensity on FLAIR images as well as some cerebellar atrophy. A reference for those who wish to know more about this rare disease is the paper by Farina *et al.* (1999).

Reference

Farina, L., Nardocci, N., Bruzzone, M. G. *et al.* Infantile neuroaxonal dystrophy: neuroradiological studies in 11 patients. *Neuroradiology* 1999; **41**: 376–380.

Case 1.10

62-year-old male patient with chronic alcoholic liver cirrhosis presents with 2-month history of declining mental status, ataxia, and hypophonic dysarthria. On examination, there is truncal ataxia as well as dysmetria in the upper extremities. The patient displayed occasional asterixis. Ultrasound examination revealed a shrunken cirrhotic liver with ascites and portal vein thrombosis.

What do you think so far?

We have already seen alcoholic cerebellar atrophy, and know that upper extremity dysmetria and dysarthria are unusual

findings. With chronic liver disease and portosystemic shunting, we also know that there is an unusual condition called "acquired hepatocerebral degeneration." This condition will be discussed more fully in the chapter on the basal ganglia. Briefly, though, it is a progressive, irreversible neurodegenerative syndrome characterized by extrapyramidal movement disorders including tremor, bradykinesia, choreoathetosis and rigidity, with possible accompanying ataxia, dysarthria, and dementia. Our patient has some, but not all of these

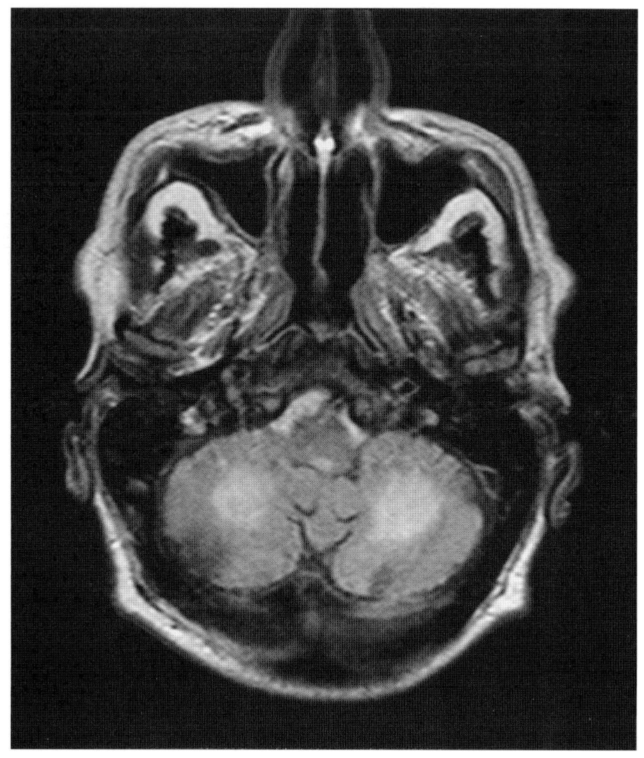

Fig. 1.27. **FLAIR axial MR image through the cerebellum.**

manifestations. Pathologically, there is vacuolar degeneration in the basal ganglia with loss of dopaminergic D2 receptors in the globus pallidus. The most common imaging correlate for acquired hepatocerebral degeneration is abnormal T1-weighted hyperintensity in the bilateral globus pallidus. Our patient did not have this.

Here, however, is the relevant MR image (Fig. 1.27).

What do you see?

There are bilateral symmetrical FLAIR hyperintensities in the deep cerebellar white matter. It turns out that this finding is part of a larger spectrum of rare manifestations of acquired hepatocerebral degeneration separate from the typical basal ganglia abnormalities described above. The changes in the deep cerebellar white matter reflect a mixture of edema and gliosis. The precise etiology is uncertain, but various hypotheses include toxic degeneration secondary to the metabolic derangements which accompany chronic liver disease, or possibly some unusual form of osmotic myelinolysis. Despite the lack of a definite pathophysiology, this set of cerebellar findings has been previously described in the literature as a rare solitary manifestation of acquired hepatocerebral degeneration (see Lee *et al.*, 1988). The predominance of cerebellar findings accounts for the clinical presentation.

Reference

Lee, J., Lacomis, D., Comu, S. *et al*. Acquired hepatocerebral degeneration: MR and pathologic findings. *American Journal of Neuroradiology* 1988; **19**: 485–487.

Case 1.11

2-year-old male patient presenting with developmental delay, increased head circumference and ataxia.

Non-contrast CT images are presented (Fig. 1.28).

What are the findings? What is your diagnosis?

There is a large posterior fossa cyst which appears to communicate directly with the fourth ventricle. There is absence of the cerebellar vermis.

Diagnosis

Dandy–Walker malformation.

The Dandy–Walker malformation is a congential anomaly, which consists primarily of agenesis or severe hypogenesis of the cerebellar vermis with a single large fourth ventricle-cisterna magna cyst that occupies much of the posterior fossa. Although there is agenesis of the vermis, the posterior fossa is usually enlarged because of the cyst. Also, despite the congenital absence of the vermis, ataxia is often not a primary feature of the presentation. Rather, the clinical presentation depends on the associated findings in the CNS. The most important of these is hydrocephalus, which is present in 80–90 percent of the patients at the time of diagnosis. The hydrocephalus is not usually present at birth, but begins to develop in the first few months of life. Other significant associated abnormalities include agenesis or hypogenesis of the corpus callosum, which occurs in about one-third of patients, and abnormalities of cellular migration in the cortex, such as heterotopic gray matter and lissencephaly (present in about

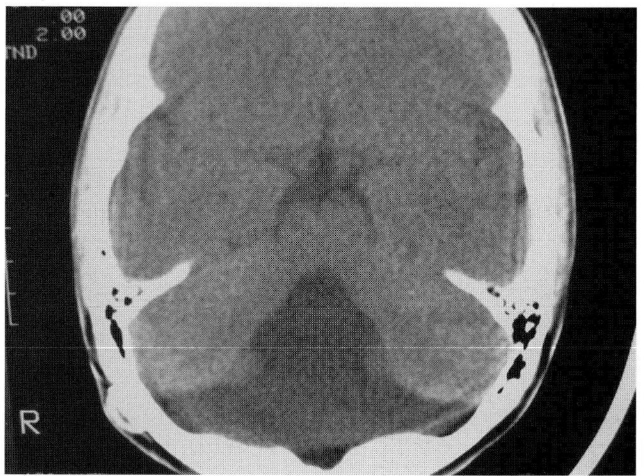

Fig. 1.28. **Axial non-contrast CT image of the posterior fossa.**

10 percent of cases). If there are no other associated abnormalities, the patient may not present until late childhood or early adulthood, and the symptoms may include ataxia as well as brainstem findings.

The diagnosis of Dandy–Walker malformation can be suggested in utero with ultrasound, and can be confirmed with prenatal MRI (Fig. 1.29).

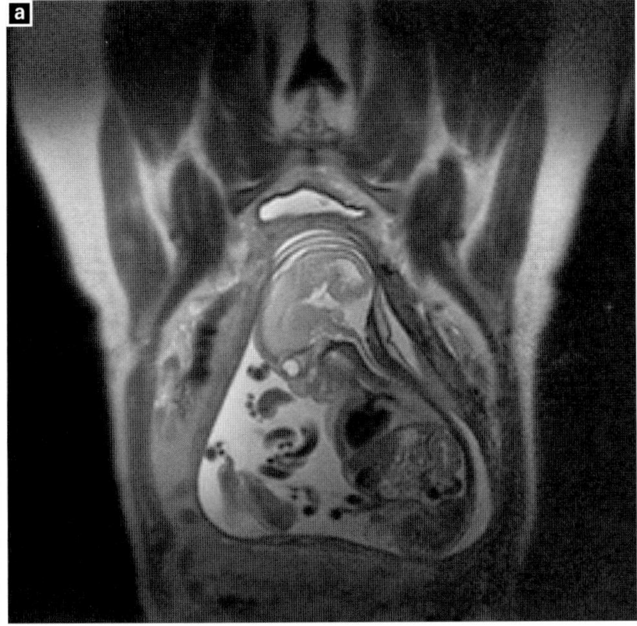
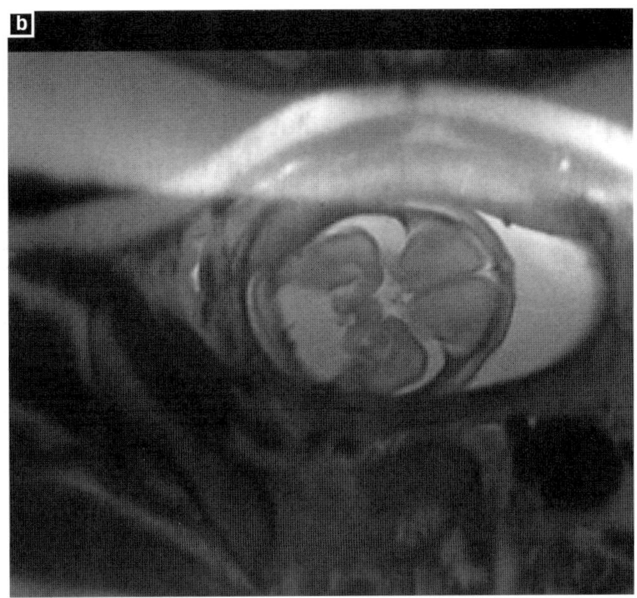

Fig. 1.29. **(a)** Coronal and **(b)** axial T2-weighted pelvic MRI images of an 8-month-old in utero fetus reveal absence of the midline cerebellar structures and a large posterior fossa cyst.

Case 1.12

2-year-old male presenting with difficulty breathing, with episodic hyperpnea, spasmodic eye movements, hypotonia, and ataxia, with developmental delay in both cognitive and physical milestones.

Relevant MRI images are presented (Fig. 1.30).

What are the findings?

The most striking feature is that the brainstem has an unusual appearance, looking like a "molar tooth" at the level of the pontomesencephalic junction on the T1-weighted axial image. It is after this feature that this group of disorders is named: "molar tooth" malformations of the cerebellum. The most famous entity in this group of disorders is Joubert syndrome, which is the diagnosis in this case. The axial T2-weighted image through the mid pons shows that the fourth ventricle has a "bat wing" appearance due to the absent vermis.

Discuss Joubert syndrome.

Joubert syndrome is a rare, probably genetic, disorder which affects approximately 1 in 100 000 children. Its most obvious imaging feature is absence or hypolasia of the cerebellar vermis, with prominent superior cerebellar peduncles. This gives the

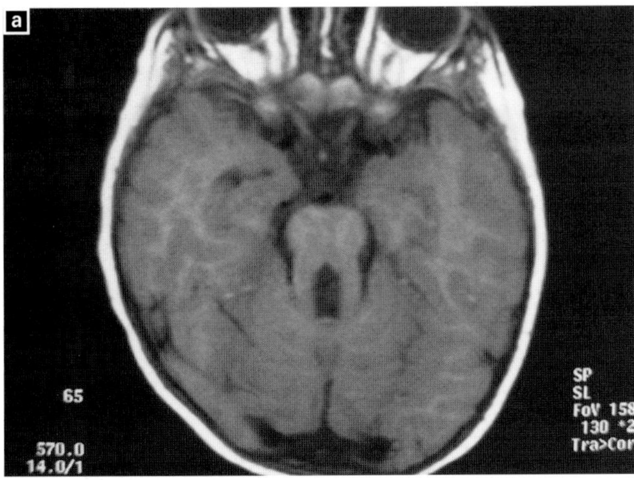
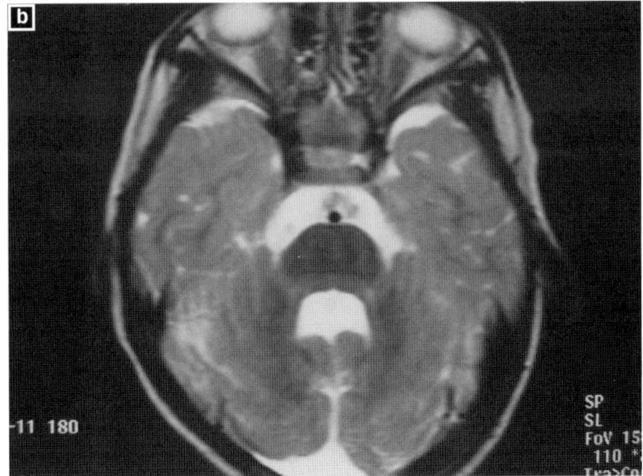

Fig. 1.30. **(a)** Axial T1- and **(b)** T2-weighted images through the pons.

brainstem its "molar tooth" appearance, and gives the fourth ventricle a batwing appearance (as above). The most prominent clinical features are those displayed by our patient, and include episodic hyperpnea, ataxia, spasmodic eye movements, as well as mild to moderate mental retardation.

After the description of this syndrome by Dr. Joubert in 1969, all "molar tooth" disorders of the cerebellum were initially referred to as Joubert syndrome. However, Joubert syndrome is better thought of as the prototype of a group of several related disorders. There are different categories of patients within this broad group. For example, some patients have renal anomalies, such as juvenile nephronothisis or multicystic dysplastic kidney, while others have ocular anomalies, such as retinal dysplasias and colobomas. Others have hepatic fibrosis and cysts, while others have extra digits. These related disorders go by such names as the Arima syndrome, Senior–Loken syndrome and COACH syndrome (see Satran *et al.*, 1999).

A very interesting feature of Joubert syndrome is a lack of decussation of the superior cerebellar peduncles, as well as lack of decussation of the corticospinal tracts. This has led some authors to speculate that the lack of decussation of these pathways may represent the primary abnormality in the central nervous system, and that the associated hypoplasia of the vermis and abnormalities of the brainstem are secondary results.

This intriguing hypothesis is supported by very recent descriptions of genetic mutations associated with some cases of Joubert syndrome. These mutations involve a gene called the AHI1 gene, which is heavily expressed in the forebrain and the hindbrain (see Ferland *et al.*, 2004 and Dixon-Salazar *et al.*, 2004). The precise function of this gene is unknown, but it is felt that it probably plays a strong role in "brain wiring," and hence defects in this gene might explain the correlation between Joubert syndrome and the lack of decussation of neural pathways mentioned above.

Discuss, in broad terms, malformations of the cerebellar vermis involving vermian aplasia or hypoplasia.

There are four main malformations of the cerebellar vermis involving aplasia/hypoplasia. The most common of these is probably the Dandy–Walker malformation which we have seen previously. This consists of partial or complete vermian agenesis, with cystic dilatation of the fourth ventricle, and an enlarged posterior fossa. The second of these is Joubert syndrome, and the related molar tooth malformations. These have vermian agenesis or hypogenesis, but without cystic dilatation of the fourth ventricle. A third condition is called rhombencephalosynapsis, and consists of vermian aplasia with midline fusion of the cerebellar hemispheres. Finally, a condition known as tectocerebellar dysraphia consists of vermian hypoplasia or aplasia with an occipital encephalocoele and rotation of the cerebellar hemispheres around the brainstem.

For those who wish to learn more about the topic of cerebellar malformations, there is an outstanding article from the University of California at San Francisco, which provides an imaging-based classification of cerebellar malformations by Patel and Barkovich. Such malformations are divided into hypoplasias and dysplasias. Each of these two broad categories is further subdivided into focal and diffuse variants. For example, "molar tooth" malformations of the cerebellum, including Joubert syndrome, fall under the focal dysplasias.

References

Dixon-Salazar, T., Silhavy, J. L., Marsh, S. E., *et al.* Mutations in the AHI1 gene, encoding Jouberin, cause Joubert syndrome with cortical polymicrogyria. *American Journal of Human Genetics* 2004; **75**(6): 979–987.

Ferland, R. J., Eyaid, W., Collura, R. V. *et al.* Abnormal cerebellar development and axonal decussation due to mutations in AHI1 in Joubert syndrome. *Nature Genetics* 2004; **36**(9): 1008–1013.

Patel, S. and Barkovich, A. J. Analysis and classification of cerebellar malformations. *American Journal of Neuroradiology* 2002; **23**: 1074–1087.

Satran, D., Pierpont, M. E., and Dobyns, W. B. Cerebello-Oculo-Renal syndromes including Arima Senior-Loken and COACH syndromes: more than just variants of Joubert syndrome. *American Journal of Medical Genetics* 1999; **86**: 459–469.

The external gross anatomy of the medulla can be viewed, to some extent, as a continuation of the spinal cord. Along the ventral or anterior surface, the median fissure of the spinal cord continues along the medulla, with the medullary pyramids on each side. The medullary pyramids are bounded laterally by the ventrolateral sulci. Lateral to these sulci are the inferior olives, which in turn, are bounded laterally by the dorsolateral sulci. The hypoglossal nerves (cranial nerve 12) exit the medulla in the ventrolateral sulci between the pyramids and olives, while the roots of cranial nerves 9, 10, and 11 exit lateral to the olives (see Fig. 2.1(a) and (b)) .

Dorsally, the gracilis and cuneatus nuclei form surface bulges known as the gracile and cuneate tubercles. The dorsal surface of the medulla forms part of the floor of the fourth ventricle, which is flanked on each side by the inferior cerebellar peduncle at the level of the medulla and the middle cerebellar peduncle at the level of the pons. The roof of the fourth ventricle is formed by the anterior (superior) and posterior (inferior) medullary velum.

The internal structure of the medulla will be described at three different levels to give a sense of the key medullary structures and their changes in orientation through the medulla. Proceeding from caudal to rostral, these levels are the level of the motor (pyramidal) decussation, the level of the sensory (lemniscal) decussation, and the level of the inferior olivary nuclei and inferior cerebellar peduncles.

Level of the pyramidal decussation

Three main sets of structures have some clinical importance at this level in the medulla. Along the ventral surface, there is the decussation of the descending pyramidal tracts. Dorsolaterally, there are the ascending spinothalamic tracts and the spinal trigeminal nucleus and tract. Dorsally, there are the gracilis and cuneatus nuclei and tracts (see Fig. 2.2).

The medullary pyramids contain the descending corticospinal and corticobulbar tracts. The corticospinal tracts represent the main pathway from the motor cortex to the spinal cord and they are responsible for the motor control of one side of the brain over the opposite side of the body. This occurs because about 90 percent of the corticospinal fibers running in the medullary pyramid decussate to the opposite side at the level of the caudal medulla, and continue as the contralateral lateral corticospinal tract. A small proportion of undecussated fibers continue inferiorly into the ipsilateral anterior corticospinal tract.

Dorsolaterally in the medulla, there is the spinal nucleus of the trigeminal nerve with the overlying spinal trigeminal tract. This is continuous with the substantia gelatinosa of the spinal cord caudally and the main sensory nucleus of the trigeminal nerve rostrally at the level of the pons. The anatomy of the trigeminal nuclei will be discussed later as part of the pons.

Adjacent to the spinal trigeminal nucleus and tract is the spinothalamic tract, mediating pain and temperature sensations from the contralateral body. It is noted that these fibers decussate one or two levels rostral to their entry into the cord, and so carry information from the contralateral body. Also, in this region of the medulla, anterior to the sensory tracts, there are the ventral and dorsal spinocerebellar tracts.

Dorsally, there are the midline nucleus gracilis and cuneatus with their respective tracts. The gracilis is located medial to the cuneatus. The gracilis and cuneatus contain fibers from both mechanoreceptors (mediating touch and vibration) as well as from proprioceptive receptors (mediating joint movement and position sense). Some fibers travel directly from the dorsal columns to the cuneatus and gracilis nuclei and then into the medial lemniscus to ultimately arrive in the contralateral thalamus. Other fibers synapse in the cord and travel indirectly through second order or third order neurons. However, they also eventually reach the medial lemniscus and then the thalamus contralateral to their side of origin.

Level of sensory (lemniscal) decussation

At this level, once again, the medullary pyramids lie ventrally in the medulla. Posterior to them, the tracts from the cuneatus and gracilis dive forward in the midline and decussate to the contralateral side, forming the medial lemnisci (see Fig. 2.3). Therefore, each medial lemniscus comes to lie directly behind

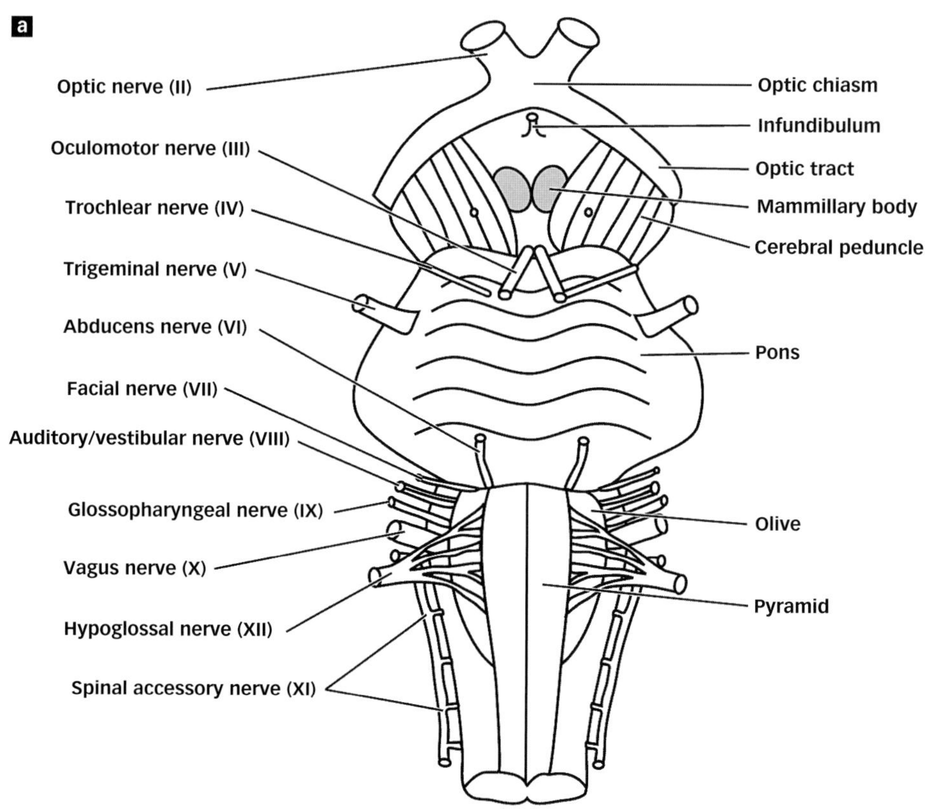

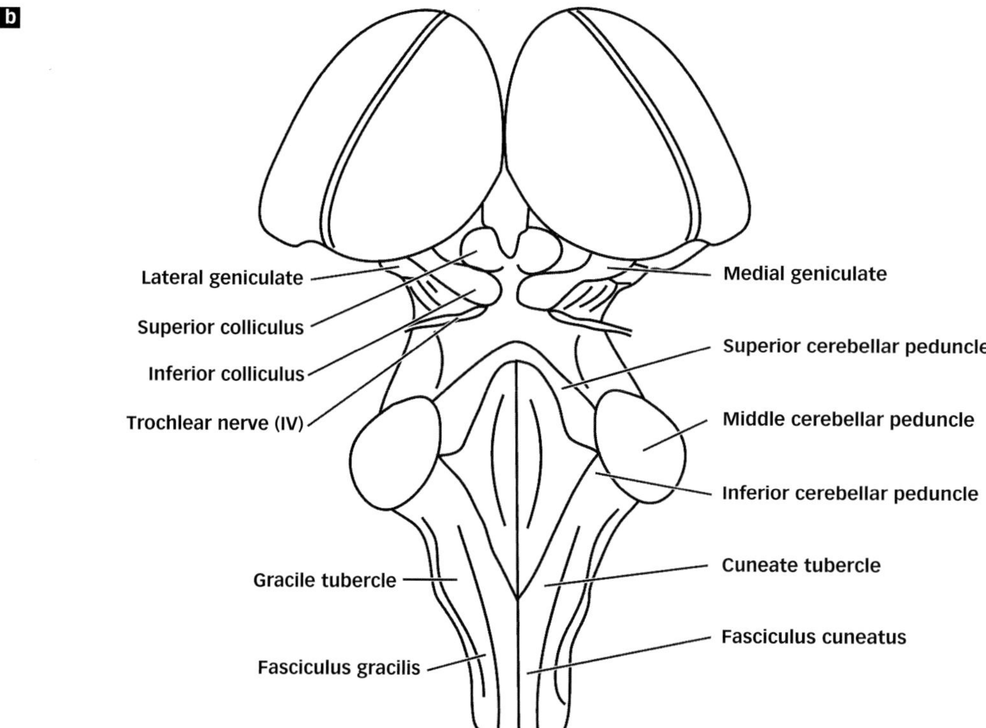

Fig. 2.1. **These figures display the major surface anatomic landmarks on the (a) ventral and (b) dorsal surfaces of the medulla respectively.**

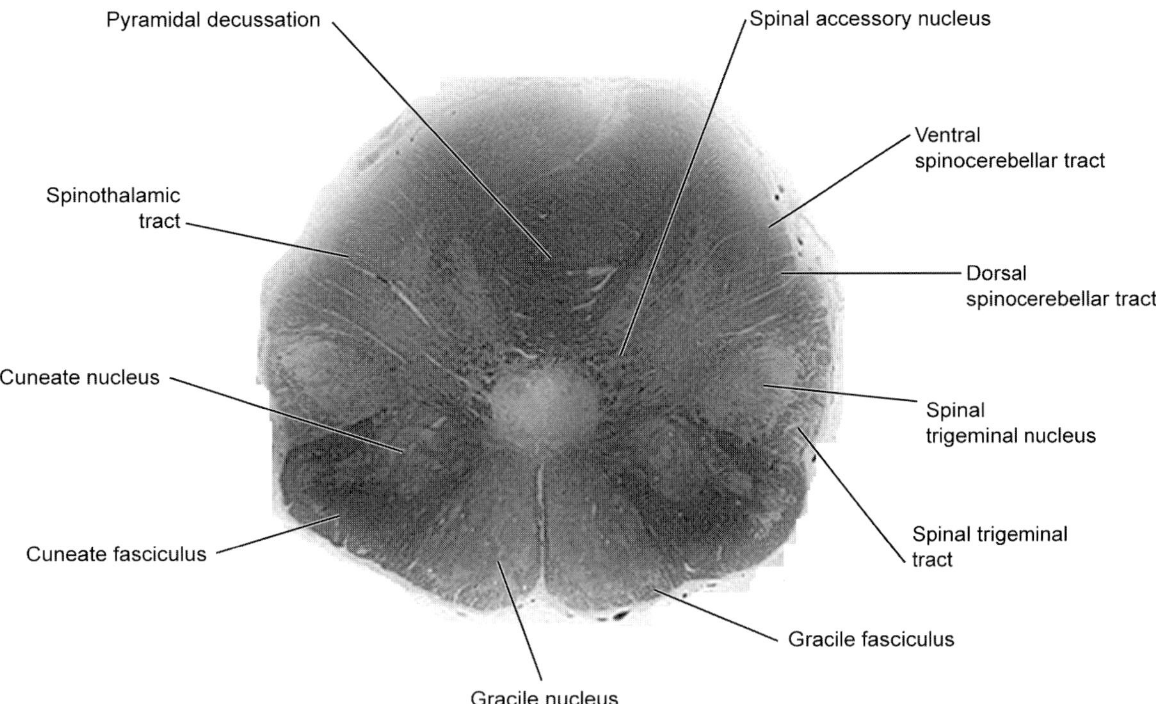

Fig. 2.2. **Axial cross-section of the medulla at the level of the pyramidal decussation. The top of the figure represents the ventral medullary surface, i.e., the same orientation as an axial MRI scan.**

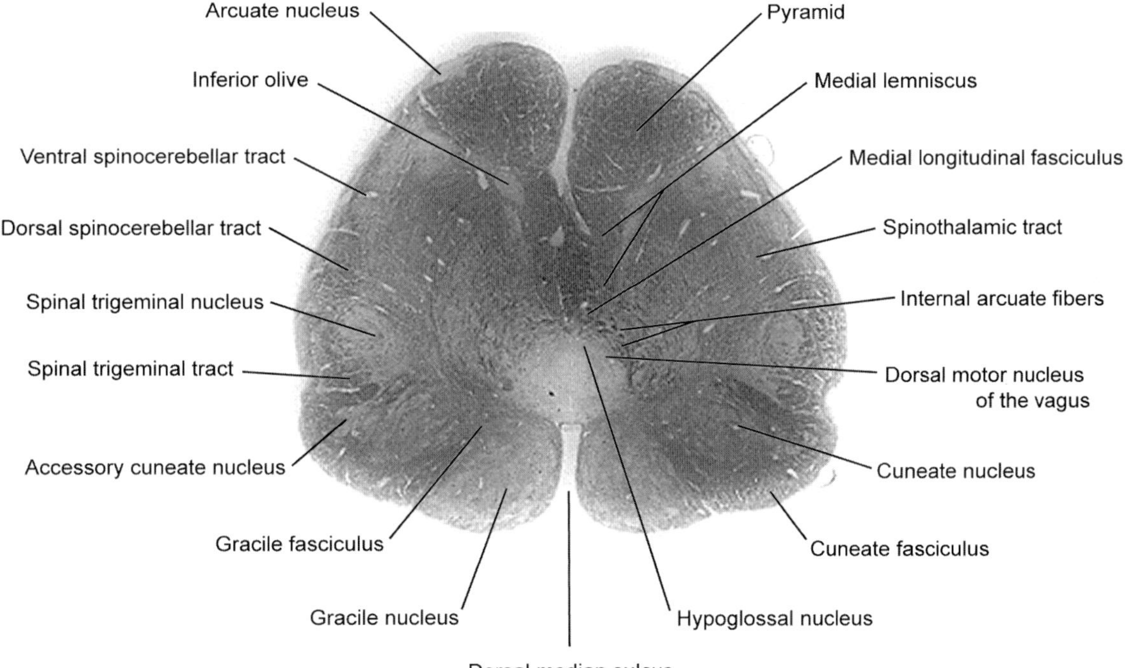

Fig. 2.3. **Axial cross-section of the medulla at the level of the lemniscal decussation. Once again, the top of the figure represents the ventral medullary surface.**

the medullary pyramid. It carries fibers from the contralateral dorsal column, and projects to the ipsilateral thalamus (right dorsal column to left medial lemniscus to VPL nucleus of left thalamus). Therefore, lesions of the medial lemniscus present with contralateral loss of vibration and proprioception.

Posterior (dorsal) to the medial lemniscus is the medial longitudinal fasciculus, which among other functions, connects the vestibular apparatus to the extraocular muscle nuclei.

In the dorsolateral medulla are once again the spinothalamic tract and the spinal trigeminal nucleus and tract. As you

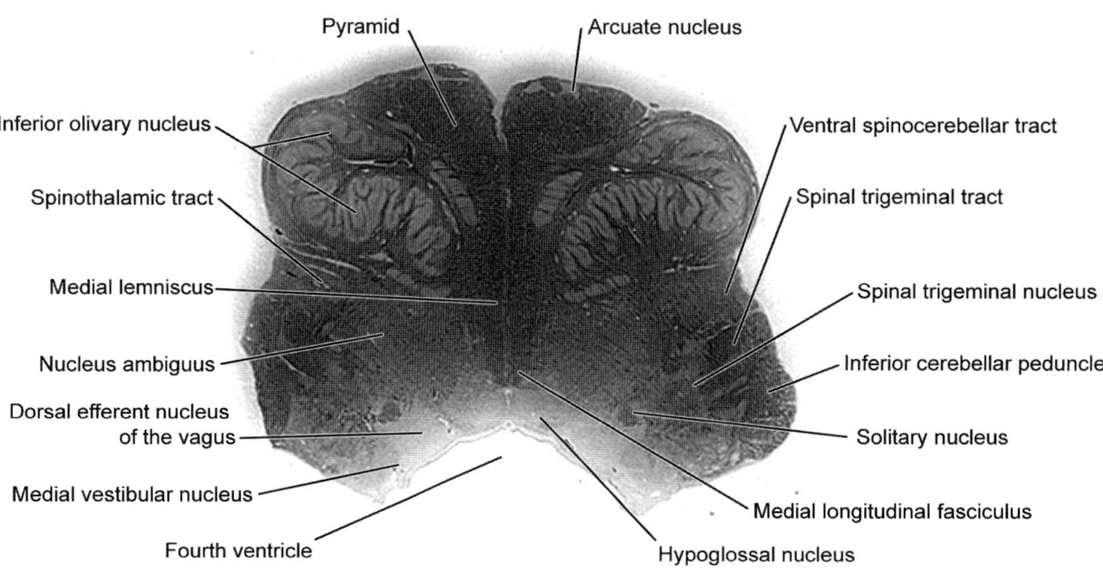

Fig. 2.4. **Cross-section of the medulla at the level of the inferior olives and inferior cerebellar peduncles (again oriented like an axial MRI).**

recall, the spinothalamic tract fibers have already decussated in the cord one or two levels above their entry point, and so also represent the contralateral body. They do not decussate again in the medulla. Along with the decussation of the dorsal columns, this underlies the mapping of sensation from one side of the body to the contralateral thalamus and cortex.

Level of the inferior olives and inferior cerebelar peduncles

Anteriorly in the medulla at this level are the medullary pyramids containing the corticospinal and corticobulbar tracts. Just dorsolateral to the pyramids, are the large inferior olivary nuclei (see Fig. 2.4).

The connections of the inferior olivary nuclei will be more fully discussed when we review the cerebellum. Briefly, the inferior olives receive inputs from the cerebral cortex, basal ganglia and spinal cord, each of which projects to both olivary complexes. Also, there is a large input to each inferior olivary nucleus from the ipsilateral red nucleus. The inferior olives provide the climbing fiber input to the Purkinjie cells of the contralateral cerebellar cortex. In a feedback circuit, they also receive significant input from the deep cerebellar nuclei.

Between the pyramids and the olives, the fibers of the 12th (hypoglossal) cranial nerves exit the medulla. Posterior to the

pyramids in the midline lie the wedge-shaped medial lemnisci which extend posteriorly to the medullary tegmentum. Posterior to the medial lemnisci in the midline are the medial longitudinal fasciculi (MLFs).

In the mid-medulla, between the pyramids and the floor of the fourth ventricle, are the multiple nuclei of the meduallry reticular formation, including the parvicellular nucleus and the magnocellular–gigantocellular nucleus. Among other functions, the reticular formation, possibly via connections with the thalamus, is important for consciousness, wakefulness and attention.

In the posterior medulla are found two of the four vestibular nuclei for the 8th cranial nerve (the medial and inferior vestibular nuclei), the spinal trigeminal nucleus and tract for cranial nerve 5, the spinothalamic tracts, the inferior cerebellar peduncles, and the descending preganglionic sympathetic fibers, called Horner's tract.

The nuclei which subserve cranial nerve 9 (glossopharyngeal), cranial nerve 10 (vagus), and cranial nerve 12 (hypoglossal) are also found in the posterior medulla. These include the hypoglossal nuclei for cranial nerve 12, and the nucleus ambiguus, the nucleus solitarius and tract, the inferior salivatory nucelus, as well as the dorsal motor nucelus of the vagus for cranial nerves 9 and 10. The anatomy of the lower cranial nerves will be discussed in more detail in the cases that follow.

Case 2.1

51-year-old male patient presents with slowly progressive dysphagia and hoarseness. The patient complains that he aspirates often while eating. Clinical testing reveals loss of the gag reflex on the right, and leftward deviation of the uvula. Careful swabbing of the back of the pharynx with a cotton swab suggests decreased sensation on the right. ENT testing reveals right vocal cord paralysis. Further neurologic testing detects some weakness in turning the head to the left against resistance, and some weakness in elevating the right shoulder against resistance. The tongue was normal, without atrophy or fasciculations, and protruded in the midline.

What cranial nerves do you think are involved? Loss of the gag reflex on the right suggests involvement of either the right 9th (glossopharyngeal) or 10th (vagus) nerves, or both. The paralysis of the right vocal cord suggests a right 10th nerve lesion. The decreased

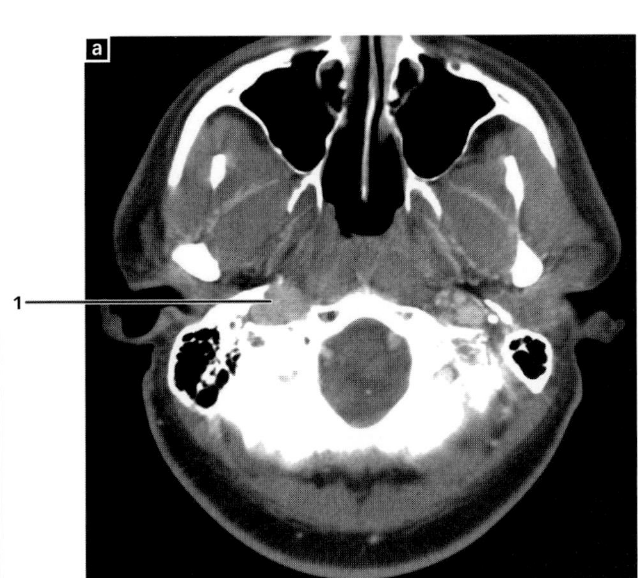
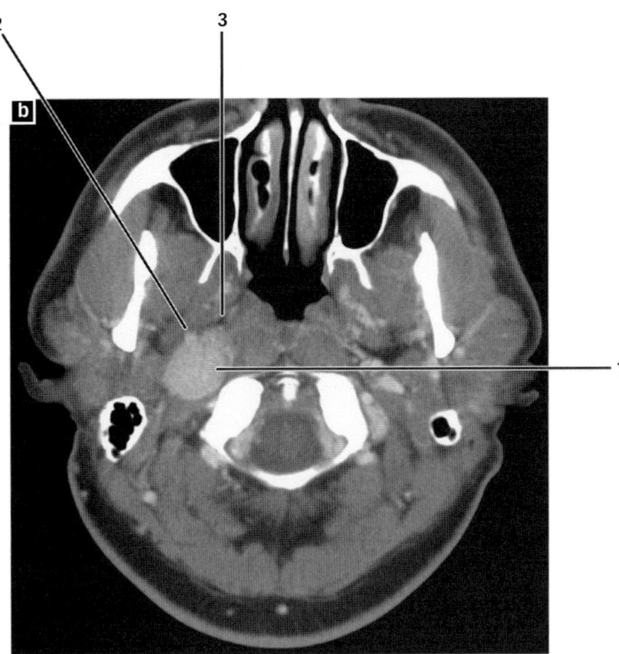

Fig. 2.5 (a),(b). **Axial post-contrast CT images show an intensely enhancing lesion (label #1) extending from the skull base inferiorly along the right carotid space, displacing the right ICA anteriorly (label #2). Note that the fatty parapharyngeal space is also displaced anteriorly (label #3).**

sensation along the pharyngeal mucosa suggests a 9th nerve lesion. Shrugging the shoulder and turning the head are functions of the trapezius and sternocleidomastoid muscles respectively. These are innervated by cranial nerve 11. Therefore, the history and physical findings strongly suggest involvement of the 9th, 10th and 11th cranial nerves.

Where do think the lesion may be located? As will be discussed below, the nuclei of the 9th and 10th nerves are in close proximity in the dorsolateral medulla, and so are often involved together. However, the nuclei of cranial nerve 11 subtending the trapezius and sternocleidomastoid muscles are actually in the cervical cord. Therefore, an intra-axial lesion would be unlikely. More likely, the lesion involves the nerves after they have exited the medulla and cervical cord and while they are traveling together. Possible locations would be in the perimedullary cistern at the level of the foramen magnum, at the level of the jugular foramen, or in the neck along the course of the carotid sheath.

Look at the images (Figure 2.5 (a) and (b)) What images are provided and what are the findings?

Two axial post-contrast CT images are provided. The left-hand image (Fig. 2.5(a)) is at the level of the skull base, and shows an enhancing lesion just below the right jugular foramen and right carotid canal. The right-hand image (Fig. 2.5(b)) is in the high cervical region, and shows an intensely enhancing mass in the right carotid space, displacing the right ICA anteriorly. The right parapharyngeal fat is displaced anteriorly as well. These findings are characteristic of a carotid space mass. It is noted that the carotid space is often also referred to as the retrostyloid parapharyngeal space, especially in neurology books. The three leading differential diagnostic possibilities for a carotid space mass are glomus tumors, schwannomas, or adenopathy. The extension superiorly to the level of the skull base and the intense enhancement make adenopathy less likely (deep jugular lymph nodes do not usually extend beyond the level of the jugulodigastric lymph node, which is the apex of the chain). Therefore, we are left with

two possibilities: glomus tumor and vascular schwannoma. Very briefly, glomus tumors are paragangliomas, which arise from neural crest paraganglion cells adjacent to nerves. They are multiple about 5 percent of the time (except if familial, where the multiplicity may be as high as 20–30%). Glomus tumors are named for the level at which they occur: *glomus tympanicum* at the level of the middle ear cavity, *glomus jugulare* at the level of the jugular foramen, *glomus vagale* at the level of the nasopharyngeal or oropharyngeal carotid space, and *carotid body tumor* at the level of the carotid bifurcation.

Glomus tumors and highly vascular schwannomas are often not separable on imaging, although schawannomas are not typically so highly vascular. In any case, both tumors are often preoperatively embolized, and resected through the same surgical approach, so making a precise diagnosis is not critical.

This was a case of glomus vagale, producing cranial nerve 9, 10, and 11 findings.

For comparison, look at the case below, in a patient with a similar clinical presentation (Fig. 2.6 (a) and (b)).

Contrast CT, and post-contrast T1-weighted MRI images are provided. Once again, there is a large mass in the right carotid space, displacing the right internal carotid artery anteriorly. As opposed to the case of glomus vagale, however, this large mass shows minimal or no enhancement on post-contrast CT. The diagnosis in this case was a 10th nerve schwannoma. Typically, schwannomas are less vascular than glomus tumors. Once again, however, it is stressed that highly vascular schwannomas do exist, and that radiographic differentiation from glomus tumors in those cases may be impossible.

Another interesting facet of this case is that, although the mass does not show significant enhancement on CT, it avidly enhances on MRI. This discordance is often a source of confusion. However, it should be recalled that there are different contrast enhancement mechanisms in CT and MRI. CT functions basically as an electron density map (really, a linear X-ray attenuation coefficient

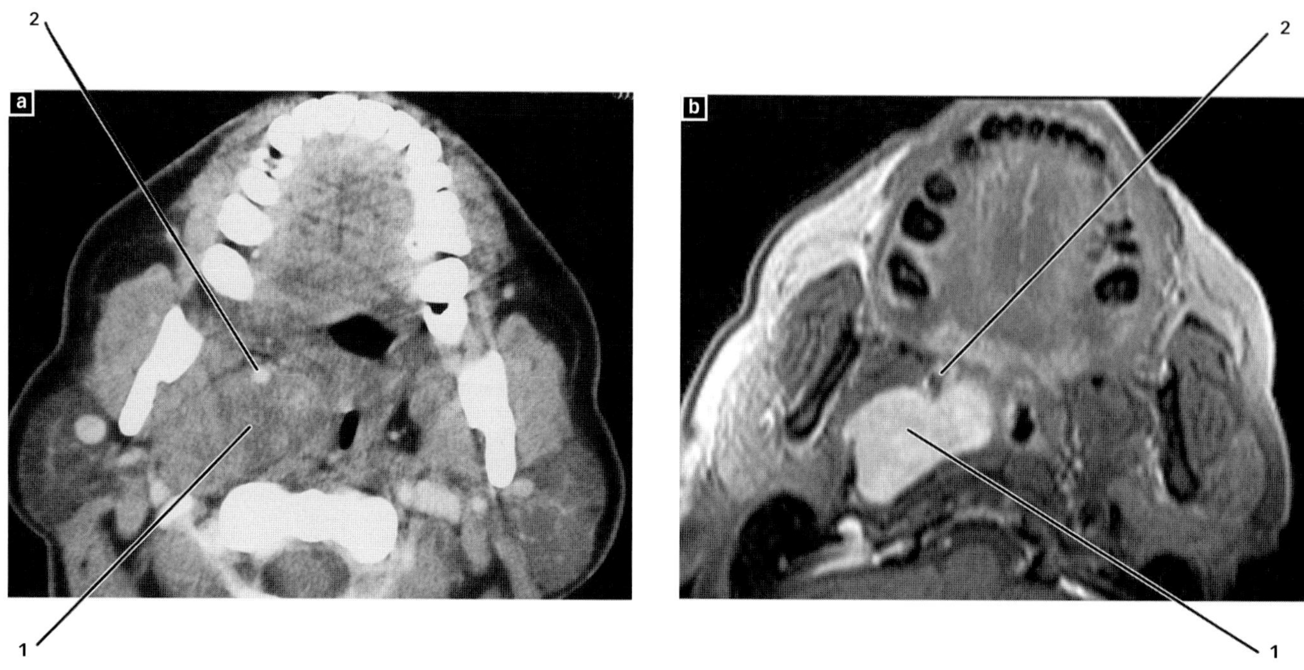

Fig. 2.6 (a),(b). **Axial post-contrast CT (right) and post-contrast T1-weighted MR images show a mass in the right carotid space (label #1). The mass displaces the right ICA anteriorly (label #2).**

map, but this is closely related to electron density), correlating brightness to the number of electrons per voxel of the CT image. What is visualized with CT contrast enhancement is the iodine contrast molecule, with its relatively high atomic number (53), and hence large number of electrons increasing the electron density per voxel. With MRI, however, only hydrogen protons are visualized. Gadolinium atoms provides "contrast enhancement" by shortening the T1 time of hydrogen protons in their vicinity, therefore causing them to appear bright on T1-weighted MRI images, in just the same fashion that protons within intrinsically short T1 time constants, such as hydrogen protons in fat, are bright on T1-weighted MRI. A smaller concentration of gadolinium is required to achieve this T1 shortening in MRI than the concentration of iodine needed to achieve appreciable increases in density on contrast CT examination. Therefore, a mass may appear as non-enhancing on contrast CT, yet as avidly enhancing on contrast MRI, as in this case.

Diagnosis

Vernet's syndrome.

Of course, you are probably thinking, "What the heck is Vernet's syndrome?" It is an eponym found in various textbooks for a syndrome which involves cranial nerves 9, 10 and 11. Vernet's syndrome is typically defined as ipsilateral loss of taste and sensation of the posterior third of the tongue, ipsilateral loss of gag reflex, ipsilateral vocal cord paralysis, and ipsilateral weakness of the sternocleidomastoid and trapezius muscles. The most common causes are tumors and skull base fractures.

Discuss the functional anatomy of the 9th and 10th nerves.

The 9th and 10th nerves are somewhat complicated, because they are both mixed sensory and motor nerves which subserve multiple modalities. Both nerves have general sensory afferent (GSA), general visceral afferent (GVA), special visceral afferent (SVA), special visceral efferent (SVE) and general visceral efferent (GVE) components, which will be described below.

To be able to perform these multiple functions, both nerves receive contributions from multiple brainstem nuclei, including the spinal trigeminal nucleus, the nucleus solitarius, and the nucleus ambiguus, which they have in common, as well as the inferior salivatory nucleus for cranial nerve 9 and the dorsal motor nucleus of the vagus for cranial nerve 10.

Parenthetically, it may seem confusing that the spinal trigeminal nucleus and tract, which are associated with cranial nerve 5 (the trigeminal nerve), also contribute to the function of other cranial nerves (7, 9 and 10). Also, it is probably confusing that one nucleus, such as the nucleus ambiguus, would contribute to both the 9th and 10th nerves. However, the medulla can be thought of as a transition zone between the spinal cord, where the deep gray matter functions as essentially one large nucleus contributing to numerous spinal nerves, and the pons and midbrain, where the deep nuclei are more discrete in their correlation with cranial nerves.

The 9th (glossopharyngeal) nerve

The 9th cranial nerve is primarily a sensory nerve. It has two ganglia (superior and inferior) located near the jugular foramen. It exits the medulla along with cranial nerve 10, and exits the skull via the jugular foramen along with cranial nerves 10 and 11 to run in the carotid sheath within the neck. It receives contributions from the spinal trigeminal nucleus, the nucleus solitarius, the nucleus ambiguus and the inferior salivatory nucleus (see Fig. 2.7).

Its separate functions, in relation to the various contributing brainstem nuclei, are listed below.

GSA component

The 9th nerve innervates part of the external auditory canal and external ear (a sensory function). These fibers have cell bodies in

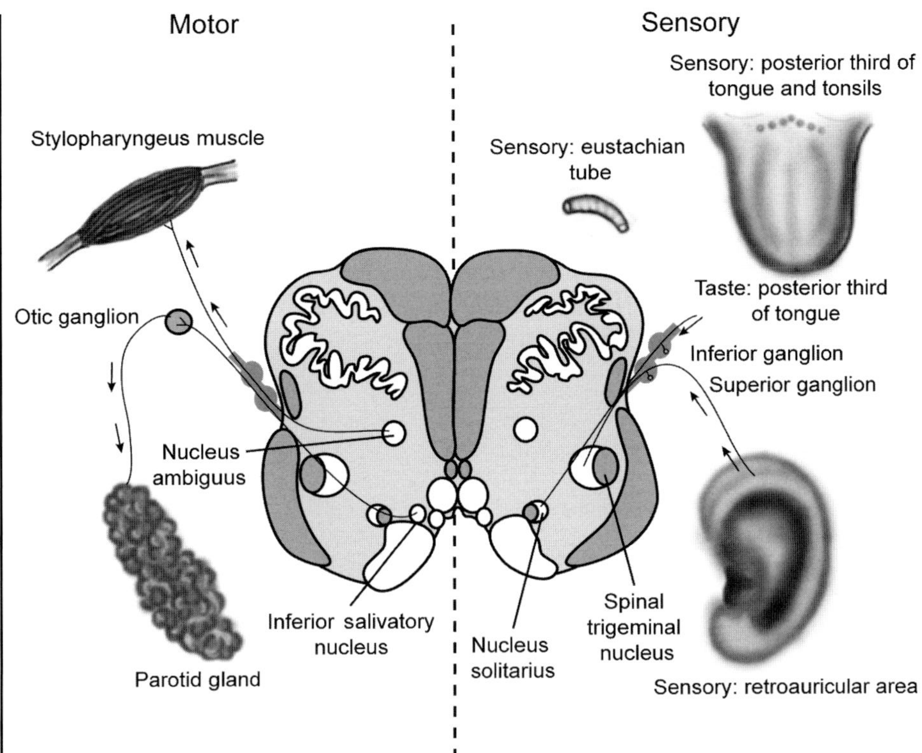

Fig. 2.7. **Anatomic diagram of the various components and functions of the 9th nerve, illustrating the contributions from various brainstem nuclei to the 9th nerve and the structures which it innervates**.

the superior ganglion of the 9th nerve, and project to the spinal trigeminal nucleus and tract.

GVA component

The 9th nerve innervates the mucous membranes of the pharynx, tonsils, and posterior tongue, as well as the middle ear cavity (a sensory function). It mediates sensations such as touch and pain. The GVA fibers have cell bodies in the inferior ganglion of the 9th nerve and project both to the nucleus solitarius as well as the spinal trigeminal nucleus and tract. It has been postulated that the pain fibers in particular project heavily to the spinal trigeminal nucleus and tract.

SVA component

This is a special sensory function of cranial nerve 9, subserving taste to the posterior one-third of the tongue. These taste fibers have cell bodies in the inferior ganglion, and project to the nucleus solitarius.

SVE component

This is the branchial motor component to the pharynx. The 9th nerve plays only a minor role in pharyngeal motor innervation, supplying only the stylopharyngeus muscle. This motor component arises from the nucleus ambiguus.

GVE component

This component consists of parasympathetic innervation of the parotid gland for salivation (the submandibular and sublingual glands are supplied by cranial nerve 7). The preganglionic parasympathetic fibers arise in the inferior salivatory nucleus, and project via the 9th nerve to the otic ganglion. Post-ganglionic fibers then supply the parotid gland.

In summary, then, the 9th nerve has many functions, but it can be considered as mainly a sensory nerve to the pharynx and posterior tongue, conveying both touch and taste, as well as causing salivation from the parotid glands.

Clinical notes

– The sensory fibers to the pharynx represent the afferent limb of the gag reflex (with the efferent limb being through the 10th nerve).
– An additional function of the GVA component of the 9th nerve is innervation of the carotid sinus and the carotid body. The fibers to the carotid sinus convey information regarding blood pressure, while the fibers to the carotid body convey information regarding blood oxygenation; both sets of information are relayed to the nucleus solitarius. Stimulation of the carotid sinus, such as by carotid massage or high blood pressure, produces a reflex reduction in heart rate. The 9th nerve is the afferent limb of this reflex, while the 10th nerve is the efferent limb.
– Glossopharyngeal neuralgia is a disorder similar in character to trigeminal neuralgia, but in the distribution of the 9th nerve. It is characterized by sharp stabbing pains at the base of the tongue or in the throat, which may be triggered by eating. Occasionally, it may be accompanied by bradycardia or even asystole secondary to a reflex stimulation of the vagus nerve. Medical therapies include carbamezapine while surgical therapies include sectioning the 9th nerve and microsurgical decompression of the 9th nerve from surrounding vessels (often the PICA). Also, and most interestingly from a neuroanatomic point of view, it is reported that sectioning the dorsomedial portion of

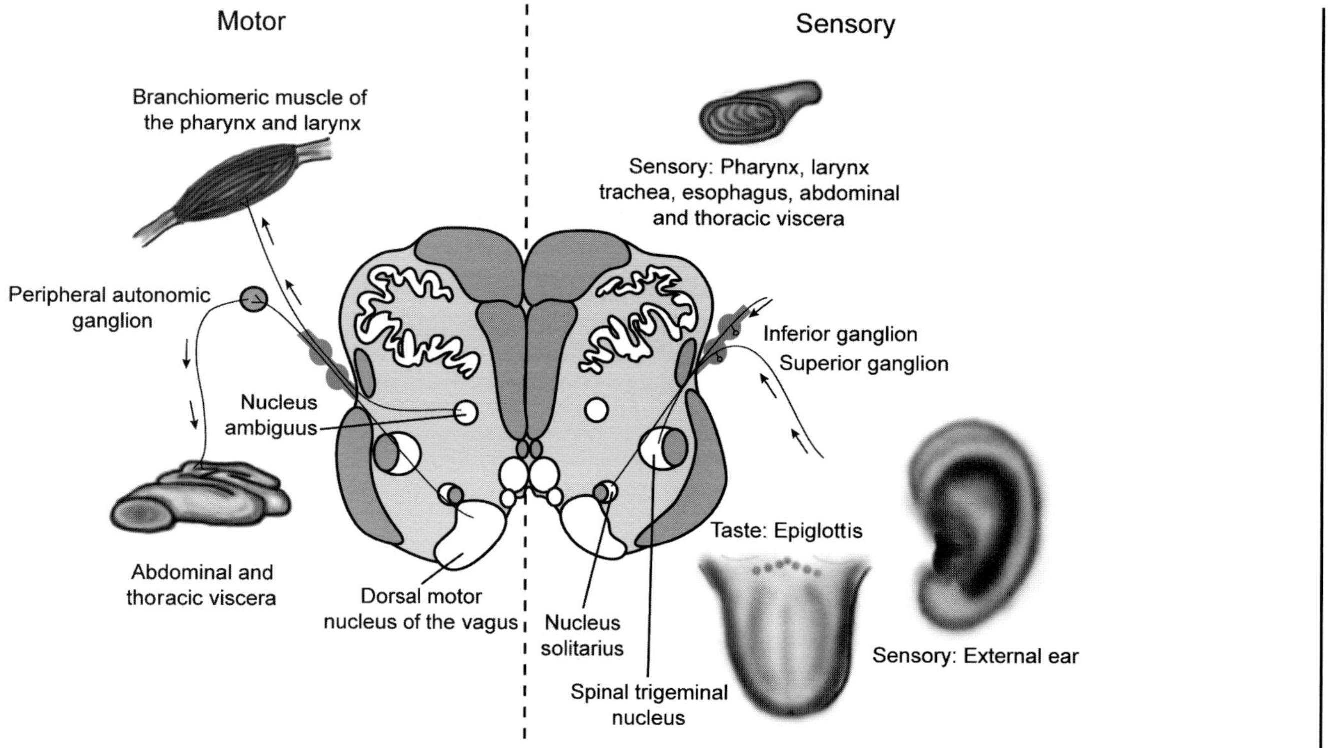

Fig. 2.8. **Anatomic diagram of the components of the 10th nerve, and the areas it supplies.**

the spinal trigeminal tract in the caudal medulla has also been used as a therapeutic alternative.
- It is reported that patients undergoing cancer chemotherapy with vincristine may develop orofacial pain secondary to glossopharyngeal nerve injury (see McCarthy and Skillings, 1992). However, it should be noted that the most common cranial nerve toxicity with vincristine is probably the oculomotor (3rd) nerves, often presenting with bilateral ptosis.

The 10th (vagus) nerve

Like the 9th nerve, the vagus (or "wandering" nerve) is a mixed sensory and motor nerve with general sensory afferent (GSA), general visceral afferent (GVA), special visceral afferent (SVA), special visceral efferent (SVE) and general visceral efferent (GVE) components (see Fig. 2.8).

Most importantly, it is the major motor nerve to the pharynx and larynx, thus serving critical functions in swallowing and talking. Also, it is the major source of parasympathetic innervation to the heart and abdominal organs.

The vagus nerve exits the medulla lateral to the olive and leaves the skull via the jugular foramen, traveling with nerves 9 and 11 in the carotid sheath. Like the 9th nerve, it has both a superior ganglion as well as an inferior ganglion (called the nodose ganglion) which are located on the vagus nerve at the level of the jugular foramen.

Its components are as follows.

SVE component

The vagus nerve innervates the muscles of the larynx and the pharynx, the striated muscles of the proximal esophagus, and the levator veli palatini and palatoglossus muscles. It provides

the efferent limb of the gag reflex. These SVE motor components arise from the nucleus ambiguus in the posterolateral medulla.

GVE component

This is the visceral motor component of the vagus nerve, and consists of preganglionic parasympathetic fibers to the heart and abdominal organs. The fibers in this component arise in the dorsal motor nucleus of the vagus in the posterior medulla. These parasympathetic fibers from the vagus nerve slow the heart rate (hence the bradycardia that accompanies vasovagal attacks), and stimulate secretions and peristalsis in the digestive system, including acid secretion from the stomach.

GVA component

This is the major sensory component of the vagus nerve, innervating the mucous membranes of the pharynx, larynx, trachea, esophagus, stomach and intestines to the splenic flexure of the colon. In this manner, the vagus nerve keeps track of visceral sensations from the abdominal organs. The cell bodies for these fibers are in the inferior vagal ganglion, otherwise known as the nodose ganglion. The central processes project to the nucleus solitarius.

GSA component

This is a minor component. The vagus innervates parts of the external ear, the tympanic membrane, and the infratentorial dura, for somatic sensations such as pain. The cell bodies for these nerve fibers are in the superior vagal ganglion, and the central processes (as with other somatic sensations) project to the spinal trigeminal nucleus and tract.

SVA component

This component is also minor. It mediates taste from the epiglottis. Again, the cell bodies are in the nodose ganglion, and the central processes project to the nucleus solitarius.

Clinical notes
- Lesions of the vagus nerve usually present with hoarseness of the voice and dysphagia, as well as loss of the gag reflex.
- The nucleus ambiguus receives bilateral cortical input. Therefore, unilateral cortical lesions, such as infarcts, do not routinely result in significant dysphagia.
- It is difficult to clinically discriminate lesions of the 9th and 10th nerves, as they are often involved together. Isolated 9th nerve lesions are rare.
- In vagus nerve lesions, it is important to assess whether dysphagia is present along with hoarseness. The SVE motor components of the vagus divide into three main branches: pharyngeal, superior laryngeal, and inferior laryngeal (from which the recurrent laryngeal nerve arises) branches. The pharyngeal and superior laryngeal branches leave the vagus nerve in the high cervical region. Therefore, low cervical lesions will leave the pharynx unaffected and the gag reflex and swallowing will be intact, but hoarseness will be present.
- The recurrent laryngeal nerve innervates the larynx, except for the cricothyroid muscle, which is innervated by the superior laryngeal nerve. The right and left recurrent laryngeal nerves take different courses. The right descends in the tracheoesophageal groove to the thoracic inlet, and runs over the right subclavian artery, and loops around it to run superiorly again into the larynx. The left recurrent laryngeal nerve descends further into the chest, looping around the aortic arch and then returning to the larynx. Therefore, lesions of the chest, such as neoplasm, aortic arch aneurysm or mediastinal adenopathy in the aortopulmonary window may produce left vocal cord paralysis without pharyngeal involvement. Thus, imaging of the neck for left vocal cord paralysis should extend to the level of the aortic arch.
- Other than infarcts or mass lesions, the vagus nerve may be affected by neuropathy from diabetes or alcoholism, by infections such as herpes simplex or herpes zoster, by basilar meningitis (either secondary to infection or sarcoidosis) as well as by demyelinating diseases, such as Guillain–Barré syndrome.
- The autonomic portion of the vagus nerve participates in the carotid sinus reflex as described above. In Guillain–Barré syndrome, there may be autonomic disturbances, with blood pressure instability secondary to demyelination of the afferent or efferent branches of the carotid sinus reflex.
- Supranuclear lesions do not commonly produce 10th nerve dysfunction because of bilateral cortical innervation. However, bifrontal or bilateral subcortical lesions which lead to pseudobulbar palsy may affect the 10th nerves as well, leading to difficulties in swallowing and speaking. Of course, the degeneration of supranuclear pathways in amyotrophic lateral sclerosis also leads to 10th nerve dysfunction.
- The motor components of the vagus also receive extrapyramidal input from the basal ganglia. Basal ganglia degeneration may lead to an unusual speech deficit known as adductor spasmodic dystonia, where the vocal cords adduct spasmodically during speech.

Describe the functional anatomy of the 11th nerve

The 11th nerve (spinal accessory nerve) is a pure motor nerve, innervating the sternocleidomastoid muscle and the superior component of the trapezius. Technically, it is classified as a special visceral efferent nerve because it innervates striated muscles that arise from the branchial arches (see Fig. 2.9).

Medulla

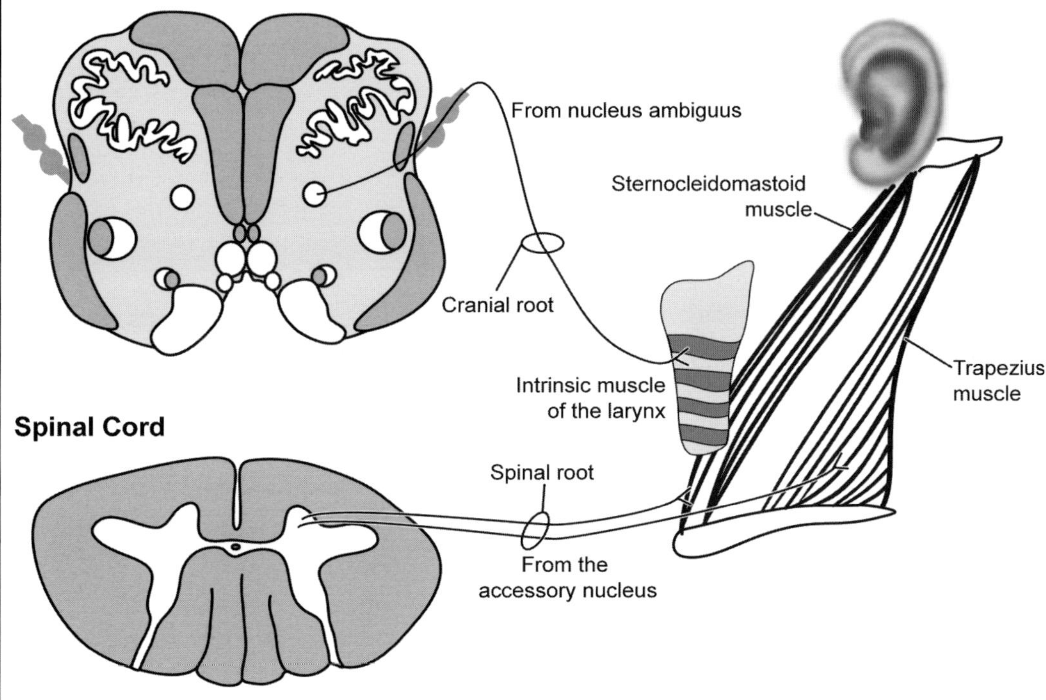

Spinal Cord

Fig. 2.9. **Components and functions of the 11th nerve.**

According to some authors, its nucleus has both cranial (medullary) and spinal components. The output of the medullary component travels with the vagus nerve and contributes the innervation to the intrinsic muscles of the larynx through the recurrent laryngeal nerve. This portion is called the ramus internus of the 11th nerve. This opinion is diagrammed in Fig. 2.9. However, in considering functional neuroanatomy from a clinical standpoint, we will side with the opinion that the cranial portion of the 11th nerve is actually a branch of the vagus (since it comes from the nucleus ambiguus and travels with the vagus) and consider that the 11th nerve has only a spinal nucleus (called the accessory nucleus), located in the high cervical cord from C1 to about C5. From this accessory nucleus, multiple slips exit the cord and coalesce to form a common trunk which runs superiorly to enter the cranial cavity through the foramen magnum. The 11th nerve then courses over the anterior lip of the foramen magnum to promptly leave the skull again, exiting through the jugular foramen with cranial nerves 9 and 10. It travels in the carotid sheath with the 9th and 10th nerves in the neck. Its fibers then diverge to supply the sternocleidomastoid muscle and the upper portion of the trapezius.

The sternocleidomastoid muscle has two heads: a sternal head which is responsible for rotating the calvarium in a contralateral direction (e.g., the left sternocleidomastoid muscle turns the head to the right), and a clavicular head, which tilts the calvarium toward the ipsilateral shoulder. The trapezius muscle elevates the shoulder. A typical way of testing the sternocleidomastoid muscle is to have the patient try to turn his head to the opposite side against resistance. Tests of the trapezius muscle include having the patient shrug his shoulder against resistance.

Damage to the 11th nerve usually occurs in the region of the foramen magnum, at the jugular foramen, or in the region of the carotid sheath.

Clinical notes:
- Interestingly, the supranuclear-cortical input to the 11th nerve nuclei is not very well understood. The 11th nerve nuclei probably receive bilateral cortical input, but from predominantly one side or the other. The portion of the accessory nucleus that controls the trapezius is predominantly supplied by the contralateral motor cortex. The input to the sternocleidomastoid muscle is predominantly from the ipsilateral cortex (a fairly unusual situation in the central nervous system). This ipsilateral innervation is probably mediated via a double decussation. The first decussation is probably somewhere in the midbrain or upper pons, and the second is in the medulla or upper cervical cord.
- Because of this predominantly ipsilateral innervation to the sternocleidomastoid muscle, sometimes with seizure foci in the cerebral cortex, the ipsilateral sternocleidomastoid muscle may be activated, turning the head contralateral to the side of the focus (as you recall, the sternocleidomastoid muscle turns the head to the opposite side).
- Because of the predominantly contralateral cortical innervation to the trapezius and predominantly ipsilateral cortical innervation to the sternocleidomastoid, there may be dissociation or crossed involvement. Thus, it has been suggested that upper brainstem lesions may lead to ipsilateral weakness of the sternocleidomastoid muscle and contralateral weakness of the trapezius.

Reference

McCarthy, G. M., and Skillings, J. R. Jaw and other orofacial pain in patients receiving vincristine for the treatment of cancer. *Oral Surgery Oral Medicine, and Oral Pathology* 1992; **74**: 299–304.

Case 2.2

64-year-old patient presents with some dysarthria. Clinical examination reveals right hemitongue atrophy and fasciculations. When the tongue is protruded, it points to the right.

What do the clinical findings suggest?

This constellation of findings is highly suggestive of a lower motor neuron lesion involving the 12th (hypoglossal) cranial nerve.

MRI images are provided (Fig. 2.10). What are the findings? What is your diagnosis?

Pre- and post-contrast T1-weighted axial MRI images reveal an enhancing mass within the right hypoglossal canal. It is ovoid in shape and slightly widens the hypoglossal canal. The leading differential diagnostic possibilities would be a 12th nerve schwannoma, or possibly a meningioma.

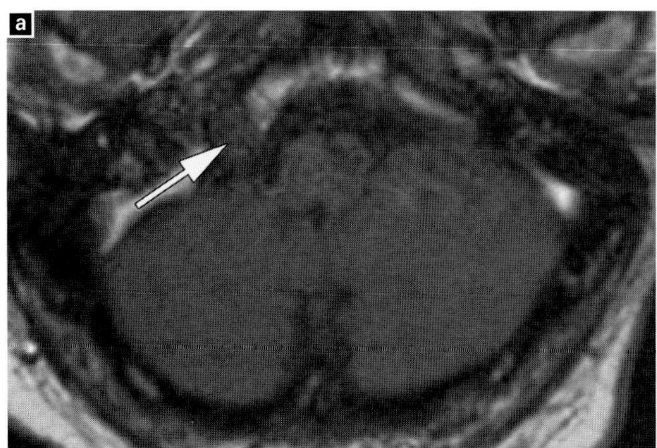
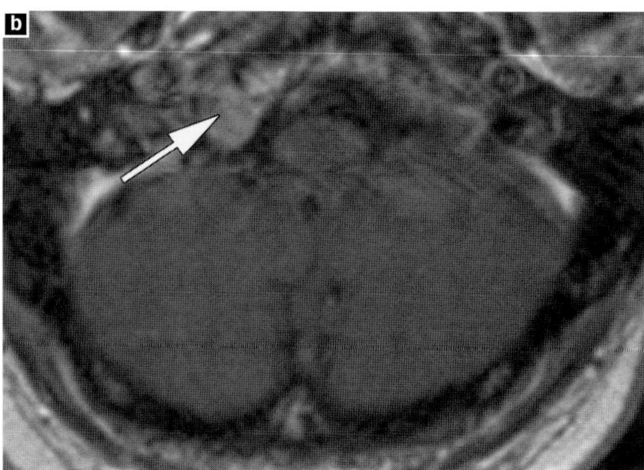

Fig. 2.10 (a),(b). **Pre- and post-contrast axial T1-weighted images show an enhancing mass expanding the right hypoglossal canal (arrow).**

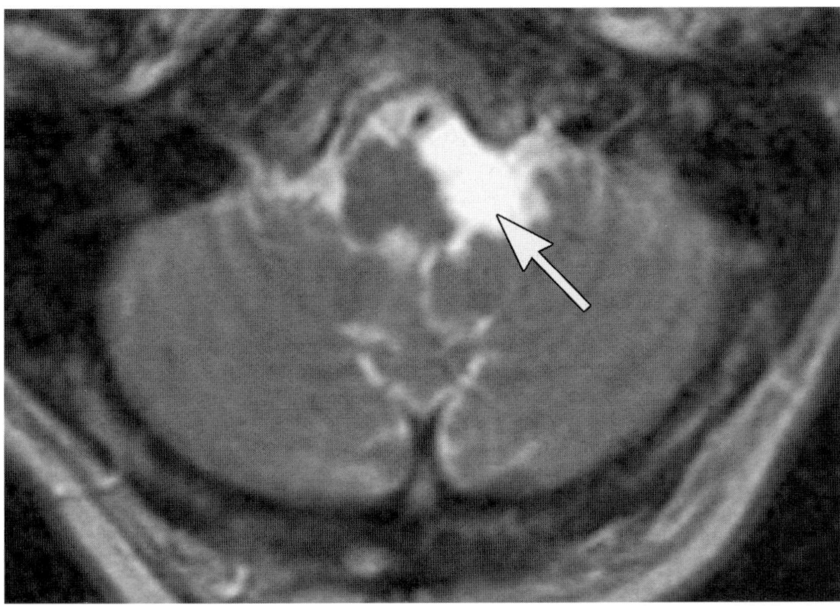

Fig. 2.11. **Axial T2-weighted image shows an arachnoid cyst in the left perimedullary cistern at the entrance to the left hypoglossal canal (arrow).**

Diagnosis

Hypoglossal schwannoma.

However, extreme care must be taken prior to making this diagnosis, and close clinical correlation is required. This is because dilated hypoglossal veins within the hypoglossal canal may mimic a 12th nerve schwannoma (see Stuckey, 1999).

Discuss the functional neuroanatomy of the 12th nerve.

The 12th (hypoglossal) nerve is a pure motor nerve. Like other pure motor nerves, the hypoglossal nuclei are located in midline of the brainstem. In this case, they are found in the posterior medulla, just anterior to the floor of the fourth ventricle.

The hypoglossal nerves leave the hypoglossal nuclei and pass anteriorly in the medulla, just lateral to the medial lemnisci, and exit the ventral medullary surface in the ventrolateral sulci between the pyramids and the olives.

The 12th nerve then travels in the perimedullary cistern, and exits the skull via the hypoglossal canal in the skull base. It descends in the neck, and passes between the internal carotid artery and the internal jugular vein.

Its main clinical interest and function is that it innervates the extrinsic muscles of the tongue, such as the genioglossus and hypoglossus muscles, which function in moving the tongue. It also innervates the intrinsic muscles of the tongue such as the superior and inferior longitudinals and the transversus muscles. Therefore, lesions of the 12th nerve cause denervation atrophy and fasciculations of the ipsilateral tongue. Also, when protruded, the tongue will point toward the side of the lesion because of the unopposed action of the normal extrinsic tongue muscles on the other side.

A little known (and probably clinically irrelevant) fact is that the 12th nerve also innervates the strap muscles like the omohyoid, sternohyoid, and sternothyroid.

Hypoglossal nerve dysfunction may occur secondary to brainstem strokes, tumors involving the nerve, infections such as basilar meningitis, carotid dissection, trauma, demyelinating diseases like Guillain–Barré, and neurodegenerative disorders like ALS.

Just for fun, an unusual cause of 12th nerve dysfunction is presented (Fig. 2.11). An axial T2-weighted MR image shows a small arachnoid cyst in the perimedullary cistern at the entrance

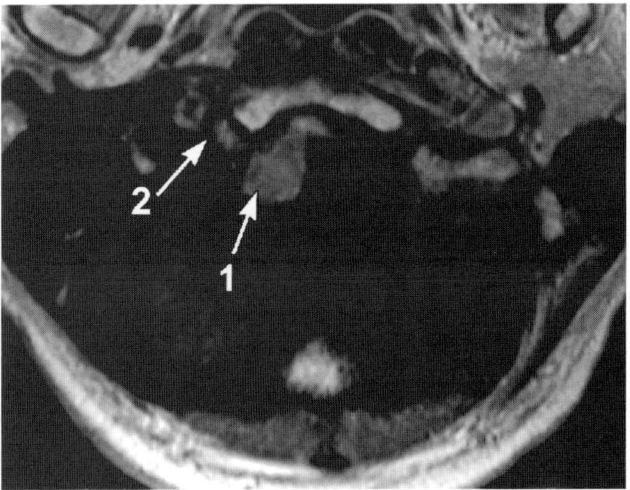

Fig. 2.12. **Post-contrast axial T1-weighted image shows a meningioma along the right anterior aspect of the foramen magnum (arrow 1). It enters the right hypoglossal canal (arrow 2).**

to the left hypoglossal canal. This 85-year-old patient presented with left hemitongue atrophy and fasciculations.

Hypoglossal nerve dysfunction may also combine with dysfunction of other cranial nerves, and this can be secondary to multiple etiologies. As described above, the hypoglossal nerve also runs with the 9th, 10th, and 11th cranial nerves within the carotid space. Therefore, lesions at the skull base or within the carotid space may cause combined cranial nerve deficits.

Look at the MRI image provided above (Fig. 2.12). What are the findings?

There is an enhancing lesion along the anterior lip of the foramen magnum to the right of midline, at the level of the hypoglossal canal. The imaging characteristics suggest a meningioma, and this patient had combined dysfunction of his right 11th and 12th cranial nerves.

Now, let us return briefly to Case 2.1 for some further correlation. In that case, a patient with a glomus vagale tumor presented

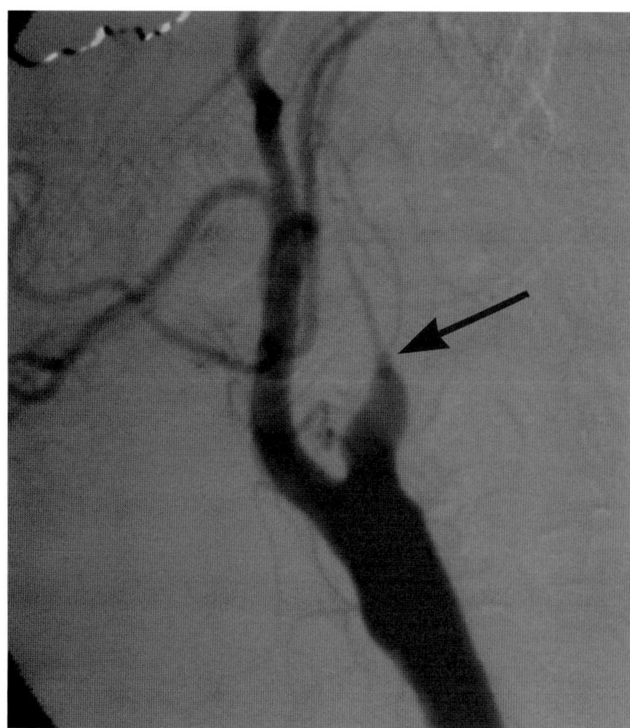

Fig. 2.13. **Right common carotid angiogram shows a carotid dissection of the right internal carotid artery beginning at the distal edge of the carotid bulb (arrow).**

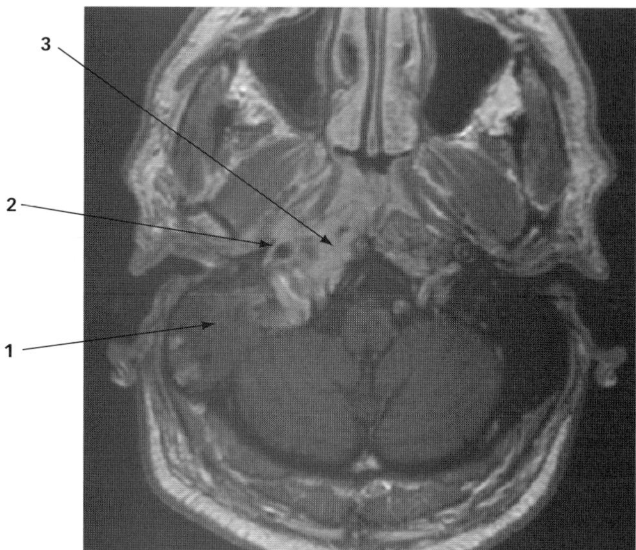

Fig. 2.14. **T1-weighted axial post-contrast image in a diabetic patient with an aggressive pseudomonas otomastoiditis shows abnormal fluid in the right mastoid air cells (arrow 1), as well as a large enhancing phlegmon in the right prevertebral and right parapharyngeal spaces (arrow 3). The right internal carotid artery is encased (arrow 2). The patient had right cranial nerve 9–12 dysfunction as well as a right-sided Horner's syndrome.**

with combined 9th, 10th and 11th nerve deficits, which is called Vernet's syndrome. Another patient is now presented for evaluation. This is a 43-year-old female patient, who presents with dysphagia, decreased gag reflex on the right, right vocal cord paralysis, weakness of the right trapezius and sternocleidomastoid muscles, as well as a peripheral right 12th nerve lesion. MRI examination of the brain (not shown) did not show evidence of skull base lesions. It was remarkable, though, for loss of the normal flow void in the right cavernous carotid artery.

Angiography of the right common carotid was performed, and is shown (Fig. 2.13). What are the findings? What is your diagnosis?

The right common carotid angiogram shows a long segment "rat-tail" stricture of the right internal carotid artery beginning at the distal edge of the carotid bulb. This appearance is classic for a carotid dissection. Cranial nerve dysfunction involving the nerves that run in the carotid space (9th–12th) is a well-described complication of carotid dissection, as apparently the blood supply to the nerves through the vasa nervosum is interrupted.

The constellation of 9th through 12th cranial nerve deficits (essentially a Vernet's syndrome plus a 12th nerve palsy) also has an eponym that is found in textbooks and case reports: the *Collet–Sicard* syndrome (see, for example, Heckmann *et al.*, 2000 or Walker *et al.*, 2003) The Collet–Sicard syndrome has also been

reported in association with skull base lesions, especially skull base fractures.

Finally, just in case you like syndromes and eponyms (and who doesn't?), we mention that the same pathologies which lead to Vernet's syndrome or the Collet–Sicard syndrome may also lead to a deficit which involves the 9th through 12th cranial nerves, as well as the sympathetic chain which travels with the internal carotid artery – a Collet–Sicard syndrome with a superimposed Horner's. An example is provided by the patient in Fig. 2.14.

Luckily, this also has an eponym for us to learn: *Villaret's* syndrome!

References

Stuckey, S. L. Dilated venous plexus of the hypoglossal canal mimicking disease. *American Journal of Neuroradiology* 1999; **20**:157–158.

Heckmann, J. G., Tomandl, B., Duhm, C. *et al.* Collet-Sicard Syndrome due to coiling and dissection of the internal carotid artery. *Cerebrovascular Diseases* 2000; **10**: 487–488.

Walker, S., McCarron, M. O., Flynn, P. A. *et al.* Left internal carotid artery dissection presenting with headache, Collet–Sicard syndrome and sustained hypertension. *European Journal of Neurology* 2003; **10** (6): 731–732.

Case 2.3

56-year-old man with history of hypertension woke up one morning with persistent vertigo. When he walked, he swayed to the right with occasional falls. He complained of dysphagia. Examination showed loss of the gag reflex on the right and leftward deviation of the uvula, among other signs and symptoms.

Where do you think the lesion is?

A combination of vertigo and ataxia to the right suggests a lesion in the right lower brainstem, most likely in the medulla involving the vestibular nuclei and their connections to the inferior cerebellar peduncle. Involvement of the vestibular nuclei results in vertigo and sometimes diplopia from damaging the otolithic portion of the vestibular nuclei. A lesion in the inferior cerebellar peduncle would cause ipsilateral ataxia and swaying to the right, also known as axial lateropulsion. Loss of the gag reflex suggests involvement of the 9th or 10th nerves or nuclei. The concomitant involvement of the vestibular nuclei suggests a brainstem location, and when taken together, these considerations place the lesion in the posterolateral portion of the medulla where all of these these structures are located.

MRI examination was performed (Fig. 2.15). *What are the findings?*

The axial T2-weighted MRI image shows a well-demarcated zone of T2-weighted hyperintensity involving the right posterolateral medulla. The appearance is consistent with an infarct.

What is the diagnosis and what is the constellation of signs and symptoms associated with this syndrome, based on the neuroanatomy of the posterolateral medulla?

An infarct of the posterolateral medulla produces the *lateral medullary* or Wallenberg's syndrome. While this syndrome is almost always due to infarction, a small number of cases are the result of hemorrhage or tumor. Most commonly, an infarct is caused by intracranial vertebral artery occlusion (80%), while the rest are attributed to occlusion of the posterior inferior cerebellar artery (PICA) or medullary branches of the vertebral artery.

The constellation of signs and symptoms comprising Wallenberg's syndrome can be deduced from the key structures within the posterolateral medulla (see Fig. 2.16), and are as follows:

– Dyspahgia and hoarseness with ipsilateral loss of the gag reflex and ipsilateral vocal cord paralysis secondary to weakness of the pharyngeal and laryngeal muscles supplied by the nucleus ambiguus. This what all the books say, and what is diagrammed below. It may be more accurate to say that the nucleus ambiguus is more medial than the other structures of the posterolateral medulla, and is most likely in a watershed zone between two vascular distributions. Therefore, Wallenberg's syndrome more likely damages the 10th nerve fascicles as they leave the nucleus rather than damaging the nucleus itself. However, we will follow convention and consider that Wallenberg's syndrome involves the nucleus ambiguus.

– Loss of pain and temperature sensation from the ipsilateral face secondary to involvement of the spinal trigeminal nucleus and tract.

– Loss of pain and temperature sensation from the contralateral body secondary to involvement of the lateral spinothalamic tract.

– Ipsilateral cerebellar ataxia, including axial lateropulsion from involvement of the inferior cerebellar peduncle.

– Vertigo, with associated nausea and vomiting, from involvement of the vestibular nuclei. There have also been reports of nystagmus, vertical diplopia and a sensation of tilting of objects in the visual field, secondary to damage to the otolithic portion of the vestibular nuclei.

– Ipsilateral Horner's syndrome from involvement of the descending sympathetic fibers destined for the intermediolateral cell column. This is a pre ganglionic form of Horner's.

– Hiccuping, of uncertain etiology, but usually attributed to involvement of the respiratory center in the medullary reticular formation.

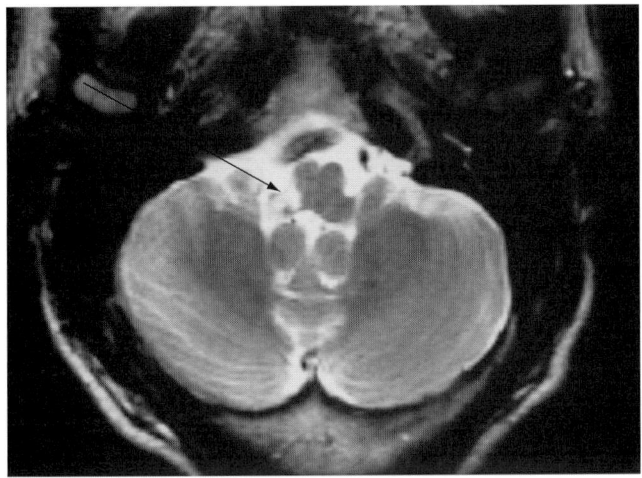

Fig. 2.15. **T2-weighted axial image shows hyperintensity in the right posterolateral medulla (arrow).**

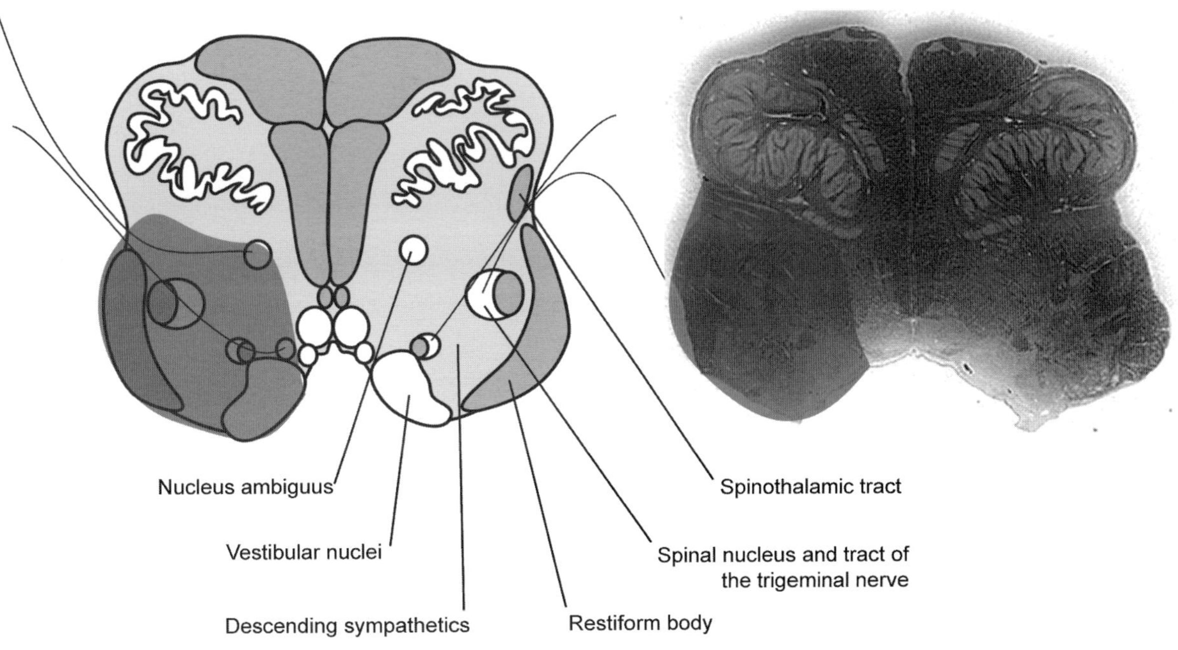

Fig. 2.16. **Schematic diagram of brainstem structures involved in Wallenberg's syndrome (see plate section for color image).**

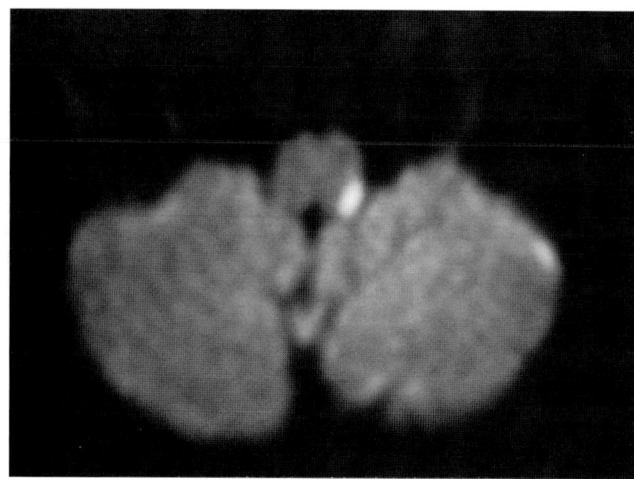

Fig. 2.17. **Diffusion-weighted images show a small infarct confined to the left dorsal aspect of the medulla, significantly smaller in volume than the infarct of Fig. 2.15, which caused the full-blown Wallenberg's syndrome shown above.**

- Abnormalities of saccades, referred to as ocular lateropulsion, are also characteristic of this syndrome, described as hypometric saccades away from the side of the lesion and hypermetric saccades towards the side of the lesion. This is probably secondary to damage of olivocerebellar fibers related to ocular movement traveling in the lateral medulla.
  Describe other variants of the lateral medullary syndrome.
- The *dorsal medullary syndrome* is a more limited form of Wallenberg's, usually caused by occlusion of the medial branch of the posterior inferior cerebellar artery, with involvement of the vestibular nuclei and the restiform body (inferior cerebellar peduncle). This produces ipsilateral limb and gait ataxia, as well as vertigo, vomiting and ipsilateral gaze-evoked nystagmus. The patient above presented with precisely these findings (Fig. 2.17). As you notice, this infarct is limited to the dorsal medulla, and therefore does not involve the nucleus ambiguus, the preganglionic sympathetic fibers, the spinothalamic tract, or the spinal trigeminal nucleus and tract.
  A nice reference regarding the spectrum of findings associated with Wallenberg's syndrome is Kim *et al.* (1994).
  Give a brief discussion of the clinical correlates of the descending sympathetic fibers in the posterolateral medulla.
  These fibers, which arise in, and descend from, the hypothalamus, run in the lateral portion of the brainstem tegmentum. They travel in the posterolateral medulla and then become the intermediolateral cell column of the spinal cord. Some of these fibers exit the cord in the low cervical region (second-order neurons) and course over the lung apex. They synapse on the superior cervical ganglion located outside the spinal canal near the cervico-thoracic junction, and then ascend as the post ganglionic (third-order neurons) sympathetic tract with the carotid artery, bifurcating with the carotid to run with both the internal

and external carotid arteries. The branches with the internal carotid cause pupillary dilatation, as well as innervate Mueller's muscle, the smooth muscle component of the upper lid, helping keep the lid open. The sympathetic branches with the external carotid artery innervate the sweat glands. Therefore, interruptions of this sympathetic pathway causes Horner's syndrome (miosis, ptosis, anhydrosis). Clinical notes to remember:

- The ptosis in Horner's is not usually as severe as that produced by third nerve lesions (Mueller's muscle plays a smaller role than the levator palebrae in elevating the upper lid; the levator is innervated by the motor portion of the third nerve).
- Since both third nerve lesions as well as Horner's syndrome cause ptosis, evaluation of the pupil helps distinguish the two. If the pupil is small (miosis), this is consistent with Horner's, while if the pupil is abnormally dilated ("blown pupil"), this is consistent with a third nerve lesion. Testing for miosis is best done in a dimly lit room, where the normal pupil dilates.
- Lesions in the cavernous sinus may affect both the third nerve and the sympathetic chain, which runs with the internal carotid inside the cavernous sinus. This gives balanced deficits, with the third nerve deficit tending to dilate the pupil, and the sympathetic palsy tending to constrict the pupil, which will then appear relatively normal; however, it will be poorly reactive to light.
- The sympathetic pathway can be affected by multiple lesions. Brainstem infarcts, such as in the lateral pontine tegmentum or more classically the posterolateral medulla, will affect the first-order neurons. Lesions at the lung apex, such as Pancoast tumors, will affect the second order neurons, while carotid dissection affects the third-order neurons. It should be recalled that dissection usually affects the internal carotid artery, and stops at the carotid bulb. Therefore, the sympathetic branches with the ECA are unaffected. While you will often hear that carotid dissection causes Horner's, only the miosis and ptosis components are present, without anhydrosis. This condition is more correctly referred to as oculosympathetic paresis.
- For those truly interested in neurophthalmology, we point out that there is something called the Cocaine test, which helps confirm Horner's. Instilling a solution of cocaine into the eyes dilates the pupils; a Horner's pupil, though, will not dilate (please do not try this at home, kids). Once the diagnosis of Horner's is made, a Paradrine (1% hydroxyamphetamine) test may be performed to distinguish pre ganglionic (first- and second-order neurons) from post ganglionic (third-order neurons arising from the cervical ganglion) Horner's. Paradrine forces the release of norepinephrine from pre synaptic vesicles, and therefore requires the third-order post ganglionic neurons to be intact in order for the pupil to dilate. If the pupil dilates, the lesion involves the first or second order neurons. If not, then the lesion is post ganglionic. There is no topical test, though, to distinguish first- from second-order neuron involvement.

Reference

Kim, J. S., Lee, J. H., Suh, D. C., and Lee, M. C. Spectrum of lateral medullary syndrome. Correlation between clinical findings and magnetic resonance imaging in 33 subjects. *Stroke* 1994; **25** (7): 1405–1410.

Case 2.4

52-year-old patient presents with acute onset of right hemiparesis. Further neurologic testing reveals decreased vibration and proprioception sense in the right body, as well as leftward deviation of the tongue.

MRI images are provided below (Figure 2.18 (a) and (b)). What are the findings? What is your diagnosis?

MRI images through the medulla at the level of the medullary pyramids demonstrate a subacute infarct in the left anteromedial

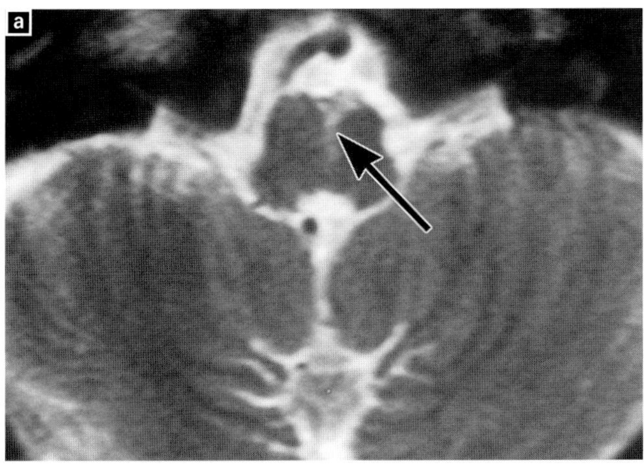

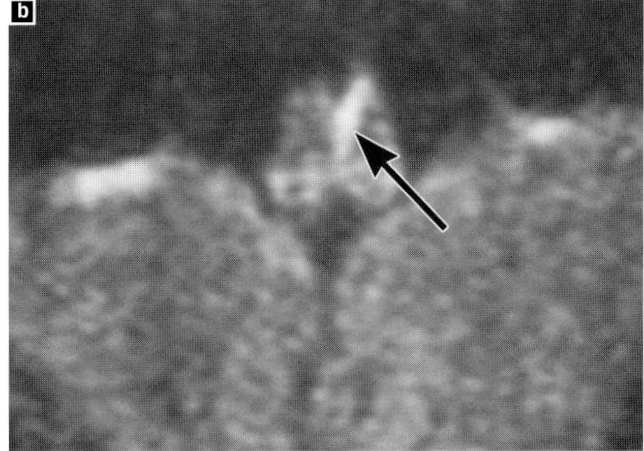

Fig. 2.18. **(a) Axial T2-weighted and (b) diffusion-weighted MRI images through the medulla at the level of the medullary pyramids are provided. There is abnormal T2-weighted and diffusion-weighted hyperintensity in the left anteromedial aspect of the medulla. Case courtesy of Dr. Noriko Salomon, UCLA Department of Radiology.**

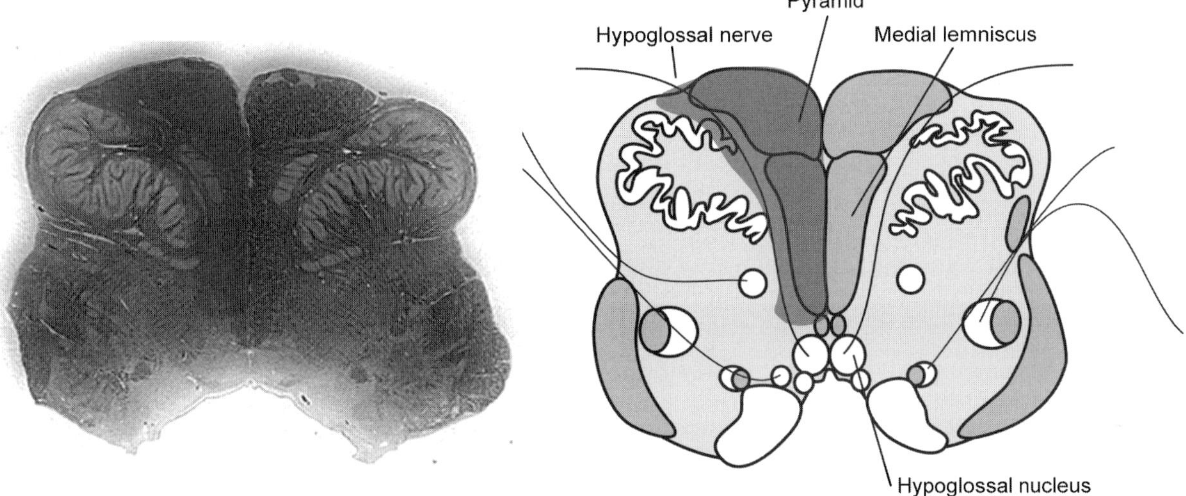

Fig. 2.19. **Schematic diagram of the structures involved in Dejerine's syndrome (see plate section for color image).**

medulla. An infarct in this location typically produces the so-called "medial medullary syndrome."

Diagnosis

Medial medullary syndrome; this is otherwise known as *alternating hypoglossal hemiparesis*, or *Dejerine's* syndrome.

Discuss Dejerine's syndrome.

From the location of the infarct in the anterior–medial aspect of the medulla, three main anatomic structures are involved, forming the constellation typically seen in this patient (see Fig. 2.19).

The corticospinal tract is involved superior to the decussation, producing a contralateral hemiparesis. Also, the medial lemniscus is involved. As described previously, this carries the fibers of the dorsal columns which have already decussated. Therefore, the patient will exhibit contralateral decreased vibration sense and proprioception. Also, the rootlets of the hypoglossal nerve will be involved, producing an ipsilateral lower-motor-neuron paralysis of the tongue. Therefore, from the contralateral body hemiparesis and ipsilateral tongue weakness, the clinical name of the syndrome is now easily understood: *alternating hypoglossal hemiparesis*. The vascular lesion typically involves either the ipsilateral vertebral artery, or the medial medullary perforators.

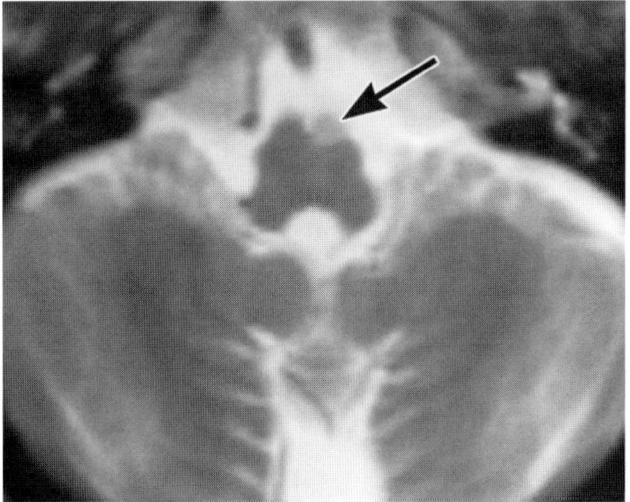

Fig. 2.20. **T2-weighted axial image shows an early subacute infarct involving only the left medullary pyramid (arrow).**

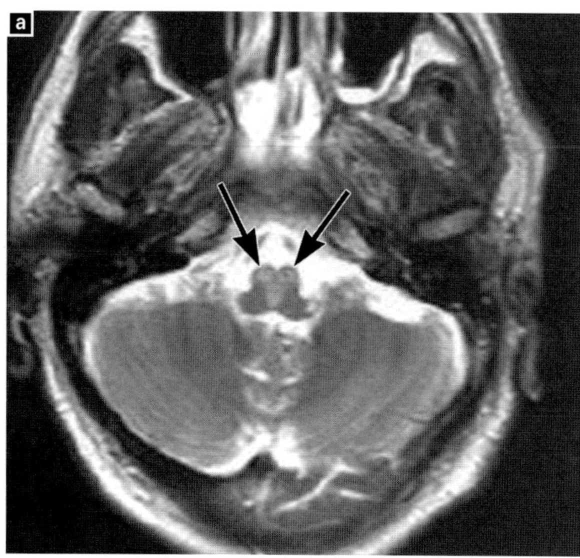 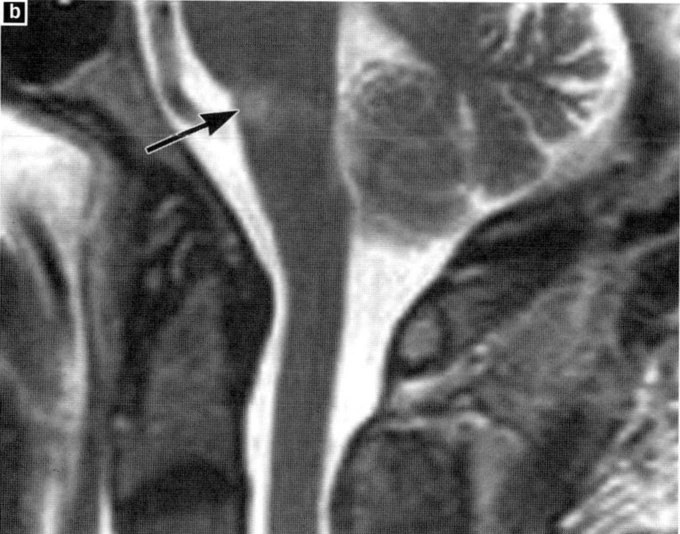

Fig. 2.21. **T2-weighted (a) axial and (b) sagittal MRI images reveal an extremely rare bilateral medial medullary syndrome. Case courtesy of Dr. Noriko Salomon, UCLA Department of Radiology.**

There are some interesting variants of the medial medullary syndrome. For example, infarcts may involve only the medullary pyramid, and not extend posteriorly to involve the medial lemniscus, or extend laterally enough to involve the rootlets of the 12th nerve. In this case, there is pure contralateral hemiparesis, such as in the MRI (Fig. 2.20).

Another interesting, and extremely rare, variant of the medial medullary syndrome is bilateral medial medullary infarcts (see Fig. 2.21 above).

This patient will exhibit quadriparesis secondary to involvement of both medullary pyramids, and generalized loss of vibration and proprioception secondary to lesions in both medial lemnisci, as well as marked weakness of the tongue, with difficulty protruding tongue due to bilateral hypoglossal nerve lesions. As expected, this would produce significant dysarthria and dysphagia.

Another interesting variant of the medial medullary syndrome occurs with more inferiorly placed infarcts which involve the anterior–medial aspect of the medulla at the level of the pyramidal decussation (see Fig. 2.22).

Such an infarct produces a very interesting syndrome, known as *cruciate hemiplegia*, or *crossed hemiparesis*, where there will be weakness of one arm and the opposite leg. This is due to the fact that the right and left corticospinal tracts, as well as the fibers for the arm and the leg contained therein, undergo differential decussation. Specifically, according to Afifi and Bergman, the left pyramid decussates first in about three-fourths of individuals, with no relationship to handedness. Also, the fibers to the upper extremity decussate first, and are located rostral to the fibers supplying the lower extremity, and more superifically as well. Therefore, a lesion between the decussation of the upper and

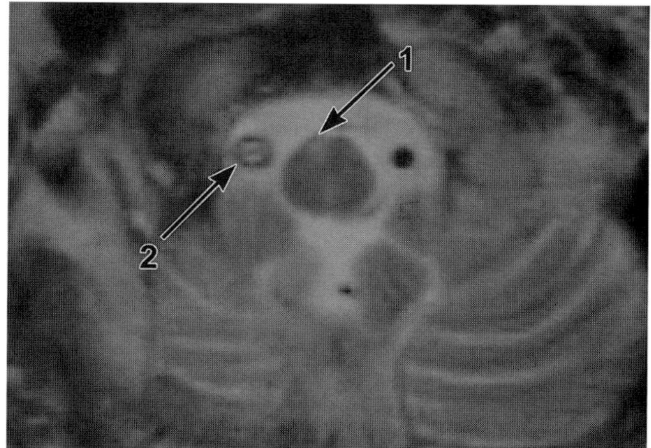

Fig. 2.22. **T2-weighted axial image shows a small infarct in the right anterior caudal medulla at the level of the motor decussation, with subtle T2-weighted hyperintensity (arrow1). Notice the thrombosed right vertebral artery with loss of the normal flow void (arrow 2).**

lower extremity can lead to the crossed paralysis described above. A concrete example would be a lesion in the right anterior caudal medulla at the level of the motor decussation. In the appropriate location, it may involve the already decussated fibers to the right arm which have come form the left corticospinal tract, as well as the uncrossed fibers of the right corticospinal tract destined for the left leg, leading to a crossed paralysis.

Case 2.5

66-year-old diabetic hypertensive patient presents with complaints of dysphagia and dysarthria, as well as vertigo and right-sided weakness. Examination reveals decreased gag reflex on the left with the uvula pointing to the right, right-sided upper motor neuron weakness, and right-sided decrease in vibration and proprioception. On tongue protrusion, the tongue points to the left. There was also mild left-sided ptosis and myosis.
Based on the signs and symptoms, where do you think the lesion is?

The patient appears to have a lesion which involves the left aspect of the medulla, giving a left-sided Horner's, involvement of

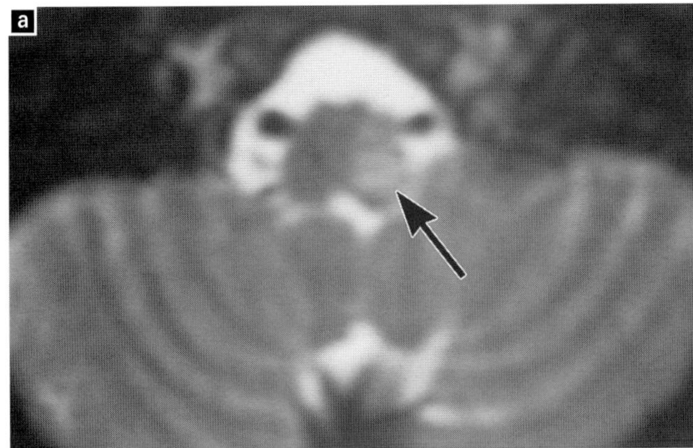

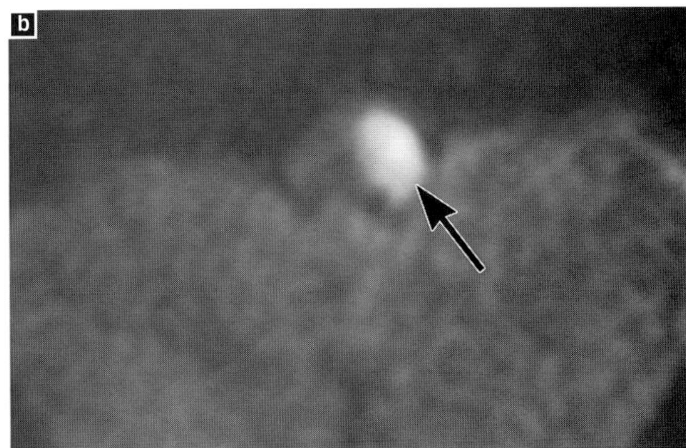

Fig. 2.23. **(a) T2- and (b) diffusion-weighted axial MRI images show a large zone of hyperintensity involving the left half of the medulla, extending from the posterolateral to the anterior medulla.**

the left nucleus ambiguus and of the vestibular nuclei. Also, there is left hypoglossal involvement, and the right-sided weakness and decreased posterior column sensation suggest involvement of the left medullary pyramid and the left medial lemniscus.

MRI images are provided above (Fig. 2.23). What are the findings? What is your diagnosis?

Axial and T2-weighted images show a large infarct involving most of the left aspect of the medulla. Both the clinical and the imaging findings are a combination of a lateral medullary syndrome and a medial medullary syndrome.

Diagnosis

Babinski–Nageotte syndrome. This unusual syndrome, also known as medullary tegmental paralysis or hemimedullary syndrome, is a combination of the medial and lateral medullary syndromes, usually due to a large infarct.

This syndrome was described by Babinski and Nageotte in 1902, with relatively few cases reported in the literature. For the interested reader, the following references may be helpful: de Freitas *et al.* (2001) and Nakane *et al.*, 1991. A rather interesting and even rarer variant of the Babinski–Nageotte syndrome (or of Wallenberg's syndrome) is reported when a similar hemimedullary infarct occurs but at a slightly lower level in the medulla, just

caudal to the level of the motor decussation. This infarct will present with a Wallenberg's-type syndrome plus *ipsilateral* motor weakness (rather than contralateral as in the Babinski–Nageotte syndrome). It is hypothesized that the corticospinal tract is involved after it has decussated, leading to ipsilateral motor weakness. Of course, this syndrome has been named as well. Any guesses? It is called *Opalski's* syndrome. That is because it was described by Dr. Opalski in 1946. Once again, for the interested reader, good references are: Montaner and Alvarez-Sabin, 1999, and Kimura *et al.*, 2003.

References

de Freitas, G. R., Moll, J., and Araujo, A. Q. The Babinski–Nageotte syndrome. *Neurology* 2001; **56**(11): 1604.

Kimura, Y., Hashimoto, H., Tagay, A. M. *et al.* Ipsilateral hemiplegia in a lateral medullary infarct – Opalski's syndrome. *Journal of Neuroimaging* 2003; **13**(1): 83–84.

Montaner, J. and Alvarez-Sabin, J. Opalski's syndrome. *Journal of Neurology, Neurosurgery, and Psychiatry* 1999; **67**(5): 688–689.

Nakane, H. Okada, Y., Sadoshima, S. *et al.* Babinski–Nageotte syndrome on magnetic resonance imaging. *Stroke* 1991; **22**(2): 272–275.

Case 2.6

61-year-old patient presents with sudden-onset dysphagia and right body numbness. On examination, the patient has a decreased gag on the left, uvula pointing to the right and lack of elevation of the left palate with phonation. ENT examination revealed left vocal cord paresis. Sensory examination revealed decreased pain and temperature sensation in the right body, with sparing of the face. There was no vertigo, nystagmus, ataxia, or motor weakness.

Where do you think the lesion is? Based on the description, the left tenth nerve is involved. However, the presence of crossed symptoms suggests a brainstem etiology. A lesion in the left medulla, involving the nucleus ambiguus and the spinothalamic tract would produce these symptoms.

An MRI is provided (Fig. 2.24). What are the findings? What is your diagnosis?

The axial T2-weighted images show a lesion in the posterior medulla, which, along with the clinical history, is consistent with an infarct. The lesion spares the dorsal or posterolateral aspect of the medulla, thus sparing the vestibular nuclei as well as the inferior cerebellar peduncle, and explaining the lack of vertigo, nystagmus, or ataxia. Also, it does not extend anteriorly enough to involve the medullary pyramid, and hence the patient had no

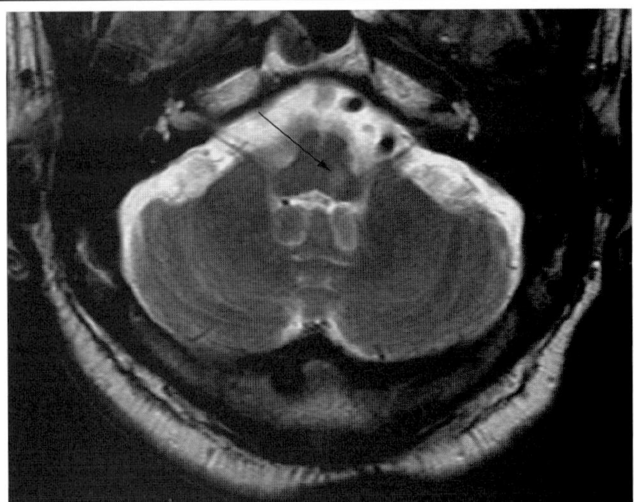

Fig. 2.24. **Axial T2-weighted MRI shows a small lesion in the left posterior medulla (arrow). Notice that the dorsal or posterolateral medulla is spared.**

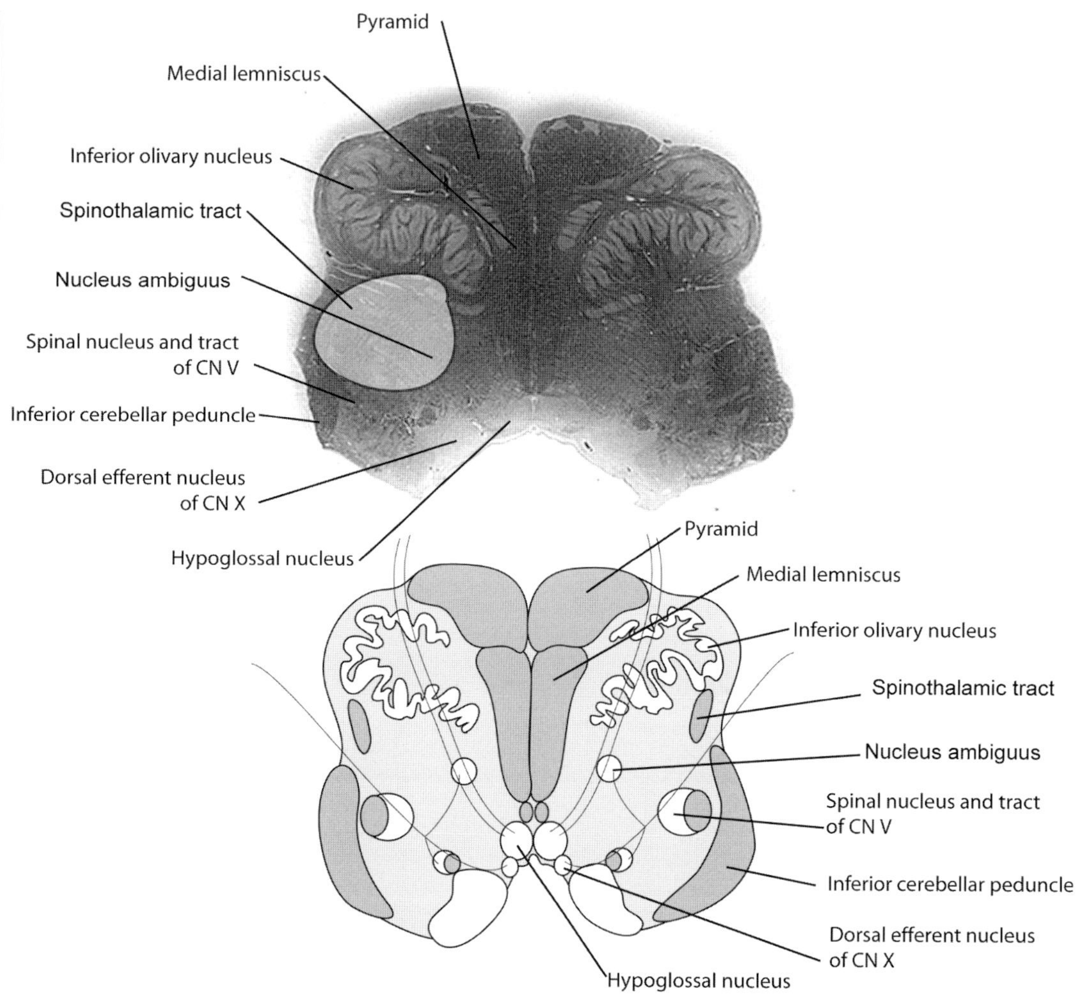

Fig. 2.25. **(a) Schematic diagram and (b) anatomic cross-section showing the main anatomic structures of the medulla. Notice the adjacency of the nucleus ambiguus and the spinothalamic tract in the "mid" posterior medulla.**

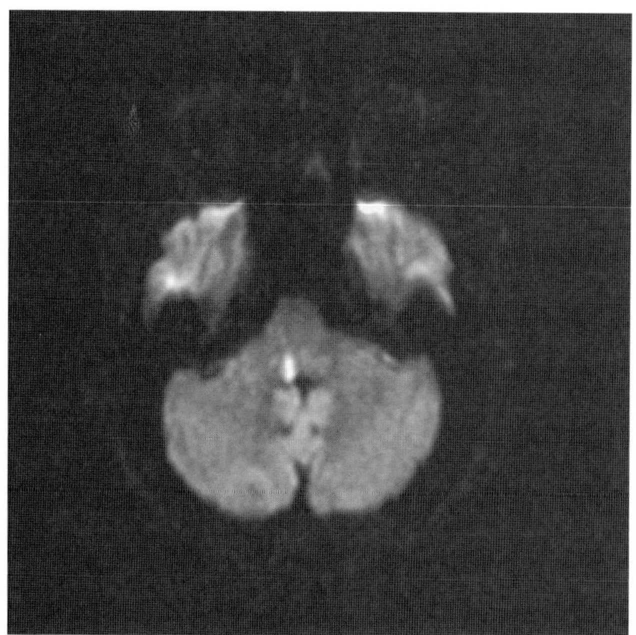

Fig. 2.26. **DWI image shows an infarct in the right posterior rostral medulla, at the level of the cerebellopontine angle cisterns.**

weakness. However, the lesion is in a good location to involve the left nucleus ambiguus and the adjacent spinothalamic tract (see diagrams, Fig. 2.25).

Diagnosis

Avellis syndrome. This is a crossed brainstem syndrome consisting of a lesion involving the nucleus ambiguus, with ipsilateral pharyngeal and laryngeal weakness, plus a contralateral body hypesthesia. Some authors also include a contralateral hemiparesis. A couple of nice references are: Kataoka *et al.*, (2001) and Takizawa and Shinohara (1996).

Another patient presents for evaluation. He complains of dysphagia and left body numbness. Examination reveals decreased gag on the right, left body pain and temperature sensory deficit and a lower motor neuron right facial droop. MRI images are presented opposite (Fig. 2.26).

Once again, an infarct is present in the posterior medulla, sparing the posterolateral aspect. As in the last case, an Avellis syndrome is present. However, since the infarct is slightly more rostral (at the pontomedullary junction), some fascicles of the facial nerve as it loops in the pontine tegmentum are involved, producing some ipsilateral facial weakness. This variant of Avellis syndrome, with ipsilateral facial nerve involvement, has been reported (Takahashi *et al.*, 2000). To the knowledge of the authors, this does not carry an eponym, so here's your chance at immortality!

A similar infarct slightly lower in the medulla produces an Avellis syndrome with an ipsilateral 12th nerve palsy. This one, alas, has been named: *Jackson's* syndrome.

References

Kataoka, S., Hori, A., Hirose, G. *et al*. Avellis' syndrome: the neurological-topographical correlation. *European Neurology* 2001; **45**(4): 292–293.

Takizawa, S. and Shinohara, Y. Magnetic resonance imaging in Avellis' syndrome. *Journal of Neurology Neurosurgery, and Psychiatry* 1996; **61**(1): 17.

Takahashi, K., Kitani, M., and Fukuda, H. [A case of Avellis' syndrome with ipsilateral central facial palsy due to a small medullary infarction] *Rinsho Shinkeigaku* 2000; **40**(4): 409–411. Japanese).

Case 2.7

52-year-old diabetic patient presents complaining of waking up with left facial numbness around the ear, right body numbness and feeling "funny" in his left upper extremity. Examination reveals decreased pain and temperature sensation in the left periauricular skin as well as the right hemibody. There is decreased proprioception in the left upper extremity as well. The left lower extremity has intact vibration and proprioception.

Where do you think the lesion is? The presence of crossed face and body symptoms immediately suggests the brainstem.

An MRI is obtained (Fig. 2.27). What are the findings? What is your diagnosis?

Diagnosis: There is a lesion along the left lateral aspect of the medulla. The appearance is consistent with an infarct, going along with the clinical history. The location of the infarct matches the patient's clinical presentation, as can be seen (Fig. 2.28).

The infarct does not extend anteriorly enough to involve the corticospinal tract, and hence there is no weakness. It does involve the caudal aspect of the left spinal trigeminal nucleus and tract, which, as described previously, would coincide with somatic sensory inputs from cranial nerves 9 and 10, and correspond with the symptoms of periauricular numbness and decreased sensation. Also, there is involvement of the left spinothalamic tract, leading to right body numbness. The infarct extends posteriorly enough to involve the nucleus and fasciculus cuneatus, producing posterior column findings in the left upper extremity, since the lesion is below the level of the lemniscal decussation. Finally, the lesion is not posteromedial enough to involve the gracilis, and so there are no posterior column findings in the left lower extremity.

To the knowledge of the authors, there is no syndrome name for this one, so here's yet another chance at immortality! However, the case underscores the point that although syndromology may be fun, there is no substitute for knowing the anatomy in neuroimaging.

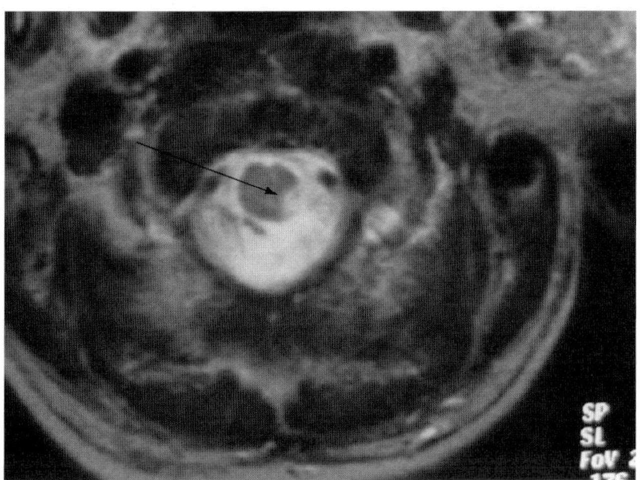

Fig. 2.27. **Axial T2 image shows a curvilinear zone of hyperintensity along the left lateral margin of the caudal medulla (arrow).**

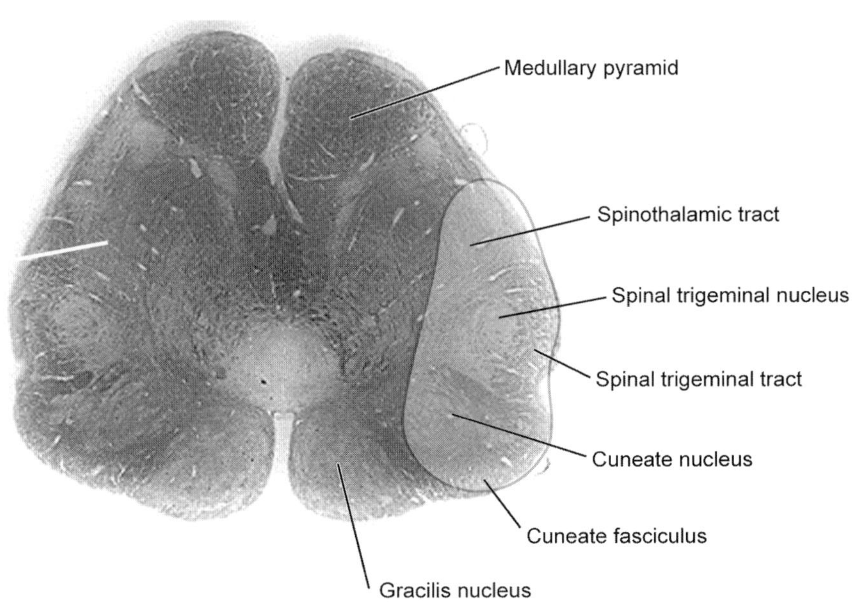

Fig. 2.28. **Labelled anatomic section showing the patient's infarct and the structures involved.**

Case 2.8

63-year-old female presents with mild ataxia, dysarthria, and ear clicking. On examination, rhythmic movements of her neck are noted, as well as rapid rhythmic movements of her palate bilaterally, known as palatal myoclonus.

Where do you think the lesion is?

Ataxia and dysarthria are rather non-specific, and may be secondary to a wide variety of lesions. The finding of palatal myoclonus is quite unusual. The symptom of ear clicking is also unusual, and is due to rhythmic snapping open and closed of the eustachian tubes. It is sometimes associated with palatal myoclonus. As you ponder the situation, the patient is called to the MR scanner.

An MRI examination is performed (Fig. 2.29). What are the findings? What is your diagnosis? Discuss this entity.

The signs and symptoms, as well as the MRI images, are consistent with the diagnosis of *hypertrophic olivary degeneration (HOD)*. This is an unusual condition, marked by a bizzare form of hypertrophic degeneration of the olivary nuclei (and so the name!). It is the result of interruption of neural inputs to the inferior olives, and hence is a type of trans-synaptic degeneration. Usually, such degeneration in the CNS is characterized by atrophy of the denervated structures. In this case, however, the degeneration takes an unusual form in that the olivary nuclei hypertrophy rather than shrink. The hypertrophy is due to a vacuolar degeneration of the denervated neurons, followed by astrocyte hypertrophy as well.

Understanding the spectrum of causes of HOD requires a brief review of the major neuronal connections of the inferior olivary nucleus. This neuronal circuit was described by Guillain and Mollaret in 1931, and has since become known as the Guillain–Mollaret triangle (see Fig. 2.30).

The Guillain–Mollaret triangle describes the connections of the dentate nucleus of the cerebellum to the contralateral red nucleus

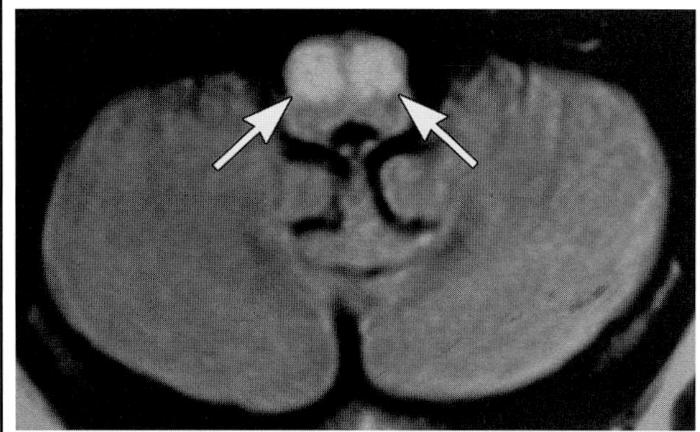 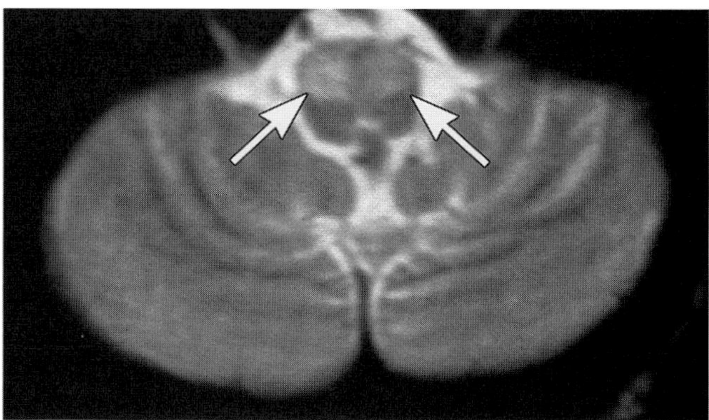

Fig. 2.29. **FLAIR and T2 axial images show marked abnormal hyperintensity and enlargement of the medullary olivary nucleii bilaterally.**

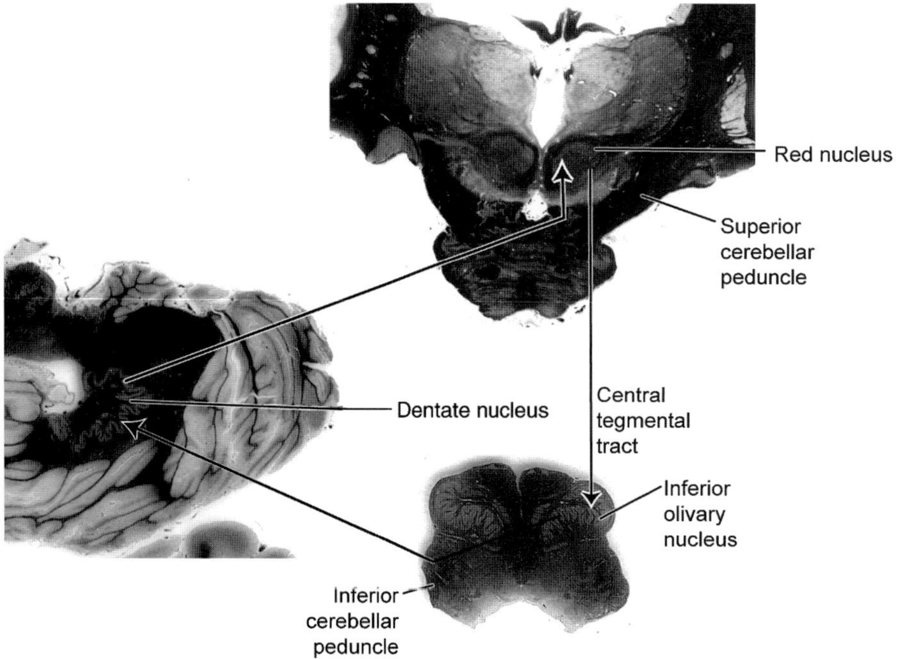

Fig. 2.30. **Anatomic sections showing the neuronal structures involved in the Guillain–Mollaret triangle. Arrows outline the pathway of neuronal impulses from the dentate nucleus of the cerebellum through the superior cerebellar peduncle to the contralateral red nucleus. The red nucleus projects via the central tegmental tract to the ipsilateral inferior olivary nucleus.**

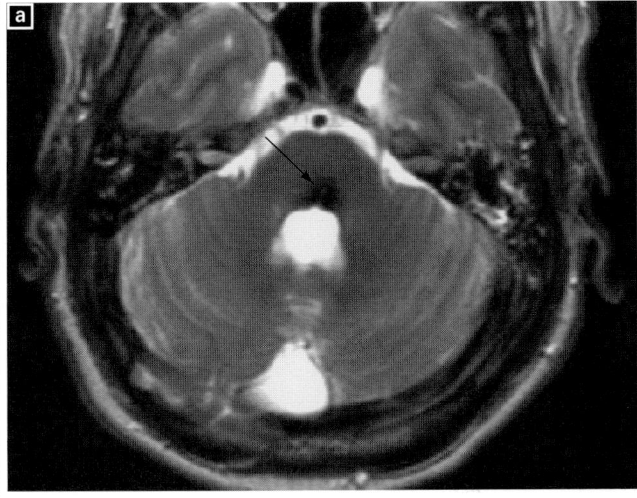 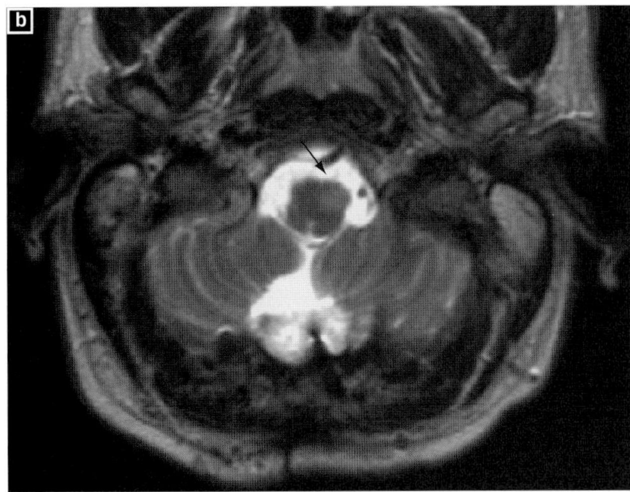

Fig. 2.31. **(a) T2 axial images show a hemosiderin-stained resection cavity in the left pontine tegmentum. (b) At the level of the medulla, T2 axial images show hypertrophic degeneration of the left inferior olivary nucleus.**

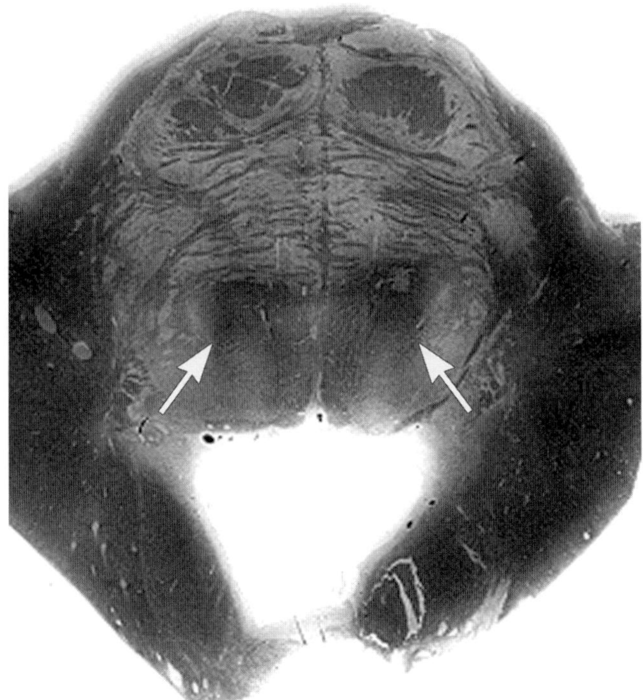

Fig. 2.32. **Anatomic brain section. The location of the central tegmental tracts is marked by arrows, and corresponds to the cavernoma resection cavity in the left pontine tegmentum.**

and inferior olivary nucleus. The dentate nucleus projects to the contralateral red nucleus via the superior cerebellar peduncle, which decussates in the midbrain. The red nucleus sends projections to the ipsilateral (to it) inferior olivary nucleus via the central tegmental tract. The inferior olivary nucleus then projects back to the contralateral dentate nucleus via the inferior cerebellar peduncle.

Having reviewed the basics of this neuronal circuit, we can now understand that there are three patterns of HOD.

(1) If a lesion occurs in the central tegmental tract, interrupting the connections between the red nucleus and the inferior olive, then there will be unilateral hypertrophic degeneration of the ipsilateral inferior olivary nucleus. Such lesions are most often infarcts or bleeds in the posterior brainstem. This pattern is illustrated by the case above (Fig. 2.31), of a 43-year-old male who had resection of a left pontine tegmentum cavernous angioma. Several months later, on follow-up MRI, he had developed hypertrophic degeneration of the left inferior olivary nucleus.

In comparing the location of the cavernoma resection cavity to an anatomic diagram (Fig. 2.32), we see that there is involvement of the central tegmental tract.

(2) If a lesion involves the dentate nucleus of the cerebellum or the superior cerebellar peduncle, then there will be unilateral hypertrophic olivary degeneration *contralateral* to the lesion.

(3) If a lesion involves both the superior cerebellar peduncle and the central tegmental tract or the decussation of the superior cerebellar peduncles, or if there are lesions in both superior cerebellar peduncles, then there will be bilateral hypertrophic olivary degeneration. One of the common causes of such lesions is severe head trauma with axonal shear injury, as in the case below (Fig. 2.33).

In this patient with massive head trauma and axonal shear injury, there is bilateral hypertrophic olivary degeneration. There is prominent hemosiderin staining involving the right superior cerebellar peduncle and dorsal right pontine tegmentum. The right central tegmental tract is slightly anterior to the hemosiderin focus in the pontine tegmentum, but may also be involved by shear injury. There is also a suggestion of minimal hemosiderin staining involving the left superior cerebellar peduncle.

Describe the clinical correlates of HOD.

Clinically, patients present with palatal myoclonus as the most characteristic sign. Other clinical manifestations can include garbled speech secondary to the palatal myoclonus, ear clicking as described above, rhythmic movements of the neck, and a slowly progressive ataxia. Sometimes, an additional symptom known as oscillopsia is noted, which is a sense of movement of the environment with head motion.

Discuss the time course of the imaging findings.

The hypertrophic degeneration of the olives manifests as enlargement and FLAIR and T2-weighted hyperintensity. In the acute stage, these findings are not present, and usually begin 3 weeks to 3 months after the onset of symptoms (see Fig. 2.34).

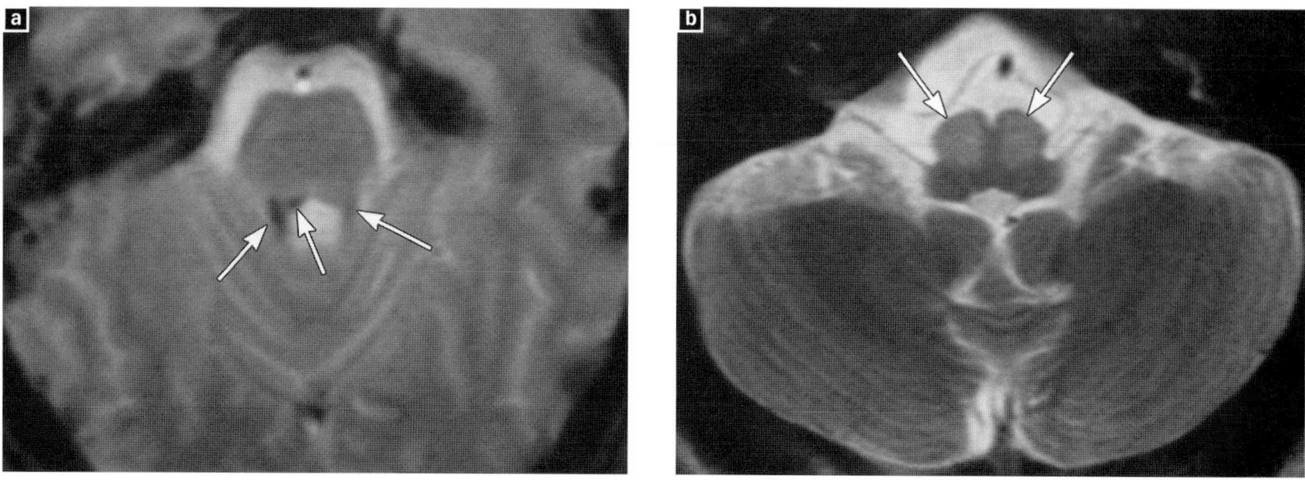

Fig. 2.33. **22-year-old six months status post-major head trauma. (a) Gradient echo T2 axial image shows hemosiderin staining involving the right superior cerebellar peduncle and the dorsal pontine tegmentum, as well as minimal hemosiderin staining of the left superior cerebellar peduncle. (b) T2 axial image shows bilateral hypertrophic olivary degeneration.**

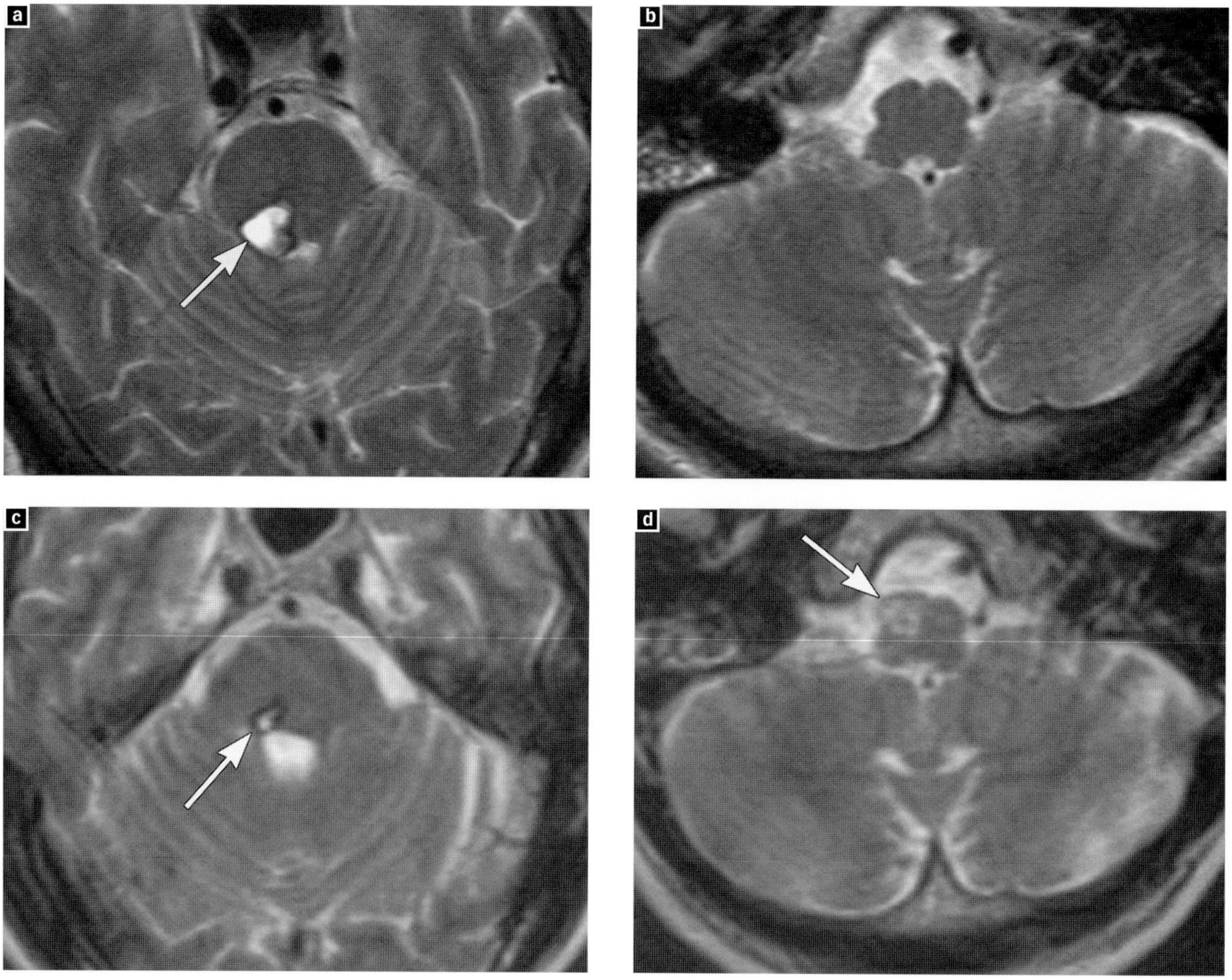

Fig. 2.34. **Axial T2-weighted images in a 42-year-old hypertensive patient 3 weeks status post-brainstem bleed. (a) There is a subacute bleed in the right pontine tegmentum. (b) The right inferior olive is normal in appearance. (c). Follow-up images at 6 months show resorption of the hematoma with a residual hemosiderin-lined cavity. (d). There has been development of ipsilateral hypertrophic degeneration of the right inferior olivary nucleus secondary to involvement of the right central tegmental tract.**

The hypertrophy reaches a maximum at 5–15 months after the injury; it corresponds to both neuronal and glial hypertrophy. In the late phases (months to years), the olivary nuclei slowly start to return to normal in size, but the T2 signal abnormalities may persist.

Are there treatment options?

Palatal tremors are sometimes resistant to therapy, and therapy is often felt unnecessary. However, 5-hydroxytryptophan and carbamazepine have been reported to be variably effective, while others have reported some success with clonazepam, tetrabenazine and trihexyphenidyl. Surgical options, including perforation of the tympanic membrane or tamponade of the eustachian tube to relieve the ear clicking are not generally considered effective.

References

Birbamer, G., Gerstenbrand, F., Aichner, F. *et al.* MR imaging of post traumatic olivary hypertrophy. *Functional Neurology* 1994; **9**: 183–187.

Kitajima, M., Korogi, Y., Shimomura, O. *et al.* Hypertrophic olivary degeneration: MR imaging and pathologic findings. *Radiology* 1994; **192**: 539–543.

Revel, M. P., Mann, M., Brugieres, P. *et al.* MR appearance of hypertrophic olivary degeneration after contralateral cerebellar hemorrhage. *American Journal of Neuroradiology* 1991; **12**: 71–72.

3 | The pons

With all due respect to Dr. Tourtellote, we have found that, with regards to the pons, it is often difficult to predict either the imaging findings from the clinical picture, or the clinical picture from the imaging findings. However, some guidelines can definitely be presented.

In studying the functional anatomy of the pons, we are caught between the relatively simple approach of the physicians of the late 1800s and the "classical pontine" syndromes which they described, and the subsequent more complex descriptions of pontine stroke syndromes, which approach the pons in terms of different vascular territories.

We believe that adopting the former approach, with an understanding of its limitations, is more conducive to both learning the relevant functional anatomy and being able to integrate this knowledge into the assessment of the more complex world of stroke presentations.

Anatomy

The functional anatomy of the pons is best understood by dividing it into two portions, a ventral "belly" of the pons, or *basis pontis*, and a dorsal *pontine tegmentum* (Fig. 3.1).

The basis pontis

The basis pontis is composed mainly of nerve fiber bundles passing through the pons, and often projecting on pontine nuclei as part of their path. These fiber bundles belong to three main fiber systems:

The corticospinal tract

Nerve fibers from the motor cortex pass through the ipsilateral half of the ventral pons on their way to the medullary pyramidal decussation. The two important facts to remember about the corticospinal tract as it travels through the pons are that:

(1) It is above the pyramidal decussation, so lesions will produce a contralateral upper motor neuron type weakness.
(2) Within the pons, the corticospinal tract is less compact than elsewhere, breaking up into multiple fascicles. Therefore, infarcts of the ventral pons sometimes produce less weakness than infarcts in other locations where the corticospinal tract is more compact, such as in the posterior limb of the internal capsule or in the medullary pyramid.

Corticobulbar fibers

These are fibers primarily from the motor cortex to cranial nerve nuclei in the brainstem. These fibers bilaterally innervate the motor nuclei of the trigeminal, facial and hypoglossal nerves. Additional terminations of the corticobulbar fibers are the red nucleus and the reticular formation.

Corticocerebellar fibers (corticopontine fibers with connections to the cerebellar hemispheres)

These are the largest group of fibers in the pons, originating from much of the cerebral cortex, but with the largest concentration being from the motor and premotor areas. These fibers, like the tracts above, arrive via the cerebral peduncles, and terminate on ipsilateral pontine nuclei. From here, axons from the pontine nuclei decussate in the basis pontis, and run transversely to enter the contralateral middle cerebellar peduncle at the lateral edge of the pons as the pontocerebellar fibers. These fibers terminate primarily on granule cells in the cerebellar hemisphere. This decussation explains why the belly of the pons, in stained sections, appears to be composed of horizontally oriented fibers. Also, the decussation of the pontocerebellar fibers in the basis pontis forms part of the famous "double decussation" characteristic of cerebellar pathways, explaining why cerebellar lesions give ipsilateral cerebellar signs and symptoms.

The pontine tegmentum

The dorsal, more primitive portion of the pons is known as the pontine tegmentum. It contains, among others, the following structures of interest to the clinician (Fig. 3.1):

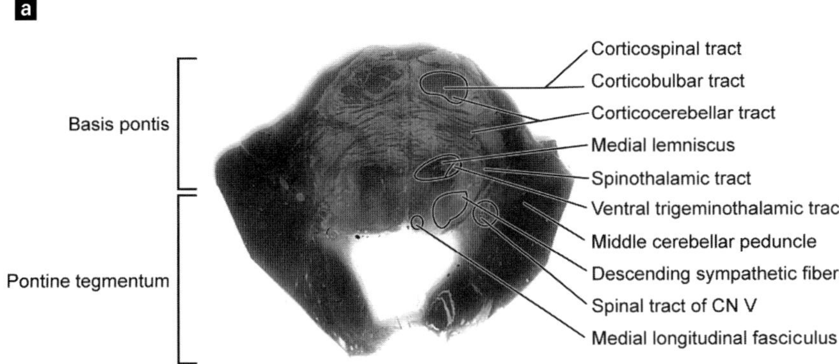

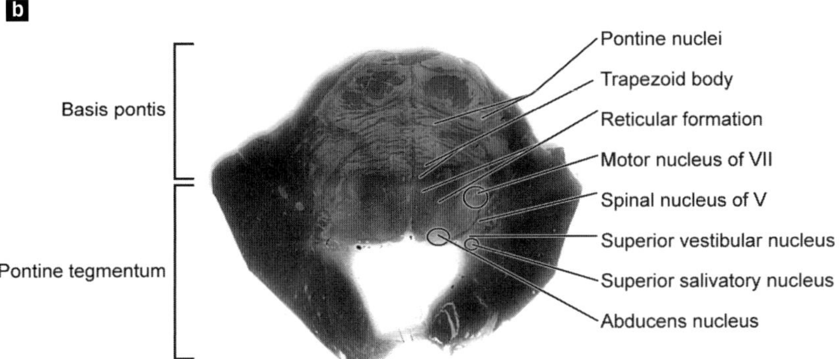

Fig. 3.1. **Anatomic sections through the pons, showing (a) the locations of the major tracts and (b) nuclei within the basis pontis and pontine tegmentum**.

The reticular formation

The pontine reticular formation is located dorsally in the pontine tegmentum, and is composed of multiple medial and lateral nuclei, the most important of which are the medially located nucleus reticularis pontis caudalis and nucleus reticularis pontis oralis. These are a continuation of medullary reticular nuclei, and give rise to the ascending reticular activating system, which plays a major role in consciousness. Therefore, lesions that destroy more than a quarter of the tegmentum may lead to an unconscious state.

The sensory lemniscal system

These structures conduct sensory information to the thalamus. They consists of the following components:

(1) Most medially are the *medial lemnisci*, which have become ovoid, flattened and oriented in a mediolateral direction. This is in distinction to their location in the medulla, where they are located anteriorly in a midline location, and are elongated in an anterior–posterior orientation. The medial lemnisci are axons from the gracilis and cuneatus nuclei, and convey proprioception, vibration and deep pressure sensations from the body. Facts to remember are:
  – These tracts have already decussated in the medulla. Therefore, lesions of the right medial lemniscus at the level of the pons, for example, will lead to loss of vibration sensation and proprioception in the left body.

  – Within the medial lemniscus, fibers from the *nucleus cuneatus (upper body)* are located medially, while those from the *nucleus gracilis (lower body)* are located laterally.

(2) Lateral to the medial lemnisci are the *trigeminal tracts*, which convey all facial sensory modalities; i.e., pain, temperature, touch, and proprioception. Please note the following:
  – The trigeminal nerve has multiple nuclei (which will be discussed). However, the ascending trigeminothalamic tract has already decussated, and therefore carries sensory information from the contralateral face.

(3) Lateral to the trigeminal tracts are the *spinothalamic tracts*, which convey pain and temperature information from the contralateral body, having decussated in the spinal cord within one or two levels of their entry into the cord.

The trapezoid body

The ascending sensory lemniscal system described above is partially embedded in the transversely oriented fibers of the trapezoid body. This arises from the cochlear nuclei, crosses the midline, and forms the lateral lemniscus in the posterolateral pons, as part of the auditory pathway. Please note that, although the nuclei for cranial nerve eight are primarily located below the ponto-medullary junction, lesions affecting the auditory and vestibular systems are commonly seen in pontine conditions. Therefore, cranial nerve eight has been placed in this chapter and will be discussed below.

The medial longitudinal fasciculus (MLF)

This small but distinctive tract runs from the medulla through the midbrain, maintaining a posterior and midline location, just anterior to the floor of the fourth ventricle and the aqueduct of Sylvius on each side of the midline. It receives input from the vestibular nuclei and connects them to the extraocular muscles to aid in the control of conjugate eye movements. It also connects the sixth nerve nucleus on one side of the brainstem with the contralateral third nerve nucleus, specifically that part which innervates the medial rectus.

The locus ceruleus

These nuclei are the major noradrenergic source to the cortex. They are located posteriorly in the pontine tegmentum, at the anterolateral margins of the fourth ventricle. Ascending fibers innervate wide areas of the brain, passing with the medial forebrain bundle to the hypothalamus, limbic system, anterior thalamus and the cortex. As we learn more, this structure will probably play a significant role in neurobehavioral medicine. For instance, the locus ceruleus is thought to play important roles in REM sleep, as well as arousal and attention. Neuronal loss in the locus ceruleus is seen in Parkinson's, Alzheimer's and

Down syndromes. Also, one model of hyperactivity attention-deficit disorder (HADD) suggests that a loss of regulation and high tonic activity of the locus ceruleus may cause HADD. In addition, there may be a link between the locus ceruleus and anxiety, as animal experiments in monkeys have shown that its stimulation produces severe anxiety. Its relationship to depression is more complex. Some models of depression posit degeneration of the locus ceruleus neurons. However, monoamine oxidase inhibitors, effective in treating depression, inhibit the locus ceruleus. This effectiveness may be mediated by ameliorating the anxiety component that often accompanies depression.

Cranial nerve nuclei

The nuclei of the fifth, sixth, and seventh cranial nerves are located in the pontine tegmentum. These cranial nerves course through the belly of the pons to exit the brainstem. The eighth cranial nerve nuclei are predominantly located just below the pontomedullary junction but will be discussed as part of the pons due to the location of their fiber tracts in the pontine tegmentum and the exit of the eighth nerves from the brainstem at the level of the cerebellopontine angle cisterns.

With this brief anatomic prelude, let us take some cases!

Case 3.1

53-year-old man presents with 1-month history of progressive left facial numbness and now with difficulty chewing.

What cranial nerve may be affected?

The history of facial numbness makes us think of the trigeminal, or fifth, cranial nerve, which subtends sensation to the face. However, the difficulty chewing is confusing, because the seventh cranial nerve innervates the muscles of the face, right? Unfortunately, not completely right. Remember, although most facial motor functions are subtended by the seventh cranial nerve, the muscles of mastication (chewing) are innervated by the motor component of the trigeminal nerve. Therefore, everything localizes to the fifth nerve.

Lesions affecting the function of the fifth cranial nerve, however, may occur at many levels in the neuroaxis. Lesions may be

supranuclear, including in the sensory cortex, corona radiata along the course of the sensory pathways, or in the facial sensory region of the thalamus (the VPM nucleus of the thalamus). Lesions may be nuclear, such as in the pons or in the medulla involving the fifth nerve nuclei, or preganglionic, ganglionic, or in the trigeminal nerve branches.

The history of gradual disease progression makes us lean away from a vascular insult and toward an inflammatory or neoplastic process.

Physical examination reveals loss to pinprick and temperature sensation across the left face, from the forehead to the mandible. The temporalis muscle is atrophic, the bulk of the masseter is diminished, and with jaw opening, the jaw tilts to the left. Both the corneal and jaw jerk reflexes are markedly diminished.

How does this affect your thinking?

The examination suggests involvement of the entire fifth nerve (all three sensory divisions and the motor division). The absence of a jaw jerk reflex and a corneal reflex suggests that the lesion is not supranuclear (in such cases, the reflexes would be brisk). Remember also that, with weakness of the masseter and pterygoid muscles, the jaw will tilt ipsilaterally to the weak side with mouth opening.

An MRI image is shown (Fig. 3.2).

What are your findings? What is your differential?

On the MRI, we see that the cisternal segment (in the prepontine cistern, after the fifth nerve exits the belly of the pons) of the left fifth nerve is swollen and diffusely enhancing (Fig. 3.2, arrow). The enhancement does not extend into the pons. However, there is some abnormal tissue in the left Meckel's cave and some mass effect in the left cavernous sinus, which bulges outward. The image suggests that the pathology involves the fifth nerve itself, and is not secondary to a mass, such as a meningioma, impinging the nerve. Also, while slightly swollen, the nerve is not mass-like, such as to suggest a fifth nerve schwannoma. Differential diagnostic possibilities for an enhancing fifth nerve would include carcinomatous meningitis,

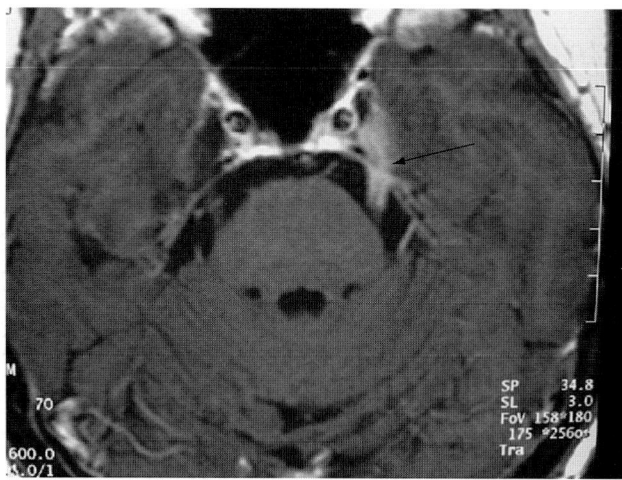

Fig. 3.2. **Post-contrast axial T1-weighted image through the pons.**

lymphoma, viral neuritis, or other infectious processes such as tuberculosis or Lyme disease, as well as non-infectious granulomatous diseases such as sarcoidosis. However, the mass effect in the cavernous sinus essentially excludes viral neuritis and Lyme disease.

Diagnosis

Carcinomatous meningitis, secondary to perineural spread of a head and neck adenoid cystic carcinoma.

Please discuss the functional anatomy of the 5th cranial nerve.

The fifth nerve is usually identified as the main sensory input of the face to the central nervous system. Aside from this main sensory function, it also has a smaller motor root, which supplies the muscles of mastication (masseter, temporalis, medial and lateral pterygoids) as well as the tensor tympani, tensor palatini, myelohyoid and anterior belly of the digastric. The motor fibers arise from the motor nucleus of the fifth nerve, at the midpontine level in the pontine tegmentum (Fig. 3.3).

The motor nucleus receives bilateral symmetric input from the motor cortex. Therefore, cortical or corticobulbar tract lesions do not paralyze the muscles of mastication. Lesions of the root or nerve, however, cause a lower motor neuron type paralysis of these muscles, with denervation atrophy. The motor fibers run with the third sensory division, or V3, of the trigeminal nerve.

The sensory portion of the fifth nerve is divided into three divisions: V1 (ophthalmic), V2 (maxillary), V3 (mandibular), each with its own course through the head and neck (Fig. 3.3). These divisions run separately in the cavernous sinus, but collect into a main nerve trunk in the prepontine cistern. The cell bodies of most of these fibers are located in the trigeminal (Gasserian) ganglion, located in Meckels's cave, just posterior to the cavernous sinus. The nerve fibers synapse in three nuclei of the trigeminal nerve in the brainstem: the main sensory nucleus, located in the pontine tegmentum, the spinal trigeminal nucleus running from the lower pons through the posterolateral medulla and down into the upper cervical cord, and a small mesencephalic nucleus in the midbrain (Fig. 3.3 and 3.4).

The sensory fibers of the fifth nerve, once they enter the brainstem, generally distribute themselves as follows: proprioceptive fibers from the mouth go to the mesencephalic nucleus and then to the thalamus. Actually, their neurons are located in the mesencephalic nucleus itself rather than in a peripheral ganglion, a fairly unique arrangement. Fibers subtending touch in each of the three divisions bifurcate, with some synapsing on the main sensory nucleus, and others traveling down the descending spinal trigeminal tract. From there, they enter the adjacent spinal trigeminal nucleus, towards its rostral and mid portions. Fibers subtending pain and temperature enter the pons, and travel downward in the spinal trigeminal tract, synapsing on the lower-most portion of the spinal trigeminal nucleus, the so-called caudal nucleus, which extends from the obex of the fourth ventricle in the medulla to the upper cervical spine.

Now, all of this sensory information has to make its way to the thalamus, and so we have to follow the output of these nuclei (Fig. 3.4). This is complex, but can be generalized as follows: most of the output of the spinal trigeminal nucleus crosses the midline, and ascends to the thalamus via the contralateral brainstem in the ventral trigeminothalamic tract, or trigeminal tract for short, which runs between the medial lemniscus and the spinothalamic tract, as described above. This ends in the ventral posteromedial (VPM) nucleus of the thalamus. Most of the output of the main sensory nucleus also crosses the midline, and joins the ventral trigeminothalamic tract. Some of the output, however, travels in an ancillary tract called the dorsal trigeminal tract, ascending ipsilaterally in an uncrossed fashion. Finally,

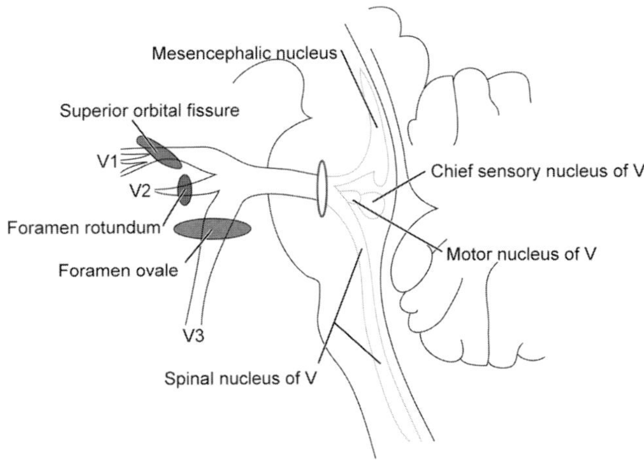

Fig. 3.3. **Anatomy of the trigeminal nerve. The sensory portion of the trigeminal nerve is composed of three divisions: V1, V2 and V3, which exit the skull through the superior orbital fissure, foramen rotundum and foramen ovale, respectively. These divisions send fibers to the three sensory brainstem nuclei of the fifth nerve: the main sensory nucleus, the mesencephalic nucleus and the spinal trigeminal nucleus. The motor component of the 5th nerve arises from the motor nucleus, and travels along with V3.**

some fibers also cross the midline and ascend in the contralateral dorsal trigeminal tract.

Some important clinical points can be extracted from this jumble of information, as follows.

Trigeminal nerve findings, such as facial sensory loss, can be caused by cortical, thalamic, capsular, brainstem, prepontine cistern, cavernous sinus, or more peripheral lesions. Some general clinical guidelines may be offered.

(1) Lesions of the 5th nerve distal to the Gasserian ganglion will typically involve preferentially one of the branches of the 5th nerve, such that the sensory loss, which should affect all sensory modalities, will preferentially involve the ophthalmic, maxillary, or mandibular (V1, V2, or V3) distributions.

(2) Lesions at the level of the Gasserian ganglion or the fifth nerve itself should involve the entirety of the face, and involve all modalities.

(3) Brainstem lesions may lead to ipsilateral facial sensory loss, from involvement of the 5th nerve as it travels through the belly of the pons, the 5th nerve main sensory nucleus in the pons, or the spinal trigeminal tract and nucleus in the lower pons and medulla. However, facial sensory findings may also occur contralateral to the lesion by involving the ascending ventral trigeminothalamic tract as part of the lemniscal sensory system. Recall that the output of the spinal trigeminal nucleus, as well as most of the output of the main sensory nucleus of the 5th nerve crosses the midline, and projects to the contralateral thalamus via the ventral trigeminothalamic tract and trigeminal lemniscus. A case of a midbrain lesion causing contralateral facial sensory symptoms is shown in Fig. 3.5. In the experience of the author, however, ipsilateral facial sensory findings are more common than contralateral facial sensory findings.

(4) Because of the somatotopic organization of the sensory fibers, such that pain and temperature fibers tend largely to project on the inferior aspect of the spinal trigeminal nucleus (caudal portion or caudal nucleus of the spinal trigeminal nucleus), it is possible to treat tic douloureux, a disabling syndrome of facial pain, by a spinal trigeminal tractotomy, where only

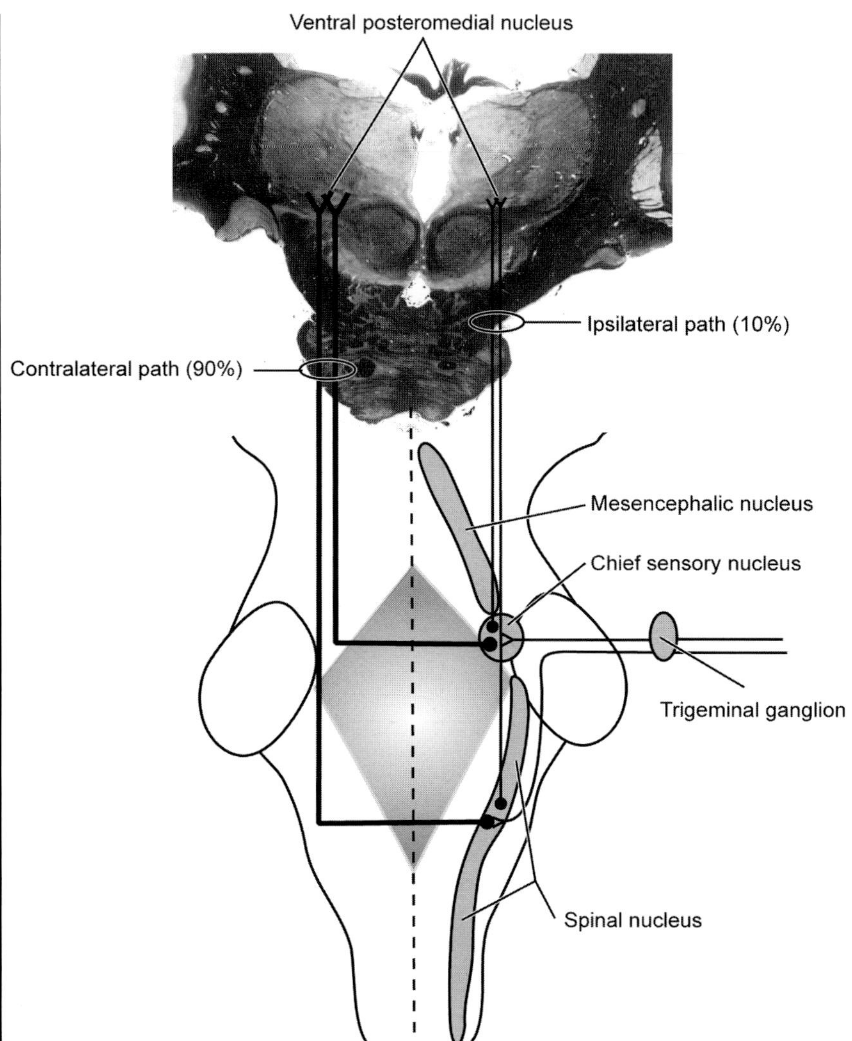

Fig. 3.4. **Output pathways of the trigeminal nuclei. Inputs to the chief sensory nucleus and the spinal trigeminal nucleus come in through the fifth nerve via the trigeminal ganglion. Most of the output (about 90 percent) from the chief sensory nucleus and the spinal trigeminal nucleus decussates to reach the contralateral thalamus via the ventral trigeminothalamic tract. There is also a small ipsilateral output component (about 10 percent). See text for further details.**

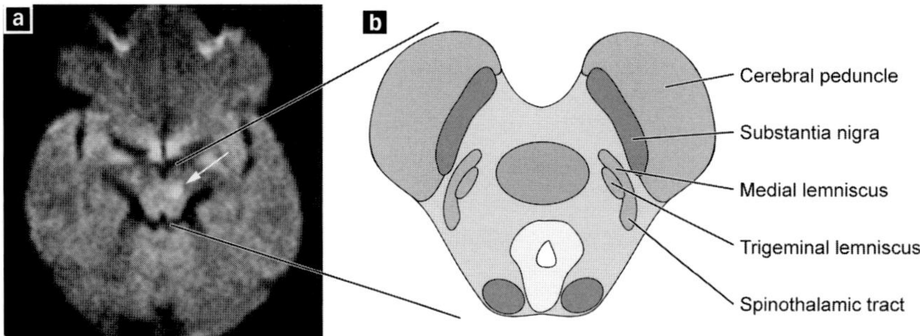

Fig. 3.5. **(a) Diffusion-weighted MRI scan shows a small midbrain infarct posterior to the substantia nigra in the region of the left trigeminal lemniscus (arrow). This patient's only symptom was right facial numbness. (b) Schematic diagram of the midbrain shows that the infarct involves the region of the left trigeminal lemniscus (and ventral trigeminothalamic tract), which is carrying information from the right-sided 5th nerve nuclei up to the left thalamus. This case illustrates that brainstem lesions may cause contralateral facial sensory findings, although ipsilateral sensory deficits are more common.**

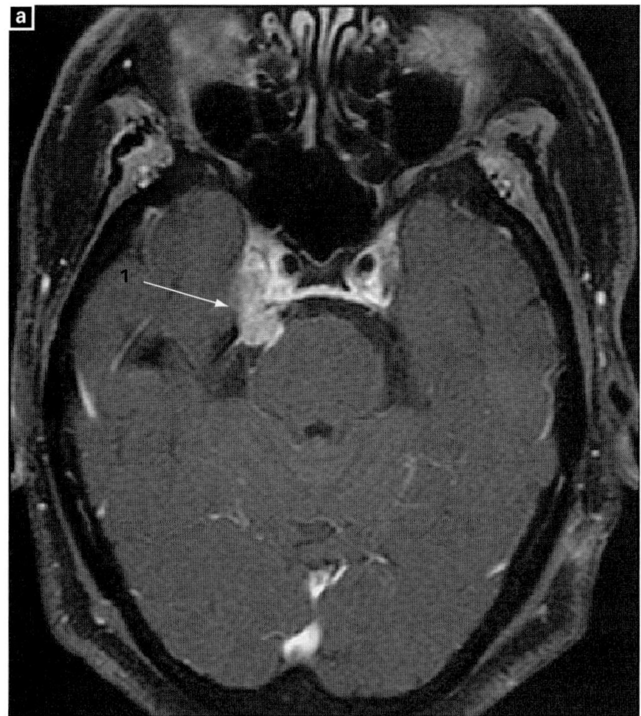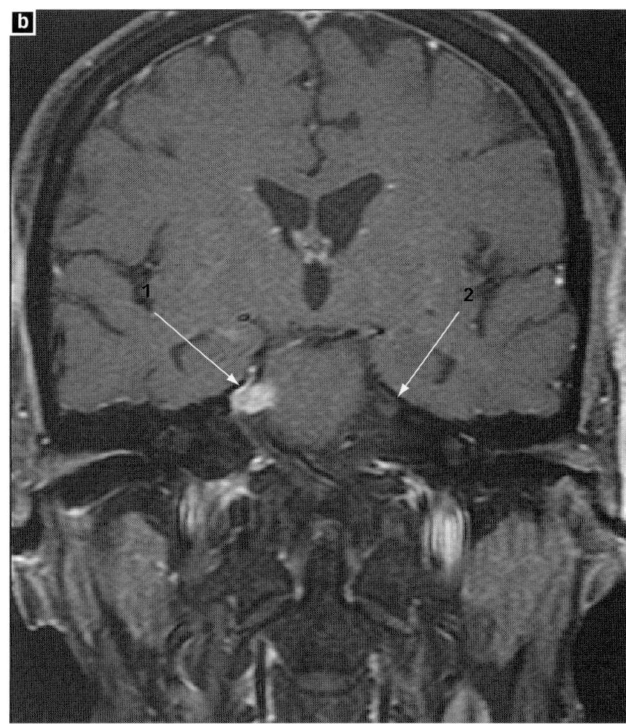

Fig. 3.6. **(a) Axial and (b) coronal post-contrast T1-weighted images show a large enhancing schwannoma involving the right fifth nerve (arrow 1). The normal left fifth nerve is shown for comparison on the coronal image (arrow 2).**

the inferior portion of the tract, at the cervicomedullary junction, is sectioned. This should leave other sensory modalities intact.

(5) It is noted that fibers for proprioception project predominantly to the mescencephalic nucleus of the 5th cranial nerve. Also, fibers for light touch divide and project both to the main sensory nucleus as well as the spinal trigeminal tract and nucleus. Since touch sensation is processed both through the main sensory nucleus in the pons and the spinal trigeminal nucleus and tract lower in the brainstem, it is difficult for single lesions of the brainstem to ablate touch sensation. Therefore, brainstem infarcts often show a dissociation of sensory modality defects, with pain and temperature sensation usually significantly more affected than other modalities. This is in distinction to more peripheral lesions, such as those of the 5th nerve itself, which should affect all sensory modalities equally. This may help in localizing the site of the lesion.

(6) It is noted that sensory fibers from the perioral region tend to project further rostral in the brainstem along the spinal trigeminal nucleus than fibers mediating sensation from the skin away from the perioral area, with a somatotopic mapping of these fibers gradually lower in the brainstem as one goes away from the region of the mouth. This may be to allow a smooth transition between cervical dermatomes and cranial nerve dermatomes to the skin most adjacent to the neck, such as the periauricular areas, and region of the angle of the mandible, with progression more rostrally in the brainstem as fibers progress toward the midline and perioral region. The clinical correlate of this arrangement is a so-called "onion-skin" sensory deficit, where lesions in the lower brainstem and upper cervical spine will spare the perioral area, where sensation remains intact. This "onion-skin" pattern of sensory loss is thus helpful in localizing a "5th nerve" lesion to the lower brainstem.

(7) The 5th nerve participates in multiple important reflexes. Only two of these are mentioned:

The corneal reflex

This represents a reflex arc between the sensory fibers of the ophthalmic division of the 5th nerve as the afferent limb, and the orbicularis oculis muscles, supplied by the seventh nerve. The 5th nerve fibers will connect to both seventh nerve nuclei. Hence, touching the cornea with sterile gauze will initiate an immediate blink reflex in both eyes. The presence of the corneal reflex verifies the integrity of the afferent 5th nerve, and the efferent seventh nerve.

The jaw jerk reflex

This reflex consists of tap on the closed but relaxed jaw at the chin, eliciting a contraction of the temporalis muscles and a "jaw jerk." The afferent limb of this reflex is the proprioceptive fiber set synapsing on the mescencephalic nucleus of the 5th cranial nerve, while the efferent limb of the reflex is the motor fiber set of the 5th cranial nerve. An intact jaw jerk would confirm the integrity of the afferent and efferent loops. If other cranial nerve five lesion symptoms are seen, an intact jaw jerk reflex would place the lesion either lower in the brainstem, or along the output sensory limb of the 5th nerve nuclei, such as the trigeminothalamic tract, thalamus, internal capsule, or sensory cortex, proximal (more central) to the reflex arc.

To round out the imaging issues of the fifth nerve, a few more sets of images are briefly presented. Fig. 3.6 presents a patient with right facial numbness who had a fifth nerve schwannoma.

Now that you are comfortable locating the fifth nerve, Fig. 3.7 presents a 62-year-old hypertensive patient with left-sided trigeminal neuralgia. MR imaging shows an ectatic vertebro-basilar system

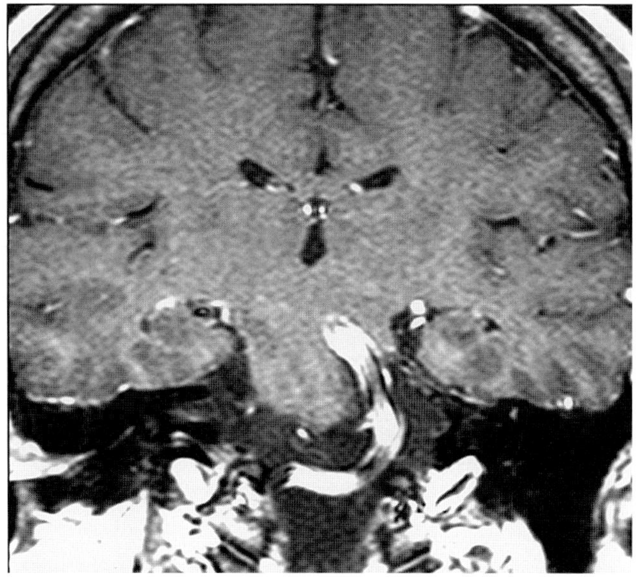

Fig. 3.7. **Post-contrast coronal T1-weighted image shows a markedly tortuous vertebro-basilar artery swinging across the course of the left fifth nerve in this patient with trigeminal neuralgia.**

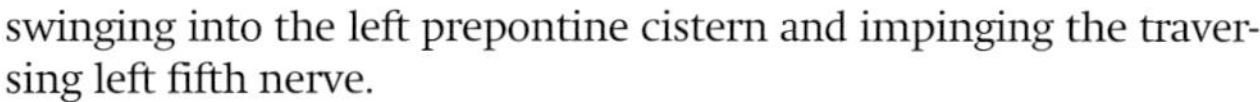

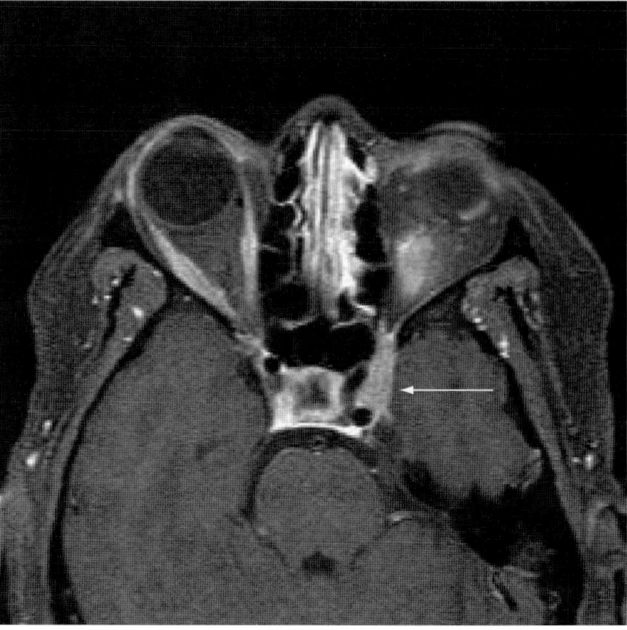

Fig. 3.8. **Axial T1-weighted fat-saturation post-contrast image shows fullness and enhancement of the left cavernous sinus (arrow). The findings are non-specific, but are consistent with Tolosa–Hunt syndrome, especially given the clinical presentation.**

swinging into the left prepontine cistern and impinging the traversing left fifth nerve.

A nice series of patients with trigeminal neuralgia (Linskey *et al.*, 1994) showed that, of 1404 with trigeminal neuralgia, 31 (2 percent) had compression of the fifth nerve by a tortuous vertebral or basilar artery, such as in our case. This subgroup tended to be older than idiopathic trigeminal neuralgia patients and to be hypertensive. Interestingly, this vertebro-basilar compression was more likely to involve the left fifth nerve (probably because the left vertebral artery is more often dominant than the right). In this series, 100 percent of patients were pain-free without medication immediately after microvascular decompression surgery, and this status was maintained at 1 year in 96 percent.

Fig. 3.8 shows another interesting case of a 46-year-old female patient who presented with painful ophthalmoplegia, with burning left retro-orbital pain, and partial third and sixth nerve palsies. A presumptive diagnosis of Tolosa–Hunt syndrome was made on the basis of imaging, and the patient responded excellently to steroids.

Tolosa–Hunt syndrome is an idiopathic inflammatory condition of the cavernous sinus which typically presents with pain in the V1 distribution from involvement of the fifth nerve, as well as paresis of the extra ocular muscles secondary to involvement of cranial nerves three, four and six in the cavernous sinus. There may also be a Horner's syndrome secondary to involvement of the sympathetic fibers in the cavernous sinus. The imaging findings are non-specific, and other entities, such as lymphoma or meningioma involving the cavernous sinus need to be carefully considered.

Reference

Linskey, M. E., Jho, H. D., and Jannetta, P. J. Microvascular decompression for trigeminal neuralgia caused by vertebrobasilar compression. *Journal of Neurosurgery* 1994, **81**(1): 1–9.

Case 3.2

62-year-old male patient presents sudden onset "double vision." Physical examination reveals that the patient is unable to adduct (medially deviate) his left eye on attempted right lateral gaze. The right eye abducted normally, but showed some beats of nystagmus.

Why can't the patient medially deviate his left eye? Where might the lesion be? What other ocular motility test may be done to help narrow the diagnosis?

The left eye is adducted by the left medial rectus muscle, which is innervated by the left third nerve. Therefore, the patient may have a problem with the left third nerve, or with the left medial rectus muscle. To explore this possibility, the patient's ocular convergence should be tested. In our patient, the left eye adducted normally with convergence.

Look at the MRI images (Fig. 3.9).
What are the findings? What is your diagnosis?

A small focus of FLAIR and DWI hyperintensity is noted in the left pontine tegmentum (arrow), just anterior to the rostral fourth ventricle at its junction with the aqueduct of Sylvius. This appearance is consistent with a small infarct involving the left medial longitudinal fasciculus (MLF), which sits just paramidline at the anterior margin of the fourth ventricle (see Fig. 3.1).

Diagnosis

Internuclear ophthalmoplegia (INO) secondary to a small pontine tegmentum infarct involving the left MLF. This disconnects the right sixth nerve (responsible for abducting the right eye) from the left third nerve (responsible for adducting the left eye) during

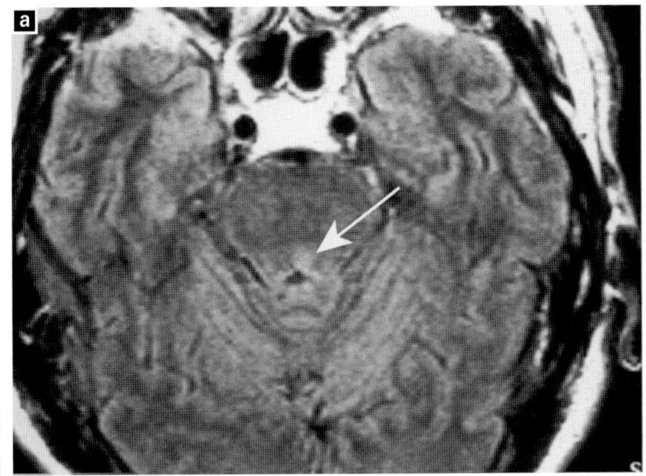
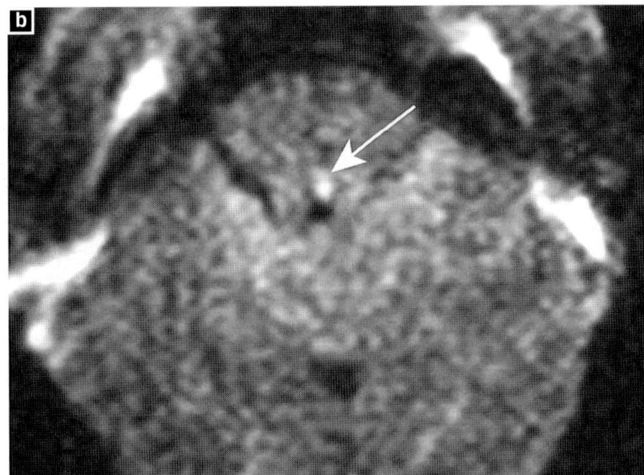

Fig. 3.9. **(a) Poor quality FLAIR and (b) DWI axial MRI images through the pons.**

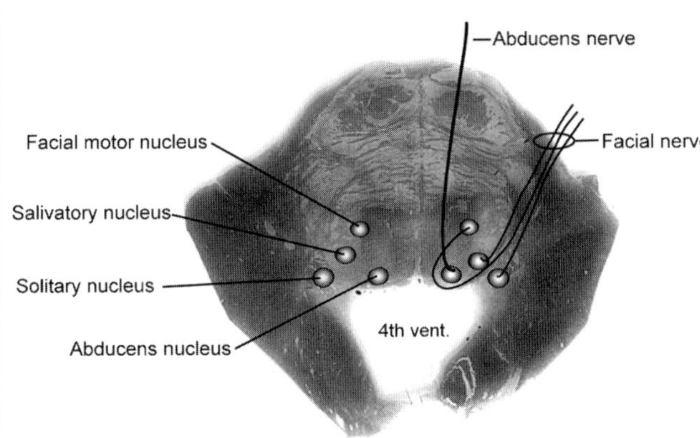

Fig. 3.10. **Anatomy of the sixth and seventh nerves. Fibers from the motor nucleus of the seventh nerve curve around the sixth nerve nucleus and form a bump in the floor of the fourth ventricle known as the facial colliculus. Note that the salivatory nucleus and solitary nucleus also contribute to the seventh nerve.**

attempted right lateral gaze. The third nerve itself is normal, so the left eye adducts during gaze convergence. Since the sixth and third nerve nuclei are disconnected from each other, and we have a problem with eye movement, we get the term "internuclear ophthalmoplegia."

Please discuss the relevant functional anatomy of the sixth (abducens) cranial nerve and the MLF.

The sixth cranial nerve innervates the lateral rectus muscle and is responsible for abducting the ipsilateral eye. The sixth cranial nerve nucleus is located in the posterior midline pontine tegmentum along the floor of the fourth ventricle. The sixth nerve nucleus has a peculiar relationship with the seventh nerve (Fig. 3.10).

The seventh nerve motor nucleus is anterolateral to the sixth nerve nucleus in the lower pontine tegmentum. Fibers leaving the seventh nerve motor nucleus course posteromedially in the pons and then posteriorly around the sixth nerve nucleus, forming the first genu of the facial nerve, before coursing anterolaterally again to exit the pons at the cerebellopontine angle cistern. This first genu of the facial nerve forms a bump along the floor of the fourth ventricle known as the facial colliculus.

The sixth nerve fibers exit the nucleus and then course anteriorly, fairly midline, through the belly of the pons, and exit the pons at the level of the pontomedullary junction. The sixth nerves then course through the prepontine cistern, and enter a small fibrous canal along the surface of the petrous apex, known as Dorello's canal. In this location, the sixth nerves are in close proximity to the trigeminal nerves.

The sixth nerves then enter the cavernous sinuses, where they run between the carotid artery and the branches of the trigeminal nerve. The sixth nerves enter the orbit to innervate the lateral rectus muscle. Therefore, before we continue, it is important to realize that, since the sixth nerve innervates only a single muscle, sixth nerve palsy may be perfectly mimicked by isolated lateral rectus muscle pathology (Fig. 3.11), a highly unusual condition.

The pattern shown in Fig. 3.11 is quite rare. While most muscle enlargement in the orbit is due to Grave's disease, isolated lateral rectus enlargement should make us strongly consider other diagnoses, as such a pattern would be rare for Grave's. Among the possibilities would be amyloid infiltration, focal orbital pseudotumor or metastatic disease. Rarely, cysticercosis of the extraocular muscles has been reported to give a similar appearance. The point here, though, is that this patient was thought to have a routine diabetic sixth nerve palsy, but an MRI was obtained "just to make sure."

A main function of the sixth cranial nerve is producing conjugate lateral gaze by abducting the ipsilateral eye. It is impossible, however, to discuss lateral gaze and the function of the sixth nerve without involving the third nerve as well. For example, for a conjugate lateral gaze to the right, the right sixth nerve needs to abduct the right eye by activating the right lateral rectus, while the left third nerve needs to adduct the left eye by activating the left medial rectus.

There are at least three conceivable distinct fashions in which this coordination between the sixth nerve and the contralateral third nerve may take place. The frontal eye fields (FEF, Brodmann's area 8) can simultaneously innervate and modulate the sixth nerve motor nucleus on one side, and the third nerve motor nucleus (subnucleus for the medial rectus) on the opposite side. Alternatively, the FEF may communicate with the third nerve nucleus, which then communicates with the contralateral sixth nerve nucleus. A third alternative is that the FEF communicate primarily with the sixth nerve nucleus, which then coordinates with the contralateral third nerve nucleus. All three alternatives would produce the required coordination between the sixth nerve nucleus and the contralateral third nerve nucleus. The question then arises as to which of the three alternatives best describes human neuroanatomy. What is your guess?

Functional neuroanatomy, in fact, most closely resembles the third alternative (see Fig. 3.12).

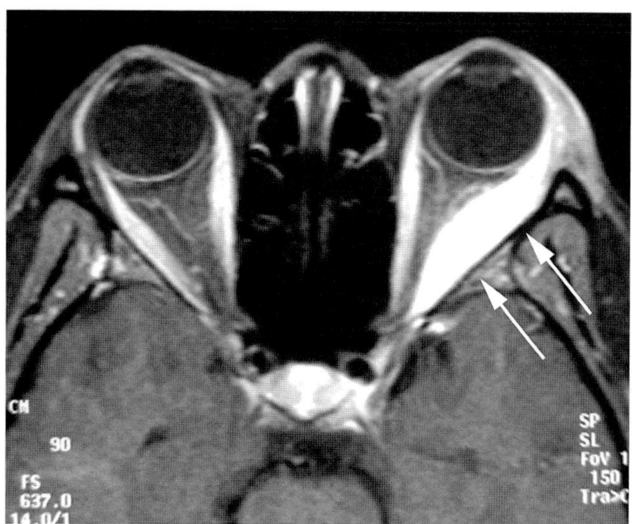

Fig. 3.11. **Axial T1-weighted post-contrast fat-saturation MRI image through the orbits shows isolated thickening of the left lateral rectus muscle.**

The left frontal eye fields project to the right (contralateral) sixth cranial nerve, which then communicates with the left (contralateral again) third nerve through the medial longitudinal fasciculus (MLF), described above. The coordination between the frontal eye fields and the sixth nerve nucleus is somewhat complex, involving a group of the nuclei in the brainstem tegmentum known as the paramedian pontine reticular formation (PPRF) (Fig. 3.12). So, let's go into a little more detail. Impulses for voluntary lateral gaze arise predominately in the frontal eye fields, a region in the superior and middle prefrontal cortex. They are modulated by impulses from the supplementary eye fields, as well as impulses from the temporal–parietal eye fields. The fibers from the frontal eye fields descend in the internal capsule, and predominately decussate in the midbrain to synapse with the contralateral PPRF, which then synapses with the sixth nerve nucleus. Therefore, the left frontal eye fields, for example, communicate with the right PPRF, which controls right lateral gaze, with abduction of the right eye, and adduction of the left eye. For simplistic functional neuroanatomy, we can consider that the left frontal eye fields push the eyes to the right side and facilitate right lateral gaze, because of a constant neural "tone" as long as the left frontal cortex is intact. Thus, when a cortical infarct involving the left frontal eye fields occurs, there is unopposed action by the right frontal eye fields, "pushing" the eyes to the left. Thus the famous dictum in neurology when talking about a cortical infarct: "the eyes look toward the side of the lesion."

The sixth nerve nucleus contains two distinct populations of cells. There are large primary motor cells, which send fibers that exit the motor nucleus, and form the sixth nerve, innervating the ipsilateral lateral rectus muscle. There are also small internuclear neurons (interneurons, for short), whose fibers exit the sixth nerve nucleus, cross the midline, and join the contralateral

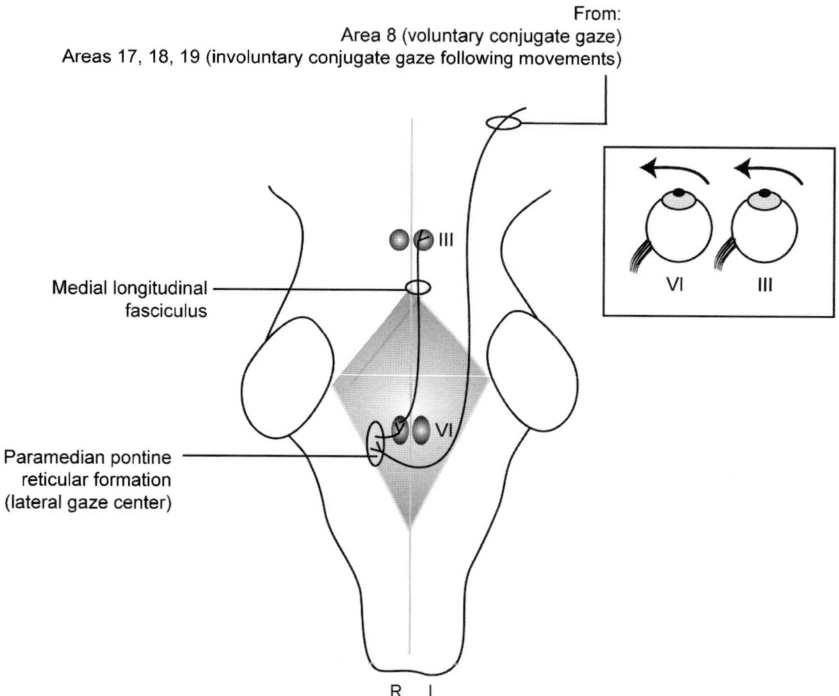

Fig. 3.12. **Anatomic diagram, illustrating function of left MLF. Left-sided cortical fibers from areas 8, 17, 18 and 19 descend in the brainstem, decussate, and synapse with the right PPRF. This sends fibers to the right VI nerve nucleus. Interneurons from the right VI nucleus cross the midline and ascend in the left MLF to synapse on the left III nucleus. This coordinates right lateral gaze, with abduction of the right eye and adduction of the left eye.**

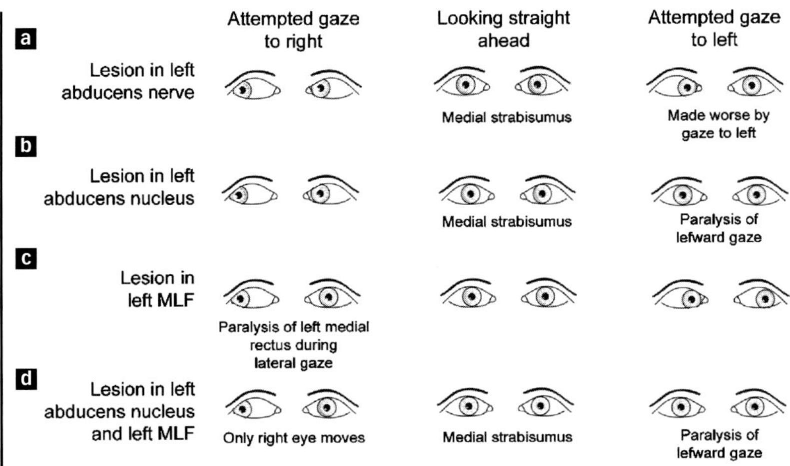

Fig. 3.13. **Illustration of gaze deficits with lesions in left sixth (abducens) nerve and left MLF. See text sections (a)–(d) for further details.**

medial longitudinal fasciculus (MLF), extending up the brainstem to innervate the contralateral third nerve nucleus, specifically the subnucleus of the medial rectus muscle (Fig. 3.12).

Understanding this anatomy allows us to delineate several separate but related lateral gaze deficits. We can use the left sixth nerve and the left MLF for concrete examples (Fig. 3.13).

(a) Left sixth (abducens) nerve palsy – in this case, the left sixth nerve is damaged after it exits the abducens nucleus. Therefore, the fibers to the left lateral rectus are disrupted, and the left eye cannot abduct (look laterally). There will be some medial deviation of the left eye from unopposed action by the left medial rectus (innervated by the left third nerve). However, the left sixth nerve interneurons, within the abducens nucleus, are intact, and enter the right MLF. Therefore, with attempted left lateral gaze, the left eye cannot look laterally, but the right eye can look medially.

The left sixth nerve may be damaged secondary to pontine infarcts that affect the nerve but spare the nucleus, secondary to diabetic small vessel disease that causes ischemic neuropathy, or secondary to trauma, since the nerve is small and travels a long course through the tough Dorello's canal.

Clinical note

Gradenigo's syndrome

This syndrome consists of an infection of the bony petrous apex, known as a petrous apicitis. Since the sixth nerve passes in Dorello's canal along the petrous apex, it is involved, and there can be a sixth nerve palsy. Also, because this is very close to Meckel's cave and the Gasserian ganglion, there may be fifth nerve symptoms, such as facial pain and headache. If the infection travels farther back along the petrous ridge, the seventh and eighth nerves may also be involved.

(b) Left lateral gaze palsy – Here, the left sixth (abducens) nerve nucleus itself is damaged. This includes both the motor neurons that innervate the left lateral rectus and the interneurons, whose axons cross the midline and enter the right MLF to communicate with the right third nerve nucleus. Therefore, with attempted left lateral gaze, the left eye still does not look laterally, but now, in addition, the right eye does not adduct (look medially).

(c) Left internuclear ophthalmoplegia (INO) – This is now easy to understand. Here, there is a lesion in the left MLF (as in our patient). Therefore, the fibers from the right sixth nerve

nucleus traveling to the left third nerve nucleus are interrupted, and the left eye does not adduct on attempted right lateral gaze. Therefore, with an INO, the eye ipsilateral to the MLF lesion will not adduct on attempted lateral gaze to the side opposite the lesion. This phenomenon is discussed in more detail below.

Clinical notes

– The eye opposite the MLF lesion (in this case, the right eye in the setting of a left INO) abducts normally, but often shows nystagmus on attempted lateral gaze. The nystagmus seen with an INO is called an abduction nystagmus. It involves the abducting eye opposite the side of the lesion producing the INO, with a rapid phase laterally. In our patient, the right eye shows beats of nystagmus with rapid phase laterally. The cause of this abduction nystagmus is unclear. It may be a gaze-evoked nystagmus with adaptation to adduction weakness in the contralateral eye, or it may be due to interruption of fibers from the vestibular nuclei to the nuclei of the extraocular muscles, which also travel in the MLF.

– With an MLF lesion, on the left in this example, the left eye cannot adduct with right lateral gaze, but will adduct with near gaze convergence.

– A unilateral INO in young adults is usually secondary to multiple sclerosis, while in older people, it is usually secondary to a small infarct. In children, it may be the presenting symptom of a tectal brainstem glioma. Bilateral INOs, on the other hand, are highly suggestive of multiple sclerosis. This is because a midline plaque in the brainstem tegmentum can involve both MLFs, which run very close to midline. Infarcts, however, tend to affect one side or the other.

– With a subtle INO, the involved eye may adduct fully, but just be slow. Therefore, the patient should be tested with saccadic eye movements (rapid repetitive lateral eye movements). A discrepancy in the velocity between the abducting and the adducting eye can be discerned.

– It is noted that patients with myasthenia gravis can present with failure of adduction of one eye and a nystagmus of the other eye, mimicking an INO. However, the dissociation of function of the medial rectus between attempted adduction with lateral gaze and with near gaze convergence typical of INO is not usually seen with myasthenia. Nonetheless, several authorities feel that any patient who presents with an isolated INO without evidence of multiple sclerosis or an infarct should have a Tensilon (edrophonium chloride) test for myasthenia.

(d) Left One and a Half – This is a funny name for a clinical syndrome, but it will make perfect sense soon. It results from a lesion that is big enough to involve the left sixth (abducens) nerve nucleus and the adjacent left MLF. Therefore, it will be a combination of a left lateral gaze palsy, where the left eye does not abduct and the right eye does not adduct on attempted left lateral gaze, and a left INO, where the left eye does not adduct on attempted right lateral gaze. The only lateral gaze function still intact is abduction of the right eye on attempted right lateral gaze. Hence, of the two lateral gaze directions, only one half of a function (right eye abduction) remains intact.

In Fig. 3.14, a DWI scan is presented with a right pontine tegmental infarct. The infarct is larger than the very small lesion in our first patient with the left INO, but still in the region of the right sixth nerve nucleus. This patient had a right one-and-a-half syndrome.

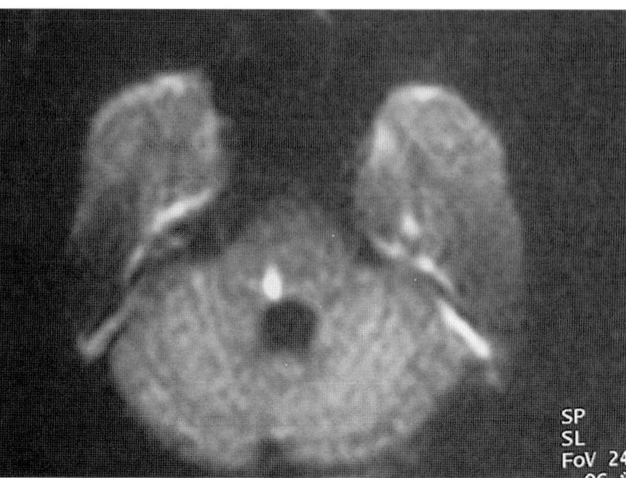

Fig. 3.14. **A DWI scan shows a right pontine tegmentum infarct. This patient has a one-and-a-half syndrome.**

Case 3.3

43-year-old male presents with a left facial palsy, which progressed over 24 hours.

What critical question regarding the facial paralysis is going through your mind? What cranial nerve might be involved? What is your differential diagnosis?

The most important question regarding a facial palsy is whether it is central or peripheral, as the differential diagnosis is quite different for the two. The former is usually due to a contralateral cerebral infarct, while the latter may be due to a variety of ipsilateral peripheral nerve lesions involving the seventh (or facial) cranial nerve. Among these, Bell's palsy would be a leading differential diagnostic consideration, since it is the most common cause of facial paralysis. The second most common cause of peripheral facial palsy is Ramsay Hunt syndrome (reactivation of varicella zoster infection involving the seventh and eighth nerves), while the third most common cause is trauma. Other causes to consider would include parotid tumor.

Careful attention must be paid to whether there is involvement of the sixth nerve, as this may indicate a brainstem etiology.

Physical examination reveals left facial paralysis. The patient cannot wrinkle his brow or close his left eye. The patient's MRI scan is presented (Fig. 3.15).

What are the findings? What is your differential now?

The coronal images show linear enhancement along the superior portion of the left internal auditory canal (arrow), without a focal mass lesion (note that the eighth nerve, just beneath the seventh, is not enhancing on the coronal image). Recall that the internal auditory canal (IAC) is divided into superior and inferior components by a septum known as the crista falciformis, and partially divided into anterior and posterior components by Bill's bar. The seventh nerve, along with the nervus intermedius, runs in the anterior–superior quadrant, while the superior vestibular division of the eighth nerve runs in the posterior–superior quadrant. Since the cochlea is anterior to the vestibule, the cochlear

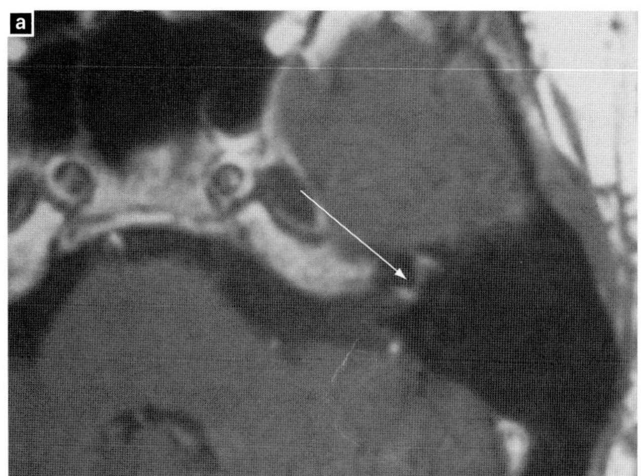
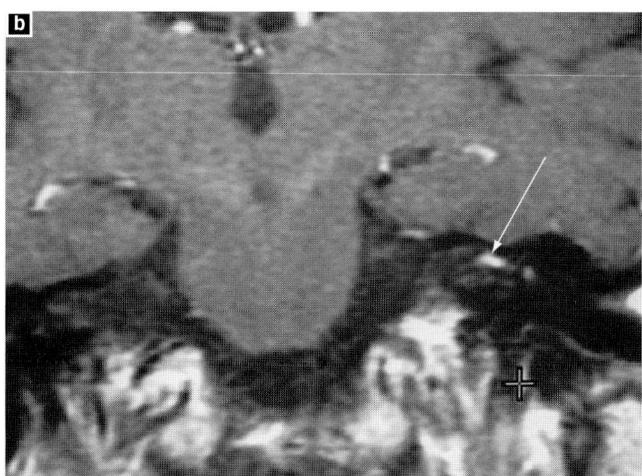

Fig. 3.15. **(a) Axial and (b) coronal T1 weighted post-contrast image.**

division of the eighth nerve resides in the anterior–inferior quadrant, while (you guessed it) the inferior vestibular division of the eighth nerve runs in the posterior–inferior quadrant. The axial image shows curvilinear enhancement along the anterior aspect of the IAC (arrow). The shape, or course, of the enhancement is characteristic for the meatal and then the labyrinthine portion of the seventh nerve as it curves into the geniculate ganglion. Bell's palsy thus remains the leading differential diagnostic possibility.

Imaging note

Enhancement of the facial nerve, *per se*, is not abnormal. In the very early days of MRI, the conventional wisdom was that the normal facial nerve did not enhance. However, as early as 1992, if not earlier, this assumption was overturned. For example, Gebarski *et al.* (1992) showed that 76 percent of clinically normal facial nerves enhanced along some segments, and that the enhancement was asymmetric between the right and left sides in 69 percent of patients. The critical fact, though, is that the cisternal portion (i.e., in the cerebellopontine angle cistern) and the intracanalicular portion (i.e., within the IAC), especially the labyrinthine portion, do not normally enhance. Thus, our patient, with enhancement in the distal intracanalicular (meatal) and labyrinthine segments is definitely abnormal.

Diagnosis

Bell's palsy.

Discuss the functional anatomy and clinical evaluation of the seventh nerve.

The 7th cranial nerve is responsible for the following functions:

(1) Motor innervation to the ipsilateral facial muscles. This is clearly the main function of the facial nerve. There is also motor innervation to the stapedius muscle, and the posterior belly of the digastric. The motor nerve fibers arise from the facial motor nucleus.

(2) Secretomotor functions to the lacrimal gland and the submandibular and sublingual glands for ipsilateral lacrimation and salivation. The parotid glands are innervated by the 9th cranial nerve. These parasympathetic fibers arise from the superior salivatory nucleus.

(3) A minor somatic sensory component, for cutaneous sensory innervation involving the anterior wall of the external auditory canal.

(4) A visceral sensory component, subtending taste to the anterior two-thirds of the ipsilateral tongue. The cell bodies for taste are part of the geniculate ganglion, and synapse in the rostral division of nucleus solitarius.

Basic anatomy of the facial nerve (Figs. 3.16 and 3.17)

Brainstem

The fibers of the facial nerve arise predominantly from the superior and inferior divisions of the motor nucleus in the pons, with additional contributions from the superior salivatory nucleus and the nucleus solitarius (see Fig. 3.10). The motor nucleus is located ventral and lateral to the abducens nucleus. Motor fibers exit this nucleus and course posteromedially, hooking around the abducens nucleus. They are joined by fibers from the superior salivatory nucleus and the nucleus solitarius, which together course ventrolaterally to exit the belly of the pons, lateral to the corticospinal tracts.

The superior division of the motor nucleus, responsible for innervation of the frontalis and orbicularis oculi muscles, receives bilateral cortical innervation from the motor cortices and premotor regions. The contralateral motor strip innervates the lower division of the motor nucleus, controlling the lower facial muscles, with corticobulbar fibers descending through the internal capsule, decussating in the pons, and reaching the contralateral 7th nerve lower motor nucleus.

Therefore, supranuclear lesions affecting the motor cortex or corticobulbar tracts produce a so-called "central" facial nerve palsy, with relative sparing of the upper facial muscles. The palsy will be contralateral to the lesion. However, lesions at the facial nerve nucleus, or distal to this, involving the facial nerve itself, produce a "peripheral" 7th nerve palsy, with involvement of all of the facial muscles, including an inability to furrow the brow, close the eyelid, or raise the eyebrow. The facial paralysis in this case is ipsilateral to the lesion.

Intracranial, outside the brainstem (Fig. 3.17)

After exiting the pons, the 7th nerve courses in the cerebellopontine angle cistern. The large motor root is accompanied by a small nerve, known as the nervus intermedius of Wrisberg, responsible for taste sensation from the anterior two-thirds of the tongue, and the minor somatic cutaneous sensory function from the anterior wall of the external auditory canal. These course in the internal auditory canal, in the anterior–superior component of the canal. In this location, the 7th nerve runs in close proximity to the 8th nerve divisions, which occupy the remaining quadrants of the internal auditory canal. At the distal end of the internal auditory canal, the facial nerve angles anteriorly, in its so-called labyrinthine portion, to the geniculate ganglion, which is the sensory ganglion of the facial nerve. Here, the greater superficial petrosal nerve is given off, which eventually courses to the pterygopalatine ganglion, and innervates the lacrimal gland.

The facial nerve then bends sharply backward in a horizontal bony canal that runs beneath the lateral semicircular canal (the tympanic portion of the facial nerve). It then makes a second sharply downward bend through a bony prominence known as the pyramidal eminence, which is just posterior to the stapes. Here, a small branch is given off to the stapedius muscle, and the facial nerve continues inferiorly through the mastoid process (vertical portion of the facial nerve). Prior to exiting the stylomastoid foramen, it gives off the chorda tympani branch, responsible for taste to the anterior two-thirds of the tongue, as well as innervation of the submandibular and sublingual salivary glands via the submandibular ganglion. The facial nerve then continues inferiorly to exit to the stylomastoid foramen. From the stylomastoid foramen, it runs in the parotid gland, where it divides into five branches, to innervate the facial muscles and posterior belly of the digastric.

Clinical notes

(1) The difference between central and peripheral 7th nerve palsy has been discussed above, and is a crucial distinction in the clinical examination of the facial nerve.

(2) Lesions which affect the facial nerve at or distal to the stylomastoid foramen produce a peripheral 7th nerve palsy affecting the upper and lower facial muscles, but preserving the remaining functions of the 7th nerve.

Lesions of the facial nerve distal to the geniculate ganglion leave lacrimation preserved, but affect taste in the anterior two-thirds of the tongue, as well as the upper and lower facial muscles. If the lesion occurs proximal to the stapedius branch, the patient will also experience hyperacusis (things will sound louder in that ear) because the function of the stapedius muscle is to maintain tension on the stapes footplate. If the stapedius is paralyzed, the excursions of the stapes footplate into the oval window become hyperdynamic, and sounds are perceived as louder on the affected side.

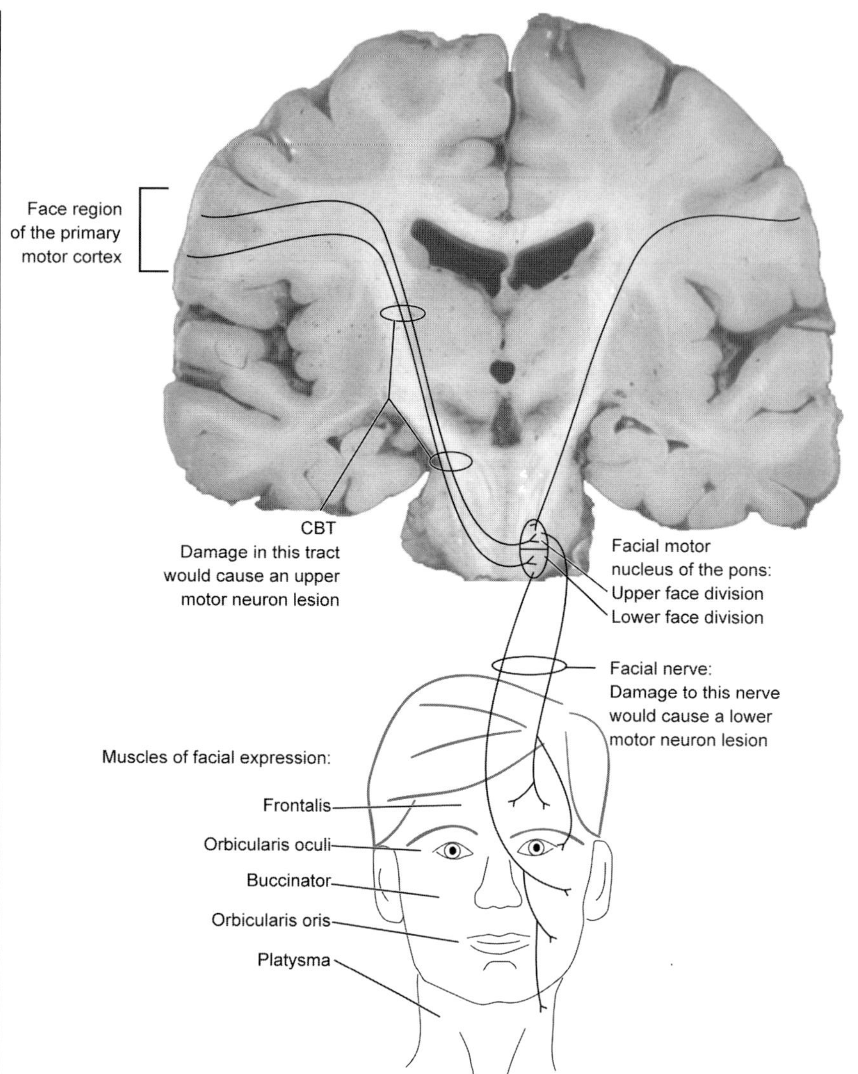

Fig. 3.16. **Cortical innervation of the facial nerve. The upper division of the motor nucleus receives bilateral cortical innervation, while the lower division receives only contralateral innervation.**

(3) These are the "classical" teachings based on the anatomy of the seventh nerve, and are further assessed by so-called topognostic tests to try to pinpoint the location of the lesion along the nerve. Among these tests is the Schirmer test for lacrimation, which involves placing filter paper along the lower conjunctival margins of both eyes and comparing the length of the strip that is wet on the side of the affected facial nerve versus the normal side. A value of less than 25 percent of normal suggests dysfunction of the greater superficial petrosal nerve. Audiologists can also perform a stapedial reflex test. Tension in the tympanic membrane of the affected side is measured after a loud sound is presented to either ear (it can be presented to the contralateral ear if there is concomitant seventh and eighth nerve dysfunction in the abnormal side). If there is appropriate tension, the stapedius branch is intact. This has some prognostic significance, since in Bell's palsy, an intact stapedius reflex indicates that complete recovery can be expected within 6 weeks. It is noted, though, that in Bell's palsy the stapedial reflex is often absent during the first two weeks, and this is not a poor prognostic sign. Taste testing in the anterior two-thirds of the tongue can be done with a swab with sugar or salt. Loss of taste (called dysgeusia) suggests a lesion proximal to the chorda tympani branch.

These topognostic tests, while neat in theory, are not very useful clinically. They are difficult to perform, and are somewhat subjective (except the stapedial reflex, which is probably prognostically useful and is more objective). Also, patients often do not know the relevant neuroanatomy, and therefore present with inconsistent lesions, such as decreased lacrimation, indicating a lesion proximal to the geniculate ganglion, but an intact stapedial reflex, suggesting a lesion distal to the stapedial branch. A useful clinical pearl, however, is that facial palsy which begins as a dysgeusia is usually due to Bell's, and some feel that no further workup is necessary.

Another group of tests to be aware of is the group of electrophysiologic tests. These are used mainly in patients with complete paralysis to help determine their prognosis. The two main tests are the nerve excitability test, and electroneuronography. The nerve excitability test involves placement

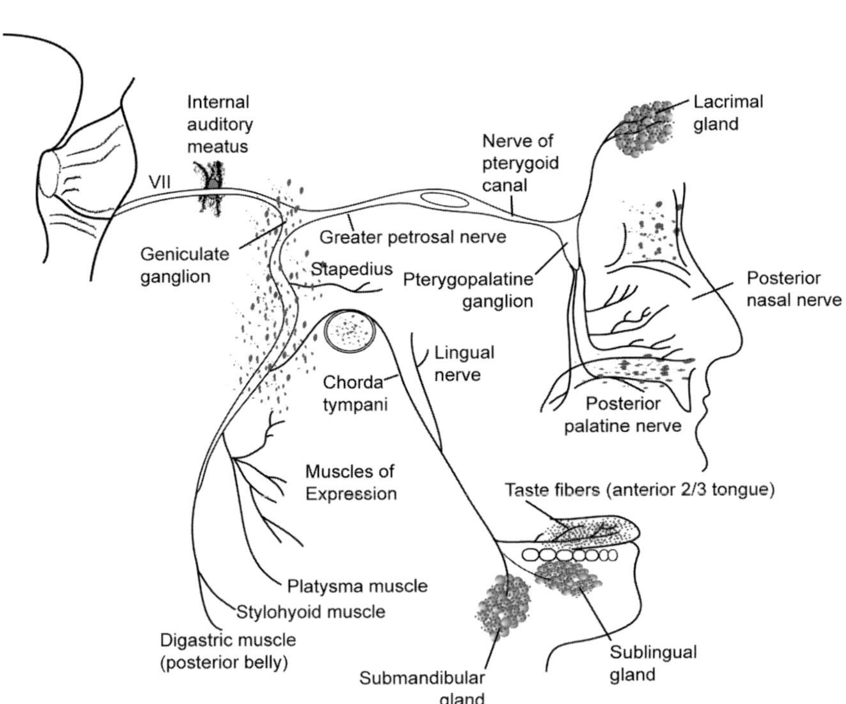

Fig. 3.17. **Anatomic diagram of the extracranial course and functions of the 7th nerve. Lacrimation is mediated through the greater superficial petrosal nerve, the stapedius reflex through the stapedius branch, and taste to the anterior two-thirds of the tongue and salivation in the submandibular gland is mediated through the chorda tympani.**

of a stimulating electrode over the stylomastoid foramen and running a current to produce a twitch on the paralyzed side of the face. The lowest current value that achieves this is labeled the threshold current, and is compared to the normal side. A difference of greater than 3.5 milliamps indicates a poor prognosis. Electroneuronography involves the measurement of evoked potentials after electrically stimulating the facial nerve at the stylomastoid foramen. The amplitude of these potentials is compared on both the paralyzed and the normal sides. If the affected side has an amplitude less than 10 percent of the normal side, this indicates a poor prognosis for recovery. Some ENT surgeons use the 10 percent cutoff to decide on surgical decompression in Bell's palsy. Decompression is otherwise a controversial practice.

(4) After injury or trauma, anomalous regeneration of the facial nerve fibers may produce several unusual manifestations. The best known of these is the "crocodile tears" phenomenon, which occurs when fibers originally destined for the salivary glands innervate instead the lacrimal gland, producing anomalous tearing while eating. Another disorder in the same vein is the "jaw-winking" phenomenon, where jaw movements cause involuntary closure of the eyelid. Also, if fibers originally destined for the orbicularis oculi muscles grow instead into orbicularis oris nerve branches, closure of the eyelids may cause a retraction of the corner of the mouth.

(5) Rare supranuclear lesions may affect the pathway eventually innervating the orbicularis oculi muscles, in a somewhat unclear fashion, leading to a condition known as "apraxia of the eyelids," where the patient loses the ability to voluntarily close the eyelids, although they continue to close reflexively in blinking, and during the corneal reflex.

(6) As stated above, the most common facial nerve lesion is Bell's palsy. This produces a peripheral facial nerve paralysis, often affecting chorda tympani branches as well. Approximately 80–90 percent of cases remit spontaneously. Recent evidence has identified herpes simplex virus genomic sequences in many of these cases, and it is now suggested that herpes simplex viral infection is the etiology of Bell's palsy.

It is noted that there is a significantly higher incidence of Bell's in pregnant females, and in diabetic patients. While this is not a clinical book, Bell's palsy is often treated with oral prednisone in a dose of 60 mg po per day for five days, tapered down by 10 mg per day for another 5 days. Also, given the link to herpes simplex, some suggest that oral acyclovir (400 mg po five times per day) may be useful.

(7) Multiple other lesions, including primary tumors of the facial nerve, such as facial nerve schwannomas, or tumors of the skull base or the parotid gland, traumatic injury, or other infectious etiologies, such as Lyme disease, or infrequently HIV, may also cause peripheral facial nerve lesions. Two illustrative cases are presented in Fig. 3.18. These are images from separate patients both with right seventh nerve palsy, both showing right seventh nerve enhancement. The lesion in the left image is secondary to lymphoma, while that in the right image is secondary to cryptococcal meningitis (note the enhancing meninges along the cerebellar sulci).

One syndrome to be familiar with is the Ramsay Hunt syndrome, most likely secondary to herpes zoster of the geniculate ganglion, spreading to the facial nerve, with vesicles visible on the tympanic membrane. The 8th cranial nerve is also often affected, with associated vertigo and deafness (Fig. 3.19).

This patient had Ramsay Hunt syndrome with vesicles on the tympanic membrane. In contrast to our Bell's palsy patient, you can see that there is enhancement of both the

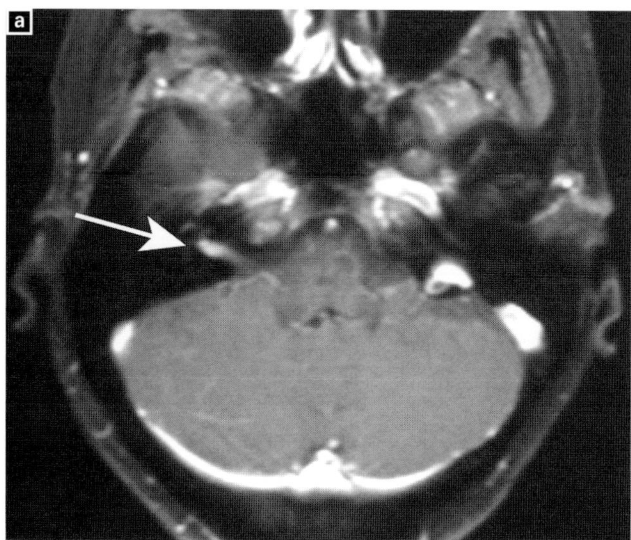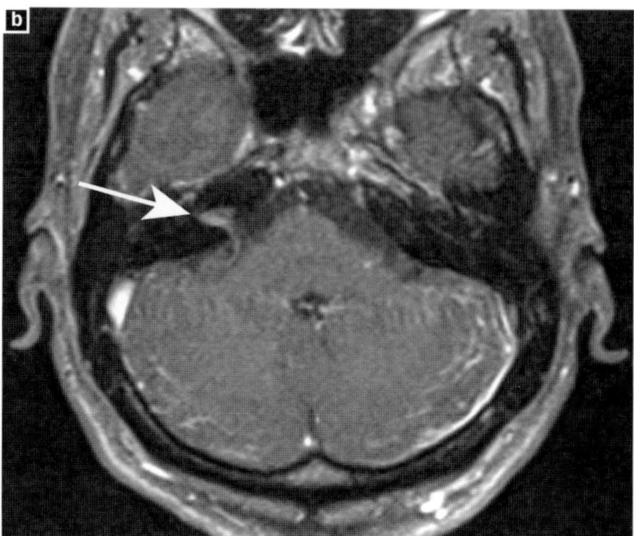

Fig. 3.18. **Axial T1-weighted post-contrast images through the internal auditory canal in two different patients with right facial nerve palsy. (a) Patient with lymphoma. There is abnormal enhancement along the right seventh nerve. (b) Patient with cryptococcal meningitis. There is abnormal enhancement along the right seventh nerve, as well as some leptomeningeal enhancement along the cerebellar sulci.**

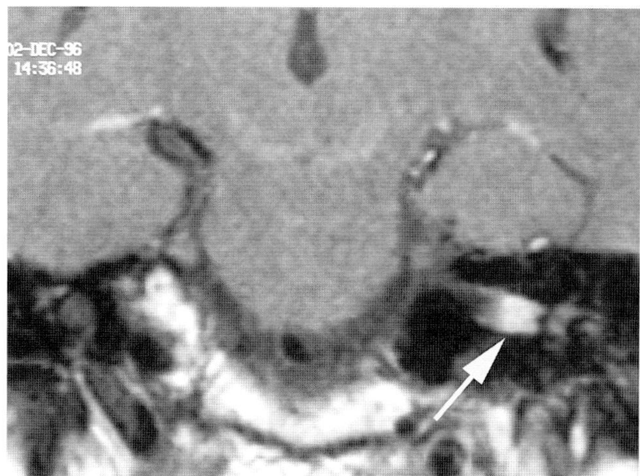
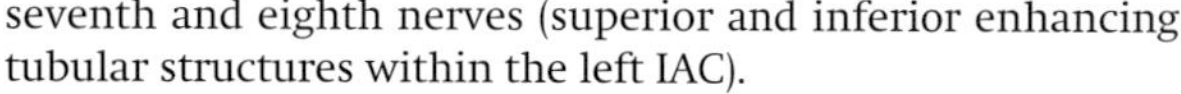

Fig. 3.19. **Coronal T1-weighted post-contrast image in a patient with left-sided Ramsay Hunt syndrome. There is enhancement along both the seventh and eighth nerves within the left internal auditory canal (arrow).**

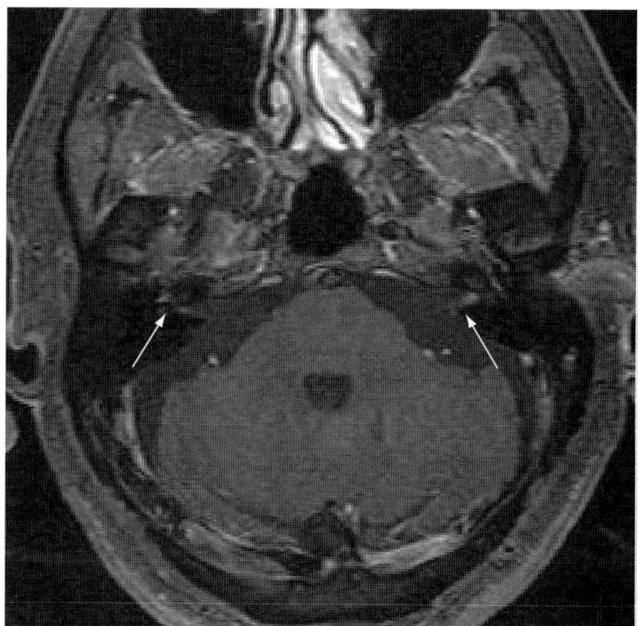

Fig. 3.20. **Axial T1-weighted post-contrast fat-saturation image through the internal auditory canal. There is subtle enhancement of both seventh nerves (arrows) in this patient with simultaneous bilateral Bell's palsy.**

seventh and eighth nerves (superior and inferior enhancing tubular structures within the left IAC).

(8) Bilateral facial weakness, known as facial diplegia, is quite unusual. Most commonly, it is a manifestation of the Guillain–Barré syndrome. It may also occur in the setting of multiple cranial neuropathies, such as with Lyme disease. One other etiology to keep in mind is sarcoidosis. In a small proportion of patients with sarcoidosis, a condition known as uveoparotid fever or Heerfordt syndrome develops, with bilateral facial weakness, but it is quite unusual for this to be simultaneous; facial nerve involvement on one side is often separated by a number of weeks from the other side. Likewise, Bell's palsy may occur bilaterally, but is extremely unusual simultaneously (Fig. 3.20).

Finally, to leave you with a zebra for gamesmanship in rounds, we mention the Melkersson–Rosenthal syndrome, consisting of a triad of recurrent facial paralysis, labial edema, and plication of the tongue.

Reference

Gebarski, S. S., Telian, S. A., and Niparko, J. K. Enhancement along the normal facial nerve in the facial canal: MR imaging and anatomic correlation. *Radiology* 1992; **183**: 391–394.

Case 3.4

44-year-old female presents with sudden onset left-sided hearing loss.

What are the two main types of hearing loss? What bedside testing can you do to help differentiate them?

This harkens back to physical diagnosis class. The first test is Weber's test, where a tuning fork is placed in the midline on the patient's forehead (remember to strike the tuning fork first to get it vibrating, otherwise nothing will happen!). Our patient hears the sound louder in the right ear. What does this mean? It indicates that either there is a conductive hearing loss in the right ear, or a sensorineural hearing loss in the left ear. We have a bit of a clue in that the patient came in saying, "I can't hear out of my left ear." That, however, should not distract us from the task at hand. The next test is the Rinne test, where the vibrating tuning fork is placed against the mastoid tip to test bone conduction and then close to the ear to test air conduction. If the patient hears better through bone than through air, this indicates a conductive hearing loss. In our patient, after the sound disappeared with the fork against the mastoid tip, she could still hear it when the fork was quickly moved next to the ear; hence, this suggests air better than bone conduction, and a left ear sensorineural hearing loss. A lesser-known test is Bing's test. In Bing's test, the vibrating fork is placed on the mastoid tip, and the examiner alternately places and removes his or her hand on the external ear to occlude it. If the patient hears a difference, this indicates normal function or a sensorineural hearing loss; if no difference is noted, it suggests a conductive loss. Our patient heard a difference with ear occlusion. Finally, we have the Schwabach's test. This requires normal hearing on the part of the examiner (eh?), since the patient will be compared to the examiner. Bone conduction is tested. If the patient hears the sound longer than the examiner, this suggests a conductive hearing loss; if the patient stops hearing the sound before the examiner, this suggests sensorineural hearing loss.

You are now convinced that there is a left sensorineural hearing loss.

What cranial nerve might be involved?

The cochlear division of the eighth cranial nerve conducts auditory impulses to the brain.

Rather than thinking too much about the differential now (after all, that's ENT's job), we obtain an MRI (Fig. 3.21).

What are the findings? What is your diagnosis?

There is an enhancing mass in the left internal auditory canal (arrow).

Diagnosis

Vestibular schwannoma. Most of these tumors arise from the superior vestibular division of the eighth nerve (therefore, the term "acoustic neuroma" is really a misnomer). Paradoxically, they tend to present with hearing loss. Counterintuitively, about 15 percent of vestibular schwannomas present with sudden onset rather than gradual hearing loss, presumably secondary to hemorrhage within the tumor.

It is noted that vestibular schwannomas may present even smaller than this case, as purely intracanalicular lesions (see Fig. 3.22). Vestibular schwannomas account for 90 percent of purely intracanalicular lesions. However, they are purely intracanicular only about 10 percent of the time. Usually, they also have a cisternal portion, and grow like an ice-cream cone into the cerebellopontine angle cistern, as in the MRI shown in Fig. 3.23.

For neuroradiologists, it is important to remember that 10–20 percent of vestibular schwannomas may present only as a mass in the cerebellopontine angle cistern, without the "cone" part which extends into the internal auditory canal. Also, the appearance may be difficult to distinguish from the next most common cerebellopontine angle mass, the meningioma (Fig. 3.24).

Several helpful distinguishing features are illustrated by the accompanying MRI. First, meningiomas don't usually extend into the internal auditory canal, but most schwannomas do, as mentioned above. Meningiomas are usually not epicentered precisely over the porous acousticus (the opening to the IAC), whereas vestibular schwannomas are. Meningiomas tend to have "dural tails," a very uncommon feature with schwannomas. Also, meningiomas tend to be broad-based to the dura, with obtuse angles to the dural margin, while schwannomas tend to have acute angles to the dura. Finally, about 10 percent of schwannomas have associated cyst formation, a very rare feature in meningiomas.

Describe the functional anatomy of the eighth nerve.

The eighth cranial nerve is made up of two components. The cochlear nerve, which subserves hearing, and the vestibular nerve, in charge of equilibrium and spatial orientation.

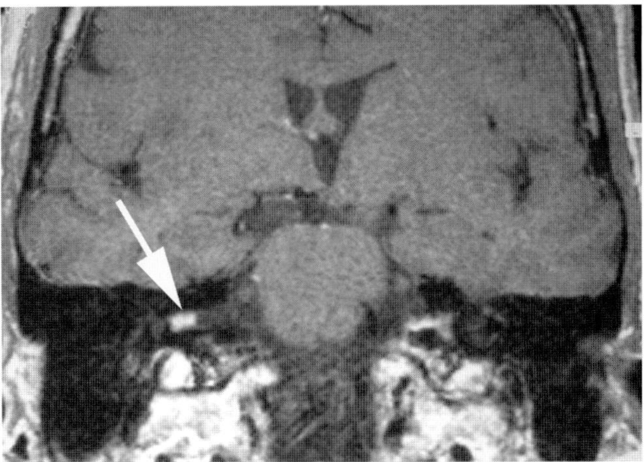

Fig. 3.21. **Axial post-contrast T1-weighted image through the level of the lower pons.**

Fig. 3.22. **Coronal post-contrast T1-weighted image of the internal auditory canals showing a small, enhancing right intracanalicular schwannoma (arrow).**

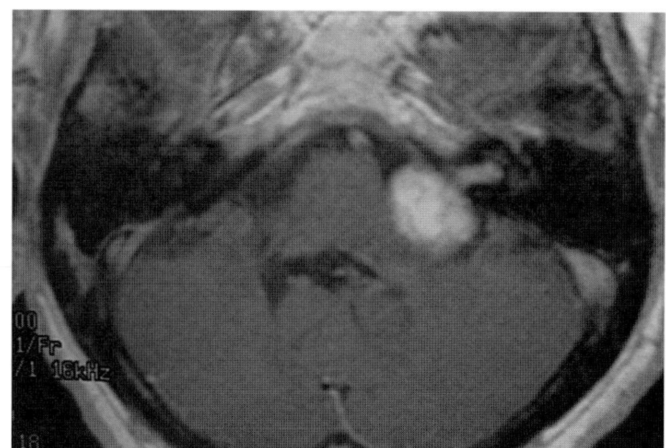

Fig. 3.23. **Axial post-contrast T1 weighted image of the internal auditory canals showing a large "ice-cream cone" vestibular schwannoma extending from the left internal auditory canal (IAC) into the cerebellopontine angle cistern. Notice enhancement within the left IAC.**

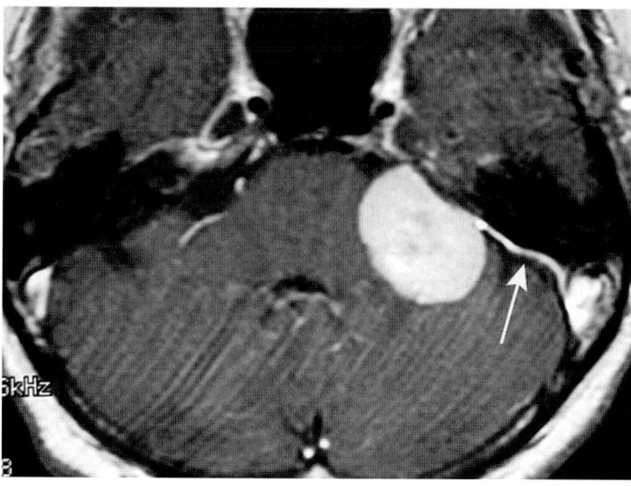

Fig. 3.24. **Axial post-contrast T1-weighted image showing a large enhancing meningioma in the left cerebellopontine angle cistern. Note that the mass is epicentered slightly above the IAC, has a broad base to the dura, and displays an enhancing "dural tail" sign (arrow).**

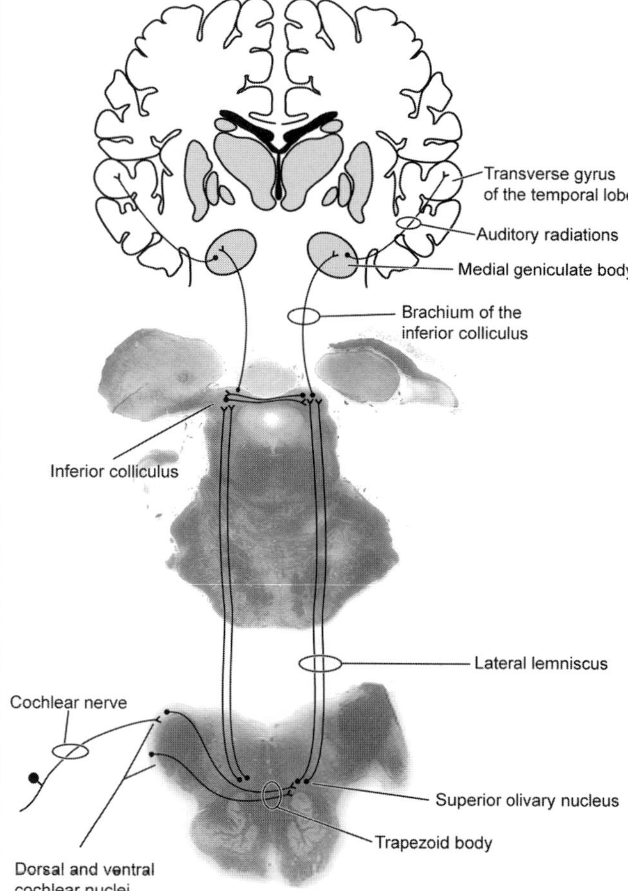

Fig. 3.25. **Anatomy of the auditory pathway. Note that most auditory fibers decussate in the trapezoid body and ascend in the contralateral lateral lemniscus.**

Cochlear division

This division has its cell bodies in the spiral ganglion, housed in the cochlea. The peripheral processes of these neurons connect with the hair cells of the organ of Corti. The central processes enter the pons, and synapse on the ventral and dorsal cochlear nuclei. From there, most of the pathway decussates in the tegmentum of the caudal pons, an anterior division going through the trapezoid body and posterior divisions running through the intermediate and dorsal auditory stria. Most of these fibers collect in the lateral lemniscus, along the posterolateral tegmentum. A few fibers from the cochlea do not decussate, and travel in the ipsilateral lateral lemniscus. From the trapezoid body, there are also efferents to and afferents from the superior olivary nuclei (bilateral connections) that are involved in sound localization. In the lateral lemniscus, fibers ascend to the inferior colliculus, and from there, to the medial geniculate body of the thalamus, and then to Heschel's gyrus, the primary auditory cortex region within the superior temporal gyrus. See Fig. 3.25.

Clinical correlates:

– Lesions in the cochlea or cochlear division of the eighth nerve can produce complete ipsilateral deafness. The MRI below shows a rare case of left cochlear enhancement on coronal and axial images in a case of viral cochleitis (Fig. 3.26).

  If you see a similar appearance, with a bright cochlea but on the precontrast T1-weighted images, think of another rare diagnosis: intracochlear hemorrhage!

  It is possible, but uncommon, for brainstem lesions which affect the cochlear nuclei to also produce ipsilateral deafness. However, such lesions are usually so large as to affect many more brainstem structures, leading to profound deficits to the point that testing hearing may become difficult.

– Proximal (more central) to the cochlear nuclei, lesions do not produce complete deafness. Most of the fibers from the cochlea ascend in the contralateral lateral lemniscus, which also includes a small number of fibers from the ipsilateral ear. Therefore a lesion in the proximal lateral lemniscus would cause contralateral greater than ipsilateral hearing loss (Fig. 3.27).

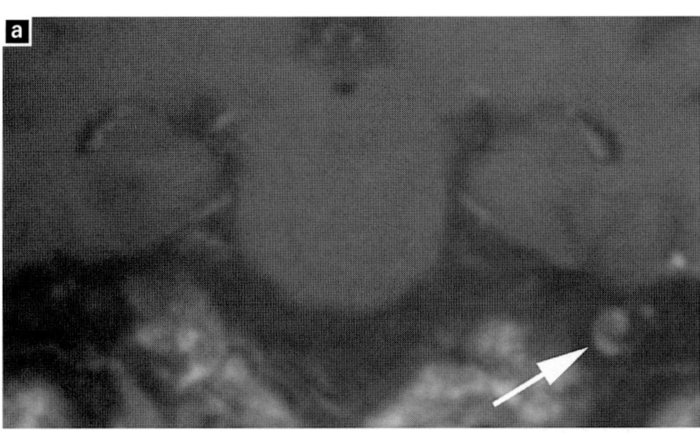 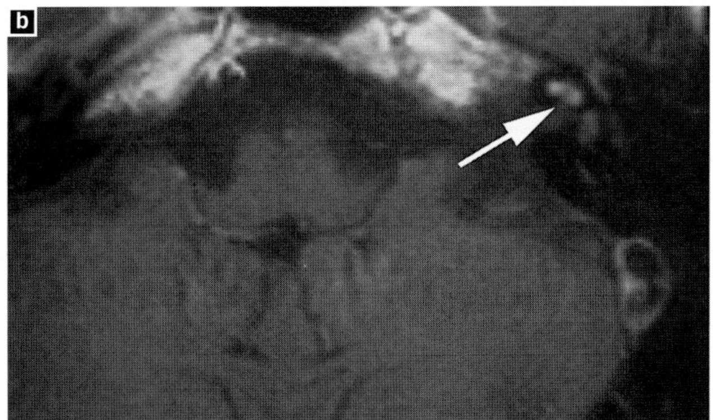

Fig. 3.26. **(a) Coronal and (b) axial post-contrast T1-weighted images show enhancement of the left cochlea (arrows) in this patient with viral cochleitis and complete left-sided deafness.**

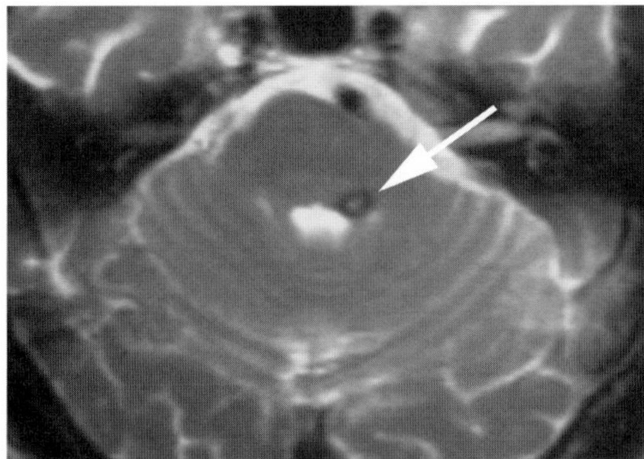

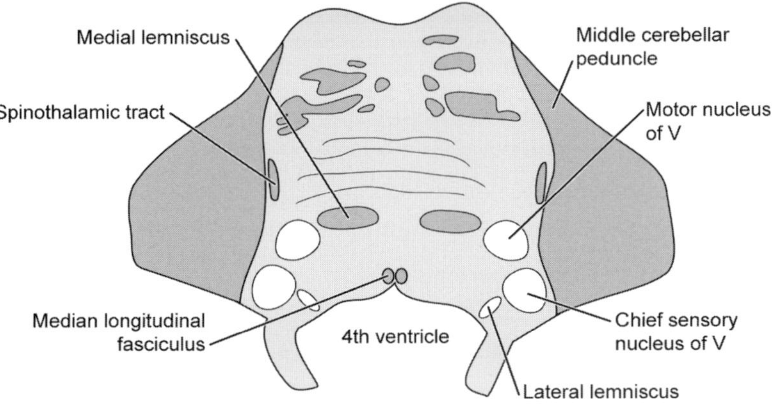

Fig. 3.27. **T2-weighted axial image shows a small hemosiderin ring in the left lateral pontine tegmentum, just anterior to the superior cerebellar peduncle (arrow). This is in the region of the left lateral lemniscus. This patient presented with a 4-month history of sudden onset right greater than left hearing loss. The provisional diagnosis was a small bleed, now chronic, probably from a cavernous hemangioma in the region of the left lateral lemniscus.**

Beyond this level, the pathway divides multiple times for essentially complete bilateral innervation. The nucleus of the lateral lemniscus projects to both inferior colliculi, which also communicate with each other (Fig. 3.25). The brachium of the inferior colliculus connects the inferior colliculus with the medial geniculate body of the thalamus, but now with fibers coming from both ears because of the multiple connections which have crossed the midline. Therefore, each auditory cortex receives fibers from both ears,

and so cortical lesions do not, in general, produce deafness. Multiple descending parts of the auditory pathway, in charge of such things as modulating the response of the organ of Corti, connecting the colliculi with the spinal cord (tectospinal tracts) to subserve the startle reflex, etc., have been omitted from the above simplified discussion.

– Non-conductive hearing loss is usually called "sensorineural" hearing loss, which includes lesions affecting the cochlea, as well as those affecting the eighth nerve and beyond. As stated above, the vast majority of such lesions will involve either the cochlea or the cochlear division of the eighth nerve, with the brainstem being involved only rarely.

- It is possible, with careful clinical testing, to separate lesions of the cochlea from lesions of the cochlear division of the eighth nerve. Clinically, cochlear hearing loss may manifest the symptoms of *recruitment* and *diplacusis*. Recruitment refers to a heightened perception of the loudness of sounds once the amplitude becomes high enough to cross the threshold of the hearing deficit. Diplacusis is a disturbed or impaired frequency discrimination, such that it is difficult to make out the words being said, although the sound is audible, or such that music sounds "out of tune."
- Some clinically relevant points in the assessment of hearing loss are presented below.
  (a) The phenomenon of recruitment can be tested specifically, and if the hearing loss is "recruiting," i.e., the deficit in the bad ear becomes less as the amplitude of the sound increases, this suggests a cochlear lesion.
  (b) A related phenomenon is that of "auditory adaptation" or "tone decay." With nerve lesions, if a tone is presented above the level of threshold and maintained, it appears to the patient to gradually decrease in loudness (auditory adaptation). With cochlear lesions, this does not happen.
  (c) Brainstem auditory evoked potentials (BAEP). This procedure uses scalp electrodes to record electrical activity following stimulation by sound. It typically produces seven "waves" in succession, each thought to correspond to a sequential relay station or integral structure in the auditory pathway (cochlear nerve, cochlear nuclei, superior olivary nuclei, lateral lemniscus, inferior colliculus, medial geniculate body, and auditory radiations, with the last two in this list being uncertain). The loss or increased latency of wave I indicates a lesion of the cochlear nerve (increased latency means a delayed appearance of the wave). Latencies between waves I and III, and waves III and V, are the most commonly assessed variables. Increased latencies are often present in multiple sclerosis, even without symptomatic hearing loss.
- Occasionally, pontine lesions have been associated with complex auditory hallucinations, known as "pontine auditory hallucinosis." Additional causes of auditory hallucinations include damage to the superior temporal auditory association areas, schizophrenia, temporal lobe epilepsy and superior olivary nucleus damage.
- Hearing loss may be caused by very loud sounds, drugs such as aminoglycosides, furosemide, high dose aspirin, or as a sequela of measles vaccination, mycoplasma pneumoniae infection, or meningitis (bacterial, fungal, tuberculous, or lymphomatous). Sudden onset unilateral hearing loss without vertigo may be secondary to vascular causes (emboli to the cochlear division of the auditory artery, a branch of the anterior inferior cerebellar artery), and when it is episodic, is often secondary to Menière's disease.
- Sudden onset of bilateral hearing loss has been described after CABG surgery, again possibly vascular in etiology, and rarely following general anesthesia for other causes.
- Vestibular schwannomas, and other tumors of the cerebellopontine angle cistern (CPA), may cause hearing loss due to direct mass effect on the cochlear nerve. Most CPA lesions (about 75 percent) are, in fact, vestibular schwannomas, while about 10 percent are meningiomas, 5 percent are epidermoids, and the rest due to miscellaneous causes.
- A rare cause of hearing loss is so-called central deafness (as distinguished from sensorineural hearing loss). One subtype of central deafness is "pure word" deafness. The patient has fluent verbal output, but very impaired comprehension. The patient can correctly identify non-verbal sounds (e.g., the ring of a telephone). This deficit usually occurs after an infarct, in the recovery phase from a Wernicke's aphasia. It is thought to be secondary to disconnection of the dominant (usually left) Heschels' gyrus from the medial geniculate and from the callosal fibers form the contralateral Heschels' gyrus as well. Another unusual syndrome is that of auditory agnosia. Here, verbal comprehension is preserved, but non-verbal sounds, like the ringing of a telephone, are no longer understood. This may occur with right hemisphere lesions alone. A variant of auditory agnosia is amusia, a selective inability to perceive music; this is thought to result from right temporal lobe lesions. Finally, there is the extremely rare cortical deafness syndrome, thought to result from emboli to both Heschel's gyri. This presents as both pure word deafness and auditory agnosia. The patient can hear sounds (e.g., a preserved startle reflex), but cannot recognize verbal or meaningful non-verbal sounds.
- There are several types of inner ear aplasia described, leading to absence or malformations of the cochlea. The most severe is Michel's anomaly (complete cochlear aplasia) and the best known is probably the Mondini malformation (incomplete development of the cochlea, with less than the normal 2 and 1/2 turns). Scheibe defect is a disorder affecting the cochlea and the saccule, with atrophy of the vestibular and cochlear nerves.
- There are numerous syndromes of congenital and early onset deafness, most of which are autosomal recessive, but some of which are autosomal dominant. An important advance in understanding in this field was the discovery of a gene known as the connexin-26 gene on chromosome 13, found in about half the cases of syndromic autosomal recessive congenital deafness, and about a third of the cases of sporadic congenital deafness. The connexin protein is a component of gap junctions, and mutations therein may interfere with potassium recycling from the hair cells of the organ of Corti to the endolymph. Another important advance has been the discovery of the cause of Pendred syndrome, an inherited disorder that accounts for as much as 10 percent of hereditary deafness. Patients usually also suffer from thyroid goiter. The disordered gene causing this syndrome was identified at NIH in 1997, and is called the PDS gene, located on chromosome 7. The normal gene makes a protein, called pendrin, that is found only in the thyroid, and appears to function in sulfate transport.

Vestibular division

The vestibular portion of the 8th nerve is divided into superior and inferior vestibular divisions, which occupy the posterior portion of the internal auditory canal, in the superior and inferior quadrants respectively, separated from the anterior compartment by Bill's bar, and separated from each other by the crista falciformis. The cell bodies of the vestibular division are in Scarpa's ganglion, which is located in the internal auditory meatus. This ganglion is composed of bipolar cells. The peripheral branches terminate in the labyrinth, composed of the lateral, superior, and posterior semicircular canals, and the utricle and saccule (Fig. 3.28).

Within the labyrinth there are hair cells covered by an otolithic membrane within the utricle and saccule, as well as specialized sensory epithelium in the lateral semicircular canals. The semicircular canals convey angular rotation, while the otoliths convey linear acceleration.

The central fibers run in the internal auditory canal, and enter the posterolateral medulla to synapse on the four vestibular nuclei, the superior, lateral, medial, and inferior or spinal (Fig. 3.29).

The vestibular nuclei are connected to the flocculonodular lobe of the cerebellum and the deep fastigial cerebellar nucleus. These

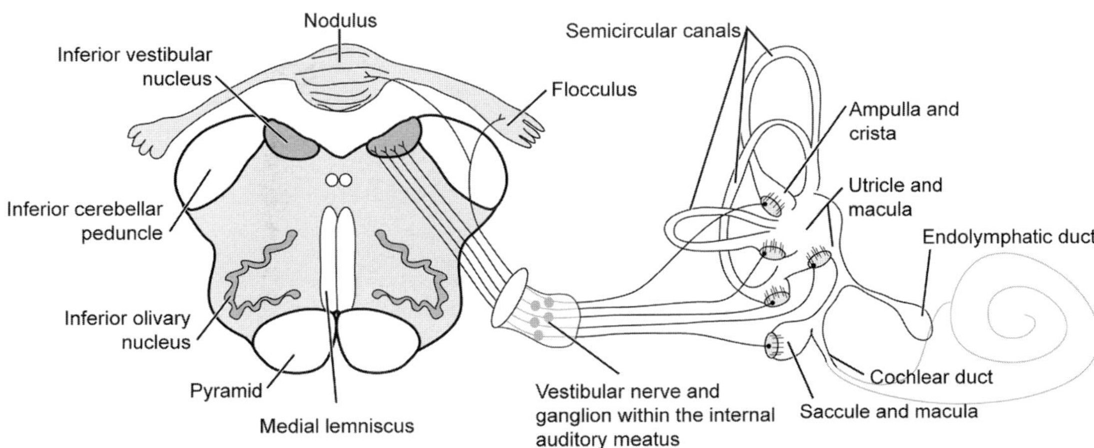

Fig. 3.28. **Anatomy of the vestibular system. Bipolar cells in Scarpa's ganglion project to the semicircular canals and to the utricle and saccule, and relay inputs to the vestibular nuclei in the brainstem and to the flocculonodular lobe of the cerebellum.**

connections are bilateral. In addition, some fibers connect with the paramedian pontine reticular formation and the abducens nucleus to control conjugate gaze. Some fibers from the semicircular canals also project directly onto the cerebellar flocculonodular lobe. Efferent fibers from the flocculonodular cerebellar cortex project ipsilaterally to the vestibular nuclei. The connections to and from the cerebellum take place predominantly via the juxtarestiform body (inferior cerebellar peduncle). Therefore, each side of the cerebellum communicates with both vestibular nuclei. Likewise, the vestibular nuclei communicate with the bilateral extraocular muscles. The vestibular nuclei also project onto the spinal cord via the uncrossed lateral vestibulo spinal tract, and the predominantly crossed but also partly uncrossed medial vestibulo spinal tract, with the axial muscles being acted upon predominantly by the medial vestibulo spinal tract and the limb muscles predominantly by the lateral vestibulo spinal tract.

Disorders of the vestibular system usually manifest as vertigo. True vertigo, with a sensation of the patient moving, or the environment moving, including a sensation of pulsion to one side, should be distinguished from pseudovertigo or dizziness. The labyrinthine system may be tested using irrigation of the ear canal with warm and cold water, known as caloric testing (Fig. 3.30).

In a normal person, when the ear is irrigated with cold water, there is nystagmus to the opposite side. For reference, when the term "nystagmus" is used, the sidedness refers to the fast component (saccade) of the nystagmus. Therefore, cold water irrigation of the left ear in a normal person will produce a horizontal nystagmus with the fast beat of the nystagmus toward the right. Warm water induces nystagmus toward the irrigated side. Therefore, caloric testing allows determination of the integrity of the labyrinthine apparatus on each side, as well as the connection between the abducens and the oculomotor nucleus. Let us discuss cold water calorics and brainstem testing (see Fig. 3.30). As the patient becomes lethargic, the fast component of the nystagmus becomes less pronounced. With stupor or obtundation (cortical depression but intact brainstem), the eyes will slowly deviate toward the side of irrigation, and remain deviated. With coma (brainstem dysfunction), the eyes do not move at all (see Fig. 3.30). You can use this test to tell if someone is truly comatose, or just faking coma because you are boring them with all of this neuroanatomy!

Now, let us briefly discuss the main causes of vertigo. An important category of vertigo is vertigo secondary to labyrinthine disease, such as Menière's disease, benign positional vertigo, and possibly viral labyrinthitis. A second category is that of vertigo caused by vestibular nerve lesions. A third category is vertigo of brainstem origin, and a fourth category is vertigo caused by cerebellar lesions, especially median lesions in the inferior posterior inferior cerebellar artery territory. Remember these four main categories of causes: labyrinthine, vestibular nerve, brainstem, and cerebellum.

Clinical notes

We'll present quite a few notes here, since vertigo is such a ubiquitous complaint.

(1) In labyrinthine disease, there is usually unidirectional nystagmus, horizontal in type, typically with a rotatory component. The direction of the nystagmus is opposite of the affected labyrinth. However, falling and past-pointing are to the side of the involved ear, so the fast direction of the nystagmus is opposite to the direction of falling.

(2) With cerebellar as well as brainstem infarcts, there is often bidirectional nystagmus, which is usually more prominent on the side of the infarct, rather than away from it. Falling is usually to the side of the lesion as well, so the falling and the predominant direction of the nystagmus tend to be toward the same side.

(3) In attempting to separate central from labyrinthine causes of nystagmus, the following clinical guidelines sum up the above: with vertigo of central origin, the nystagmus is often horizontal bidirectional, but may be vertical or rotatory, and is often worsened by attempted visual fixation. Nystagmus of labyrinthine origin is usually unidirectional, horizontal with a rotatory component, and is lessened or inhibited by visual fixation.

(4) Purely vertical nystagmus indicates a lesion in the brainstem rather than in the labyrinth. Downbeat nystagmus has been described in paramedian lesions of the craniocervical junction, while upbeat nystagmus may occur in lesions adjacent to the perihypoglossal nuclei, or in the pontomesencephalic tegmentum.

(5) Menière's disease is characterized by episodic paroxysmal attacks of vertigo. It is unusual for the disease to occur without associated tinnitus and deafness. Therefore, isolated vertigo is an unusual presentation. However, there is isolated episodic deafness without vertigo in Menière's disease, known as cochlear Menière's syndrome.

(6) With brainstem or cerebellar lesions, there is usually no deficit in hearing, as the vestibular and cochlear pathways diverge in the brainstem. However, labyrinthine lesions,

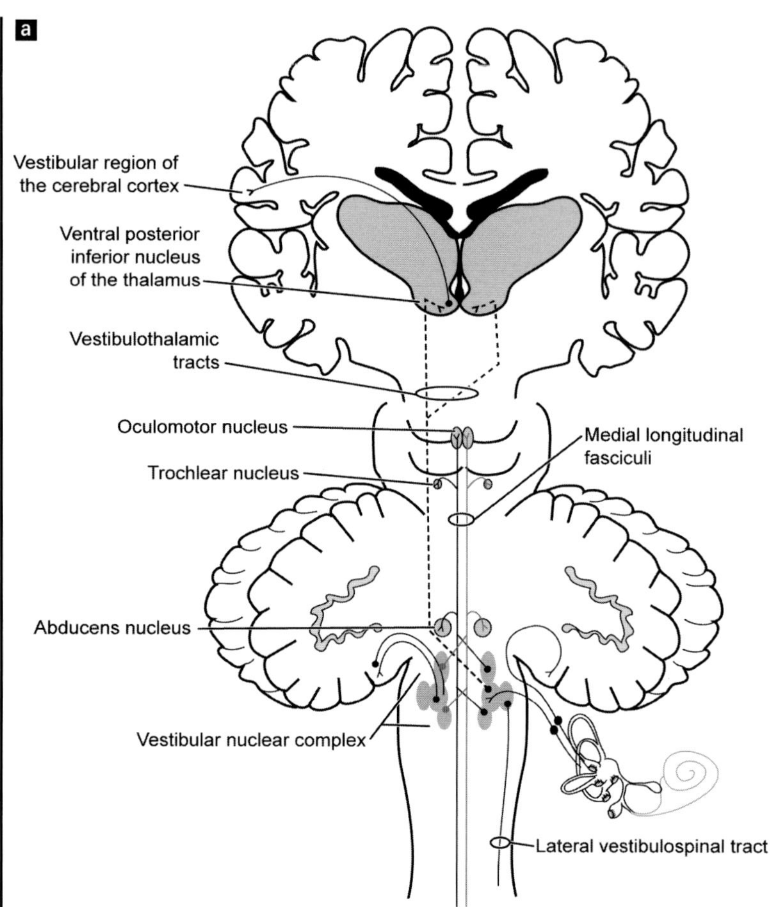

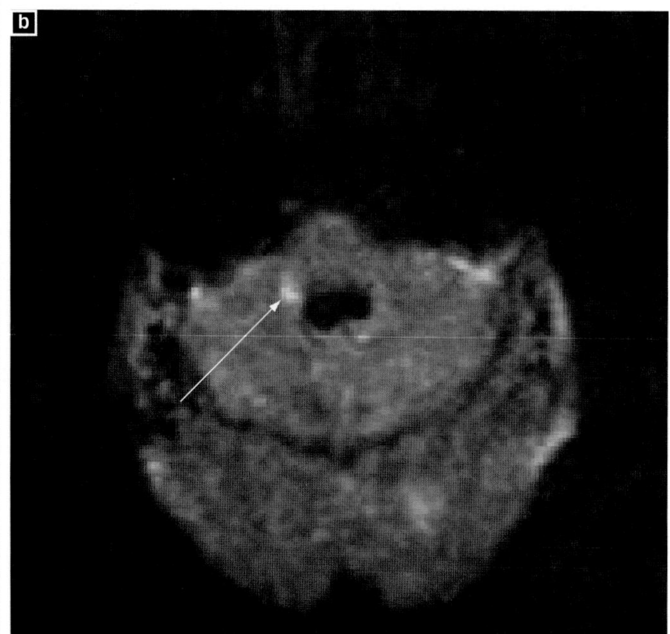

Fig. 3.29. **(a) Schematic illustration of the central connections of the vestibular nuclei. Vestibular nuclei give inputs to the ascending MLF and extra-ocular muscles to help coordinate ocular tracking as well as vestibulo-ocular reflexes. The vestibular nuclei also project to the anterior horn cells of the spinal cord via vestibulospinal tracts to mediate postural reflexes and help coordinate gait and limb motion. (b) Poor-quality axial DWI image in a patient who presented with acute vertigo and bidirectional nystagmus, more prominent to the right. There is a small infarct in the right brainstem tegmentum at the pontomedullary junction in the location of the right vestibular nuclei (arrow).**

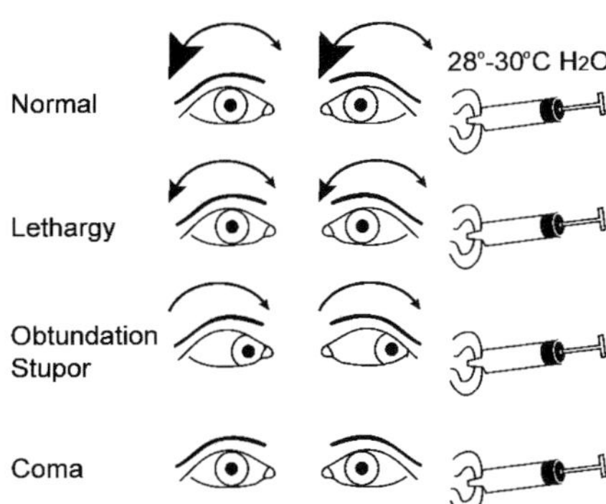

Fig. 3.30. **Schematic illustrating cold water calorics in testing the vestibular apparatus and brainstem. The large arrow indicates the direction of the fast phase of the nystagmus. With cortical depression but an intact brainstem (obtundation/stupor), the fast phase of nystagmus is lost, and the eyes slowly deviate toward the irrigated ear and remain there.**

such as Menière's disease, or vestibular nerve lesions, such as vestibular schwannoma, or Ramsay Hunt syndrome, often involve hearing as well.

(7) With cerebellar and brainstem infarcts, falling to one side or experiencing a horizontal nystagmus may be present just like with vestibular lesions. However, the presence of limb ataxia, dysarthria, or other cranial nerve involvement (except the seventh nerve), such as involvement of the nucleus ambiguous, will help to distinguish central lesions from vestibular nerve or labyrinthine lesions.

(8) Benign positional vertigo is characterized by paroxysmal vertigo that occurs with changes in head position. There is usually some latency of onset with rapid change in head position, a reversal of the direction of nystagmus (upbeat versus downbeat on lying down or sitting up), and fatigability of the nystagmus with repetition of the head movements to elicit the nystagmus. Diagnostic maneuvers to elicit the vertigo in benign positional vertigo include laying the patient down quickly with the head hanging over the edge of the examining table, and then rotating the head. This is known as the Dix–Hallpike maneuver.

(9) Other types of vertigo may consist of a single severe sudden-onset attack, without auditory involvement, but with ablation of labyrinthine function to one side, which does not recover. This may be secondary to occlusion of the labyrinthine division of the internal auditory artery, and labyrinthine hemorrhage has been reported by MRI in a few of these patients.

Case 3.5

55-year-old hypertensive male presents with a sudden onset of a right sixth nerve palsy, mild right facial weakness and left body hemiplegia. Clinical examination determines that the seventh nerve palsy is "peripheral." In other words, the patient could not wrinkle his brow, indicating that both the upper and lower motor divisions are damaged.

Where would you locate the lesion?

As a general rule, crossed lesions, with facial involvement on one side and body involvement on the other, imply that the

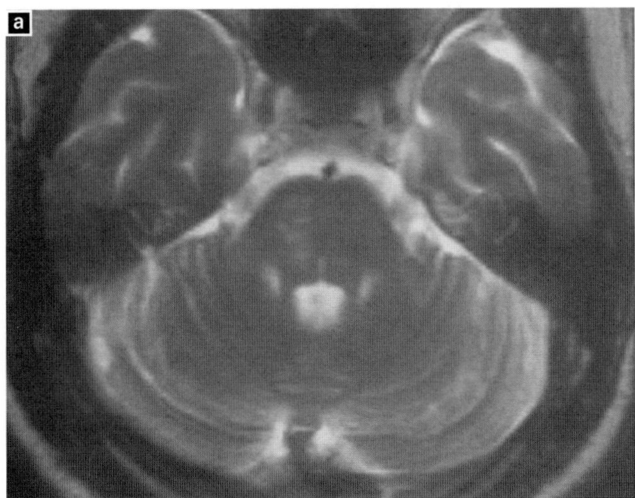

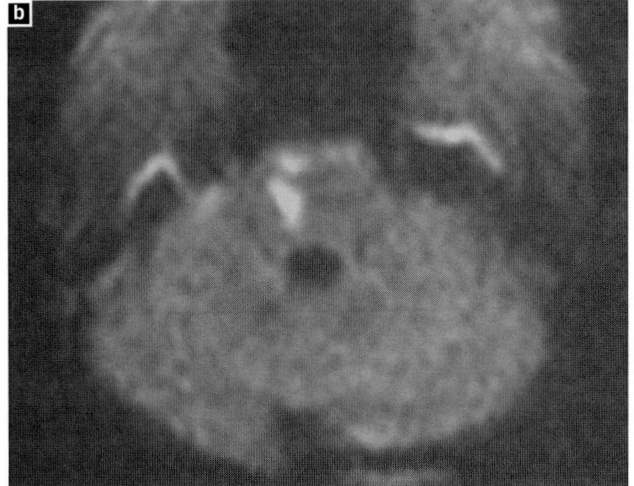

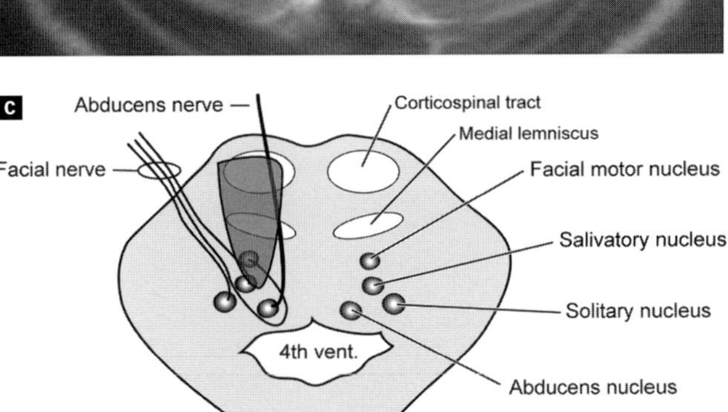

Fig. 3.31. **(a) T2-weighted axial image, with very subtle wedge-shaped T2 hyperintensity in the right aspect of the belly of the pons. (b) Diffusion weighted image demonstrating abnormal hyperintensity in the same zone, consistent with a subacute infarct. (c) Anatomic diagram of the pons illustrating the structures involved by the infarct.**

lesion is in the brainstem. In this case, we need a lesion that would involve the right seventh nerve, the right sixth nerve but not the nucleus (no lateral gaze palsy), and the right corticospinal tract. These considerations would locate the lesion in the caudal basis pontis.

MRI images are provided (Fig. 3.31A–B). What are the findings? What is your diagnosis?

There is a subacute infarct in the right aspect of the belly of the pons, extending posterolaterally enough to catch the seventh nerve fascicles, medially enough to involve the sixth nerve fascicles, and anteriorly enough to involve the right corticospinal tract.

Diagnosis

Millard–Gubler syndrome.

This syndrome, described by Millard and Gubler in the 1850s, is characterized by ipsilateral (to the lesion) facial nerve palsy and contralateral body weakness. It may also include a sixth nerve palsy. This syndrome is also known as the caudal basal pontine syndrome. While usually considered a vascular syndrome, any appropriately located lesion in the pons can produce the syndrome. This is illustrated by the case presented in Fig. 3.32.

If the belly of the pons (basis pontis) lesion occurs more rostrally, the patient might have ipsilateral fifth nerve (both sensory and motor) deficits, and contralateral hemiparesis (Fig. 3.33). This is called the "rostral basal pontine syndrome." Thankfully, it does not have an eponym!

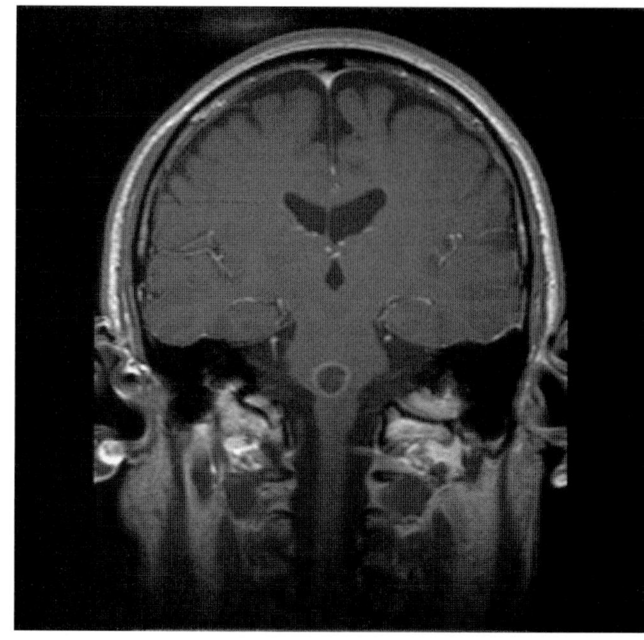

Fig. 3.32. **Coronal T1-weighted post-contrast image shows a ring-enhancing metastatic lesion in the right caudal basis pontis in this patient with a Millard–Gubler syndrome. This 57-year-old male presented with progressive right sixth nerve palsy, mild peripheral right seventh nerve findings, and left body weakness.**

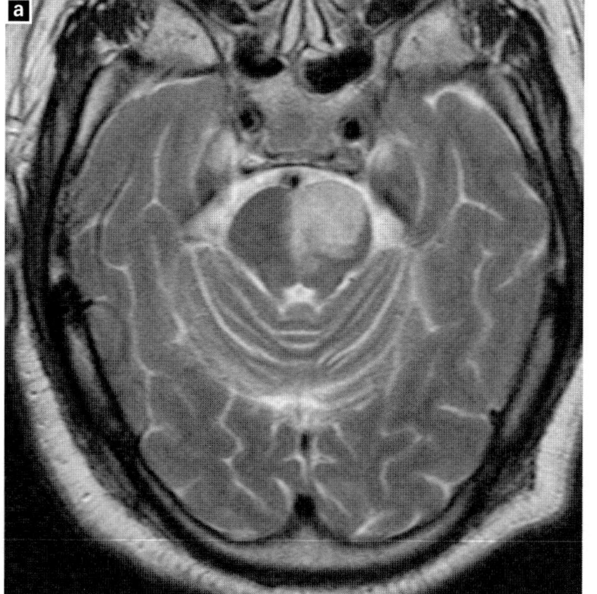

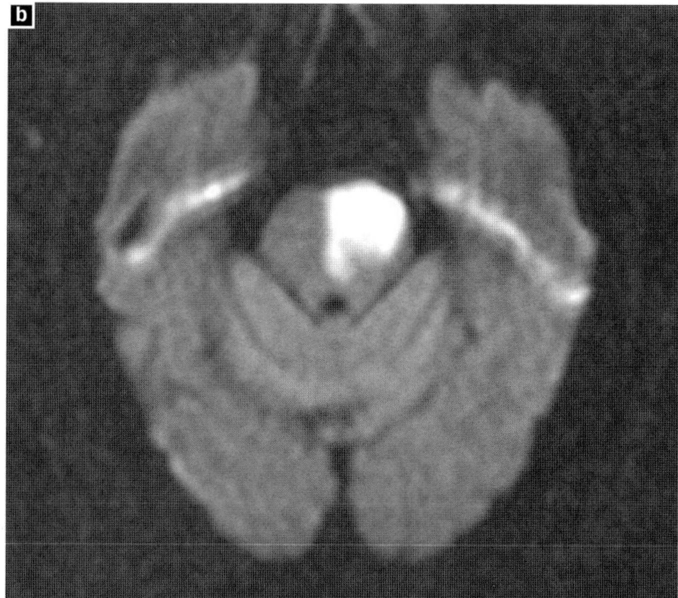

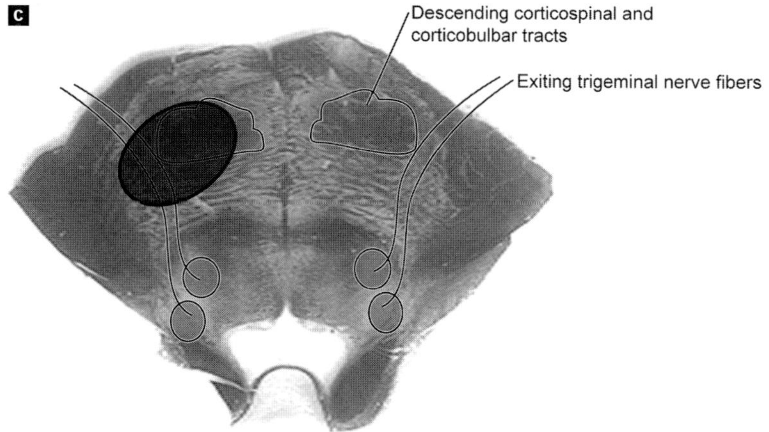

Fig. 3.33. **(a) Axial T2 image and (b) DWI image showing a large left rostral pontine infarct in this patient with left fifth nerve motor and sensory deficits as well as dense right-sided hemiparesis. (c) Anatomic diagram showing the structures involved in producing the rostral basal pontine syndrome.**

Case 3.6

49-year-old diabetic hypertensive male who presented with right hand "clumsiness" and significant dysarthria.

Look at the accompanying MRI (Fig. 3.34). What are the findings? What is your diagnosis?

Diagnosis: *Based on the description, we would say the patient has a "dysarthria–clumsy hand" syndrome (or DCHS).*

This is a lacunar stroke syndrome that usually manifests with loss of fine motor control and mild weakness of the hand contralateral to the stroke as well as an often profound dysarthria. An additional component may be an upper motor neuron or central facial weakness also contralateral to the lesion. The classic description of the culprit is a lacunar infarct in the belly of the pons, at the junction of the rostral one-third and the caudal two-thirds. The same syndrome may be seen with infarcts in the posterior limb of the internal capsule. A recent paper (Arboix *et al.*, 2004) finds that DCHS accounts for about 1.6 percent of acute strokes and about 6 percent of lacunar strokes. Defying the classical descriptions, this paper finds that internal capsule strokes are a more common cause of DCHS than basis pontis infarcts.

Two other related stroke syndromes of the basis pontis (as opposed to the pontine tegmentum) are described below.

Pure motor hemiparesis

This is secondary to involvement of the corticospinal tract in the basis pontis with contralateral upper motor neuron weakness.

Ataxic hemiparesis

This syndrome is classically described as presenting with contralateral body weakness more pronounced in the lower extremity, with an accompanying ataxia. This is due to involvement of both the corticospinal tract (which is broken up into

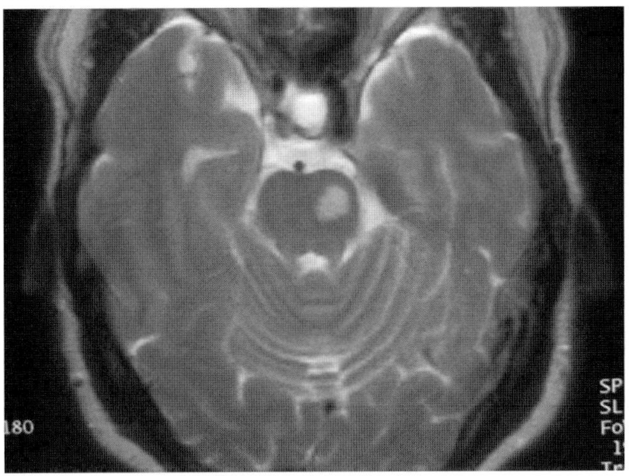

Fig. 3.34. **T2-weighted axial image shows a subacute infarct in the left basis pontis (DWI image, not shown, was markedly hyperintense in this region).**

multiple fascicles within the pons, which rejoin in the medullary pyramid) and the corticocerebellar fibers running through the basis pontis.

References

Arboix, A., Bell, Y., Garcia-Eroles, L. *et al.* Clinical study of 35 patients with dysarthria-clumsy hand syndrome. *Journal of Neurology Neurosurgery and Psychiatry* 2004; **75**: 231–234.

Case 3.7

67-year-old patient who over 1 day developed quadraparesis, facial muscle weakness, aphonia (inability to speak), and loss of lateral gaze. However, the patient was conscious, and would respond to questions with vertical movement of his eyes, which were preserved.

Look at the accompanying MRI images (Fig. 3.35). What are the findings? What is your diagnosis?

There are large bilateral lesions in the belly of the pons on the T2-weighted axial image, consistent with infarcts. The circle of Willis MRA gives a frontal view of both internal carotids. Anything missing? If you said the basilar artery (which in this projection will be seen in the midline between the ICAs), you are correct. Notice that there is no flow void in the basilar on the T2 axial image.

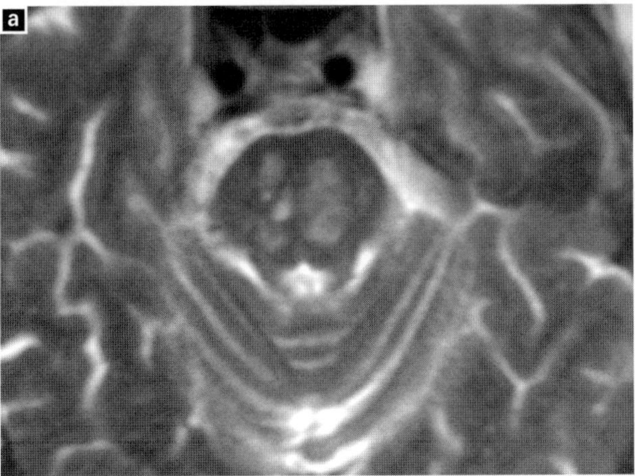
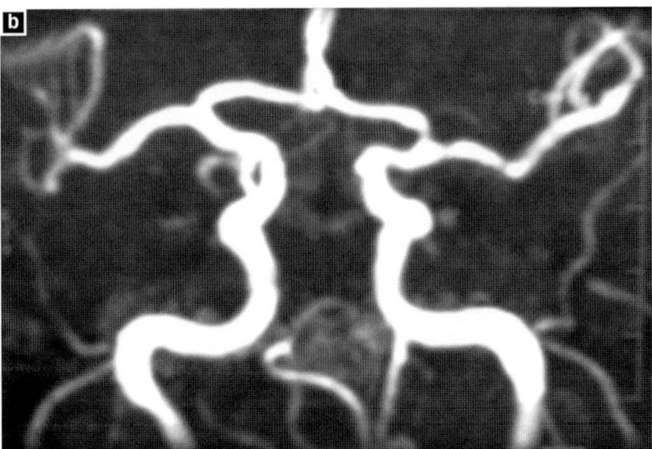

Fig. 3.35. **(a) T2-weighted axial MRI image through the pons. (b) Time-of-flight MR angiogram through the circle of Willis. See text for findings.**

Diagnosis

The "locked-in" syndrome.

This syndrome occurs secondary to severe infarcts in the basis pontis to both sides of midline. The paralysis of motor activity in the body occurs secondary to the interruption of the corticospinal tracts, while aphonia is secondary to loss of the corticobulbar fibers going to the tenth nerves (the tenth nerve controls the larynx, as you remember). The patient is conscious, because the reticular formation in the pontine tegmentum is spared. Vertical gaze is spared because the vertical gaze centers are in the midbrain. Lateral gaze is lost presumably due to interruption of the fibers from the frontal eye fields to the paramedian pontine reticular formation (PPRF) adjacent to the sixth nerve nuclei, which coordinates lateral gaze.

Case 3.8

64-year-old male presents with right body hemiplegia, left peripheral (lower motor neuron) facial nerve palsy and left conjugate gaze palsy.

Where do you think the lesion is?

Based on crossed body and face findings, we immediately localize the lesion to the brainstem. We know that the sixth you are now confused, because that means you remember the description of Millard–Gubler syndrome, which seems identical. In fact, according to some authors, the syndromes are synonymous. However, there is a subtle difference. Millard–Gubler is a syndrome of the belly of the pons, involving the sixth nerve fibers, and producing a sixth nerve palsy, where the ipsilateral

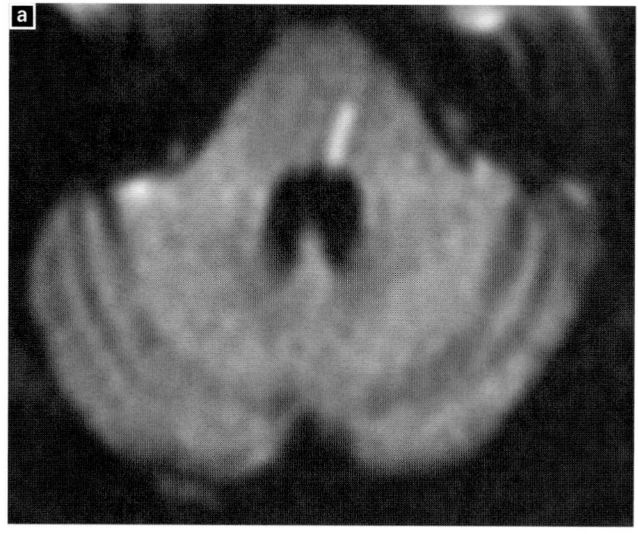

Fig. 3.36. **(a), (b) Two contiguous DWI images through the caudal pons.**

and seventh nerves run close to each other, and that a conjugate gaze palsy (as opposed to a sixth nerve palsy which involves the sixth nerve fascicles) needs to involve the sixth nerve nucleus/ PPRF. Therefore, we need a lesion in the pontine tegmentum, medial enough to involve the sixth nerve nucleus and PPRF. It can also, therefore, involve the seventh nerve as it wraps around the sixth nerve nucleus, giving a peripheral facial palsy. The lesion also needs to extend anteriorly enough to involve some of the fascicles of the corticospinal tract.

Look at the MRI scans (Fig. 3.36). What are the findings? What is your diagnosis?

Two contiguous DWI images show an infarct in the caudal pons, involving the pontine tegmentum and extending anteriorly into the belly of the pons at the level of the pontomedullary junction.

Diagnosis

Raymond–Foville syndrome.

This is the syndrome described above. It is caused by a lesion (often an infarct) of the pontine tegmentum, causing ipsilateral (to the lesion) peripheral facial nerve palsy and conjugate gaze palsy, as well as contralateral body hemiplegia. Hopefully,

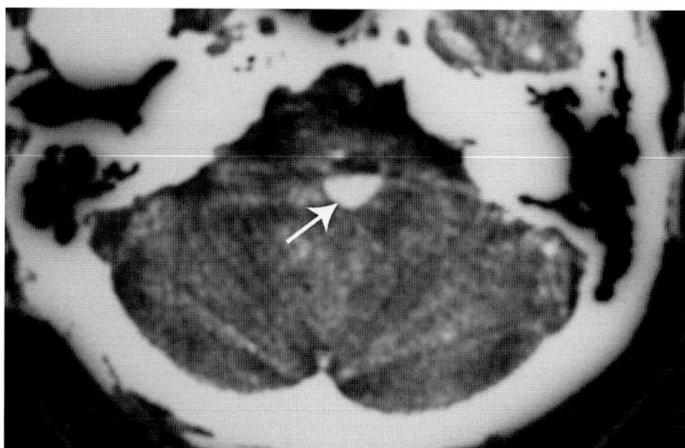

Fig. 3.37. **Axial non-contrast CT shows a hemorrhage with a blood–fluid level involving the left pontine tegmentum and the basis pontis (arrow) in this patient with a Raymond–Foville syndrome. The blood–fluid level represents red cells that have settled to the bottom and plasma on top. Why not just a round clot? Because the patient has just been thrombolyzed.**

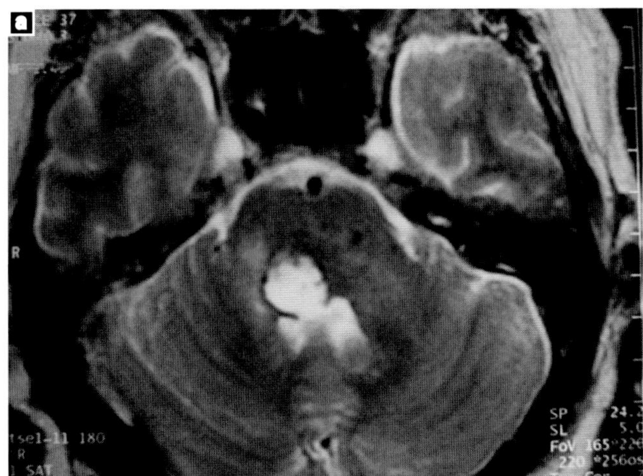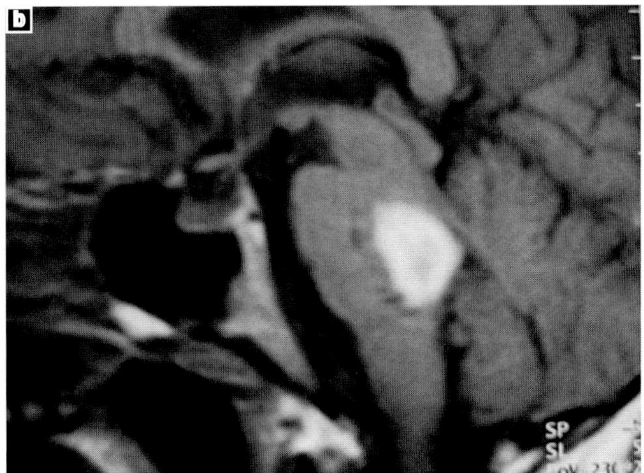

Fig. 3.38. **(a) T2-weighted axial and (b) T1-weighted sagittal images show a subacute hemorrhage in the right caudal pons involving the pontine tegmentum and the basis pontis in this patient with a right-sided Raymond–Foville syndrome. The bleed is bright on T1 and T2, indicating blood in the extracellular methemoglobin phase.**

eye will not abduct with lateral gaze. However, Raymond–Foville is a syndrome of the pontine tegmentum, involving the sixth nerve nucleus and the PPRF, therefore producing an ipsilateral conjugate or lateral gaze palsy, wherein the ipsilateral eye does not abduct and the contralateral eye does not adduct.

Some authors claim that the classical pontine syndromes, such as Raymond–Foville, do not really exist. However, please also look at the two cases below.

(1) A 60-year-old male received intravenous TPA for an acute myocardial infarction. Shortly thereafter, he developed a left-sided Raymond–Foville syndrome (see Fig. 3.37).
(2) In a similar case, a 55-year-old hypertensive male presented with a Raymond–Foville syndrome after a brainstem bleed affecting the caudal tegmentum (Fig. 3.38).

If you had not heard of Raymond–Foville syndrome before, you can now honestly say that you've seen case after case after case!

Case 3.9

56-year-old diabetic hypertensive male who presented complaining of left body numbness. Sensory testing revealed generalized left body decrease in pinprick and temperature sensation. Proprioception and vibration appeared intact.

Where would you localize the lesion?

That's a hard one. The symptoms and signs point to the spinothalamic tract somewhere along its course, from the medulla through the midbrain, or possibly a thalamic lesion. A cortical lesion in the sensory strip would be unlikely, because the leg sensory area is parasagittal in the anterior cerebral artery territory, while the arm area is over the convexity, in the middle cerebral artery territory, and all sensory modalities project to it.

Which side of the brain should the lesion be on?

The findings are left body, and so the lesion should be on the right, since the spinothalamic fibers decussate in the cord, one or two levels above or below their entry point, as previously mentioned. By the time we reach the medulla, the tract is already crossed.

Look at the MRI images (Fig. 3.39). What are the findings? What is your diagnosis?

The T2-weighted image shows a small infarct in the right pontine tegmentum, at the level of the superior cerebellar peduncles. The infarct is similar in location to the lesion we have already encountered in Case 2 (see Fig. 3.9), which involved the MLF. However, carefully comparing, we see that the epicenter of this lesion, while still in the pontine tegmentum, is slightly anterior and lateral to the prior MLF lesion. It turns out that this is the location of the spinothalamic tract (Fig. 3.39(b)).

There is no syndrome name here, just the neuroanatomy! However, so as not to disappoint you, we point out a few related syndromes of the pontine tegmentum.

(1) Raymond–Chenais–Cestan syndrome, or the rostral tegmental pontine syndrome. This is a more rostral version of Raymond–Foville, involving the pontine tegmentum and extending to the basis pontis. The structures in the pontine tegmentum that are involved are the MLF, leading to internuclear ophthalmoplegia, and the spinothalamic tract and the medial lemniscus, leading to contralateral hemisensory loss. Involvement of corticopontine fibers leads to an ipsilateral ataxia, while involvement of the corticospinal tract fascicles leads to a contralateral hemiparesis.
(2) Marie–Foix syndrome, or extreme lateral pontine tegmental syndrome. This is very similar to the above, except that the lesion is more lateral in the tegmentum, so that the MLF and the medial lemniscus are not involved. The spinothalamic tract may be involved if the lesion extends medially enough. Thus, the manifestations are an ipsilateral cerebellar ataxia from the interruption of fibers that are going to enter the brachium pontis (middle cerebellar peduncle), and a contralateral hemiparesis secondary to involvement of the corticospinal tract, plus–minus a contralateral pain and temperature sensory deficit secondary to involvement of the spinothalamic tract (Fig. 3.40).
(3) There have been descriptions of a rare syndrome known as the "dorsolateral tegmental pontine syndrome," which involves an infarct of the pontine tegmentum in the region of the spinothalamic tract, coupled with a contralateral infarct involving the posterolateral medulla, in the region of the medullary portion of the spinothalamic tract. This produces a syndrome of sensory loss over the whole body to pain and temperature, but with preservation of vibration and proprioception. There is usually some component of ataxia as well, due to interruption of corticocerebellar fibers.

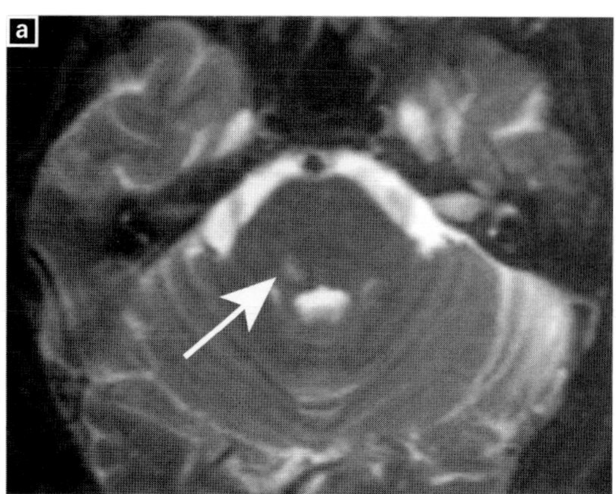

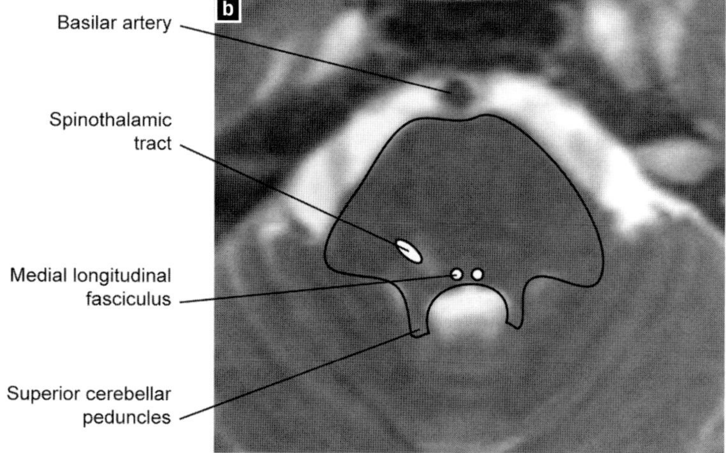

Fig. 3.39. **(a) Axial T2-weighted image shows a small T2 hyperintense lesion, consistent with a small infarct, in the right pontine tegmentum. (b) The accompanying diagram shows the relevant neuroanatomic structures in the region.**

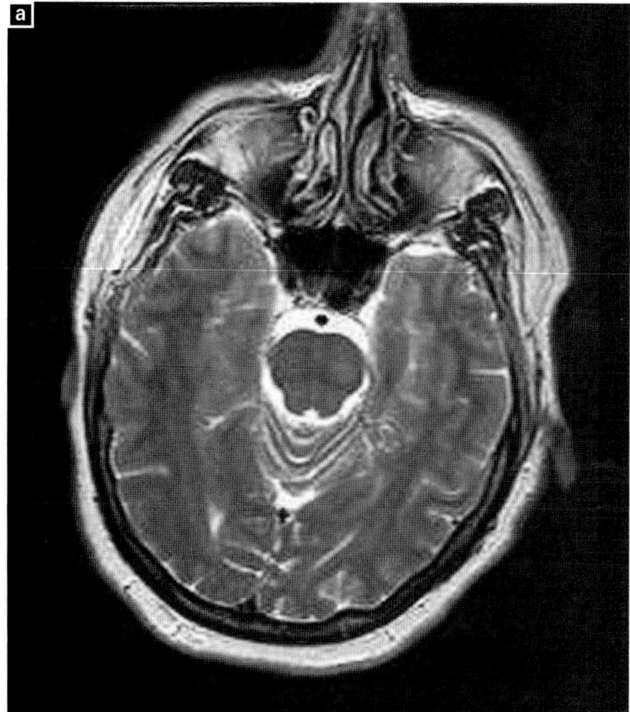

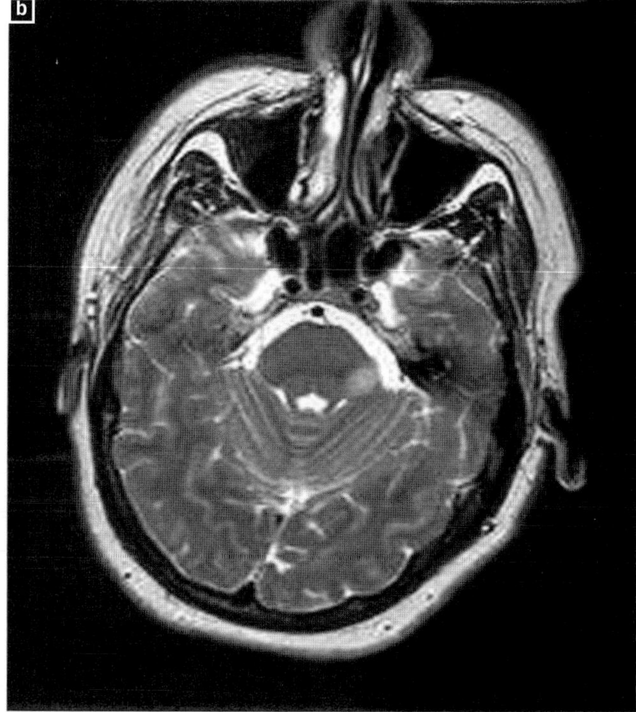

Fig. 3.40. **(a), (b) Contiguous T2-weighted axial images showing an unusual infarct in the far lateral left pontine tegmentum and lateral basis pontis in this patient with left-sided cerebellar ataxia, right-sided weakness, and right-sided pain and temperature sensory loss – components of the Marie–Foix syndrome. There was no evidence of INO or loss of vibration-proprioception sense.**

Case 3.10

52-year-old malnourished alcoholic patient presents with hypo-natremia. The patient was found unresponsive. Brainstem testing showed no response to cold calorics.

What is your differential? Look at the MRI scan (Fig. 3.41)? What are the findings, and what is your diagnosis?

This sounds like a classic case of "central pontine myelinoly-sis," a condition of osmotic demyelination usually affecting the pons and classically associated with over-rapid correction of hyponatremia. The MRI examination shows diffuse abnormal T2 weighted hyperintensity involving the belly of the pons. Looks like a slam dunk diagnosis!

Diagnosis

Massive pontine infarct.

Unfortunately, if you've ever watched an NBA game, even the pros sometimes miss slam dunks. Before we proceed, please look at the MRI below (Fig. 3.42) on a similar patient with a history of alcohol abuse and hyponatremia with an Na of 102 mEq/L. The

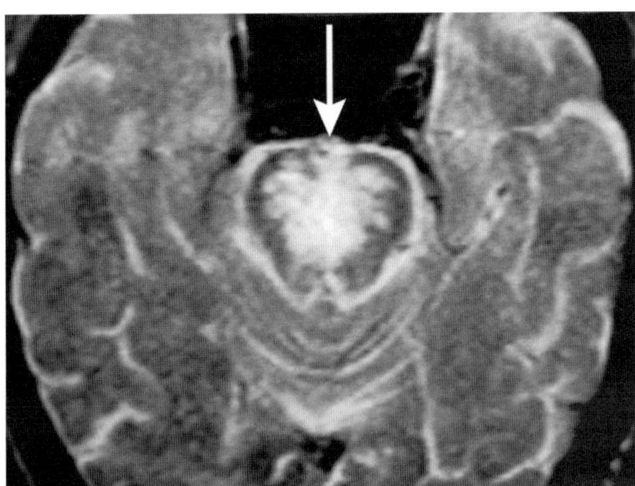

Fig. 3.41. **T2-weighted axial image through the pons. See text.**

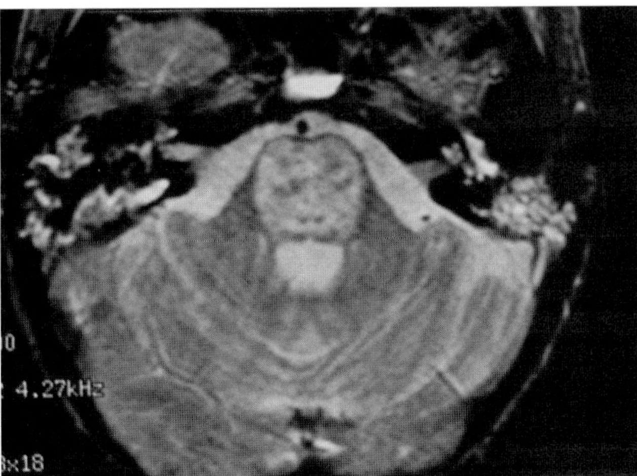

Fig. 3.42. **Axial T2-weighted images shows diffuse, sharply marginated hyperintensity in the belly of the pons, with a thin spared outer rim as well as central "owl eyes." This appearance is classic for central pontine myelinolysis.**

patient's Na was corrected to 135 mEq/L in the first 24 hours. Over the course of the next 3 days, the patient became dysarthric and then unresponsive.

This (Fig. 3.42) is a case of central pontine myelinolysis (CPM). Now let us compare the two cases. What does the second case have that the first does not? Answer: a basilar artery flow void! In Fig. 3.41, the arrow indicates the missing basilar artery flow void (see also Fig. 3.35). The first case (Fig. 3.41) has "rough" edges to the hyperintensity in the belly of the pons. In the second case (Fig. 3.42), the hyperintensity on T2 is sharply marginated with a thin spared outer rim along the belly of the pons. Also, centrally, there are dots, or "owl eyes" of T2 isointensity appearing dark within the bright belly of the pons. These represent relative sparing of the corticospinal tracts. These are the classic findings of central pontine myelinolysis. Just to show you how classic these findings are, another case of CPM is shown. This patient (Fig. 3.43) was markedly hyponatremic in the setting of liver fail-ure. The hyponatremia was corrected too rapidly, and the patient became unresponsive.

What is the cause of central pontine myelinolysis (CPM)?

The answer here is unclear. Initially, around 1980, investigators suggested that CPM was caused by over-rapid correction of hypo-natremia, and this has been the conventional wisdom, passed on from father to son. However, more recent work seems to suggest that the situation is more complex. Some have suggested that it is not due to too rapid a correction, but to delay in starting therapy, which may lead to respiratory insufficiency. Others have sug-gested that it is secondary to overcorrection of hyponatremia beyond normal levels. Still others have linked it to correction of Na levels by more than 25 mEq/L in a 24–48 hour period. For reference, a review in the *Annals of Internal Medicine* suggests that correction rates should not exceed 10 mEq/L in 24 hours (see Laureno *et al.*, 1997).

Reference

Laureno, R. and Karp, B. I. Myelinolysis after correction of hyponatremia. *Annals of Internal Medicine* 1997; **126**: 57–62.

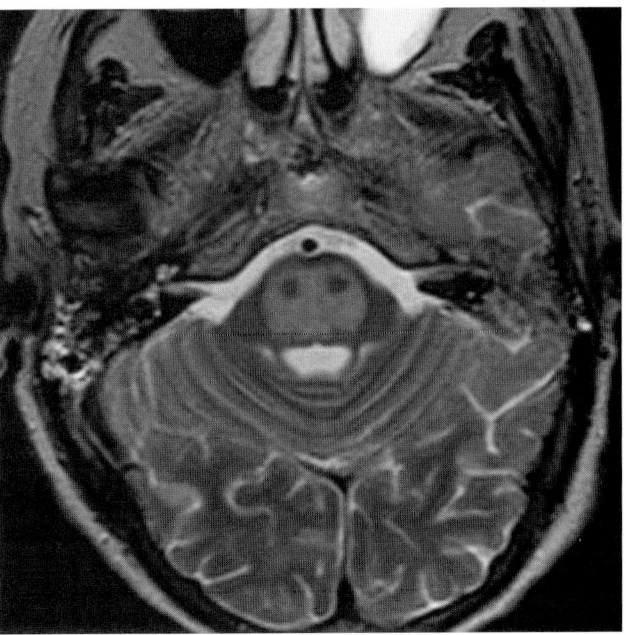

Fig. 3.43. **Axial T2-weighted image showing the classic findings of CPM discussed in the text.**

Summary and conclusions

Let us briefly recap the pontine syndromes we have seen and talked about thus far.

Syndromes of the basis pontis

Millard–Gubler
Rostral basal pontine syndrome
Pure motor hemiparesis
Ataxic hemiparesis
Dysarthria–Clumsy Hand syndrome
Locked-in syndrome

Syndromes of the pontine tegmentum

Raymond–Foville syndrome
Raymond–Chenais–Cestan syndrome
Marie–Foix syndrome

Despite the neat compartmentalization of pontine syndromes shown in the above cases and text, it is time for us to state that real life is often not so neatly compartmentalized. There are several reasons for this.

The original classical descriptions of the pontine syndromes by Millard, Gubler, Raymond, Foville, Cestan and others occurred in the mid 1800s to the early 1900s, when knowledge of functional neuroanatomy was just beginning to approach its current complexity. For example, the existence of such structures as the medial longitudinal fasciculus was only being hypothesized when Raymond and Cestan were making their original descriptions.

While today much of the pontine pathology we see is related to strokes, the original descriptions were usually due to tuberculomas, hemorrhage, or syphilis. Stroke syndromes are more complex because the vascular territories of the pons, and hence the anatomic distribution of pontine infarcts, do not match the more focal deficits caused by tuberculomas or syphilitic gummas. Therefore, in the world of infarcts, you will hear and read time and time again that the classical pontine syndromes do not exist. We do not quite agree with that statement, but certainly grant that they are uncommon, especially, for example, the full spectrum of the Marie–Foix syndrome.

Regardless of how one classifies pontine stroke syndromes, one concludes that there is significant overlap of signs and symptoms between stroke groups, and that it is not possible to neatly compartmentalize infarcts and isolate weakness to one group, ataxia to another, sensory loss to a third, etc.

Because of the presence of deep perforators from the basilar, the basis pontis and the tegmentum are often both involved by a single infarct, and so the division of pontine syndromes into those of the basis pontis and those of the tegmentum is also artificial.

So what to do now? Probably the best approach is to first be aware of the blood supply of the pons, and then be aware of a couple of classifications of pontine stroke syndromes. Just to clarify, when the term ipsilateral is used, it is with reference to the side of the lesion in the brainstem.

Blood supply to the pons

The pons is supplied by the basilar artery or its branches via three main types of vessels (named after Foix and Hillemand): paramedian branches, and short and long circumflex. The paramedian arteries supply the medial basis pontis and anterior and medial portion of the tegmentum. The short circumflex arteries supply the ventrolateral pons. The long circumflex arteries arise from the basilar and the superior and anterior inferior cerebellar arteries and supply the lateral edge of the pons as well as the posterior part of the tegmentum (Fig. 3.44).

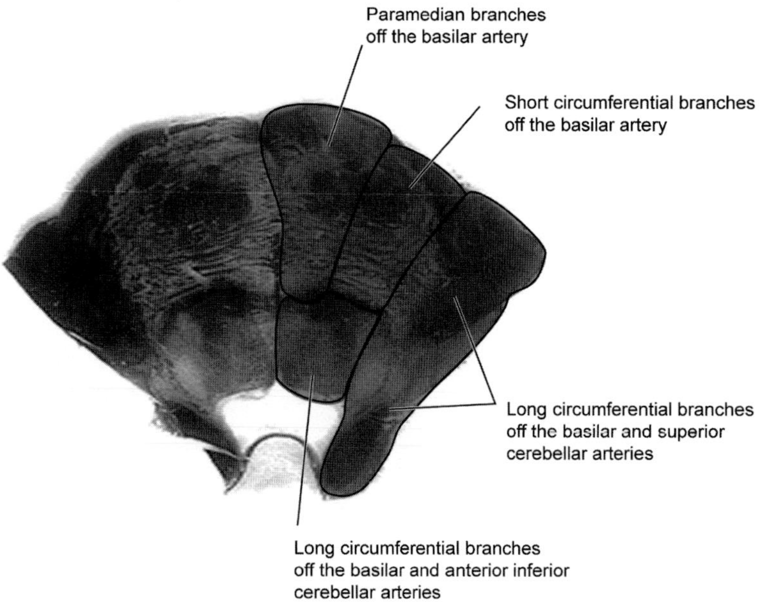

Fig. 3.44. **Schematic diagram showing the blood supply of the pons (see plate section for color image).**

Classification systems of pontine stroke

I. Superior, middle, lower and medial or lateral. This is the classification used in the textbook *Neurology in Clinical Practice: Principles of Diagnosis and Management*, by Bradley, Daroff, Fenichel, and Mardsen. It divides pontine stroke syndromes into the following groups:
   - Superior medial pontine syndrome (arterial territory: median branches of the basilar artery). This can present with ipsilateral ataxia, internuclear ophthalmoplegia (MLF), and myoclonus of the palate pharynx and vocal cords (? central tegmental tract to inferior olive), and contralateral motor weakness (corticospinal tract).
   - Superior lateral pontine syndrome (arterial territory: branches from superior cerebellar artery). This can present with: ipsilateral ataxia, ipsilateral Horner's syndrome (preganglionic sympathetic fibers), facial hemianesthesia, and masticator motor weakness (nuclei and fibers of cranial nerve five), as well as contralateral hemianesthesia and loss of vibration and proprioception (medial lemniscus, trigeminothalamic tract, spinothalamic tract).
   - Middle medial pontine syndrome (arterial territory: median branches of the basilar artery). This can present with ipsilateral ataxia, conjugate gaze paresis to the side of the lesion (PPRF or sixth nerve nucleus), internuclear ophthalmoplegia (MLF), and contralateral weakness (corticospinal tract).
   - Middle lateral pontine syndrome (arterial territory: long lateral branches of the basilar artery). This can present with contralateral hemisensory loss (spinothalamic tract) and ipsilateral ataxia, paralysis of muscles of mastication (fifth motor nucleus), facial hemianesthesia (spinal trigeminal tract and nucleus), and Horner's syndrome.
   - Inferior medial pontine syndrome (arterial territory: median branches of the basilar artery). This presents with contralateral weakness (corticospinal tract), contralateral impairment of proprioception and tactile sense over half the body (medial lemniscus), ipsilateral paresis of conjugate gaze (sixth nerve nucleus), lower motor neuron facial palsy (fibers of seventh nerve at the facial colliculus or in the tegmentum), and one-and-a-half syndrome (sixth nerve nucleus and MLF).
   - Inferior lateral pontine syndrome (arterial territory: anterior inferior cerebellar artery). This may present with contralateral loss of pain and temperature over the body, possibly including the face (spinothalamic and trigeminothalamic tracts) and ipsilateral deafness (eighth nerve), facial paralysis (seventh nerve), ataxia, impaired sensation over face (spinal trigeminal tract).
II. Ventromedial, ventrolateral and tegmental. Drs. Bassetti, Bogousslavsky, Barth, and Regli advanced this classification in a paper titled "Isolated Infarcts of the Pons" (*Neurology*, **46**: 165, January 1996). The classification scheme is based on four main arterial territories: anteromedial pontine arteries (ventromedial infarcts), anterolateral pontine arteries (ventrolateral infarcts), lateral pontine arteries (tegmental infarcts) and posterior pontine arteries (tegmental infarcts).
   - Ventromedial pontine infarcts are in the territory of the anteromedial pontine arteries (paramedian arteries of Foix and Hillemand), which supply the medial portion of the corticospinal tract and medial portion of the tegmentum, such as the medial lemniscus, and cranial nerve nuclei. These infarcts tend to present with significant contralateral hemiparesis, often accompanied by dysarthria and ipsilateral ataxia (ataxic hemiparesis). Some of the patients also have contralateral lower extremity ataxia. Many patients will also show symptoms or signs of tegmental involvement, such as eye movement disorders, and lemniscal sensory loss, but the tegmental involvement is usually transient.
   - Ventrolateral pontine infarcts are in the territory of the anterolateral pontine arteries (branches of the paramedian arteries and short circumflex arteries of Foix and Hillemand), which supply the lateral portion of the corticospinal tracts, and portions of the medial tegmentum. These patients present with a constellation of findings, including ataxic hemiparesis with dysarthria, ataxic hemiparesis, dysarthria–clumsy hand, and cranial nerve palsies. However, the hemiparesis is milder than ventromedial infarcts. The hemiparesis and ataxia are contralateral to the lesion. Most patients show mild symptoms of tegmental involvement, and some patients also experience vertigo.
   - Tegmental infarcts are in the territory of the lateral pontine arteries (branches of the short circumflex and medial branches of the long circumflex arteries of Foix and Hillemand, such as arising from the anterior inferior cerebellar artery and superior cerebellar artery). These patients present with vertigo, diplopia, eye movement disturbances, cranial nerve palsies, especially 6th and 7th cranial nerves, and body, or face and body sensory loss involving the lemniscal or spinothalamic tracts. Some motor deficits are present, but they are usually mild. Bilateral tegmental infarcts are often characterized by acute pseudobulbar palsy, somnolence, facial or abducens palsy, and unilateral or bilateral sensorimotor dysfunction.

   From these various classifications, several conclusions may be drawn.
(1) In our mind, the best approach is a knowledge of the relevant clinical neuroanatomy of the basis pontis and pontine tegmentum, with an ability to correlate lesions visualized on MRI with the corresponding structures and the expected symptoms and signs.
(2) In general, infarcts of the basis pontis tend to present with involvement of the corticospinal tract, leading to motor weakness, which is more pronounced with ventromedial than ventrolateral basis pontis infarcts. There is also involvement of the cortico cerebellar fibers, often leading to an ataxia, again predominantly ipsilateral to the motor weakness. There may be involvement of the sixth cranial nerve

along its course in the basis pontis, leading to ipsilateral sixth nerve palsy, and possibly also involvement of the 7th nerve along its course within the basis pontis, leading to ipsilateral lower motor neuron facial palsy, such as in the Millard–Gubler syndrome.

However, it is important to remember that basis pontis infarcts may interrupt corticobulbar fibers, including those to the 7th nerve. Thus, it is in fact more common to have homolateral body and facial weakness (i.e., on the same side), rather than a crossed brainstem syndrome with contralateral body weakness and ipsilateral facial weakness, as in original descriptions of Millard–Gubler.

(3) As infarcts become more lateral in the basis pontis, the motor weakness becomes less pronounced. Contralateral hemisensory loss becomes more pronounced, as does cerebellar ataxia. Ventrolateral infarcts may also give 5th nerve findings, including both fifth nerve motor weakness and impaired sensation over the ipsilateral face, as well as a Horner's syndrome.

(4) Infarcts of the tegmentum often present with eye movement disorders, including conjugate gaze palsy, from involvement of the sixth nerve nucleus, internuclear ophthalmoplegia, one-and-a-half syndrome (possibly associated ipsilateral peripheral 7th nerve findings), and mild contralateral motor weakness, such as the Raymond–Foville syndrome. Also, sensory lemniscal findings, such as contralateral body pain and temperature loss from involvement of the spinothalamic tract, contralateral body proprioception loss from involvement of the medial lemniscus, ipsilateral or contralateral facial anesthesia from involvement of the spinal trigeminal tract and nucleus (ipsilateral to the lesion), or 5th nerve nucleus or nerve fibers (ipsilateral to the lesion), or the ascending trigeminothalamic tract (contralateral to the lesion).

4 | The midbrain

MICHAEL F. WATERS *Clinical Stroke Program, Cedars-Sinai Medical Center, LA, USA*

Midbrain anatomy

The midbrain is derived from embryonic mesencephalon, one of the three primary vesicles present in the embryonic neural tube. Grossly, it is bounded caudally by diencephalic structures (hypothalamus, thalamus) and caudally by the pons (embryonic rhombencephalon). The gross external features of the midbrain allow for ready identification. Ventrally, two large fiber bundles, the cerebral peduncles, mark the inferior surface. Ventromedially, the paired oculomotor nerves emerge from the interpeduncular fossa. Dorsally, the midbrain is identified by the quadrageminal plate, consisting of a pair of rostral elevations, the superior colliculi, and a second pair of smaller caudal elevations, the inferior colliculi. Just caudal to the inferior colliculi, the trochlear nerves exit. The interior of the midbrain is generally divided into three regions. This includes: (1) the tectum, a mixture of gray and white matter dorsal to the central canal, including the surface structure known as the quadrageminal plate (the paired eminences superior and inferior colliculi), (2) the tegmentum, the largest portion of the midbrain including the central gray matter, ascending and descending tracts, reticular nuclei, cranial nerve nuclei, locus ceruleus, and the red nucleus, and (3) the basis, containing the substantia nigra, and the cerebral peduncles fibers. It is useful to consider the cross-sectional anatomy of the midbrain at the levels of both the inferior and superior colliculi.

Anatomy of the caudal midbrain

The tectum of the caudal midbrain is dominated by the inferior colliculus nuclei, which are composed of an oval mass of small- and medium-sized neurons organized as a central nucleus, pericentral nucleus, and external nucleus. The central nucleus is a laminated mass of neurons which function in auditory relay pathways, with high frequency sounds represented ventrally and low frequency sounds represented dorsally. The pericentral nucleus is a thin dorsal layer receiving contralateral monaural input directing auditory attention.

The external nucleus, a group of neurons surrounding the central nucleus laterally and ventrally participates in acousticomotor reflexes. Afferent connections include the lateral lemniscus, contralateral inferior colliculus, ipsilateral medial geniculate body, auditory cerebral cortex, and cerebellum (Fig. 4.1).

Efferent connections from the inferior colliculus include the medial geniculate body, contralateral inferior colliculus, superior colliculus, lateral lemniscus, and cerebellum (Fig. 4.2).

The midbrain tegmentum consists of ascending and descending tracts, as well as multiple nuclear groups. Let's begin our discussion with the tracts. The largest fiber tract is the brachium conjunctivum, arising from the deep cerebellar nuclei (dentate and interposed), decussating at this level, and either terminating in the red nucleus, or bypassing it to terminate in the ventrolateral thalamic nucleus. These fibers form the superior cerebellar peduncle. Another important tract originating in the spinal cord is the paired medial lemniscus. This tract lies in the lateral aspect of the midbrain and conveys discriminative touch and kinesthesia from the periphery to the ventral posterolateral nucleus of the thalamus (VPL). In close proximity runs the trigeminal lemniscus, originating from the head region and heading to the ventral posteromedial nucleus of the thalamus (VPM). The spinothalamic tracts run laterally, dorsal to the medial lemniscus, and convey pain and temperature information from the periphery to the VPL. The lateral lemniscus, running lateral and dorsal to the spinothalamic tract is made up of auditory fibers. Medially, the medial longitudinal fasciculus (MLF) runs dorsally in a paramedian position carrying information governing eye movements. Just lateral to the MLF is the central tegmental tract, which provides connections from the basal ganglia and midbrain to the inferior olive. Lastly, the rubrospinal tract carries fibers connecting the red nucleus to the spinal cord (Fig. 4.3).

Multiple important nuclear groups are found at the level of the inferior colliculus. The mesencephalic nucleus contains the cell body of the unipolar neurons which convey proprioceptive information from the muscles of mastication.

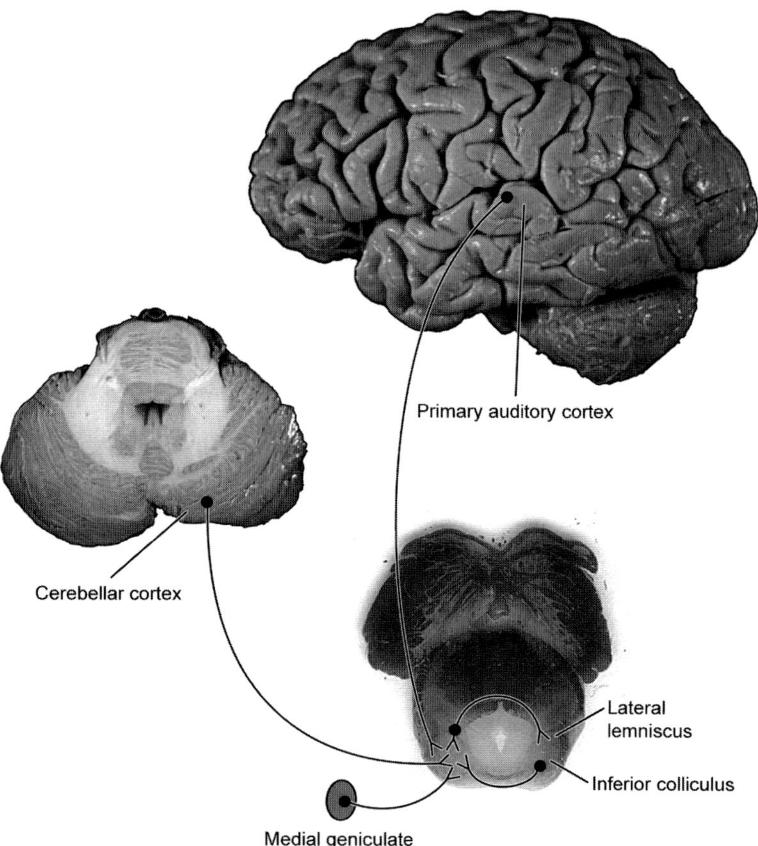

Fig. 4.1. **Afferent connections of the inferior colliculus.**

Between the substantia nigra and interpeduncular nucleus is the nucleus parabrachialis pigmentosus consisting of the ventral extension of the tegmental area of Tsai. The dorsal tegmental nucleus, found in the central gray matter in close proximity to the dorsal raphe nucleus, receives fibers from the interpeduncular nucleus and projects to autonomic nuclei in the brainstem and reticular formation. The ventral tegmental nucleus receives input from the hypothalamic mammillary bodies and participates in circuitry regulating emotion and behavior. Two cholinergic nuclei, the pedunculopontine and dorsal tegmental nuclei also lie in the tegmentum. The pedunculopontine nucleus receives cortical, pallidal, and nigral input and projects back to the substantia nigra and thalamus. It is involved in locomotion. The dorsal raphe nucleus is located in the ventral periaqueductal gray matter projecting serotonergic fibers to the substantia nigra, striatum, and cortex. The parabigeminal areas are additional cholinergic neurons projecting to, and receiving input from, the superior colliculi, which respond to visual stimuli. The locus ceruleus lies at the edge of the central gray matter and sends wide-ranging noradrenergic projections to the thalamus, hypothalamus, telencephalon, cerebellum, spinal cord, and brainstem sensory nuclei. These projections occur in three main fiber bundles including the central tegmental tract, the dorsal longitudinal fasciculus, and the medial forebrain bundle (Fig. 4.4).

In the ventral area of the central gray matter at the level of the inferior colliculus lies the nucleus for cranial nerve i.v. (trochlear nerve). It is situated nearly midline, ventral to the cerebral aqueduct. Axons emanating from the nucleus course dorsal and slightly caudal to wrap around the cerebral aqueduct, decussating in the superior medullary velum. The trochlear nerve exits the brainstem on the dorsal surface of the midbrain, caudal to the inferior colliculus. It wraps anteriorly around the cerebral peduncle, passing between the superior cerebellar and the posterior cerebral arteries lateral to the oculomotor nerve. The nerve then courses anteriorly in the subarachnoid space along with the oculomotor nerve until it pierces the dura covering the roof of the cavernous sinus. In the cavernous sinus, the nerve runs along the lateral wall then enters the orbit through the superior orbital fissure. The nerve courses medially along the roof of the orbit then divides into several branches to innervate the superior oblique muscle (Fig. 4.5).

It is responsible for somatic motor function supplying efferent innervation to the superior oblique muscle of the eye. This muscle affects inward rotation (intorsion) as well as downward and lateral movement of the eye. There are several unique features of the trochlear nerve including: smallest cranial nerve (approximately 2400 axons), the longest intracranial course, only cranial nerve with complete decussation, and only cranial nerve to exit the brainstem dorsally.

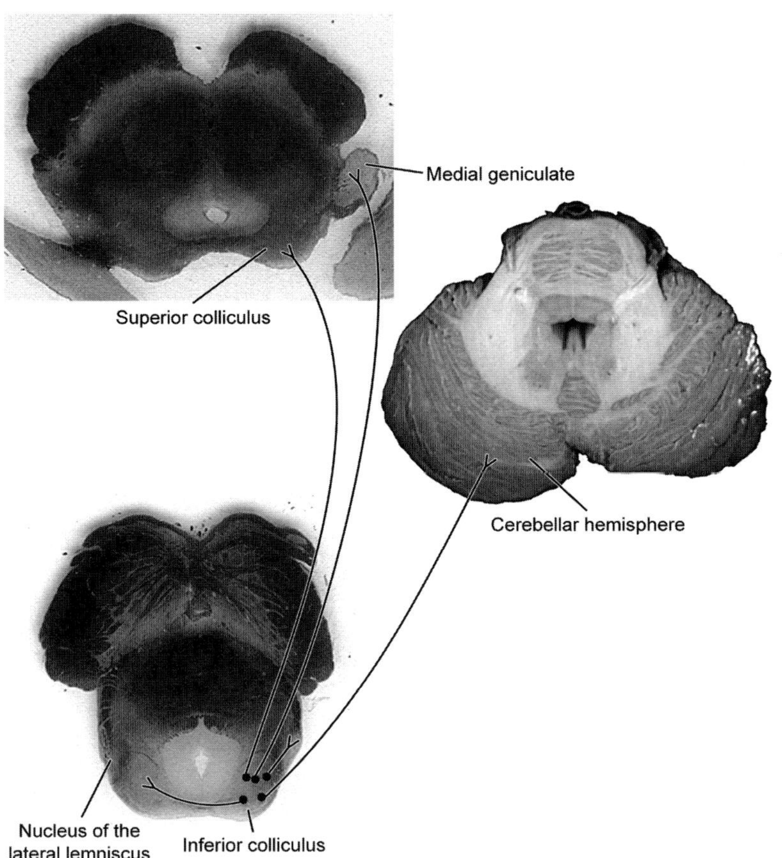

Fig. 4.2. **Efferent projections of the inferior colliculus.**

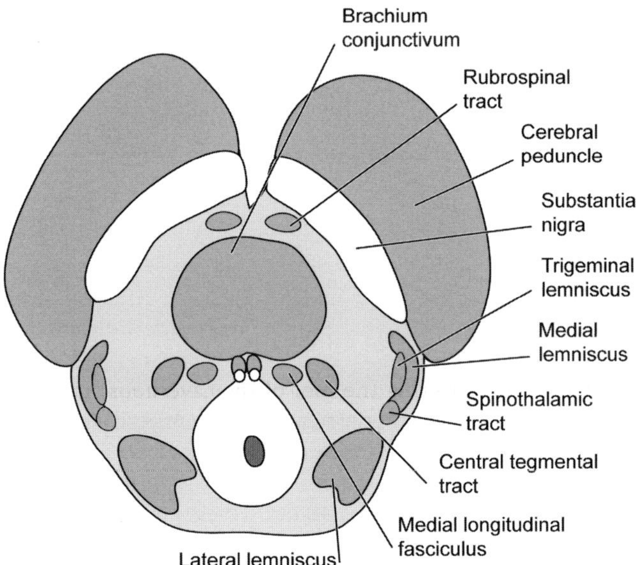

Fig. 4.3. **White matter tracts in the caudal midbrain.**

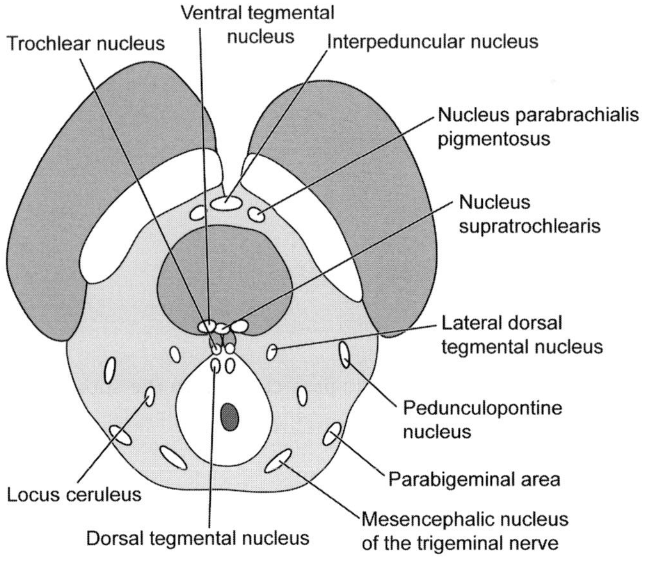

Fig. 4.4. **Nuclei of the caudal midbrain.**

The basal portion of the mesencephalon, at the level of the inferior colliculi is made of the cerebral peduncles and the substantia nigra (Fig. 4.6).

The cerebral peduncles are large fiber bundles, which merge caudally in the basis pontis as the longitudinal fibers of the pons. Rostrally, before becoming the cerebral peduncles, these fibers were the internal capsule. The peduncles can roughly be divided into thirds, with the inner made up of corticobulbar and corticospinal fibers somatotopically arranged medially to laterally as face, arm, trunk, and leg. On

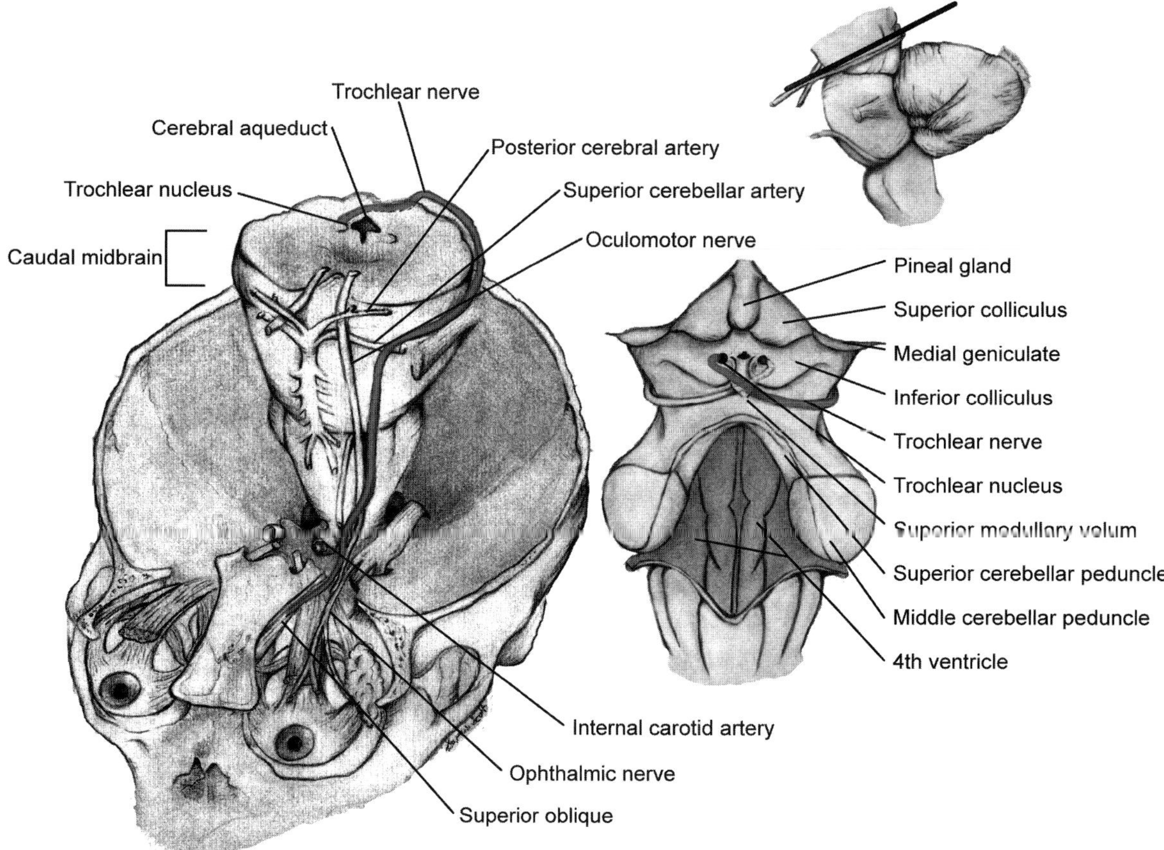

Fig. 4.5. **Course and innervation of the trochlear nerve.**

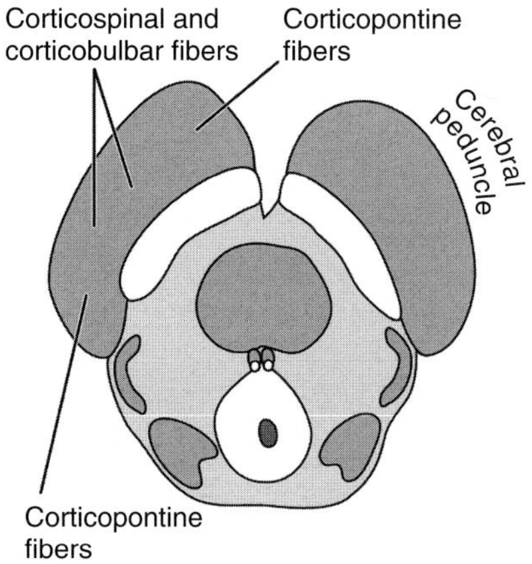

Fig. 4.6. **Tracts in the cerebral peduncle.**

either side of the corticobulbar/corticospinal bundles are corticopontine fiber tracts originating from the frontal cortex (medially) and the occipital, parietal and temporal cortex (laterally). Lying dorsomedial to the cerebral peduncles, but lateral to the tegmentum, is a pigmented mass of neurons referred to as the substantia nigra. This area is divided into the dorsally located zona compacta, where melanin-containing neurons send dopaminergic axons, and the ventrally located zona reticulata. The substantia nigra possesses extensive interconnections and plays a key role in several important pathologies including Parkinson's disease, Huntington's disease, and multisystem atrophy. Afferent connections include the neostriatum, cerebral cortex, globus pallidus, subthalamic nucleus, and tegmentonigral tracts. Efferent projections include the nigrostriate, -cortical, -pallidal, -rubral, -thalamic, -subthalamic, -tegmental, -collicular, and -amygdaloid tracts (Fig. 4.7).

Anatomy of the rostral midbrain

The tectum at this level is occupied by the nucleus of the superior colliculus. This is a laminated mass of neurons that play key roles in controlling eye movements and visual reflexes. Key functional features of the superior colliculus include a visual space map in the superficial layers which project to motor program maps in the deep layers encoding vector signals. These tracts initiate motor programs to effect start-to-goal eye positioning. Afferent signals to the superior colliculus include the cortex, retina, spinal cord, inferior colliculus, and the tectospinal, -pontocerebellar, -reticular, and -thalamic tracts.

The tegmentum at this level contains both fibers of passage and important nuclear groups. Most of the fiber bundles and tracts are similar as discussed in the section on the level of the inferior colliculus. The exception to this is the lateral

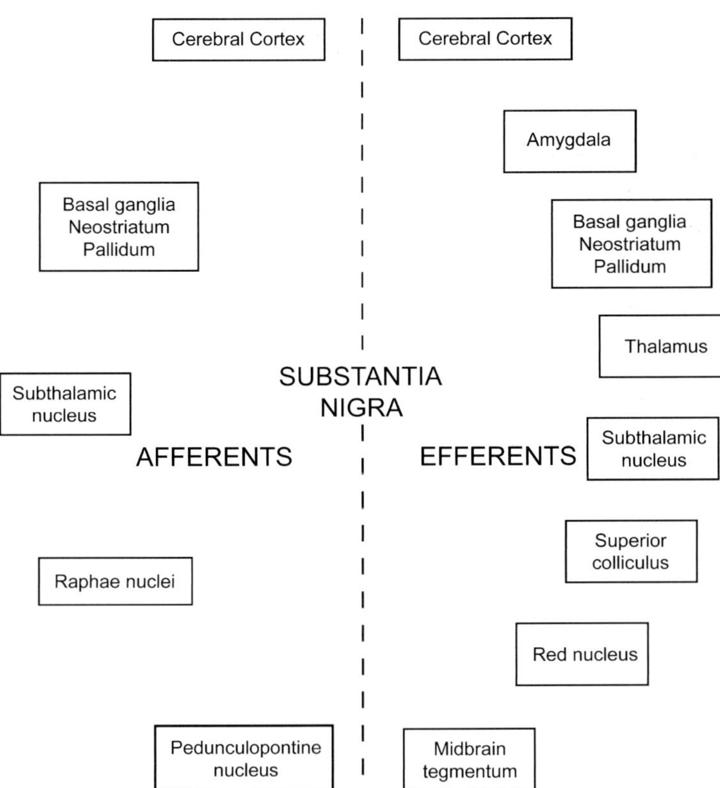

Fig. 4.7. **Inputs and outputs of the substantia nigra.**

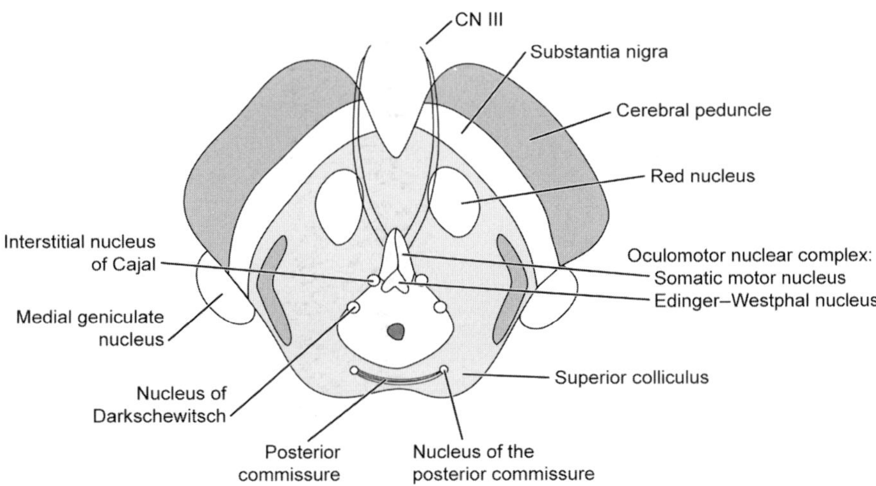

Fig. 4.8. **Location of the red nucleus and surrounding nuclei of the rostral midbrain.**

lemniscus, which terminates in the inferior colliculus. Principal nuclear groups include the red nucleus and the nucleus of the third cranial nerve.

The red nucleus, so named due to its rich vascularization and reddish hue on fresh preparations, is located near the midline medially to the substantia nigra (Fig. 4.8). It has extensive interconnections including afferent input from the deep cerebellar nuclei and cerebral cortex. Efferent projections include the spinal cord, cerebellum, reticular formation, and inferior olive.

The oculomotor nucleus is located in the midbrain at the level of the superior colliculus. It is situated nearly midline, ventral to the cerebral aqueduct and receives input from several principal sources including the cerebral cortex, cerebellum, mesencephalon, pons, and medulla. It consists of a lateral

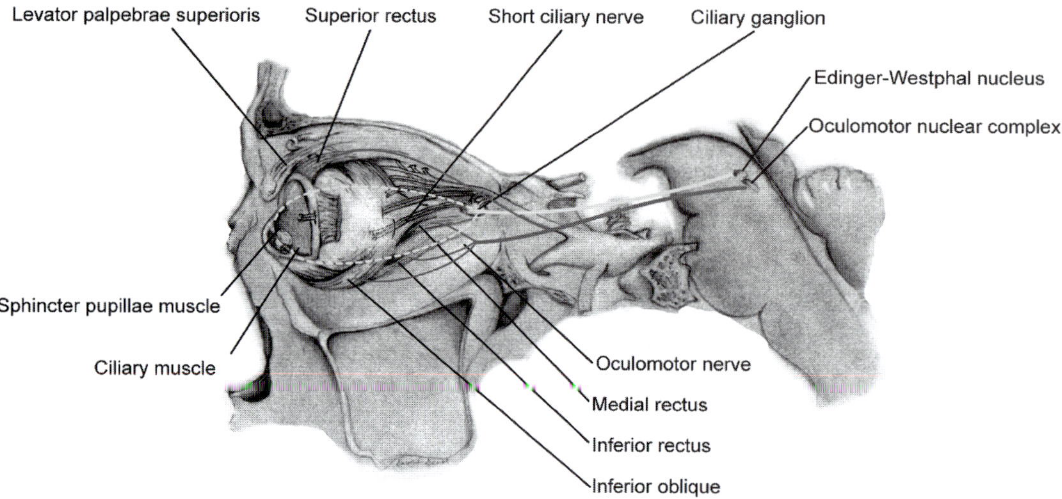

Fig. 4.9. **Course of the parasympathetic fibers originating from the Edinger–Westphal nucleus.**

somatic motor column and a medial visceral cell column. The oculomotor nuclear complex consists of three subnuclei: (1) the lateral subnucleus, which supplies the ipsilateral inferior rectus, inferior oblique, and medial rectus, (2) the medial subnucleus, which supplies the contralateral superior rectus, and (3) the central subnucleus, which provides bilateral innervation to the levator palpebrae superioris. The lower motor neuron axons course through the midbrain tegmentum ventrally through the red nucleus and the medial aspect of the cerebral peduncles exiting the brainstem in the interpeduncular fossa between the midbrain and pons. These fibers coalesce with fibers from the parasympathetic fibers of the Edinger–Westphal nucleus to form the oculomotor nerve (CN III). CN III then passes between the superior cerebellar and the posterior cerebral arteries and courses anteriorly in the subarachnoid space, passing through the dura with CN IV into the cavernous sinus. In the cavernous sinus, the nerve divides into inferior and superior divisions. The inferior division supplies the inferior oblique, inferior rectus, and medial rectus muscles. The superior division supplies the superior rectus and the levator palpebrae superioris.

The Edinger–Westphal nucleus is located in the midbrain dorsal to the oculomotor complex. The preganglionic (lower motor neuron) axons course ventrally through the midbrain with the somatic motor axons. Following their exit from the brainstem, they course with the third cranial nerve through the middle cranial fossa, cavernous sinus, and superior orbital fissure to enter the orbit. In the orbit, the fibers leave the nerve and terminate in the ciliary ganglion. Postganglionic axons leave the ganglion and course with the sympathetic fibers to enter the eye near the optic nerve. The axons then run anteriorly along the eyeball between the sclera and choroid to terminate in the ciliary body and iris where they innervate the ciliary and constrictor pupillae muscles (Fig. 4.9).

Somatic motor function is supplied by efferent innervation to the levator palpebrae superioris, superior rectus, medial rectus, inferior rectus, and inferior oblique muscles of the eye. These muscles affect lid elevation, downgaze, medial gaze, upgaze, and inward torsional gaze respectively. Visceral motor function is supplied by parasympathetic innervation to the constrictor pupillae and ciliary muscles via the ciliary ganglion. These muscles affect pupil size and lens shape respectively. The visceral motor component also mediates both the pupillary light reflex as well as the accommodation reflex. In the light reflex, light entering the eye sends an afferent signal along the optic nerve, which relays in the pretectal area to provide bilateral innervation to the Edinger–Westphal nuclei. This, in turn affects bilateral pupillary constriction when light is shone in either or both eyes. The accommodation reflex, which adapts the eye for near vision, combines increased lens curvature, pupillary constriction, and convergence of the eyes.

Midbrain blood supply

The vascular supply of the midbrain is complex, though the majority is serviced via the basilar (paramedian perforators), superior cerebellar (SCA), and posterior cerebral (PCA) branches. Vascular supply zones may be roughly divided rostro-caudally into three levels: (1) pretectal, (2) superior colliculus, and (3) inferior colliculus. Axially, the midbrain may be divided into medial and lateral zones. At the level of the pretectum, the paramedian branches of the basilar artery supply the medial zone. The more lateral zones are supplied primarily by the PCA. At the level of the superior colliculus, the lateral zones receive the majority of their vascular supply from the PCA, though the superior colliculi themselves are supplied principally by the SCA. The basilar artery supplies the medial zone. At the level of the inferior colliculi, the lateral zones are supplied by the SCA, whereas the medial zones are once again principally supplied by paramedian branches of the basilar artery (Fig. 4.10).

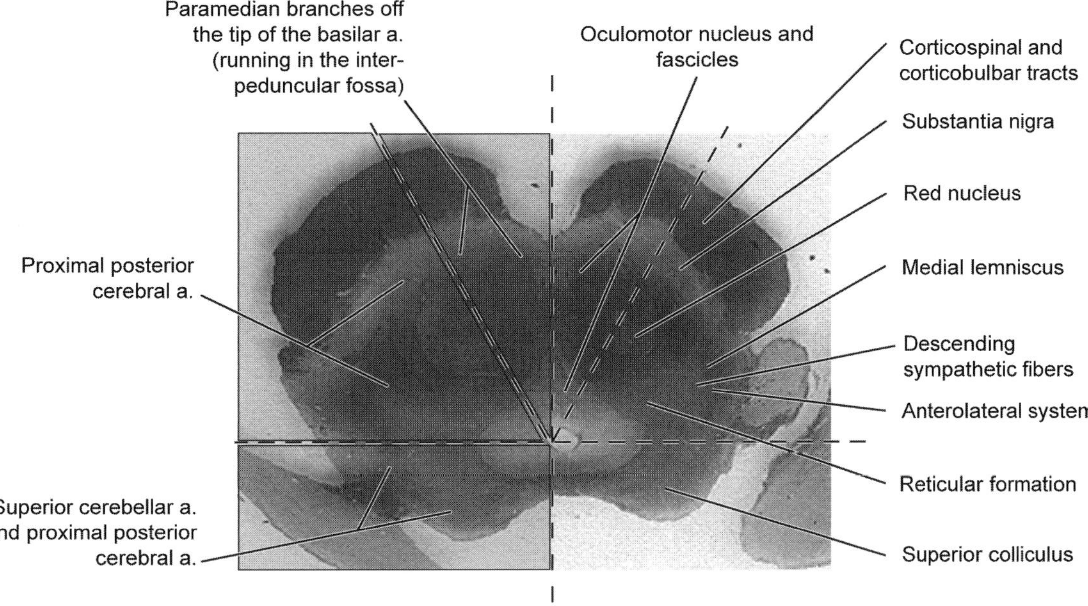

Fig. 4.10. **Vascular distribution of the midbrain (see plate section for color image).**

Case 4.1

52-year-old man comes to your office with a past medical history significant for diabetes, hypertension, coronary artery disease, and remote lymphoma treated and in remission. He is now reporting an approximate 2-week history of progressive left eye pain and double vision. In particular, he states that the diplopia is much more pronounced when looking to the right. Moreover, he reports blurred vision in his left eye even with his glasses on, though his acuity in the right eye remains sharp. In asking him to elaborate, he states that this problem has actually been going on for nearly a year, though historically it was intermittent and resolved spontaneously. For the headache, he took over-the-counter analgesics with good relief. For the past 2 weeks, his symptoms have not abated, and the eye pain persists despite taking 2400 mg of ibuprofen daily.

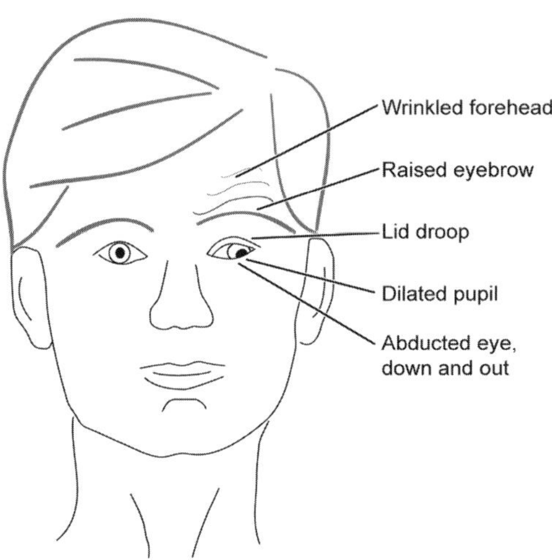

Fig. 4.11. **Eye and facial signs for the patient in Case 4.1.**

On examination, asymmetry with respect to his eyes is immediately apparent. Attempts at fixed primary gaze reveal a downward and laterally deviated left orbit. Moreover, he has moderate left lid ptosis with a raised eyebrow and wrinkled forehead on the left. Closer inspection reveals a dilated left pupil that is sluggishly reactive to light. Interestingly, the consensual response on the right is intact, though the opposite is not true (Fig. 4.11).

Based on the present exam, where would you localize the lesion?

This patient's history and physical exam are compatible with a palsy of the third cranial nerve. Given the longstanding symptoms with recent exacerbation, one would suspect a slow, insidious process such as a mass lesion, indolent infection, or metabolic derangement. To assist in localization, let's review the anatomy of the third cranial nerve.

Recall that the oculomotor nucleus is located in the midbrain at the level of the superior colliculus. Lower motor neurons course through the red nucleus and cerebral peduncles exiting ventrally into the interpeduncular fossa. Here, fibers from the parasympathetic Edinger–Westphal nucleus join superficially to form the oculomotor nerve (CN III). Its course immediately encounters a common site of pathology, as it is sandwiched between the posterior cerebral (PCA) and superior cerebellar (SCA) arteries. PCA aneurisms often present as third nerve palsies, and this gentleman's presentation is not entirely inconsistent with this. However, his complaint of eye pain is somewhat atypical for this pathology, though this is an important diagnosis and should be considered in the differential. After progressing anteriorly, CN III travels through the cavernous sinus, another common site of pathology (Fig. 4.9). However, recall that the cavernous sinus also contains branches of the trigeminal nerve (V1 and V2), as well as the trochlear (CN IV) and abducens (CN VI) nerves. It would be atypical for this man to have an isolated third nerve palsy referable to cavernous sinus pathology. Finally, the nerve travels through the superior orbital fissure and splits into superior and inferior divisions innervating the following structures:

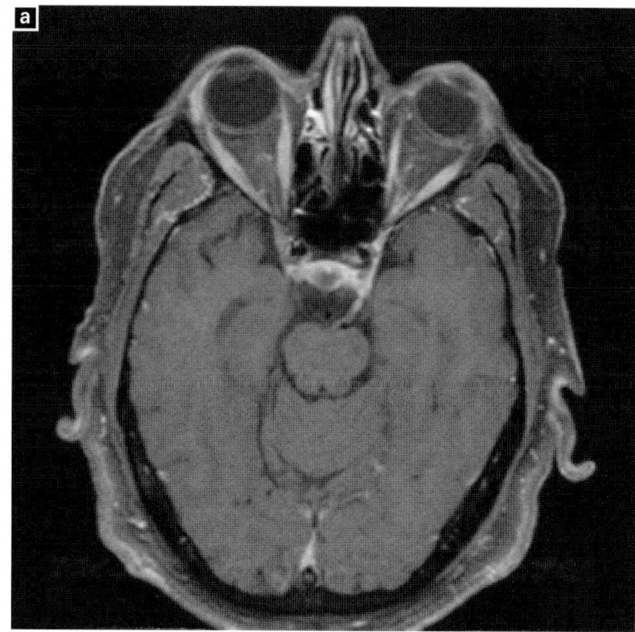

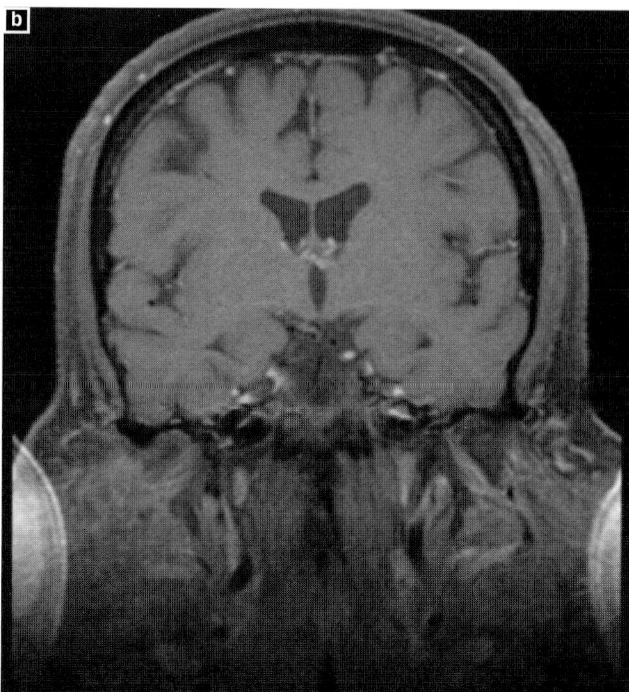

Fig. 4.12. **Axial and coronal post-contrast fat-saturation images through the brainstem revealing enhancement of the left third nerve.**

Superior division
   Superior rectus – elevation and intorsion
   Levator palpebrae superioris – elevates the eyelid
Inferior division
   Inferior rectus – depression and intorsion
   Inferior oblique – elevation and extorsion
   Medial rectus – adduction
The parasympathetic fibers of the Edinger–Westphal nucleus innervate the pupillary constrictor muscles. The fact that these fibers course on the periphery of CN III can provide important diagnostic clues. When a third nerve palsy involves the pupil, a compressive/surface pathological process should be suspected immediately. When a third nerve palsy spares the pupil, a metabolic derangement such as diabetes becomes more likely.

MRI examination is presented above (Fig. 4.12). What does the imaging reveal?

This man has diffuse, linear enhancement of his left CN III. This pathology is consistent with all of his presenting signs and symptoms. Given his history of lymphoma, the most likely diagnosis is carcinomatous lymphomatosis of the third cranial nerve. A lumbar puncture to evaluate cytology would be helpful in establishing this diagnosis.

Case 4.2

65-year-old woman with past medical history significant for poorly controlled hypertension, diabetes, and coronary artery disease, was brought into the emergency department after falling and striking her face. In obtaining more details, it is discovered that she fell after becoming markedly weak on her left side. On your examination, she is able to lift her left arm off the gurney, but remains unable to support her weight with her left leg. She has a contusion on the left side of her face, though careful inspection reveals facial weakness on that side including drooping of the mouth and flattening of the left nasolabial fold.

On further testing, it becomes obvious that, in addition to her facial weakness, initially masked by the contusion, she is having difficulty moving her right eye, and is reporting double vision on attempts to gaze to the left. Careful inspection reveals a down and out deviation of the right eye, drooping of the eyelid, and a dilated, non-responsive right pupil.

Based on the present exam, where would you localize the lesion?

This case is interesting in that it presents with clear involvement of cranial nerves in conjunction with upper motor neuron plegia. This clinical condition is often referred to as the "Syndrome of Weber," after Sir Herman David Weber, a German–English physician who first described it in 1863 (Fig. 4.13). Thoughtful consideration of midbrain anatomy is

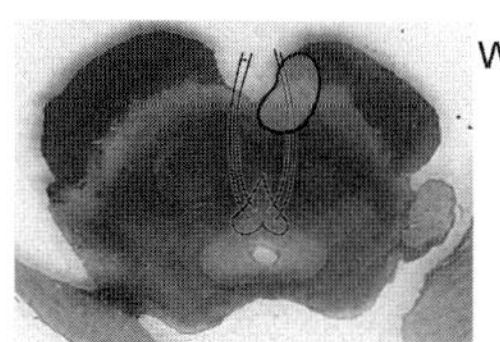

Fig. 4.13. **Overview of Weber syndrome and anatomical localization.**

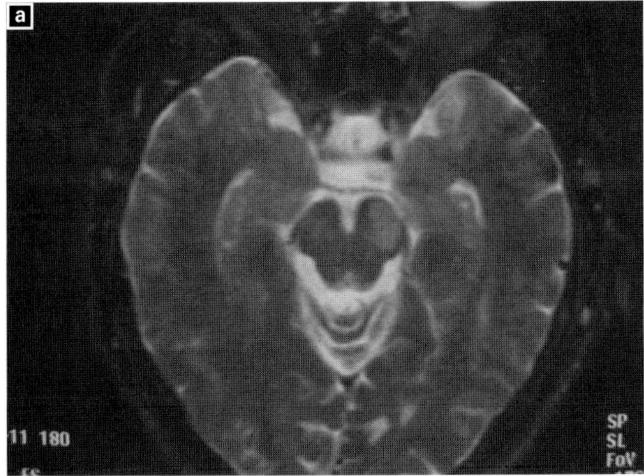 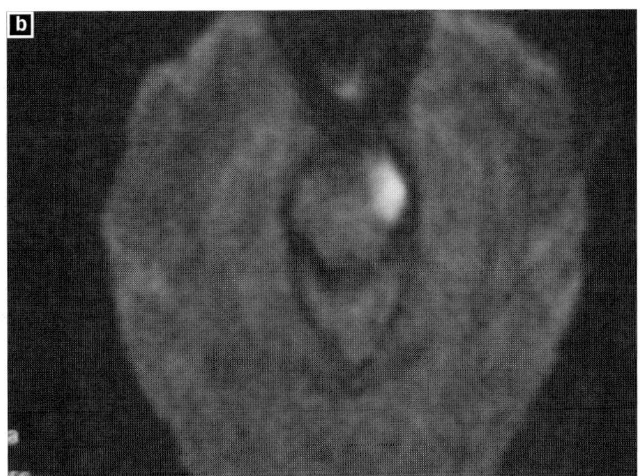

Fig. 4.14. **(a) Axial T2 and (b) DWI images revealing a subacute infarct involving the left cerebral peduncle.**

invaluable in localizing the lesion. Involvement of CN III or its nucleus on the right side would explain the eye deviation, diplopia, ptosis, and afferent pupillary defect. Given the additional pathology you find on exam, it is extremely unlikely to be a CN III nerve lesion, and more likely involves the nucleus or fibers as they course through the midbrain. Further, you know that the nucleus of CN III lies very proximal to the red nucleus. If a lesion involved this area, you may expect a tremor as part of the presentation. However, you can explain the contralateral weakness by involvement of the corticospinal tracts, as they pass through the midbrain (Kim and Kim, 2005). In fact, at this level of the midbrain, the dorsal aspect consists of the cerebral peduncles, which, among other tracts, contain the corticospinal tracts serving the face, arm, and leg (Fig. 4.13).

The pattern of weakness you observed in the face is referred to as lower facial weakness. That her forehead is relatively spared is a consequence of the bilateral cortical innervation of the upper face. When you observe a "peripheral" facial palsy involving both the lower and upper face, a lesion of the facial nerve (CN VII) is usually the culprit.

MRI imaging is presented above (Fig. 4.14). What does the imaging reveal?

These three images reveal an acute infarct involving the midbrain. The pattern of hyperintensity is consistent with dysfunction of corticospinal tracts coursing through the left cerebral peduncle, as well as rootlets of cranial nerve three as they exit the midbrain ventrally. The vascular distribution of this acute infarct likely involves the posterior cerebral and/or posterior communicating artery.

Reference

Kim, J. S. and Kim, J. Pure midbrain infarction: clinical, radiologic, and pathophysiologic findings. *Neurology* 2005; **64**(7): 1227–1232.

Case 4.3

52-year-old woman with diabetes and hypertension presented to your office after several months of progressively worsening blurred vision and difficulty in walking. She describes an indolent course and cannot recall with precision the exact onset. However, she can recall an event approximately 2 to 3 months ago when she was stepping onto a curb with her left leg, misjudged the height, and fell. Following that incident, she feels as if her vision has not been "right," and notes occasional double vision. She admits to poor dietary discretion and diabetes control and has felt that her symptoms were due to this. However, she is now barely able to ambulate independently, has developed a significant tremor, and continues to have difficulty with her vision.

At examination, the patient was found to have dense, pupillary-involving palsy with an inferolateral deviation of the globe and a dense ptosis. The patient was also mildly dysarthric, with some slurred speech. Cerebellar function testing with finger-to-nose and heel-to-shin exercises was intact on the right but compromised by significant tremor on the left. Moreover, the patient showed disturbances in gait with unsteadiness, broad-based stance, swaying, short, irregular steps with variable amplitude and occasional high-stepping (especially with the left leg), and difficulty initiating locomotion. The patient was unable to attempt tandem gait. Sensory testing revealed markedly diminished vibratory and proprioception in the left arm and leg, as well as some diminution of temperature and pin-prick sensation. You observe no evidence of truncal ataxia while the patient was sitting. No stooping or shuffling was seen during the patient's gait, and no evidence of masked facies or resting tremor was present.

Based on the present exam, where would you localize the lesion?

The overall clinical picture for this patient is very interesting, and includes pathology involving the oculomotor nucleus or nerve, locomotor systems, posterior column sensation, and cerebellum or red nucleus (tremor). The most likely localization

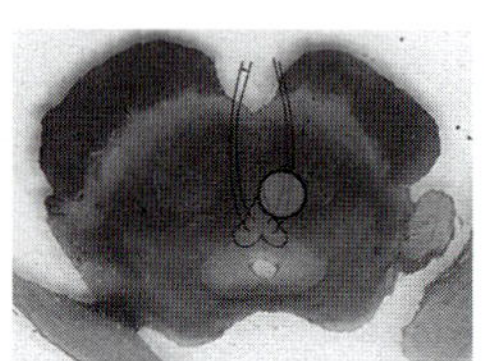

Fig. 4.15. **Overview of Benedikt syndrome and anatomical localization.**

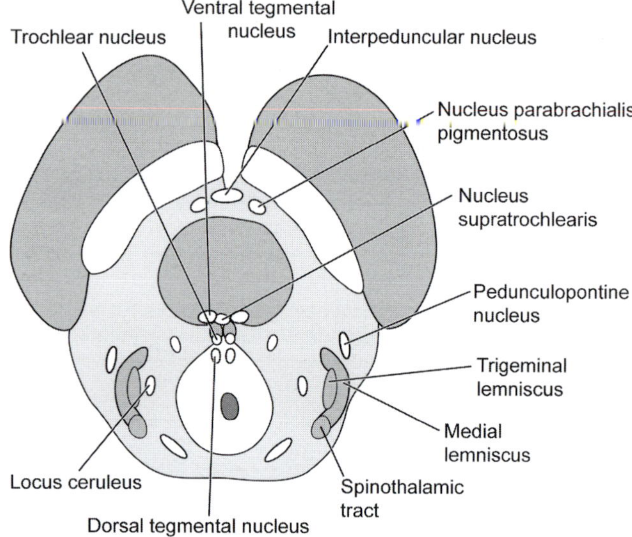

Fig. 4.16. **The location of the pedunculopontine nucleus in relation to the spinothalamic tract and medial lemniscus.**

placing all of these pathways in proximity is the tegmentum of the mesencephalon at the level of the superior colliculus. Recalling the anatomy of this location, one can assign oculomotor pathology to the rootlets of CN III, the hemianesthesia to the fibers of the medial lemniscus and to a lesser extent the spinothalamic tracts, and the tremor to the red nucleus (Fig. 4.15).

Taken alone, these symptoms are described as the "Syndrome of Benedikt," after Moritz Benedikt, an Austrian physician who described it as a vascular syndrome in 1889.

However, this case is more interesting in that it was not an abrupt onset (as would be expected in a vascular syndrome), and the difficulties with ambulation seem to be disproportionate with what would be expected for the above listed systems. Recollection of other key structures in the immediate vicinity reveals a nuclear group known as the pedunculopontine nucleus, which has been described as important in locomotion (Bhidayasiri *et al.*, 2003; Hathout and Bhidayasiri, 2005). At the level of the inferior colliculus, this lies in close proximity to the spinothalamic tract and medial lemniscus, further clarifying this woman's symptomatology (Fig. 4.16).

Because of the slow but relentless progression of her disease course, a mass lesion at the level of the superior colliculus, with caudal extension to the level of the inferior colliculus, may be expected.

MRI images are presented below (Fig. 4.17). What does the imaging reveal?

Other common clinical pathologies involving midbrain nucleus extra ocular movements not illustrated in these cases include the following.

CN III

– Vascular

    (a) Aneurysms of the posterior cerebral or superior cerebellar artery may compress the oculomotor nerve
    (b) Infarction in the basal midbrain may damage either the nucleus or axons of the oculomotor nerve.

– Inflammation

    Any inflammatory processes (especially tuberculous meningitis) located in or around the optic chiasm, temporal lobes, or pons, may specifically affect the oculomotor nerve.

– Temporal lobe herniation

    Any condition effecting downward herniation may cause the tentorial notch to displace the cerebral peduncle and compress the oculomotor nerve.

– Cavernous sinus pathology

    Multiple pathologies of the cavernous sinus, including infection, venous thrombosis, and mass lesions may affect the oculomotor nerve as it passes through the sinus.

Clinical correlates

    – Lower motor neuron lesions of the oculomotor nerve may effect any or all of the following clinical symptoms
        (a) divergent gaze resulting in diplopia
        (b) ptosis
        (c) midriasis
        (d) down and out deviation of the eye
        (e) inability to accommodate

CN IV

– Vascular

    Aneurysms of the posterior cerebral or superior cerebellar artery may compress the trochlear nerve.

– Inflammation

    Inflammatory processes may affect the trochlear nerve.

– Cavernous sinus pathology

    Multiple pathologies of the cavernous sinus, including infection, venous thrombosis, and mass lesions may affect the oculomotor nerve as it passes through the sinus.

Clinical correlates

    – Lower motor neuron lesions of the trochlear nerve may effect vertical diplopia which is most pronounced on contralateral downward gaze. Patients may present with a head tilt towards the non-paretic nerve to compensate for the action of the paralyzed superior oblique.

Reference

Bhidayasiri, R., Hathout, G., Cohen, S. N., and Tourtellotte, W. W. Midbrain ataxia: possible role of the pedunculopontine nucleus in human locomotion. *Cerebrovascular Diseases* 2003; **16**(1): 95–96.

Hathout, G. M., and Bhidayasiri, R. Midbrain ataxia: an introduction to the mesencephalic locomotor region and the pedunculopontine nucleus. *American Journal of Roentgenology* 2005; **184**(3): 953–956.

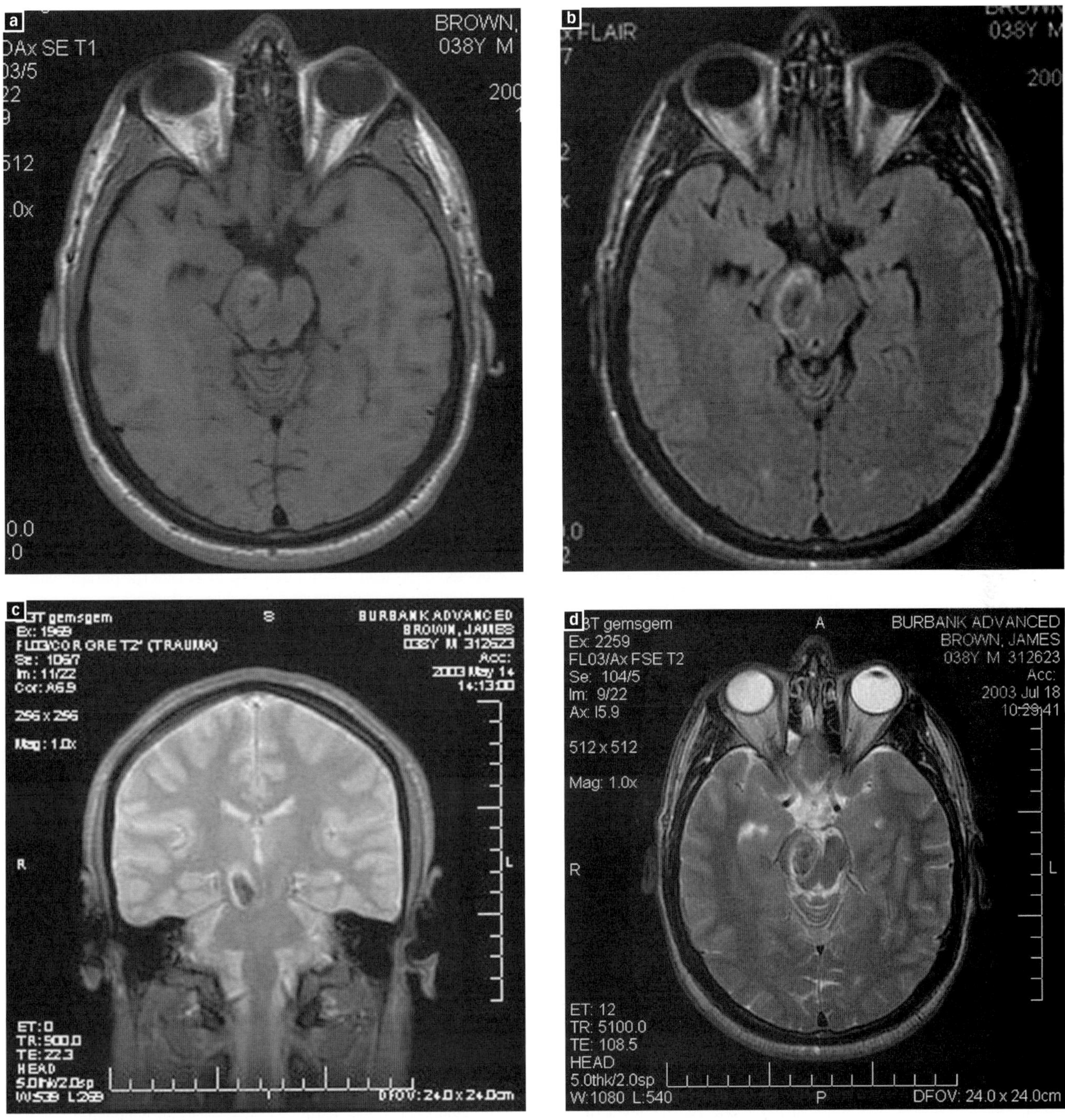

Fig. 4.17. **(a)** T1 axial, **(b)** FLAIR axial, **(c)** GRE T2 coronal, and **(d)** T2 axial images through the midbrain are provided. There is an ovoid lesion, isointense on T1, slightly hypointense on T2, and blooming on the GRE sequence, consistent with an unusual cavernous hemangioma in the right midbrain.

Case 4.4

You are called to evaluate Mr. M in the emergency department. The patient is a 66-year-old man with a past medical history of Type-II diabetes, coronary artery disease, peripheral vascular disease, and chronic myelogenous leukemia with complaints of visual problems and incoordination. The ED physician reports to you that he has gait difficulties and restricted eye movements.

These difficulties began abruptly, and were noticed immediately, as the gentleman was driving during symptom onset. He was suddenly aware of diplopia and restricted gaze in attempting to navigate traffic.

In the ED, your exam reveals dysmetria on finger-to nose testing with the right arm. The arm ataxia is accompanied by a slight tremor that worsens when the gentleman approaches your finger and his nose. This incoordination is also seen in the right leg, both when you request that he perform heel-to-shin exercise, and on attempts to walk. His natural gait shows poor foot placement and cadence limited to the right leg. He is unable to tandem walk without assistance, again due to difficulties involving his right leg.

Mr. M states that part of his problem with walking is due to his double vision. On careful oculomotor exam, you detect an inability to adduct the left eye when instructed to look rightward. He reports that this attempt exacerbates his diplopia. In addition, he

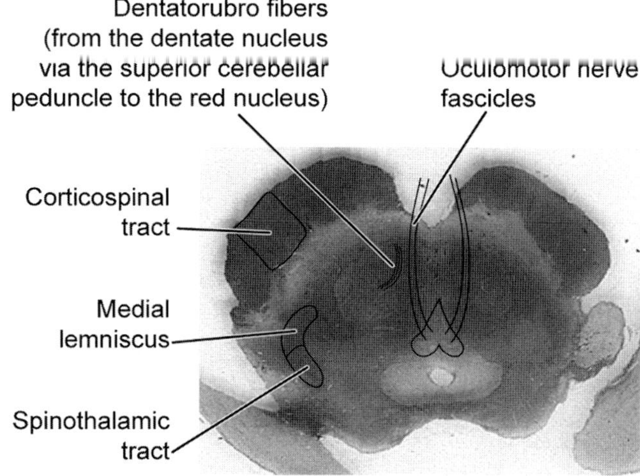

Fig. 4.18. **Affected structures in Case 4.4.**

has difficulty looking superiorly with his left eye. Downgaze is intact and pupillary movements to direct and consensual light, and convergence are intact bilaterally.

Based on the present exam, where would you localize the lesion?

The constellation of symptoms presented is known as Claude syndrome (Asakawa *et al.*, 2003) and includes pathology referable to the left oculomotor nerve or nuclei and coordination centers involving the right hemibody (Fong, 2005). Given the acute and simultaneous onset of his symptoms, one would predict a single lesion as causative, and suspect stroke as the etiology. The most likely site of localization is the rostral midbrain (Seo *et al.*, 2001). The affected anatomical structures may be seen in Fig. 4.18.

A stroke in this area may involve the neuroanatomic structures including cranial nerve III, explaining the eye findings, and the red nucleus, and/or brachium conjunctivum, explaining the incoordination. It is likely that the brachium conjunctivum is involved given the description of the tremor. Tremors that worsen when the target is approached, known as intention tremor, are often referable to cerebellar pathology.

MRI images are presented (Fig. 4.19). What does the imaging reveal?

Recall the neuroanatomy of the midbrain at the level of the oculomotor nucleus (Figs. 4.8, 4.10, and 4.20).

Importantly, recognize that, though the oculomotor nucleus itself lies close to the midline, the fibers of CN III run through the red nucleus and proximal to the brachium conjunctivum (superior cerebellar peduncle). It is notable, on exam, that the patient exhibits no pathology regarding nuclei governing other extra ocular movements, and especially pupillary defects. Remember that the parasympathetic fibers from the Edinger–Westphal nucleus do not join the nerve proper until their exit from the midbrain. Therefore, an infarct involving the territory of the proximal posterior cerebral

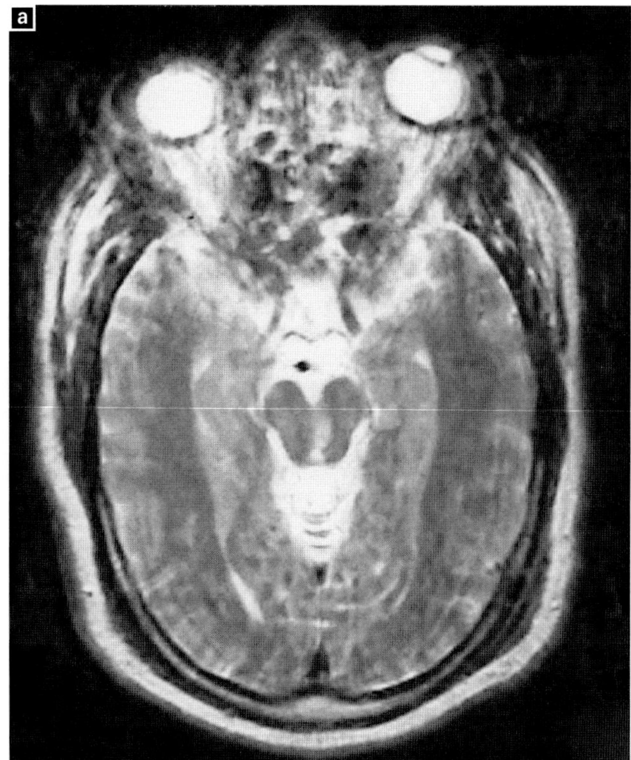

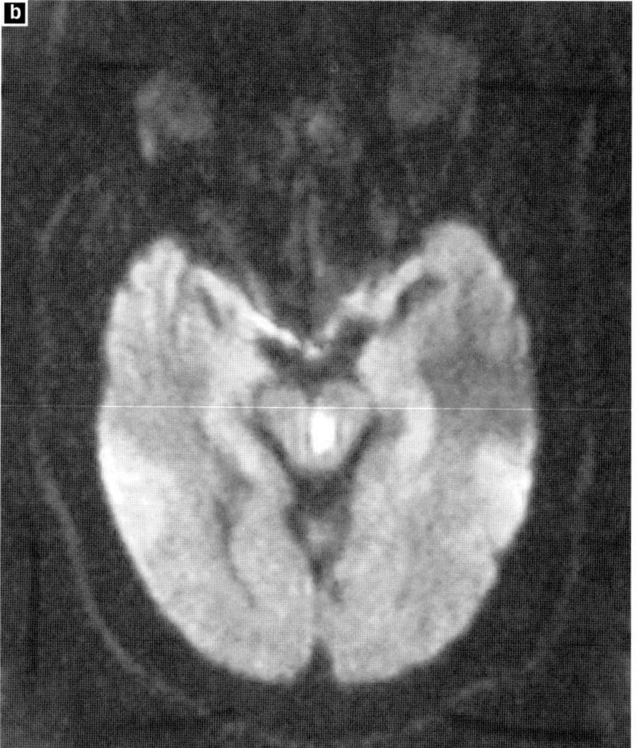

Fig. 4.19. **(a) Axial T2 and (b) DWI images through the midbrain, with significant motion artifact. There is a subacute infarct in the left midbrain tegmentum, extending from the aqueduct of Sylvius through the red nucleus.**

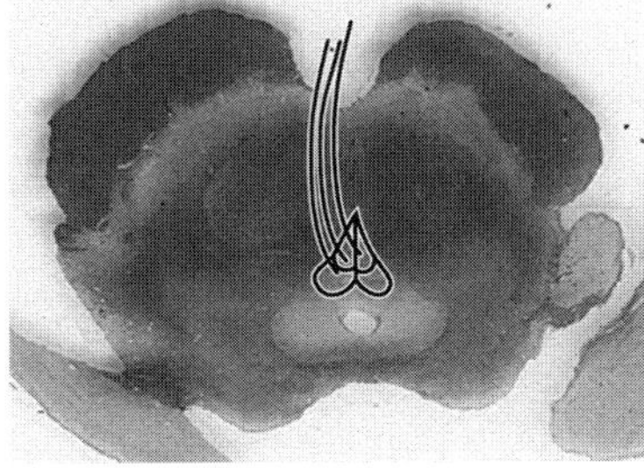

Fig. 4.20. **The location of the fibers exiting the oculomotor nuclear complex and the structures they innervate.**

artery, or alternatively, paramedian branches of the top of the basilar artery, would affect the anatomical structures implicated in this gentleman's clinical pathology.

References

Asakawa, H., Yanaka, K., and Nose, T. MRI of Claude's syndrome. *Neurology* 2003; **61**(4): 575.

Fong, C. S. Claude's syndrome associated with supranuclear horizontal gaze palsy caused by dorsomedial midbrain infarction. *Acta Neurologia Taiwan* 2005; **14**(3): 147–150.

Seo, S. W., Heo, J. H., Lee, K. Y. *et al*. Localization of Claude's syndrome. *Neurology* 2001; **57**(12): 2304–2307.

Case 4.5

50-year-old engineer, previously in good health, reports incoordination, difficulties with vision, and ataxia slowly progressing over the past several months. Approximately 1 week ago he had presented to a local clinic with an acute onset of vertigo and vomiting (lasting 1 to 2 hours), after which he was relatively unresponsive and remained so for about 24 hours. Initially, it was thought that he had contracted a severe gastroenteritis with fluid loss. However, upon regaining consciousness, he was unable to open his eyes or keep his balance while walking. Vomiting and vertigo did not recur. There was no history of fever, trauma, or headache. Plain non-contrast CT of the head was unremarkable, though his failure to return to his baseline prompted a transfer to your hospital.

On your examination, his speech was slurred but he had no evidence of aphasia. Both eyes were infra and abducted suggesting bilateral third nerve (or nuclei) lesions. There was sustained horizontal nystagmus when he attempted to look at an object at the extreme right or left. His pupils were round, unequal, and not reactive to either light or accommodation. Finger-to-nose and heel-shin tests elicited an intention tremor. His gait was ataxic, wide-based, and lurching. The neurologic exam was otherwise normal.

Based on the present exam, where would you localize the lesion?

The combination of bilateral third nerve lesions and ataxia suggests lesion of the dorsal midbrain. This combination of signs and symptoms is referred to as the Nothnagel Syndrome (Derakhshan *et al.*, 1980). This is based on Nothnagel's remark in 1879 in a review of clinico-pathological data of lesions involving the quadrageminal plate. Nothnagel's concluding remarks on the syndrome were: "Bilateral, symmetrical lesions of specific branches of the oculomotorius indicates involvement of lamina quadrigemia, especially if there is no concomitant alternate paralysis of extremities ... It appears that with lesions of posterior gemini there are disturbances of balance and coordination that are very similar to those seen with lesions of the cerebellum. However, this point is not indisputable."

The close proximity of the oculomotor nuclear complex and the decussation of the superior cerebellar peduncles within the dorsal midbrain constitute the accepted anatomic basis of this syndrome.

MRI images are presented (Fig. 4.21). What does the imaging reveal?

These images reveal an enlarged quadrageminal plate likely representing a tectal glioma. This enlargement would be consistent with bilateral involvement of the third nerve roots and/or nuclei. The lack of pupillary constriction either in response to light or accommodation suggests involvement of the Edinger–Westphal nucleus and its fibers. This can be appreciated by reviewing the anatomy of each reflex. In the afferent limb of the light reflex, neural activity is transmitted from the retina through the optic nerve and optic tract to the pretectal region in the midbrain. Following synapse on neurons in the pretectal area, impulses are transmitted through the posterior commissure to both Edinger–Westphal nuclei in the oculomotor complex. Efferent parasympathetic preganglionic fibers travel along CN III to the orbit. There, they project to neurons of the ciliary ganglion. Postganglionic fibers originating from the ciliary ganglion directly innervate the sphincter pupillae and ciliaris muscles effecting pupillary constriction (Fig. 4.22).

Functionally, the Edinger–Westphal nucleus effects bilateral pupillary constriction when light is shone in either eye separately. The receiving eye represents the direct response, whereas the contralateral eye represents the consensual response. This is possible because of pretectal projections to both oculomotor nuclei.

In this particular case, your patient fails to constrict either pupil with a direct or consensual response. This suggests either a lesion of one optic nerve or a bilateral lesion involving the Edinger–Westphal nuclei or their efferent fibers. To further localize the lesion, it is helpful to attempt elicit an accommodation-convergence reflex. This reflex is employed when viewing objects at a close distance and involves: (1) accommodation of the lens, described as a thickening of its convexity to sharpen focus, (2) contraction of the bilateral medial recti to converge the eyes into alignment, and (3) bilateral pupillary constriction to aid in regulating the depth of field. It is thought that the afferent pathway for this reflex originates in the retina and projects to the occipital cortex. The efferent limb projects to the oculomotor nuclei after synapsing in the pretectal nucleus and/or superior colliculi (Figs. 4.23 and 4.24).

This pathway is distinct from the pathways forming the light reflex (light near dissociation), a fact that can be clinically demonstrated in a condition known as Argyll Robertson pupil. In this condition, caused by syphilis, a patients' light reflex is lost, whereas the accommodation-convergence reflex remains intact.

Detailed clinical descriptions of the Nothnagel syndrome are rare, partly due to the rarity of its occurrence. Although the occurrence of cerebellar damage in this patient remains a possibility, the cerebellar findings can also be explained by tegmental midbrain damage. Tegmental lesions can disrupt the decussation

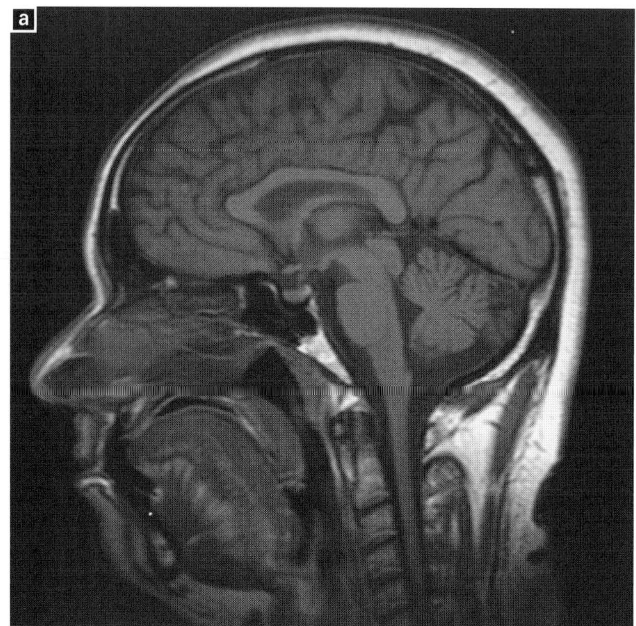
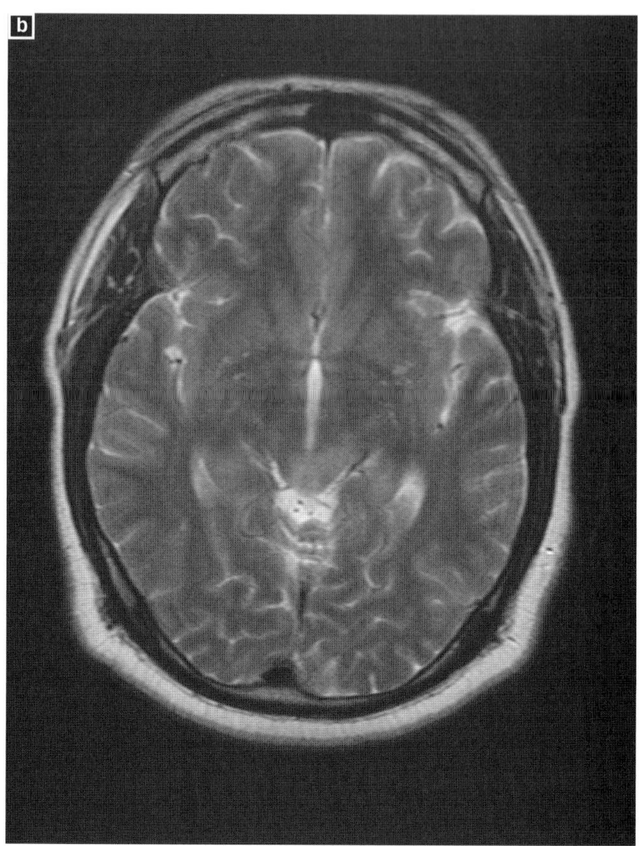

Fig. 4.21. **(a) Sagittal T1 and (b) axial T2-weighted images through the brainstem reveal marked enlargement of the midbrain tectum on T1 with abnormal hyperintensity on T2.**

of the superior cerebellar peduncles causing either ipsi- or contralateral ataxia. Partial ophthalmoplegia, ataxia and dysarthria in the absence of a cerebellar lesion, have been reported in patients with vascular lesions involving this region (Cogan, 1974; Jacobs *et al.*, 1973; Reagan, 1978). The occurrence of nystagmus in the presence of a complete third nerve palsy can be explained by phasic contraction, followed by relaxation, of the unopposed lateral rectus muscle in each eye.

References

Cogan, D. G. Paralysis of downgaze. *Archives in Ophthalmology* 1974; **91**: 192–199.

Derakhshan, I., Sabouri-Deylami, M., and Kaufman, B. Bilateral Nothnagel syndrome. Clinical and roentgenological observations. *Stroke* 1980; **11**(2): 177–179.

Jacobs, L., Anderson, P. G., and Bender, M. B. The lesion producing paralysis of downward but not upward gaze. *Archives of Neurology* 1973; **28**: 319–323.

Nothnagel, H. Corpora Quadrigemina. In *Gehirnkrankheiten, Eine Klinische Studie*, 1879; Berlin, Verlag: Von August Hirschwald, 204–220.

Reagan, T. J. Combined nuclear and supranuclear defects in ocular motility: a clinico-pathologic study. *Archives of Neurology* 1978; **35**: 133–137.

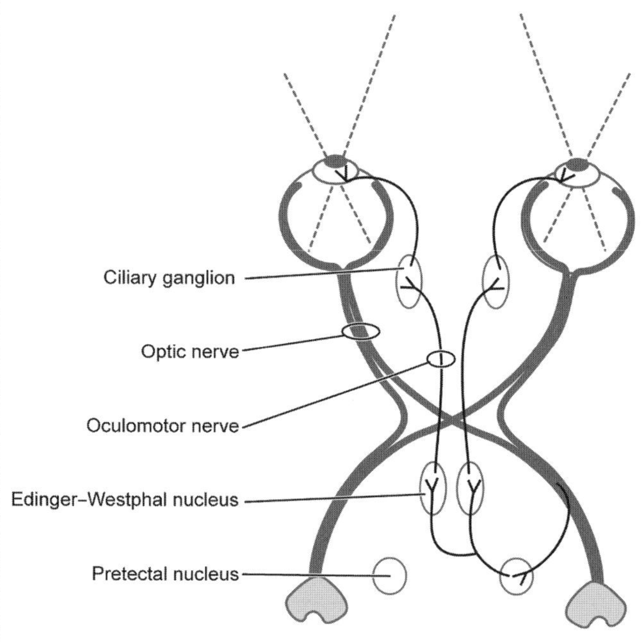

Fig. 4.22. **The pupillary light reflex.**

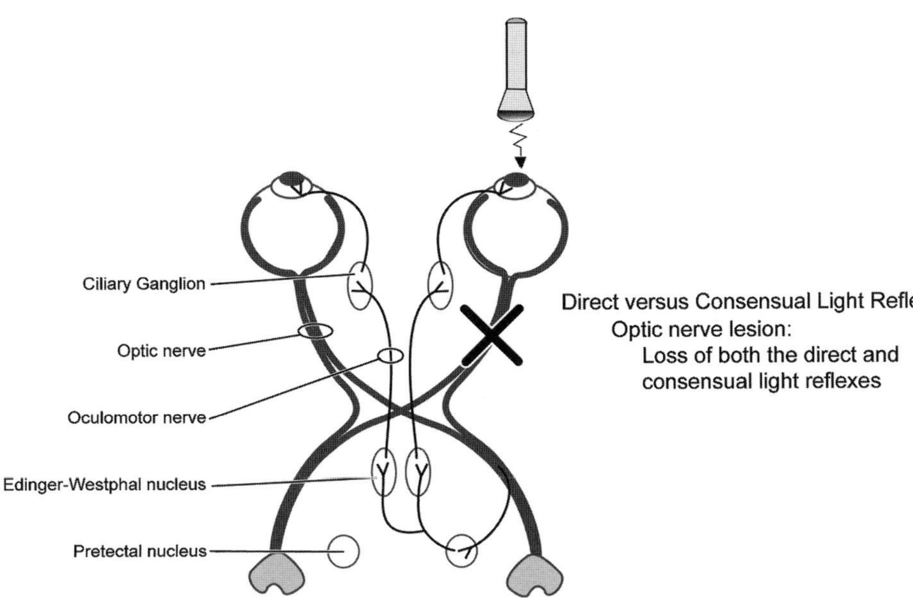

Fig. 4.23. **Optic nerve lesion affecting the pupillary light reflex. Note the loss of both the direct and consensual light reflex when the light is shone in the affected eye.**

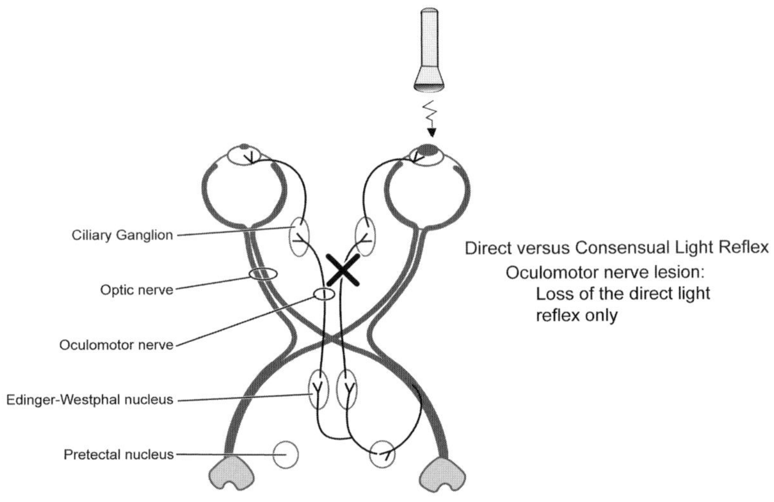

Fig. 4.24. **Oculomotor nerve lesion. Note that light shone in the affected eye results in loss of the direct but not the consensual light reflex.**

Case 4.6

28-year-old librarian comes to your office reporting an approximate 6-month history of headache. She states that she has headaches fairly frequently, mostly associated with job stress, thus she did not think too much of them at the time. Initially, they responded to over-the-counter analgesics, but this has not been the case for the last several months. Other than tension type headaches, this is unusual for her. She has no other significant past medical history, takes no other medications, and has no known allergies.

On further questioning, she states that the headaches have a throbbing character, occasionally waking her up at night, and tend to be severe in the early AM. There is clearly an exacerbation of the pain on coughing, sneezing, or Valsalva. She states that sitting upright helps alleviate the pain, standing and walking around even more so. However, she has quit exercising as any strenuous physical activity also increases the pain intensity.

She has been tolerating these symptoms until recently, upon noting another peculiar phenomenon. Specifically, she reports

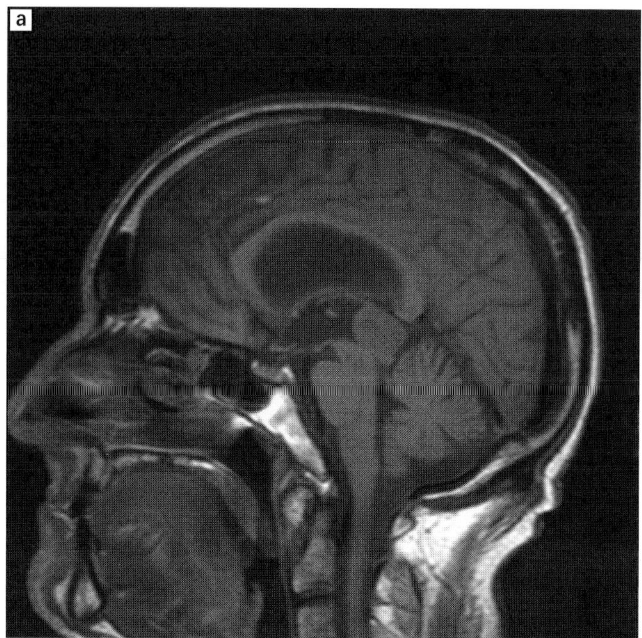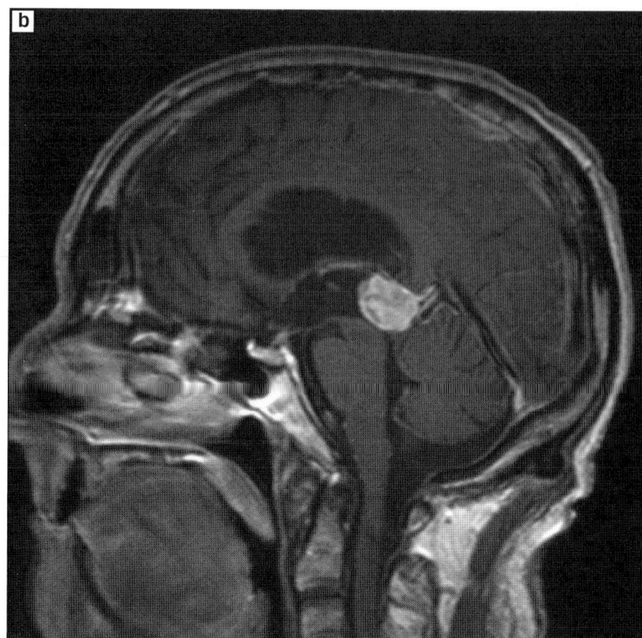

Fig. 4.25. **(a)** Pre- and **(b)** post-contrast sagittal T1-weighted images through the brainstem show a large enhancing mass involving the pineal gland and impinging the midbrain tectum.

that she is now having difficulties returning books to the upper shelves. Any shelves above her head give her difficulty, and she notes having to lean her head back in an effort to identify the correct area for replacing books. At first, she thought this unusual, though the result of her headaches. But now, she tells you that she is also unable to see stoplights as she approaches the intersection unless she tilts her head back in similar fashion.

There are several notable findings on your examination. Her ophthalmic examination is significant for evidence of papilledema with blurred disc margins and reduced venous pulsations. Moreover, she has bilateral, symmetric midriasis, with 5 mm pupils poorly reactive to light. Interestingly, her pupils did constrict during accommodation. Her horizontal eye movements were intact, as was downgaze. However, when asked to look up, either voluntarily or with target pursuit, she was unable to do so. Attempts at upgaze elicited a peculiar finding of lid retraction, in combination with convergence nystagmus.

On the basis of the presenting symptoms, as well as your examination, where would you localize the lesion?

The key symptoms and signs in this patient include her headache, midriasis with light-near dissociation, impaired upgaze, and lid retraction with convergence-retraction nystagmus. This patient has classic Parinaud syndrome. The most typical lesion location for this syndrome involves the dorsal midbrain and pretectal area. Given the slowly progressive course, an expanding neoplasm would be a likely etiology.

What does the imaging reveal (Fig. 4.25)?

The mid-sagittal MRI clearly demonstrates a large, enhancing midline lesion with clear compression of the rostrodorsal midbrain. This is likely to be a tumor of the pineal gland, for example, a pineocytoma. In sorting the signs and symptoms with the neuroanatomy, it is likely that the headache is due, at least in part, to partially obstructive hydrocephalus. Ventricular dilatation can clearly be appreciated in these mid-sagittal images. This is also supported by the positional nature of her symptoms, as well as its exacerbation with an increase in intra-abdominal/thoracic

pressure. Let's consider the remainder of her examination. First, she exhibits severely impaired vertical gaze. Unlike control of horizontal eye movements, which are principally controlled in the pons and brainstem, vertical gaze control is mediated in the rostral midbrain, near the mesencephalic–diencephalic junction.

When eyes are affected bilaterally, as in this case, it is believed the localization resides in the posterior commissure where upgaze fibers from the interstitial nuclei decussate en route to the oculomotor nuclei (Michielsen *et al.*, 2002). Further, your examination reveals light-near dissociation, a phenomenon describing the condition when pupils constrict in response to accommodation more than to light. The classic description of this phenomenon is in neurosyphilis (Argyll–Robertson pupil). However, nothing in the history would suggest this as an etiology, and it has also been described in midbrain compression syndromes, which fits this case perfectly. Though the precise mechanisms are not known, the likely localization is also compression of the posterior commissure, as fibers from the optic tract travel through this structure prior to synapsing in the Edinger–Westphal nuclei. Your patient's lid retraction on upgaze (Collier sign) and convergence nystagmus, also localizes to the pretectal area.

Though MRI is not definitive in diagnosing the pineal gland tumor type, it remains an important diagnosis. A variety of pathologies involving the pineal gland may give rise to Parinaud syndrome (also known as pretectal syndrome or, with the addition of anisocoria, Koerber–Salus–Elschnig syndrome). Various histological types of tumors arise in the pineal region, most commonly pineal parenchymal tumors and germ cell tumors (Hirato and Nakazato, 2001). Parenchymal tumors are divided into pineocytoma (Fig. 4.25), pineal parenchymal tumor with intermediate differentiation, and pineoblastoma (Patil *et al.*, 1995). Pineocytomas are well differentiated. In contrast, pineoblastomas are embryonal tumors resembling primitive neuroectodermal tumors (PNET). Although pineal cysts are tumor-like lesions, and not true neoplasms, they are occasionally difficult

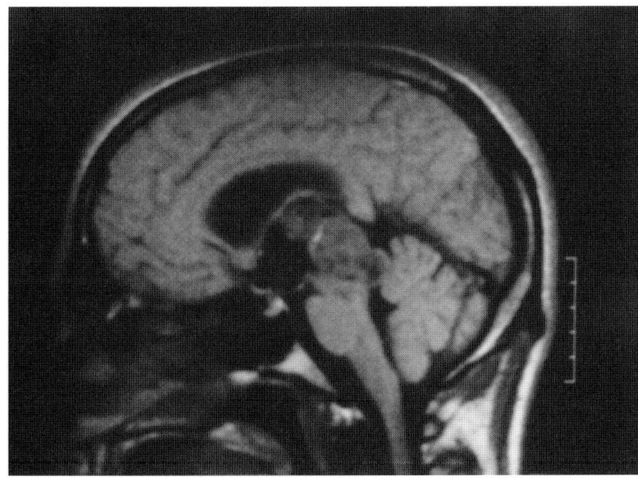

Fig. 4.26. **Poor-quality pre-contrast sagittal T1-weighted image through the brainstem shows a large, heterogeneous mass involving the pineal gland in this patient with pineal teratoma.**

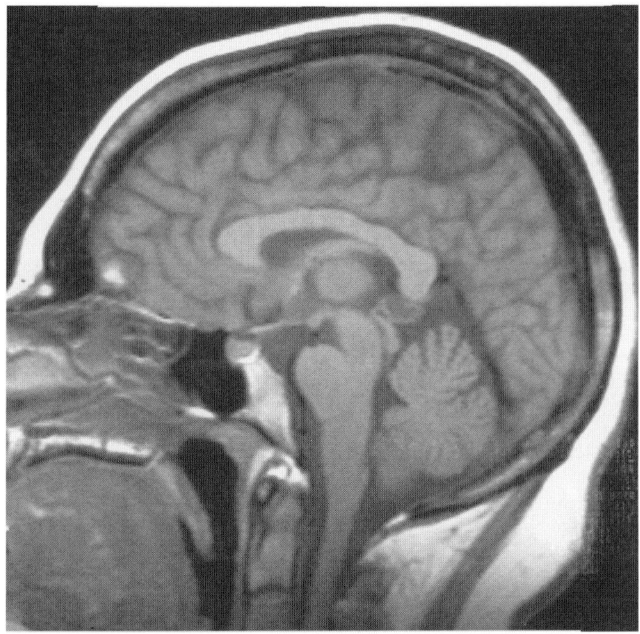

Fig. 4.27. **Sagittal T1-weighted image reveals a small pineal cyst. This was asympomatic, as such cysts usually are.**

to distinguish from pineocytoma and astrocytoma. From a therapeutic aspect, a precise differential diagnosis is critical. The pineal region is the most common site of the brain in which germ cell tumors occur. The most frequent presenting symptom is due to increased intracranial pressure (90 percent), followed by Parinaud syndrome or diplopia (50 percent) (Cho *et al.*, 1998). The overall mean survival time with pineal tumors is 66 months and the 3-year survival rate is 84 percent with minimal post-treatment complications (Jouvet *et al.*, 2000). Pineal region tumors can be approached safely and effectively surgically. Their prognosis is dependent on the pathologies and treatment modalities. Though not arising from the pineal gland, similar symptomatology may be seen

from tumors arising in the tectal plate (Daglioglu *et al.*, 2003; Ternier *et al.*, 2006; Stark *et al.*, 2005). As treatment and prognosis differ, appropriate imaging studies are imperative in evaluating tumor origin.

Although rare, teratomas of the pineal gland have also been described. Growing teratoma syndrome is a mixed germ cell tumor with a secreting portion that responds to chemotherapy and a non-secreting portion of mature teratoma that continues to grow despite chemotherapy (Hanna *et al.*, 2000). Findings may include elevation of the tumor marker HCG (human chorionic gonadotrophin) in CSF and serum. Following chemotherapy, MRI may show an increase in tumor size with morphologic modifications (Fig. 4.26) despite normalization of HCG in CSF and serum. MRI often demonstrates that the tumor has a heterogeneous signal enhancement. Therapeutic approaches to these tumors include surgical resection and radiotherapy.

In addition to neoplastic pathologies involving the pineal gland, pineal cysts can form and create pathologies such as hydrocephalus, Parinaud syndrome, Collier sign and Koerber–Salus–Elschnig syndrome. Although pineal cysts are incidental findings in as many as 4 percent of magnetic resonance imaging studies, symptomatic pineal cysts are fairly rare (Maurer *et al.*, 1990). When symptomatic, manifestations typically include hydrocephalus from aqueductal stenosis with resultant headache and syncope (Michielsen *et al.*, 2002; Maurer *et al.*, 1990) (Fig. 4.27).

In one study series, 17 of 21 symptomatic pineal cysts were shown to contain hemorrhagic products, leading these investigators to conclude that intracystic bleeding may be the principal feature distinguishing symptomatic from asymptomatic cysts (Musolino *et al.*, 1993).

References

Cho, B. K., Wang, K. C., Nam, D. H. *et al.* Pineal tumors: experience with 48 cases over 10 years. *Childs Nervous System* 1998; **14**: 53–58.

Daglioglu, E., Cataltepe, O., and Akalan, N. Tectal gliomas in children: the implications for natural history and management strategy. *Pediatric Neurosurgery* 2003; **38**: 223–231.

Hanna, A., Edan, C., Heresbach, N., Ben Hassel, M., and Guegan, Y. Expanding mature pineal teratoma syndrome. *Case report. Neurochirurgie* 2000; **46**: 568–572.

Hirato, J. and Nakazato, Y. Pathology of pineal region tumors. *Neurooncology* 2001; **54**: 239–249.

Jouvet, A., Saint Pierre, G., Fauchon, F. *et al.* Pineal parenchymal tumors: a correlation of histological features with prognosis in 66 cases. *Brain Pathology* 2000; **10**: 49–60.

Maurer, P. K., Ecklund, J., Parisi, J. E., and Ondra, S. Symptomatic pineal cyst: case report. *Neurosurgery* 1990; **27**: 451–454.

Michielsen, G., Benoit, Y., Baert, E., Meire, F., and Caemaert, J. Symptomatic pineal cysts: clinical manifestations and management. *Acta Neurochirurgiea (Wien)* 2002; **144**(3): 233–242; discussion 242.

Musolino, A., Cambria, S., Rizzo, G., and Cambria, M. Symptomatic cysts of the pineal gland: stereotactic diagnosis and treatment of two cases and review of the literature. *Neurosurgery* 1993; **32**: 315–320.

Patil A. A., Good R., Bashir R., Etemadrezaie H. Nonresective treatment of pineoblastoma: a case report. *Surgical Neurology* 1995; **44**: 386–390; discussion 390–391.

Stark, A. M., Fritsch, M. J., Claviez, A., Dorner, L., and Mehdorn, H. M. Management of tectal glioma in childhood. *Pediatric Neurology* 2005; **33**: 33–38.

Ternier, J., Wray, A., Puget, S., Bodaert, N., Zerah, M., and Sainte-Rose, C. Tectal plate lesions in children. *Journal of Neurosurgery* 2006; **104**: 369–376.

5 | The basal ganglia

"Things should be made as simple as possible – but no simpler."
Albert Einstein

The coordination of movement in the central nervous system is a complex phenomenon, involving the integration of the corticospinal system with the guiding and modulating influences of the basal ganglia and the cerebellum, among other structures. In the broad scheme, we may distinguish four general types of motor disorders:

(1) Paralysis or weakness of voluntary movement.
(2) Hypokinesis without significant weakness.
(3) Hyperkinetic involuntary movements, such as choreoathetosis.
(4) Incoordination of movement (ataxia).

The second and third categories above have been equated with damage to the basal ganglia, and used to be called extrapyramidal movement disorders. This term, coined around 1912 by S. A. K. Wilson (of Wilson's disease fame), has since fallen into some disfavor, because the movement disorders associated with lesions of the basal ganglia are still expressed or mediated through the corticospinal tract. We, however, believe that it still provides a useful way to refer to movement disorders associated with the basal ganglia.

This chapter will explore some aspects of the functional neuroanatomy of the basal ganglia. Following this, we will review the neuroradiology of some pathologies of the basal ganglia. In doing so, we will undoubtedly fall short of Professor Einstein's maxim, probably by oversimplifying rather than by failing to simplify enough. Our excuse for this is threefold:

(a) While much has been learned in the past two or three decades about the functional neuroanatomy of the basal ganglia, in many cases a precise correlation between lesions and the resultant movement disorders still eludes us. That is probably because the function of the basal ganglia depends on a fine balance between inhibitory and excitatory pathways, using multiple neurotransmitters. This balance also involves a set of complex variables, including discharge rates and firing patterns of basal ganglia neurons, and a synchronization between the different components of the "extrapyramidal" movement system. Subtle disturbances in this balance then manifest in the various movement disorders which have come to be associated with basal ganglia lesions.

(b) It has become clear that the basal ganglia function in more than just motor control, with additional functions relating both to cognition and emotion now receiving increased attention.

(c) Even if our understanding of basal ganglia clinicopathologic correlation were quite specific, unfortunately, the neuroradiology of the various pathologic entities is not. The basal ganglia may be affected by lesions such as infarcts, bleeds, tumors, or infections. Also, they may undergo neurodegeneration as part of a variety of disorders. These degenerative changes (when they have associated imaging findings) have limited manifestations: atrophy and signal abnormalities. The signal abnormalities, as we shall see, tend to be abnormal T2-weighted hyperintensity (a fairly non-specific response), but may also be abnormal T2-weighted hypointensity, or less commonly, abnormal T1-weighted hyperintensity. In other words, among the numerous disorders which involve the basal ganglia, many are not easily detectable by imaging, while others have very similar imaging manifestations. Therefore, close clinical correlation becomes a key aspect of evaluating the patient who presents with a movement disorder.

With these caveats in mind, it should still be possible to make some useful points about the functional neuroanatomy of the basal ganglia, as well as the neuroradiology of many basal ganglia disorders.

Definition and nomenclature of the basal ganglia

The term "basal ganglia," from the clinical viewpoint of this chapter, will refer to the following structures: caudate nucleus, putamen, nucleus accumbens septi, globus pallidus, subthalamic nucleus, and substantia nigra (pars compacta and pars reticulata).

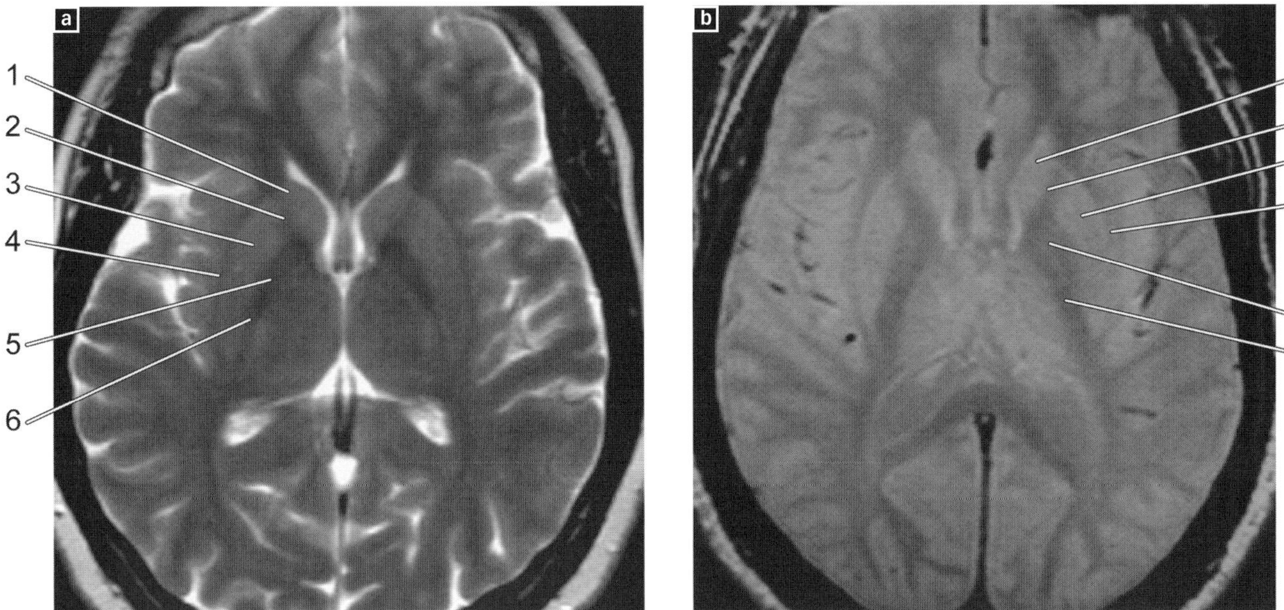

Fig. 5.1. **(a) Axial T2 and (b) proton density MRI images showing the normal anatomy of the basal ganglia. The caudate nuclei (arrow 1) invaginate the frontal horns of the lateral ventricles and are medial to the anterior limbs of the internal capsule (arrow 2). The putamen (arrow 3) is just medial to the external capsule (arrow 4). On the T2-weighted images, it is difficult to separate the globus pallidus (arrow 5) from the posterior limb of the internal capsule (arrow 6), but the structures are better delineated on the proton density image. The reason it is hard to separate them on T2 is that the posterior limb is dark because it is white matter, while the globus pallidus is dark because it has a higher iron content.**

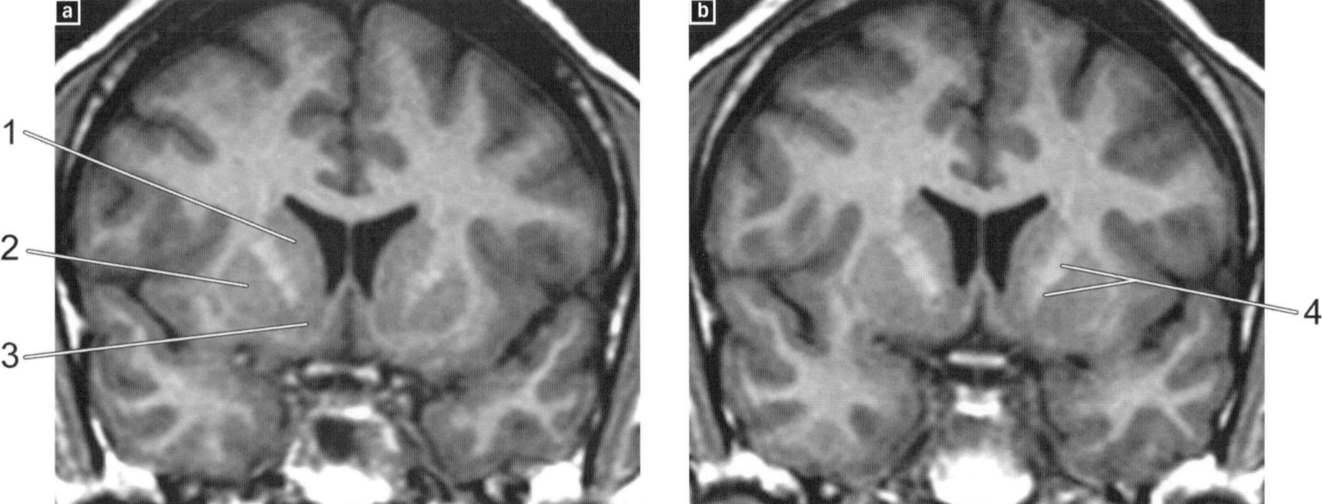

Fig. 5.2. **(a), (b) Coronal thin-slice T1-weighted images show the junction of the caudate head (arrow 1) with the anterior aspect of the putamen (arrow 2) in the region of the nucleus accumbens (arrow 3), a part of the ventral striatum. Arrow 4: anterior limb of internal capsule.**

The caudate nucleus is located medial to the internal capsule, and the caudate head indents the frontal horn of the lateral ventricle. The putamen is located lateral to the internal capsule, just medial to the external capsule. The caudate and the putamen share a common embryologic origin and are histologically identical. Small bridges of gray matter cross the anterior limb of the internal capsule to connect them, giving a sort of striated appearance. Thus, together the caudate and the putamen are called the *striatum*. At the anterior and inferior edge of the striatum, the head of the caudate is actually continuous with the anterior edge of the putamen. This area of continuity is called the *nucleus accumbens septi* (nucleus accumbens for short). Along with adjacent parts of the caudate, putamen and basal forebrain, the nucleus accumbens forms a separate functional division of the basal ganglia known as the *ventral striatum* (see Figs. 5.1 and 5.2).

The globus pallidus is emryologically and histologically distinct from the putamen. Anatomically, the globus pallidus is

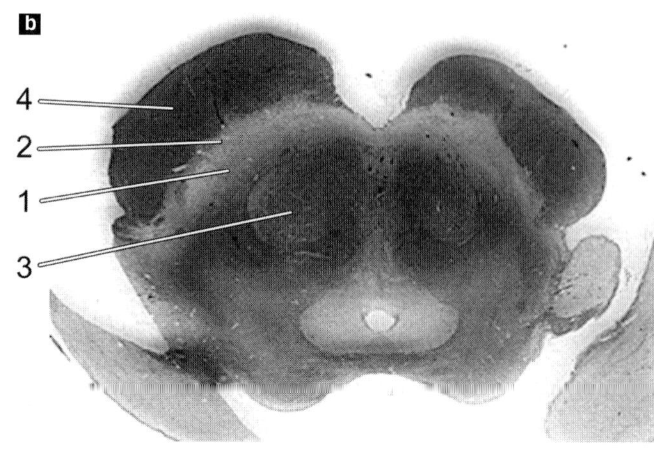

Fig. 5.3. **(a) Axial T2-weighted image of the midbrain of a showing the normal anatomy of the substantia nigra. The zona compacta of the substanti nigra (SNc) is seen as a relatively bright band (arrow 1) between the more ventral dark zona reticulata (SNr) (arrow 2) and the more dorsal dark red nucleus (arrow 3). Both the SNr, as an analog of the globus pallidus internal (GPi), and the red nucleus, have relatively high iron concentrations, making them hypointense on the T2-weighted images. Ventral to the SNr are the crural fibers of the cerebral peduncle (arrow 4). (b) A myelin-stained section through the midbrain for comparison.**

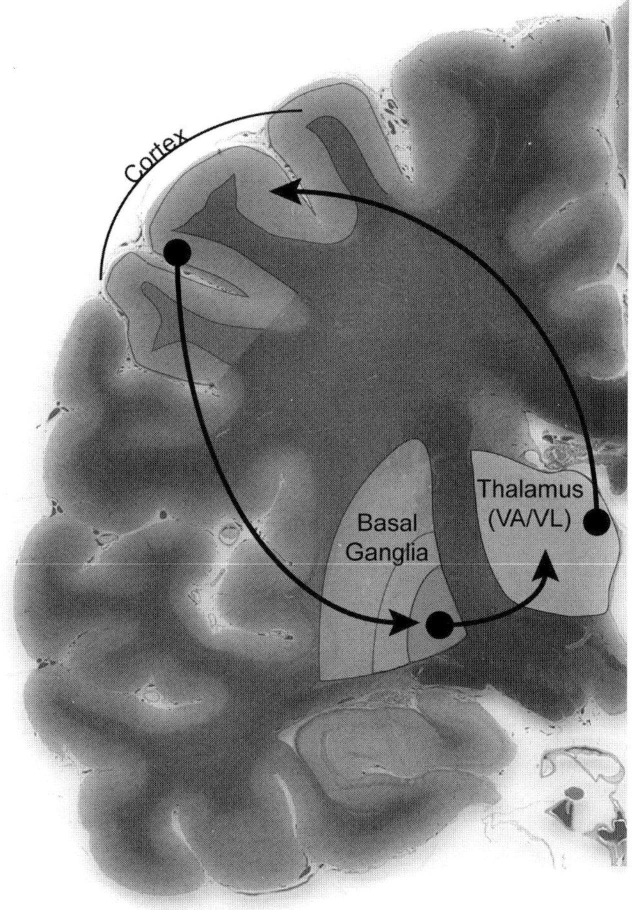

Fig. 5.4. **Connections of the basal ganglia. In very simplistic terms, the cortex projects to the basal ganglia, which project back to the cortex via the thalamus.**

just medial to the putamen. The lateral edge of the globus pallidus is separated from the putamen by a thin band of myelinated fibers called the lateral medullary lamina. The globus pallidus itself is divided into an external, or lateral, segment (globus pallidus externa or GPe) and an internal, or medial, segment (globus pallidus interna or GPi), which are separated from each other by the medial medullary lamina. Taken together, the putamen and the globus pallidus look like a wedge, and are referred to as the *lentiform nucleus*.

The substantia nigra is located in the midbrain, within the cerebral peduncles (Fig. 5.3). It is composed of two parts: a more ventral *pars reticulata* (SNr) and a more dorsal *pars compacta* (SNc). The SNr functions almost as an extension and an analog of the internal segment of the globus pallidus, known as the GPi, and will not be emphasized much in this chapter.

A general overview of basal ganglia connectivity

The basic scheme of basal ganglia connectivity is fairly straightforward. The basal ganglia function as part of a loop, where they receive inputs from the cortex and output back to the cortex (Fig. 5.4).

There are, in fact, multiple parallel cortex–basal ganglia loops, which will be touched upon shortly. For now, the main motor loop (which is thought to be integrally involved in the movement disorders associated with Parkinson's disease and Huntington's disease) will be used as the prototype for this simplified model of basal ganglia function.

The cortex–basal ganglia–cortex loop explains how the basal ganglia are able to impact motion. Although there are essentially no direct connections between the basal ganglia and the anterior motor horn cells of the spinal cord, the basal ganglia, prior to and during motor activity, receive massive inputs from the motor, sensory and premotor cortex. The response to these inputs is modulated by inputs from the SNc and the thalamus. The basal ganglia then output back to these same areas of cortex via the motor nuclei of the thalamus (the VA and VL). This output to the motor and premotor regions helps scale and focus motion, facilitating desired motions while suppressing unwanted motor activity, and helping to regulate the initiation, velocity and amplitude of the various components involved in complex movements.

A few facts about basal ganglia neurons

Prior to painting this picture in more detail, it is necessary to briefly describe the neuronal makeup of the striatum, which functions as the receptor field for cortical inputs and inputs from the SNc. The striatum is composed mostly of spiny neurons. These are also called projection neurons, because they will project outward, carrying the output of the striatum. These neurons use gamma-aminobutyric acid (GABA) as their principal neurotransmitter, and are hence inhibitory in function. The spiny neurons receive extensive "extrinsic" inputs from the cortex in the form of corticostriatal fibers, which predominantly use glutamate as their neurotransmitter, and are hence excitatory in function. The spiny neurons also receive extrinsic input from the SNc in the form of dopaminergic neurons. It turns out that there are at least six different types of dopamine receptors on the spiny neurons of the striatum and in the CNS in general, numbered D_1 through D_6. However, these have been grouped into two main families: D_1-like and D_2-like. In the striatum, the preponderance is of D_1 and D_2 receptors, while the other receptor groups predominate elsewhere. In this way, dopamine from the pars compacta of the substantia nigra is able to modulate the response of the striatum to cortical inputs, and to ultimately impact the motor pathway.

The spiny neurons also receive some "intrinsic" input from other spiny neurons, and a smaller population of striatal cells known as aspiny neurons. Some of the aspiny neurons use acetylcholine as their neurotransmitter, while others use GABA.

A slightly more detailed view of basal ganglia connectivity

The motor, premotor, supplementary motor, sensory, and sensory association areas of the cortex send inputs to the putamen, which are somtatotopically organized as face, arm, and leg fibers. These inputs, as described above, are excitatory. The putamen simultaneously receives modulating dopaminergic inputs from the SNc through the nigrostriatal pathway. In response to these inputs, the putamen outputs to the internal segment of the globus pallidus (GPi). The GPi then sends inhibitory GABA-ergic fibers to the VA and VL nuclei of the thalamus. These fibers need to cross the posterior limb of the internal capsule, and do so in the form of two fiber bundles, the *ansa lenticularis* and the *lenticular fasciculus*, which then join together to form the *thalamic fasciculus*, which enters the thalamus. The motor nuclei of the thalamus complete the loop by

sending excitatory fibers back to the motor and premotor cortex through the internal capsule.

The putamen, as noted above, outputs to the GPi. However, it does so in two distinct ways: via direct projections from the putamen to the GPi (known as the direct pathway) and via an indirect pathway. In the indirect pathway, the putamen projects to the external segment of the globus pallidus (GPe), which projects to the subthalamic nucleus (STN), which then projects to the GPi. Thus, the presence of a direct pathway and an indirect pathway turn the cortex–BG–cortex loop into two functional loops.

The direct pathway (Fig. 5.5): cortex–putamen–GPi–thalamus–cortex

In the direct pathway, impulses travel from the putamen directly to the internal segment of the globus pallidus, hence the name "direct pathway."

By looking at Fig. 5.5, we can trace out the function of the direct pathway, working backwards. The GPi sends inhibitory signals to the thalamus, which has excitatory output to the cortex. Thus, unregulated, the GPi would have a net inhibitory effect on the cortex. The putamen, however, sends inhibitory impulses to the GPi, thus lessening the inhibitory effect of the GPi. Therefore, the *direct pathway* has a net *excitatory* effect on the cortex. Or, more correctly, it facilitates neuronal activity in the motor cortex (remember we're using the motor loop as our prototype for BG connectivity).

The indirect pathway: cortex–putamen–GPe–STN–GPi–thalamus–cortex

In the indirect pathway, impulses make their way from the putamen to the GPi indirectly, via connections through the globus pallidus externa and the subthalamic nucleus (STN).

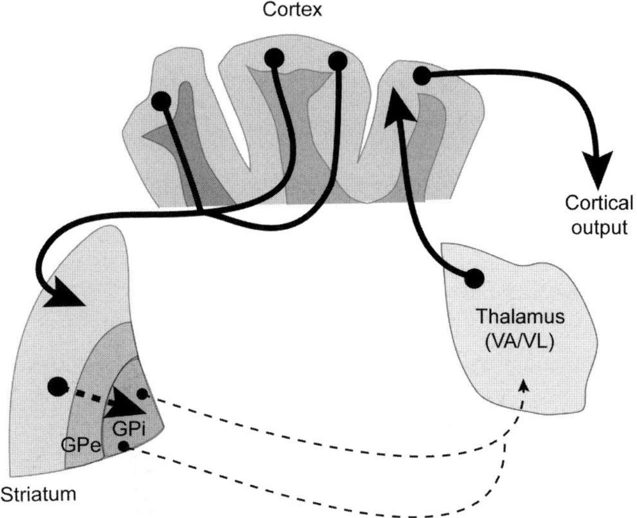

Fig. 5.5. **Diagram of the direct pathway. Excitatory pathways are solid, while inhibitory pathways are dashed. The thickness of the lines indicates the strength of the output.**

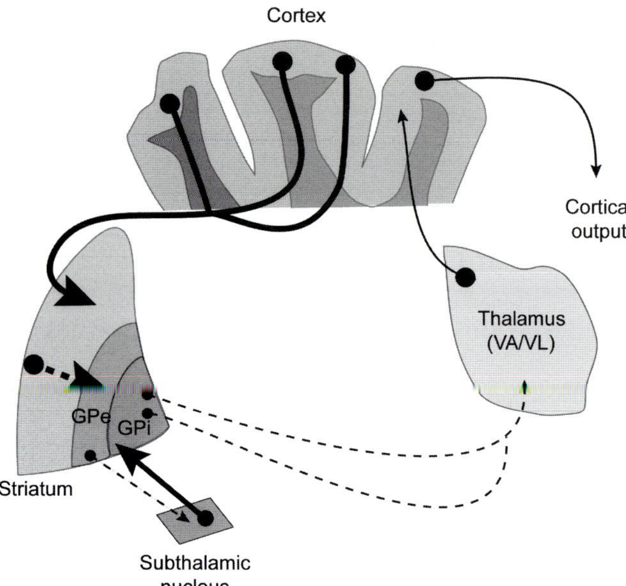

Fig. 5.6. **Diagram of the indirect pathway. Excitatory pathways are solid, while inhibitory pathways are dashed. The thickness of the lines indicates the strength of the output.**

By looking at Fig. 5.6, we can likewise trace out the effect of the indirect pathway.

The subthalamic nucleus (STN) sends excitatory signals to the GPi, thus increasing its inhibitory effect on the cortex. The GPe sends inhibitory impulses to the STN, so would lessen the inhibitory effect of the STN-GPi, and have a net excitatory effect on the cortex. However, the putamen sends impulses which inhibit the output of the GPe, thus ultimately inhibiting neuronal activity in the cortex. Therefore, the *indirect pathway* has a net *inhibitory* effect on the motor cortex.

Minor outputs of the basal ganglia motor loop

The major output of the GPi is to the thalamus, functioning to inhibit the excitatory thalamocortical circuit. However, there are also several other minor outputs, which may play a role in the clinical manifestations of movement disorder syndromes:

Pedunculopontine nucleus

There is some output of the GPi to the pedunculopontine nucleus of the midbrain. This nucleus has multiple connections and a variety of functions, among which is its involvement in the so-called mesencephalic locomotor region of the midbrain, which helps modulate gait. It receives its main input from the GPi (and the related SNr). Two main subdivisions of the PPN have been recognized: a pars compacta of the PPN (PPNc), located in the caudal part of the nucleus, and a second part known as the pars dissipatus (PPNd). Most of the PPNc neurons are cholinergic. The PPNd has a higher proportion of glutaminergic neurons. Neuropathologic studies in humans demonstrate a significant loss of cholinergic neurons in the PPNc in patients with progressive supranuclear palsy, idiopathic

Parkinson's disease and combined Parkinson's and Alzheimer's disease. The pedunculopontine nucleus also seems to play a role in such functions as sleep, motivation, and attention. Several movement disorder syndromes show disturbances in these spheres as well, and disruptions in this circuit may underlie some of the disturbances seen in Parkinson's disease (see, for example, Pahapill, P. and Lozano, A. The pedunculopontine nucleus and Parkinson's disease. *Brain* 2000; **123**: 1767–1783).

Superior colliculus

Outputs of the GPi also project to the superior colliculus, linking the basal ganglia to the spinal cord via the tectospinal tract, and to brainstem centers relating to head and eye movements via the tectoreticular tract. This connection may underlie some of the oculomotor manifestations of extrapyramidal movement disorders.

Other cortex–striatum loops and other basal ganglia functions

While we have used the motor loop through the putamen as our prototype for studying basal ganglia functional neuroanatomy, it is important to note that there are other cortex–basal ganglia loops which subtend other aspects of basal ganglia function. We will consider three striatal regions around which these loops are centered: the putamen, the caudate, and the ventral striatum.

In broad terms, while the putamen receives inputs from the motor cortical regions and is involved in movement, the caudate nucleus functions as the input field of the striatum for outputs coming from the association areas of the frontal lobes. The caudate also receives modulating dopaminergic axons from the SNc. The caudate then projects back to the prefrontal areas through the GPi and thalamus. Thus, the caudate nucleus is much more involved in cognitive tasks than motor tasks, and probably plays a significant role in the cognitive manifestations of Parkinson's disease and Huntington's disease.

The ventral striatum, meanwhile, receives its major inputs from limbic cortex, and outputs back to limbic cortex. Thus, the ventral striatum plays a role in emotional and drive-related behaviors, and the limbic cortex–ventral striatum loop may be involved in some of the psychiatric manifestations of basal ganglia disorders. This loop is also thought to be involved in Tourette's syndrome.

Neuroanatomists have further refined the generalizations above by discovering at least five separate cortico-striato-thalamo-cortical loops. The motor loop has been discussed above, and is centered on the putamen. Other loops include the following.

Dorsolateral prefrontal loop

This loop is centered on the caudate, with inputs from the dorsolateral prefrontal cortex and posterior parietal cortex. The caudate outputs back to these regions via the GPi and and the thalamus. The thalamic nuclei of this loop are the ventral anterior and dorsomedial nuclei.

Oculomotor loop

This loop is also centered on the caudate. Cortical inputs to the caudate come from the frontal eye fields and dorsolateral frontal lobes. The caudate outputs to the GPi, which projects to the ventral anterior and dorsomedial nuclei of the thalamus. The thalamus then projects back to the frontal eye fields.

Lateral orbitofrontal loop

This loop is connected similarly to the oculomotor, but with cortical inputs to the caudate (and cortical outputs of the thalamus) originating in the lateral orbitofrontal cortex.

Limbic loop

Projections from the anterior cingulate gyrus, medial orbitofrontal cortex, and the temporal lobe, including the hippocampal formations, input to the ventral striatum, which projects to the dorsomedial nucleus of the thalamus. The dorsomedial nucleus, in turn, projects back to the anterior cingulate and medial orbitofrontal cortices.

Like the motor loop, each of these loops has a direct pathway to the GPi, and an indirect pathway to the GPi through the GPe and the subthalamic nucleus. The direct pathway functions to facilitate or excite neuronal activity in the target cortex, while the indirect pathway inhibits the excitatory thalamocortical connections to the target cortex, thus having a net inhibitory effect on the cortex.

While we are still a long way from detailed understanding, we can now begin to fathom the multiple facets of disorders such as Parkinson's disease or Huntington's disease, and appreciate that they are not just motor disorders, but that they also have prominent cognitive and emotional components.

Now, let us take some cases.

Case 5.1

55-year-old male presents with a 2-year history of progressive left arm stiffness and a 1-year history of some difficulty walking, with dragging of the left foot. He has also begun to notice some right arm stiffness. He has been experiencing increased difficulty with routine tasks, such as buttoning his shirt. Examination reveals some cogwheel rigidity of the elbow, as well as a resting tremor of the left hand. There is some decrease in facial expression, and gait testing reveals a decreased left arm swing and some dragging of the left foot, and mild rigidity of the right wrist and elbow.

What is your differential?

The patient presents with bilateral but asymmetric rigidity, left-sided bradykinesia, and a resting tremor. The picture could be consistent with parkinsonism, especially early Parkinson's disease. However, in the early stages, it may still be non-specific.

Describe briefly the main clinical features of Parkinson's disease.

Parkinson's disease is characterized by four main clinical features:

– *resting tremor*: this is the most common clinical feature, seen in nearly 70 percent of the patients. It may be present in one or more limbs, with a frequency of 4–6 cycles per second. In the hand, it often assumes a characteristic "pill-rolling" movement.
– *bradykinesia*: this indicates slowness of movement
– *rigidity*: this typically assumes a "cogwheel" character when passive movement is attempted.
– *postural instability*: this is typically a late feature of Parkinson's disease.

Other clinical features include a stooped posture, masked facies, a shuffling gait, speaking in a low voice (hypophonia) and making small letters while writing (micrographia).

It is noted that asymmetery of the signs and symptoms is *highly characteristic* of early Parkinson's diease.

The age of onset is typically in the 50s and 60s. Onset before age 25 is unusual, but 5–10 percent of patients will have disease onset before age 40.

How is the diagnosis made?

The diagnosis of Parkinson's disease is a clinical one. There are, in general, no blood tests or imaging tests by which to make the diagnosis. The most reliable predictors are asymmetry of symptoms, presence of a resting tremor, and a positive response to levodopa.

What causes Parkinson's disease?

The proximate cause is a marked degeneration of the dopaminergic neurons of the pars compacta of the substantia nigra. When 60–80 percent of these neurons are lost, the symptoms of Parkinson's disease begin to appear. The primary causes (i.e., why do the dopaminergic neurons of the SNc degenerate?) remain elusive, but some comments will be made below. Tremendous research on possible environmental factors has failed to yield any definite environmental cause, other than MPTP, the heroin/mepiridine analog accidentally synthesized in an illicit drug laboratory. This has been shown to cause degeneration of the dopaminergic neurons of the SNc essentially identical to Parkinson's disease. Interestingly, cigarette smoking and coffee drinking have been shown to decrease the risk of Parkinson's disease (finally some good news for the chain-smoking coffee-holics in the crowd!).

Regarding the role of genetics, there has been some extremely interesting work over the past decade, with isolation of several "Parkinson" genes, which cause Parkinson's disease in certain small subsets. Among these are a mutation in the alpha-synuclein gene on chromosome 4q21–23 (also called the PARK1 gene). This mutation is extremely rare, but may open the door to some understanding of the pathophysiology behind Parkinson's. PARK2 through PARK10 genes or loci have also been described very recently. Several of these mutations have to do with a protein degradation pathway in cells known as the ubiquitin proteasome pathway. Genetic defects in this pathway appear to result in abnormal protein accumulation, which may lead to cell damage.

Discuss the functional neuroanatomy of the basal ganglia in the setting of Parkinson's disease.

As stated, Parkinson's disease involves the loss of dopaminergic inputs from the pars compacta of the substantia nigra to the putamen. These dopaminergic inputs have two functions:

(a) They normally *stimulate* the *direct* pathway described above. That is because the direct pathway projection neurons of the putamen have a preponderance of D1 dopamine receptors, for which dopamine functions as an excitatory neurotransmitter.

(b) However, dopaminergic inputs to the putamen tend to *inhibit* the function of the *indirect* pathway. That is because there is a predominance of D2 receptors in the putaminal projection neurons of the indirect pathway, and dopamine has an inhibitory effect on neurons with D2 receptors.

Both by stimulating the direct pathway (which is excitatory to motor cortex) and inhibiting the indirect pathway (which is inhibitory to motor cortex), the dopaminergic input from

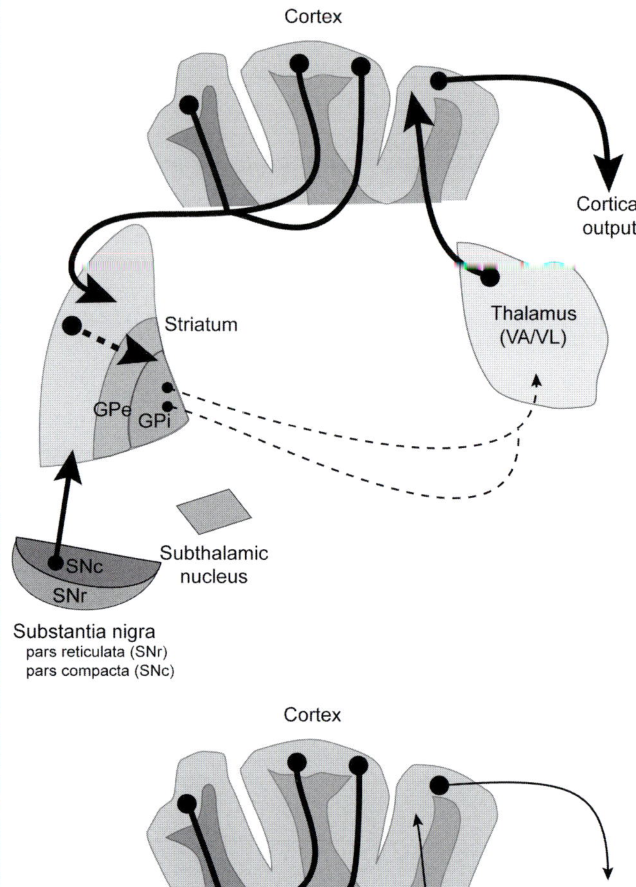

Fig. 5.7. **Top: normal function of the direct pathway, with D1 input to the putamen from the SNc. Bottom: loss of D1 dopaminergic neurons of the SNc in Parkinson's disease leads to net decreased activity in the direct pathway. This is due to decreased inhibition of the GPi by the GPe. With less inhibitory inputs coming to it, the GPi is more free to send inhibitory outputs to the thalamus. Excitatory pathways are solid, while inhibitory pathways are dashed. The thickness of the lines indicates the strength of the output.**

the SNc to the putamen functions to facilitate motor cortex activity.

With Parkinson's disease (see Figs. 5.7 and 5.8), there is degeneration of the dopaminergic neurons of the SNc. This has two synergistic effects: it diminishes the excitatory input to the direct pathway, and diminishes the inhibitory input to the indirect pathway (thus increasing activity in the indirect pathway). Both of these effects lead to a net inhibitory effect (compared to baseline) in the motor cortex. Once again, this is because the direct pathway has a net excitatory effect on the motor cortex, while the indirect pathway has a net inhibitory effect on the motor cortex. Thus, when the direct pathway output is diminished and the indirect pathway output is enhanced, both of these factors tend to have a net inhibitory effect on the motor cortex. This is thought to underlie the bradykinesia and rigidity characteristic of Parkinson's disease.

Discuss the pathologic hallmarks of Parkinson's disease.

As mentioned, there is significant loss of the dopaminergic neurons of the SNc, as well as loss of the neuromelanin normally found in the SNc. Within the remaining neurons, there are characteristic inclusions known as Lewy bodies. These are eosinophilic hyaline cytoplasmic inclusions, characteristic of, but not completely exclusive to, Parkinson's disease. They may be the result of neuronal damage.

Although outside our scope, briefly describe the neurochemistry of Parkinson's disease.

Parkinson's disease is a primary dopamine deficiency. Dopamine is made from tyrosine, through the action of the enzyme tyrosine hydroxylase, which hydroxylates tyrosine into L-DOPA. This is the rate-limiting step in the synthesis of dopamine. L-DOPA is acted upon by an aromatic amino acid decarboxylase, and turned into dopamine. Dopamine, once formed, is metabolized by two enzymes: monoamine oxidase B (MAO-B) which acts inside the neuron, and catechol-O-methyltransferase, which acts outside the neuron.

Dopamine is also deactivated by reuptake into the neurons via a dopamine transporter.

Even this rudimentary review allows us to understand a bit about the major categories of drug therapy for Parkinson's disease:

- *Levodopa*: this is L-DOPA, the precursor of dopamine. Dopamine itself does not cross the blood–brain barrier. Therefore, its precursor, levodopa, is administered as an oral medication to help increase the low levels of brain dopamine. Levodopa is taken up by the CNS and synthesized into dopamine.
- *Dopamine agonists*: these medications "substitute" for dopamine and activate the dopaminergic neurons of the striatum. Some of these are bromocriptine, pergolide, ropinirole, and pramipexole.
- *Inhibitors of MAO and COMT*: These limit the breakdown of dopamine, thereby increasing available levels. These include such medications as selegiline, tolcapone, and enacapone.
- *Anticholinergics*: As mentioned in the introductory section, the striatum also contains cholinergic neurons. Therefore, in some sense, the decrease of dopaminergic input to the striatum may be viewed as a relative excess of acetylcholine. Therefore, anticholinergics may also have a role to play in Parkinson's therapy.

It is also important to remember that drugs which antagonize dopamine, or act as dopamine blockers, can induce parkinsonism. Such drugs include numerous antipsychotic/neuroleptic medications, such as chlorpromazine or haloperidol. Also, the gastrointestinal motility drug metochlopramide causes dopamine antagonism.

Finally, understanding something about the neurochemistry of dopamine allows us to touch upon one of the leading hypotheses of the causes of neuronal degeneration in Parkinson's disease: the

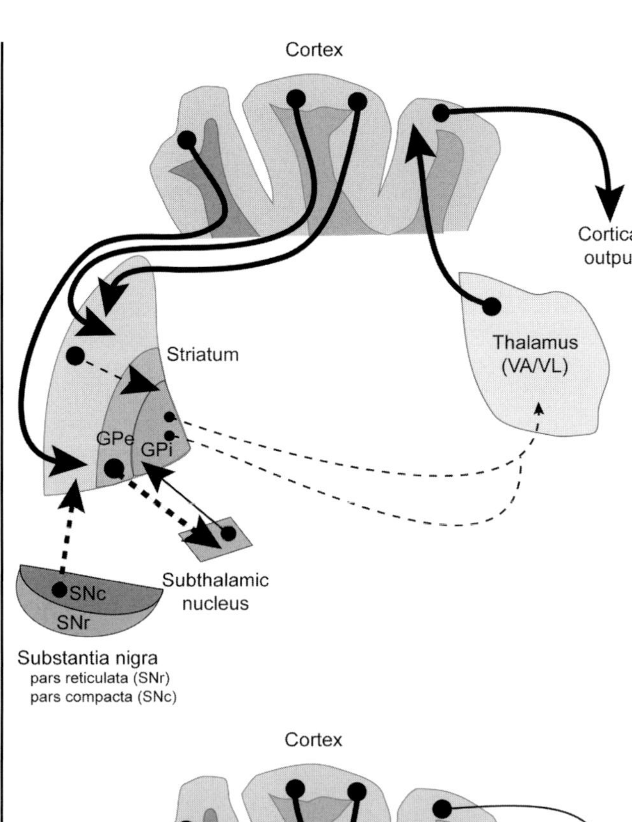

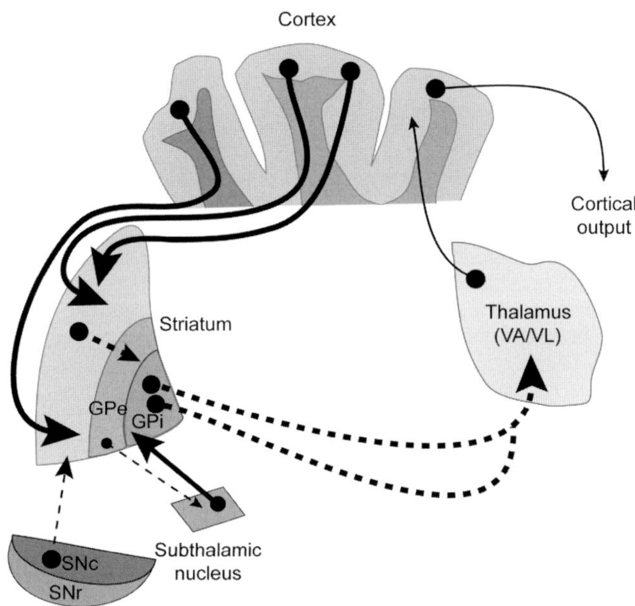

Fig. 5.8. **Top: normal function of the indirect pathway with D2 input to the putamen from the SNc. Bottom: loss of D2 dopaminergic neurons in Parkinson's disease leads to net increased activity in the indirect pathway. Decreased D2 inhibition of the dopaminergic receptor fields in the putamen causes more inhibitory inputs to the GPe. This lessens its inhibitory effect on the STN. The STN now more strongly excites the GPi, which send stronger inhibitory signals to the thalamus. Excitatory pathways are solid, while inhibitory pathways are dashed. The thickness of the lines indicates the strength of the output.**

dopamine oxidative stress hypothesis. As stated, dopamine is broken down by MAO-B. One of the products of this oxidative breakdown is hydrogen peroxide. The hydrogen peroxide is normally cleared by a glutathione. If the glutathione protective mechanism is overwhelmed, hydrogen peroxide can be reduced by the addition of an electron to a reactive hydroxyl free radical, which can cause cellular damage. The oxidation reactions above are facilitated by the presence of iron, which contributes electrons, as well as by copper and manganese.

It has been found that glutathione is indeed decreased in the brains of Parkinson's disease patients. Also, there is an increase of iron in the SNc of Parkinson's disease patients. The link between the glutathione–oxidative stress mechanism, the new information about "Parkinson's genes" and the role of the ubiquitin proteasome pathway is not clear at present.

Look at the MRI images of our patient. Images through the substantia nigra are presented and compared to a normal control (Fig. 5.9). Describe the anatomy of the midbrain in the normal control. What are the findings in the patient with Parkinson's disease? What is the role of imaging in the diagnosis of Parkinson's disease?

The late appearance of images in this case presentation should clue us in that MRI does not play a significant role in diagnosing Parkinson's disease. However, multiple studies have been published on the MR imaging of Parkinson's disease, with the main abnormality noted on MR imaging being a decrease in the width of the SNc (see Figure 5.10 and see, for example, Duguid *et al.*, 1986)

Less commonly, small areas of T2 hyperintensity can be noted in the SNc (see, for example, Braffman *et al.*, 1988), but this is a difficult call due to the presence of perivascular (VR) spaces in the midbrain which are also hyperintense on T2.

It must be noted, though, that significant overlap exists between normals and abnormals, such that MRI is not a particularly useful diagnostic tool. In fact, a recent and careful study of MR imaging of the SN failed to find a difference in the width of the SNc between Parkinson's patients and controls (Oikawa *et al.*, 2002).

There are, however, rare circumstances when the substantia nigra specifically is involved by other pathology, and in these circumstances, MRI imaging is very useful. One such rare circumstance is involvement of the substantia nigra by Japanese encephalitis, leading to parkinsonism (see Fig. 5.11(a) and Pradhan *et al.*, 1999). We note that Japanese encephalitis does not usually present in this fashion, and that this is a rare manifestation. Another rare disease which may specifically involve the substantia nigra is St. Louis encephalitis. Rather than rigidity and bradykinesia, though, these patients tend to present with fever and severe tremors (see Fig. 5.11(b) and Cerna *et al.*, 1999).

Much interesting work is being done in PET imaging of movement disorders, especially Parkinson's disease. At this time, such work is considered investigational, but seems very promising. PET is able to provide neurochemical assessments of dopamine in the brain, using various dopamine analogs. This is generally done using either presynaptic or postsynaptic dopaminergic ligands.

Assessing presynaptic dopaminergic function can be done using [18F]-6-fluoroDOPA, which is a DOPA analog. It gets metabolized to [18F]-fluorodopamine and is stored in presynaptic dopaminergic nerve endings. Other presynaptic ligands target the dopamine transporter protein complex, thus assessing the amount of dopamine reuptake in the presynaptic nerve endings as an indirect measure of their density. Finally, a new ligand called ^{11}C dihydroteterabenazine (DTBZ) is aimed at the type 2 vesicular monoamine transporter, expressed by neurons using dopamine. It can be used to assess dopaminergic function in the striatum.

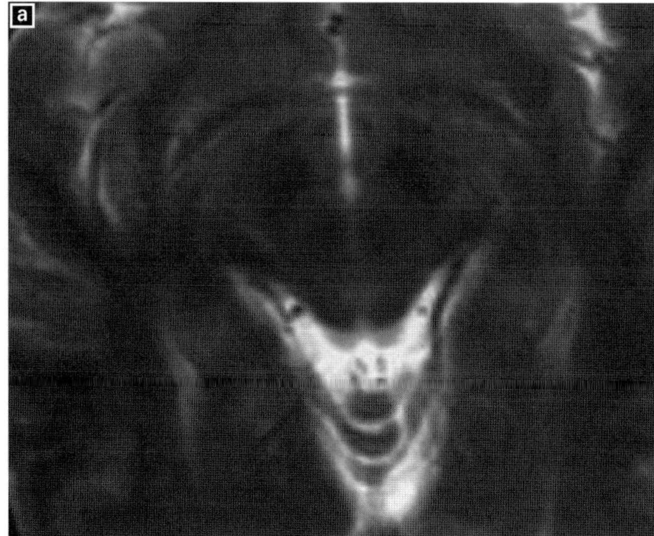
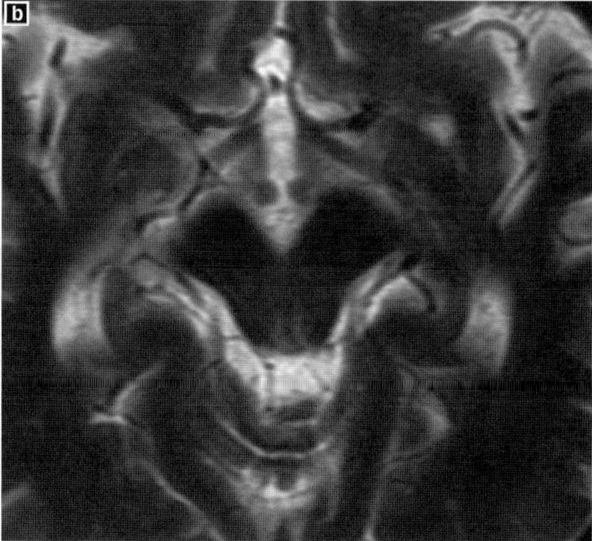

Fig. 5.9. **(a) T2-weighted axial images a normal subject. The zona compacta of the substantia nigra (SNc) is the bright band just anterior to the dark red nucleus. The dark band anterior to the SNc is the zona reticulata of the substantia nigra (SNr). As you recall, the SNr is an analog of the GPi, and so also contains iron, making it dark on T2-weighted images. (b) T2 axial image from our patient. Note loss of the SNc, with the dark of the SNr directly abutting the red nucleus.**

Postsynaptic ligands have also been developed to assess the concentration of D1 and D2 receptors in the striatum. These include [^{11}C]-raclopride, used to assess D2 receptors. It has been found that, in idiopathic Parkinson's disease, there is decrease in presynaptic dopamine concentration, but an upregulation in postsynaptic D2 receptors. This may be a reaction to the lack of dopamine, which is inhibitory to neurons with D2 receptors. Parkinsonism-plus syndromes, on the other hand, often show degeneration of both the presynaptic and postsynaptic dopaminergic neurons, with decreased D1 and D2 receptor uptake. Therefore, in the future, PET may be able to help separate Parkinson's disease from parkinsonism-plus syndromes. For an excellent review article on the current status of PET imaging in movement disorders, see Bohnen *et al.*, 2003.

Discuss some of the non-motor problems which are part of Parkinson's disease.

As described in the introduction to this chapter, there are several cortex–basal ganglia loops. While motor symptoms are the most prominent part of Parkinson's disease, it is known that dopamine levels decrease in the caudate as well as the putamen (although the decrease *is* more pronounced in the putamen). Therefore, it is reasonable to suggest that there may be disturbances that go beyond the motor component in diseases which involve the basal ganglia. These disturbances involve both cognitive and emotional faculties. Thus, depression has been estimated to occur in nearly 50 percent of Parkinson's disease patients, while progressive dementia occurs as a late feature in as many as 30 percent of patients. Also, sleep disturbances are very common in Parkinson's disease patients. Other disturbances involve autonomic regulation, with over 50 percent of patients having symptoms such as constipation, impotence, dizziness with orthostatic hypotension, and disturbances in sweating. It must be stressed, however, that not all of these non-motor problems are related to the basal ganglia. As Parkinson's disease progresses, cell loss begins to affect other regions of the brain beyond the dopaminergic neurons, including the hypothalamus, cholinergic neurons of the nucleus basalis of Meynert (a major cholinergic relay center of the forebrain), and sympathetic and parasympathetic neurons, as well as cortical neurons.

Discuss some of the complications of long-term drug therapy in Parkinson's disease.

Levodopa is the key element of medical therapy for Parkinson's disease. As you recall, this is a dopamine precursor (dopamine itself does not cross the blood–brain barrier, and so cannot be peripherally administered). Levodopa administration in healthy individuals probably does not have significant side effects. However, the inexorable progress of neuronal degeneration in Parkinson's disease, along with levodopa therapy, leads the patient through clinically predictable stages wherein medical therapy gradually becomes less effective.

Early in the course of disease, most patients achieve good control of their symptoms with levodopa. Levodopa is usually mixed with a peripheral decarboxylase inhibitor (PDI) to lessen peripheral conversion to dopamine. This allows a greater concentration of levodopa to reach the CNS (and helps lessen the nausea which peripheral conversion to dopamine produces). Although the levodopa/PDI concentrations have a fairly short half-life (typically about 2.5 hours), patients in the early phase of the treatment usually experience a stable response during the day. This is presumably due to the ability of the remaining dopaminergic neurons in the SNc to store and slowly release the dopamine which they have manufactured from levodopa. This period of stable response usually lasts 3 to 5 years.

Between about 4 and 8 years (roughly speaking), patients begin to notice two main effects:

(1) A wearing off of the levodopa effect only a few hours after each dose, gradually leading to pronounced "on" and "off" periods where the levodopa is working, and then when it stops, respectively. This pattern is known as "motor fluctuations."

(2) Patients begin to notice involuntary choreiform twisting movements at the time when the levodopa effect is at its peak. This is known as "peak-dose dyskinesia." The term "dyskinesia" refers to the involuntary choreiform movements.

Patients who begin to experience motor fluctuations can often be treated by increasing the dose or frequency of levodopa/PDI administration, by the addition of selegiline (a dopamine agonist), or by the addition of a COMT inhibitor.

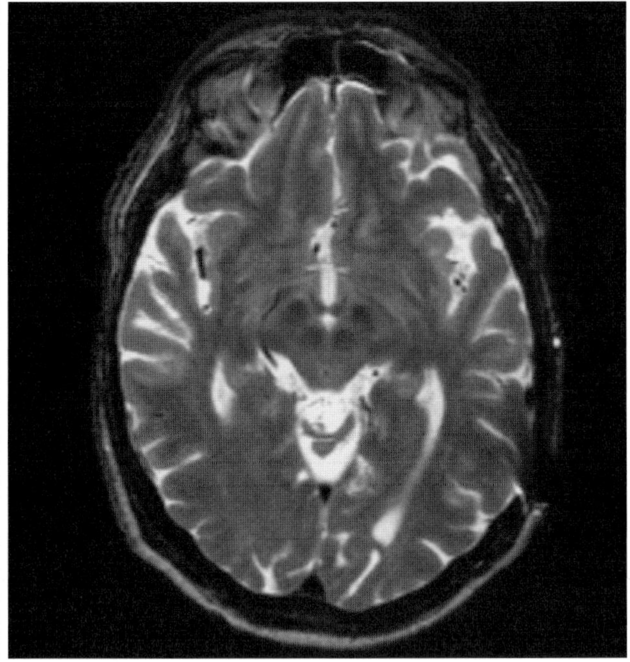

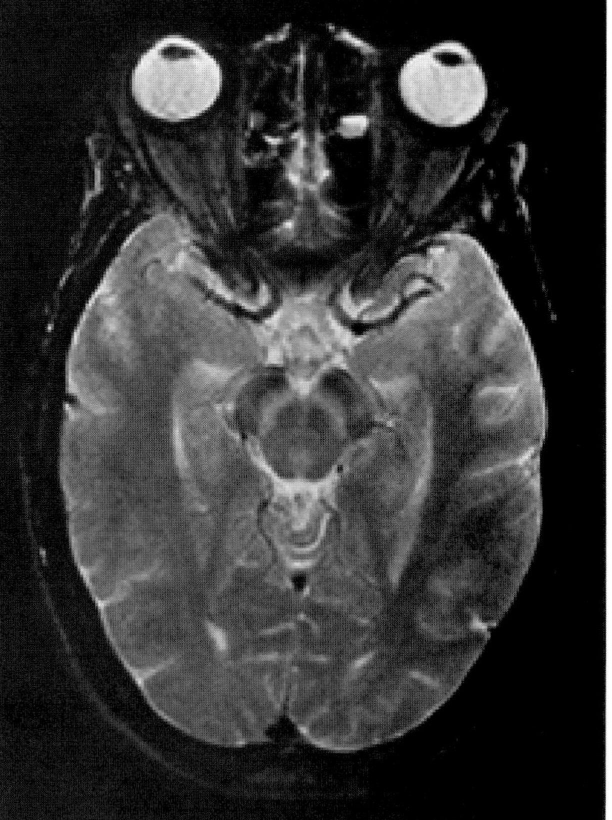

Fig. 5.10. **T2 axial image showing subtle narrowing of the SNc in a patient with Parkinson's disease.**

However, patients who have both significant motor fluctuation with increasing "off" periods, as well as significant peak-dose dyskinesia, present an especially difficult clinical challenge, because dyskinesia limits the ability to increase levodopa dosing.

When it becomes very difficult to find a medical treatment regimen that achieves an acceptable balance between motor fluctuations and dyskinesia, such patients are often referred for surgical therapy.

References

Bohnen, N. I., and Frey, K. A. The role of positron emission tomography imaging in movement disorders. *Neuroimaging Clinics of North America* 2003; **123**: 791–803.

Braffman, B. H., Grossman, R. I., Goldberg, H. I., *et al.* MR imaging of Parkinson disease with spin-echo and gradient-echo sequences. *American Journal of Neuroradiology* 1988; **9**: 1093–1099.

Cerna, F., Mehrad, B., Luby, J. P., *et al.* St. Louis encephalitis and the substantia nigra: MR imaging evaluation. *American Journal of Neuroradiology* 1999; **20**: 1281–1283.

Duguid, J. R., De La Paz, R., and DeGroot, J. Magnetic resonance imaging of the midbrain in Parkinson's disease. *Annals of Neurology* 1986; **20**: 744–747.

Oikawa, H., Sasaki, M., Tamakawa, Y. *et al.* The substantia nigra in Parkinson disease: proton density-weighted, spin-echo and fast short inversion time inversion-recovery MR findings. *American Journal of Neuroradiology* 2002; **23**: 1747–1756.

Pradhan, S., Pandey, N., Shashank, S. *et al.* Parkinsonism due to predominant involvement of substantia nigra in Japanese encephalitis. *Neurology* 1999; **53** (8): 1781–1786.

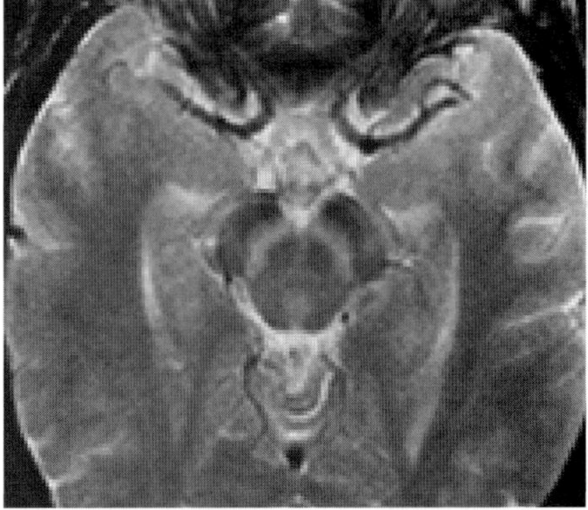

Fig. 5.11. **(a) T2-weighted axial image showing marked abnormal hyperintensity in the SNc in a case of Japanese encephalitis and parkinsonism. (Reproduced from Pradhan, S., Pandey, N., Shashank, S. *et al.* Parkinsonism due to predominant involvement of substantia nigra in Japanese encephalitis. *Neurology* used with permission.)**
(b) T2-weighted axial image showing abnornmal T2 hyperintensity in the SNc in a patient with St. Louis encephalitis and severe tremors (small arrows). (Reproduced from Cerna, F., Mehrad, B., Luby, J.P., *et al.* St. Louis encephalitis and the substantia nigra: MR imaging evaluation. *American Journal of Neuroradiology* used with permission.)

Case 5.2

66-year-old patient with Parkinson's disease. Patient has disabling right upper extremity and right lower extremity tremors.
A T1 axial MRI image is shown (Fig. 5.12). What are the findings? Briefly discuss surgical treatment in Parkinson's disease.

In the last case, we discussed the problems encountered with long-term medical therapy in Parkinson's disease. Patients with advanced disease may benefit from surgical therapy, and it is important to have at least some familiarity with the various surgical options.

Initial surgeries for Parkinson's disease (in the early 1940s) consisted of lesions of the motor cortex or corticospinal tract in an effort to alleviate tremor and rigidity. Tremor was indeed reduced, but at the expense of hemiparesis. A few years later, lesions of the basal ganglia were found to significantly improve tremor, rigidity, and bradykinesia, but had mortality rates in the range of 10 percent. In the 1950s, stereotactic techniques for pallidotomy were introduced, initially using plaster casts and pneumoencephalograms to obtain coordinates for lesioning the basal ganglia. Also, thalamotomy was attempted, and found superior to pallidotomy for controlling tremor. These treatments reached a peak in the 1960s, but then sharply declined due to the introduction of levodopa therapy.

In the 1980s, however, there was a resurgence of interest in surgical therapy for a variety of reasons: the limitations of medical therapy began to become apparent in late-stage disease, the idea of adrenal implants was introduced, and an improved understanding of the neuroanatomy of the basal ganglia suggested that surgical options should be re-evaluated.

At present, there are three main types of surgery:

(1) Implants to replace dopaminergic neurons. In the early 1980s, this was attempted using autologous adrenal medullary tissue. However, over the long term, the grafts did not take, and this procedure is no longer used. This was followed by transplants of fetal mesencephalic cells. Initial results have been promising, but this is considered experimental, and will not be discussed further.

(2) Ablative lesions.

(3) Deep brain stimulators.

The second and third options are widely practiced, with the trend shifting toward deep brain stimulators (DBS). The purpose of both of these surgical approaches is to inactivate neurons within the target zone. Ablation achieves this by physical destruction of the neurons, usually through thermocoagulation, while DBS implantation does it by an electrical disruption of normal neuronal function. This is sometimes a point of confusion among students, who often think that the purpose of deep brain stimulation is to stimulate the neuronal function within a given target zone – not so. It is simply a temporary, adjustable electrical disruption, rather than a physical ablation. It is performed by passing a stimulating electrode into the target zone under stereotactic imaging guidance. This is connected with a subcutaneous wire to a battery-driven stimulator placed in the chest wall or supraclavicular fossa similar to a pacemaker. The stimulation parameters can be adjusted to maximize clinical benefit.

There are three main targets for surgical treatment: the GPi, the thalamus (see Fig. 5.12), and the subthalamic nucleus (STN). Each of these will be discussed, with the main point being that there are somewhat different benefits to be obtained at each target site.

GPi

Surgical pallidotomy makes some sense in light of the previously presented model of basal ganglia neuroanatomy in Parkinson's. As explained previously, loss of dopamine diminishes inhibition of the GPi via the direct pathway, and increases stimulation of the GPi via the indirect pathway, leading to an increase in the activity of the GPi, which in turn inhibits the excitatory thalamocortical pathway, thus inhibiting the motor cortex. Lesioning the GPi, or disrupting its function with DBS placement, would thus lessen the GPi's inhibitory input to the thalamus.

Initial attempts at pallidotomy tried placing anterodorsal lesions in the GPi, without much success. However, pallidotomy now focuses on lesioning the posteroventral aspect of the GPi. It has been found that pallidotomy in this location is successful at

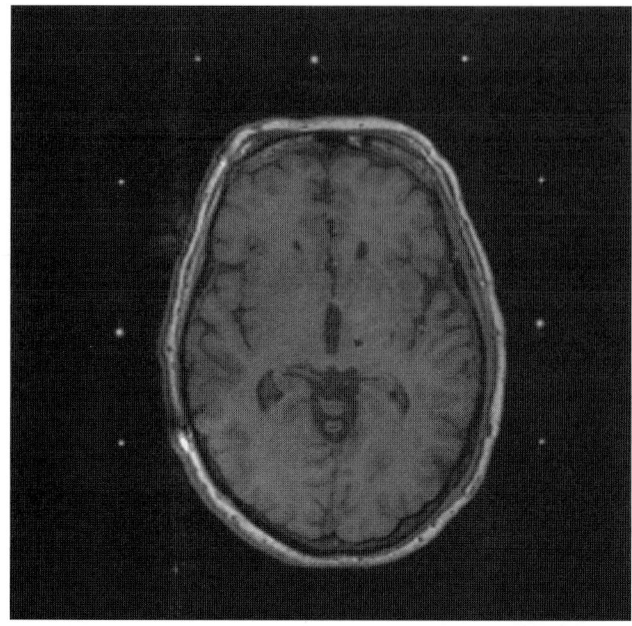

Fig. 5.12. **The MRI mages show the tip of a deep brain stimulator lead in the region of the left thalamus. Microelectrode stimulation was used to place the stimulator lead into the ventral intermediate (VIM) nucleus of the thalamus. A stereotactic frame is seen around the patient's head.**

relieving many features of Parkinson's disease, predominantly contralateral to the side of the lesion. Pallidotomy is most successful at relieving drug-induced dyskinesia, with success rates in the range of 90 percent. This allows increases in the dose of levodopa. Pallidotomy also improves rigidity, bradykinesia, and tremor. Various reports have shown improvements in the Unified Parkinson's Disease Rating Scale (UPDRS) of 30–60 percent. Pallidotomy is currently recommended in patients who are young and cognitively intact, with significant drug-induced dyskinesias, who have bradykinesia, rigidity, and tremor. It is noted that postural and gait disturbances are not as significantly improved by pallidotomy. It is difficult to assess the complication rate of bilateral pallidotomy, but there is concern that there may be a high incidence of speech impairment.

DBS of the GPi is still somewhat investigational, but it may provide a safer alternative for patients who have had pallidotomy on one side and do not want the possible risks of bilateral pallidotomy (see Fig. 5.13).

STN

There has been rapidly increasing interest in DBS of the STN as an alternative to pallidotomy or DBS of the GPi. Once again, this is sensible in light of the simple neuroanatomic model we have presented. The STN stimulates the GPi, increasing its inhibitory output to the VA and VL nuclei of the thalamus. Inhibition of the STN, therefore, leads to decreased output of the GPi, and disinhibition of the thalamus. The preliminary experience with DBS of the STN suggests that it is quite effective in ameliorating most or all aspects of Parkinson's, including tremor, bradykinesia, drug-induced dyskinesia, and posture and gait problems. In one report comparing DBS of the STN with DBS of the GPi, the improvement in the motor portion of the UPDRS was significantly better for DBS of the STN. Thus, DBS of the STN has become one of the most popular surgeries for Parkinson's diease (see Fig. 5.14 and Krack *et al.*, 1998).

Thalamus

Thalamotomy or DBS of the thalamus are both surgical options in practice today, again with increasing popularity of DBS because it is a "reversible" and somewhat adjustable procedure. The ventral intermediate nucleus (VIM) of the thalamus is the most common target for thalamotomy or DBS. The critical fact to know about thalamic surgery (DBS or thalamotomy) is that it is considered effective only in controlling tremor, but not in improving the other symptoms of Parkinson's, such as rigidity, bradykinesia, gait disturbance, or drug-induced dyskinesia. Alleviation of tremor occurs in 80–90 percent of patients, according to some

reports, and patients with disabling tremors, despite optimal medical therapy are considered the appropriate candidates for thalamic surgery.

There is a relatively high complication rate for bilateral thalamotomy, often with significant dysarthria or dysphagia. Thus, bilateral DBS, or thalamotomy on one side and thalamic DBS on the other are considered superior to bilateral thalamotomy.

Understanding the benefit of surgical lesions to the thalamus is difficult using our model of basal ganglia function. After all, the purpose of surgical intervention in the GPi or the STN is to lessen the inhibitory effect of the GPi on the thalamus, and to disinhibit the thalamocortical pathway. Therefore, it is paradoxical that surgical or electrical ablation of the thalamus would be productive. According to our model, such lesions would worsen, not improve, motor function. Various explanations for this paradox have been proposed. As surgical intervention has been largely an empirical art, we will not discuss the various theories put forth to resolve this paradox, but instead refer the interested reader to the excellent review article article by Mardsen and Obeso, 1994.

Of course, this has been a very abbreviated and incomplete summary of a complex and important area. The interested reader is referred to the additional sources in the References section, which provide excellent literature-based summaries of the current state of surgical treatment for Parkinson's disease.

References

Hallett, M., Letivan, I., and the Task Force on Surgery for Parkinson's Disease. Evaluation of Surgery for Parkinson's Disease – A report of the Therapeutics and Technology Assessment Subcommittee of the American Academy of Neurology. *Appendix B of Continuum*, 2004, **10**, (3).

Hauser, R., and Zesiewicz, T. *Parkinson's Disease: Questions and Answers*. 2nd edn. Merit Publishing International, 1997.

Krack, P., Pollack, P., Limousin, P. *et al.* Subthalamic nucleus or internal pallidal stimulation in young onset Parkinson's disease. *Brain* 1998; **121**: 451–457.

Mardsen, C. D. and Obeso, J. A. The functions of the basal ganglia and the paradox of stereotaxic surgery in Parkinson's disease. *Brain* 1994; **117**: 877–897.

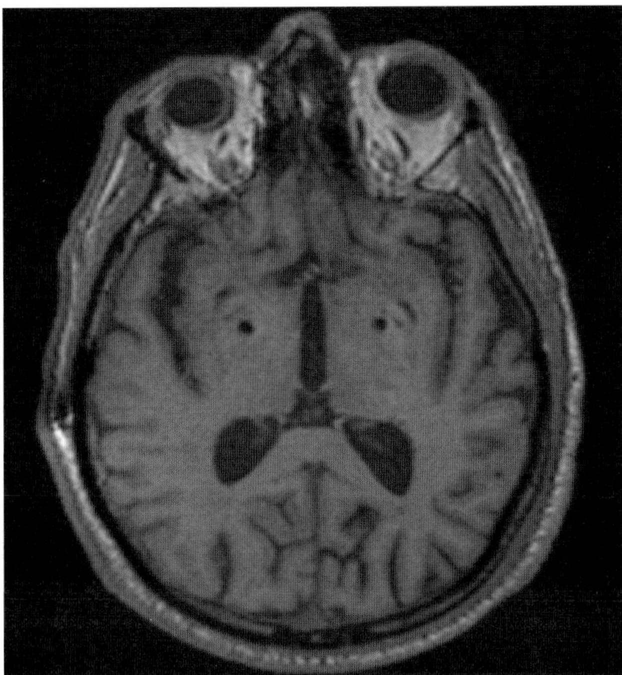

Fig. 5.13. **T1 axial image showing bilateral GPi deep brain stimulator leads in a patient with Parkinson's disease and significant drug-induced dyskinesia.**

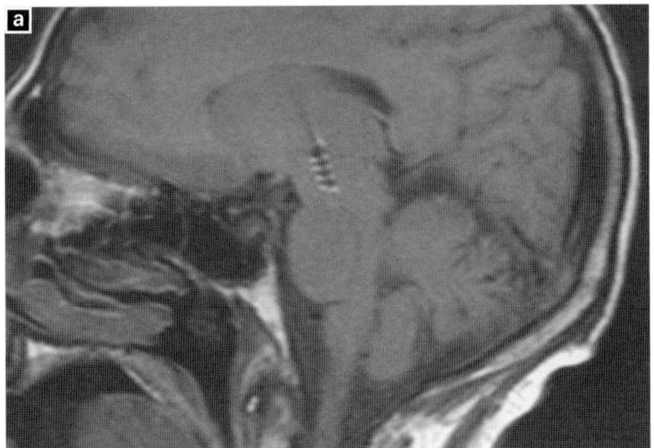

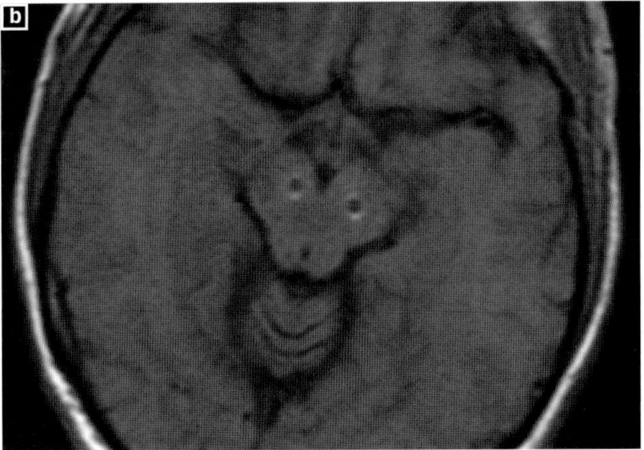

Fig. 5.14. **(a)** T1 sagittal and **(b)** T1 axial images showing bilateral DBS leads in the STN. Notice that the STN projects over the substantia nigra on axial images.

Case 5.3

58-year-old male patient with 1-year history of gait disturbances with postural instability, urinary frequency and impotence. Examination shows symmetric bradykinesia and rigidity without significant tremor, dysarthria or hypophonia. A trial of levodopa did not produce significant therapeutic benefit. The patient exhibited mild hyperreflexia and extensor plantar responses, as well as mild dysmetria.

The patient seems to have some parkinsonian features. Discuss a way to approach the differential diagnosis of parkinsonism.

A patient who presents with the parkinsonian features of rigidity and bradykinesia prompts consideration of a vast list of differential diagnostic possibilities. A nice way to organize our thinking is along the lines of the diagram in Fig. 5.15 into primary and secondary parkinsonian disorders, with the primary disorders further divided into Parkinson's disease and the atypical parkinsonian disorders.

The secondary causes of parkinsonism, such as medications, strokes, or infections, must be carefully excluded by history, clinical correlation, and imaging. As the choice narrows to a primary parkinsonian syndrome, clues that one is not dealing with Parkinson's disease, but rather one of the atypical parkinsonian disorders, include the following:
– lack of response to levodopa in the early stages of the disease,
– the presence of bradykinesia and rigidity in the absence of tremor,
– the presence of autonomic signs and symptoms, such as impotence, urinary disturbances and orthostatic hypotension,
– early postural instability,
– early speech disturbance,
– presence of cerebellar findings,
– early onset of dementia,
– marked symmetry in bradykinesia and rigidity early in the disease process,
– pyramidal signs,
– ocular signs such as impaired vertical gaze.

Briefly discuss the categories of secondary parkinsonism.

There is a long list of so-called "secondary" causes of parkinsonism. These include medications, toxins, infarcts, trauma, normal pressure hydrocephalus, infections, and certain heredodegenerative disorders such as Wilson's disease or Hallervorden–Spatz syndrome.

Medications

As discussed earlier, medications which either block or deplete dopamine, such as neuroleptics, antiemetics or reserpine may produce parkinsonian features. Lithium and tricyclic antidepressants can also cause extrapyramidal symptoms.

Toxins

As discussed earlier, MPTP is the best example in this category, although essentially no longer seen. Manganese toxicity, carbon monoxide, and methanol are also on this list.

Infarcts

Basal ganglia infarcts may produce bradykinesia and rigidity on the contralateral side, but usually without tremor. Also, there have been isolated reports of unilateral tremor caused by thalamic infarcts (e.g., Ferbert, A., and Gerwig, M. Tremor due to stroke. *Movement Disorders* 1993; **8**: 179–182), but tremor as a result of stroke is quite uncommon.

Trauma

Best known in boxers, repeated head trauma may cause dementia and parkinsonism, with degeneration of the dopaminergic neurons of the SNc.

NPH

The bradykinesia and gait apraxia of NPH may mimic Parkinson's diease, although there is typically no associated tremor.

While not in the category of secondary parkinsonisms, one other entity should be explicitly mentioned to avoid clinical confusion: essential tremor. This is a familial autosomal dominant condition with variable penetrance. There is usually a postural tremor of the upper extremities which is relatively symmetric, without bradykinesia or rigidity. It is mentioned here because there are many discussions in the literature about whether there is a relationship between Parkinson's disease and essential tremor, and because it is a disorder which is sometimes treated with thalamic deep brain stimulators.

Briefly discuss the categories of atypical parkinsonism.

As molecular biology has evolved, this list has been reorganized several times. At the time of this writing, there are four main entities generally recognized as the "atypical parkinsonisms." These are:
(1) Multiple system atrophy (MSA)
(2) Dementia with Lewy bodies (DLB)
(3) Progressive supranuclear palsy (PSP)
(4) Corticobasal degeneration (CBD)

These four entities are classified into two broad categories based on the type of intracellular protein aggregates or inclusions which characterize them. The first category is the *synucleinopathies*, composed of MSA and DLB. These disorders (like Parkinson's disease) have intracellular inclusions which contain alpha-synuclein. The second category is the *tauopathies*, composed of PSP and

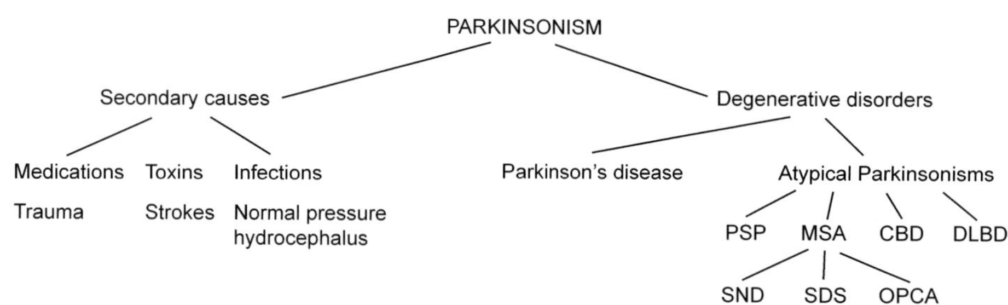

Fig. 5.15. **The differential diagnosis of parkinsonism. PSP, progressive supranuclear palsy. MSA, multiple system atrophy. CBD, corticobasal degeneration. DLBD, diffuse Lewy body disease. SND, striatonigral degeneration. SDS, Shy–Drager syndrome. OPCA, olivopontocerebellar atrophy.**

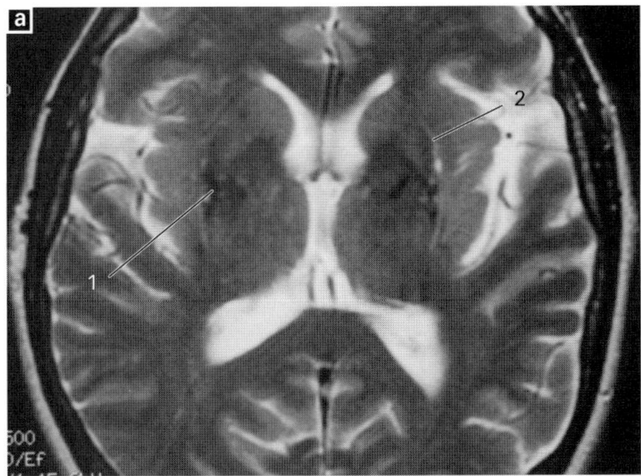
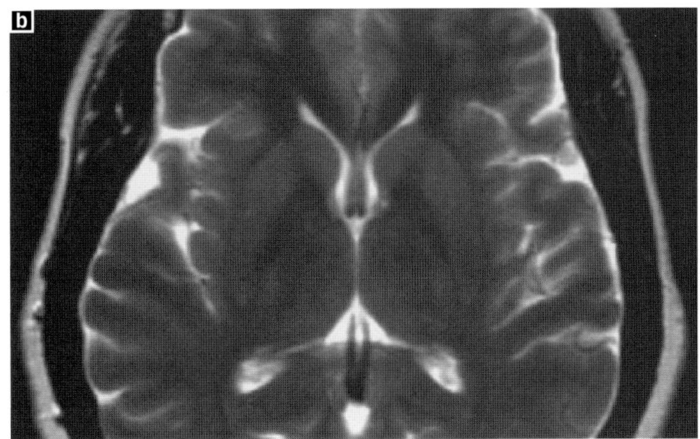

Fig. 5.16. **T2-weighted axial images are presented. Our patient (left, image (a)) shows hypointensity of the poterolateral putamen bilaterally (now darker than the globus pallidus, arrow 1), with a thin rim of T2 hyperintensity along the outside of the dark lateral putaminal margins (arrow 2). Also, there is some atrophy of the putamina bilaterally. In the normal patient (right – image (b)), the putamen is clearly brighter than the globus pallidus, and is uniform in signal without lateral margin darkening or a thin rim of lateral margin T2 hyperintensity.**

CBD. Some authors also add to this group an entity called fronto-temporal dementia with parkinsonism linked to chromosome 17 (FTDP-17). These disorders (like Alzheimer's disease) contain intracellular inclusions, which have tau protein aggregates. Of course, there are significant differences among these entities, and the above is but one method of classification.

The atypical parkinsonisms, also known as the Parkinson-plus (or parkinsonism-plus) syndromes, show a poor response to medical therapy and have, in general, a worse prognosis than Parkinson's disease.

It is difficult to be precise about the preponderance of Parkinson-plus syndromes as compared with Parkinson's disease. As a rough guide, the Baylor College of Medicine Parkinson's Disease Center and Movement Disorders Clinic, in a review of 2052 of their patients, reported that about 12 percent of their parkinsonian patients were felt to be in the Parkinson-plus category (see Stacy and Jankoric).

Let us return to our patient. Look at the MRI images provided (Fig. 5.16). On the left is our patient, and on the right is a normal comparison. What are the findings? Putting these together with the clinical presentation given above, what is your diagnosis?

Our patient presented with parkinsonian features but with prominent early postural instability, as well as pyramidal system findings, autonomic findings of impotence and urinary frequency, and a suggestion of some cerebellar findings. Hence, the patient showed involvement of multiple systems.

Diagnosis

Multiple system atrophy.

This Parkinson-plus syndrome originally used to be three separate syndromes: Shy–Drager's syndrome (SDS), striatonigral degeneration (SND), and olivopontocerebellar atrophy (OPCA), sporadic type. However, in the late 1960s, Graham and Oppenheimer noted that there was significant overlap in the clinical findings of these three syndromes, and suggested that they be categorized as variants of a single syndrome: multiple system atrophy. They were quite precient in doing this. Advances in molecular biology have since shown that all three groups of patients show a characteristic cytoplasmic inclusion in the glial cells, particularly in the oligodendrocytes, known as a glial cytoplasmic inclusion (GCI). The fact that GCIs are present in the brains of patients with SDS, SND, and sporadic OPCA but not in normal brains or other categories of parkinsonism, is strong evidence that these entities should indeed be grouped as a single syndrome.

The GCIs are composed of ubiquitin, alpha synuclein, and a host of other proteins. The composition shares some similarity to that of Lewy bodies in Parkinson's disease and DLB, but there are also significant differences. Chief among these is that the GCIs are found in the glial cells, whereas Lewy bodies are found in neurons. The GCIs are associated with neuronal loss in the SNc, locus ceruleus, putamen, inferior olives, pontine nuclei, intermediolateral cell columns of the spinal cord, and the Purkinjie cells of the cerebellum, reflecting the multiple systems involved.

Thus, multiple system atrophy is defined as an idiopathic progressive neurodegenerative syndrome of adults which involves four main systems:

- extrapyramidal system, leading to parkinsonism, with rigidity and bradykinesia.
- autonomic system, leading to such findings as impotence, orthostatic hypotension, urinary disorders, loss of sweating, and constipation.
- pyramidal system, often leading to hyperreflexia and extensor plantar responses.
- cerebellar system, leading to both gait and limb ataxia, cerebellar dysarthria, and sometimes gaze-evoked nystagmus.

Its prevalence is estimated to be between about 4 and 16 per 100 000 depending on the source of the estimate, but it is clearly much lower than the prevalence of Parkinson's disease, which averages about 200 to 300 per 100 000.

Almost all patients have both parkinsonian features as well as autonomic disturbances. About 50 percent of the patients will also show cerebellar signs at some point during the course of their disease.

The most suggestive clinical clues that one is dealing with MSA rather than Parkinson's disease is the lack of response to levodopa, and the presence of autonomic and cerebellar findings. Additional clues, as mentioned, include pyramidal signs, rapid disease progression, and early postural instability. Nonetheless, sometimes the diagnosis is difficult, and it is estimated that up to 10 percent of patients diagnosed with Parkinson's disease actually have MSA.

It is also important to point out that past descriptions of MSA as being composed of three separate syndromes are not without basis or merit. The clinical picture of MSA is not uniform, and there is often a predominance of either parkinsonian signs or

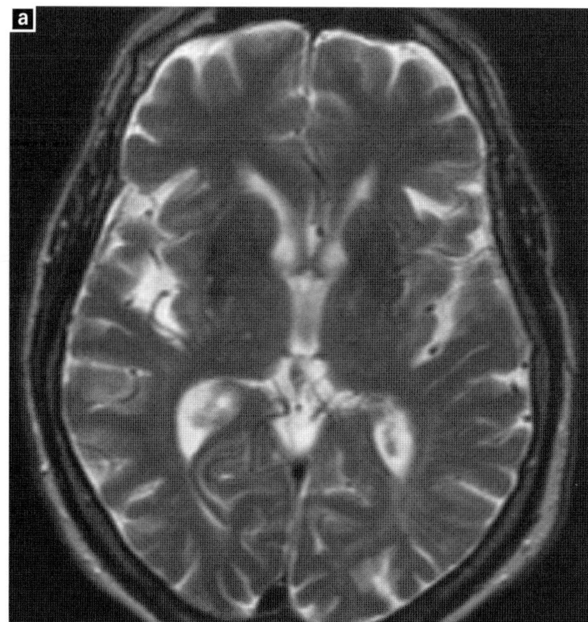

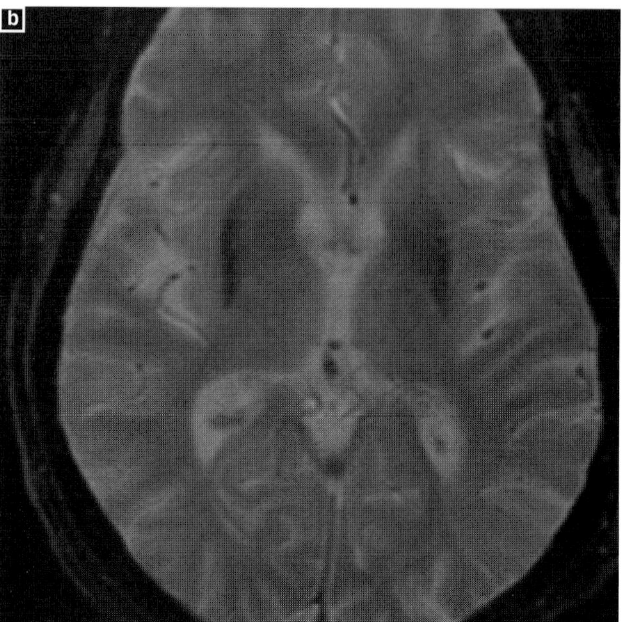

Fig. 5.17. **Spin-echo T2 (a) and gradient echo T2 (b) images in a patient diagnosed with MSA-P. The darkening of the posterolateral putamen and the signal inversion between the putamen and the globus pallidus is more pronounced on the gradient echo images. Note the slit-like hyperintensities along the posterolateral putaminal margins on the spin-echo T2 images adjacent to the dark zones.**

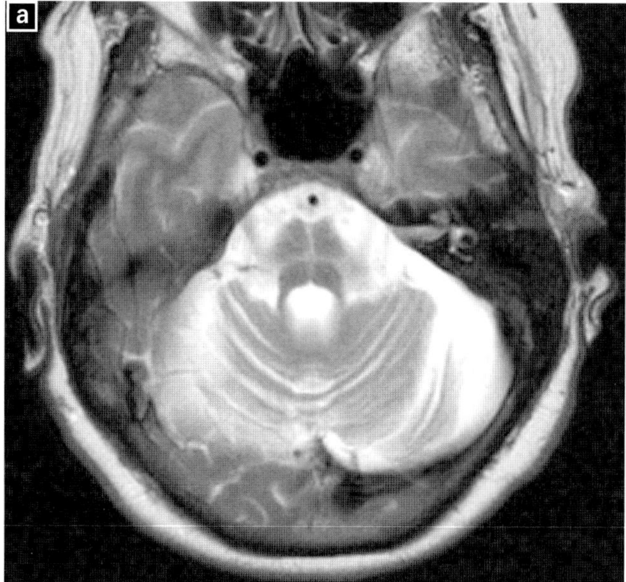

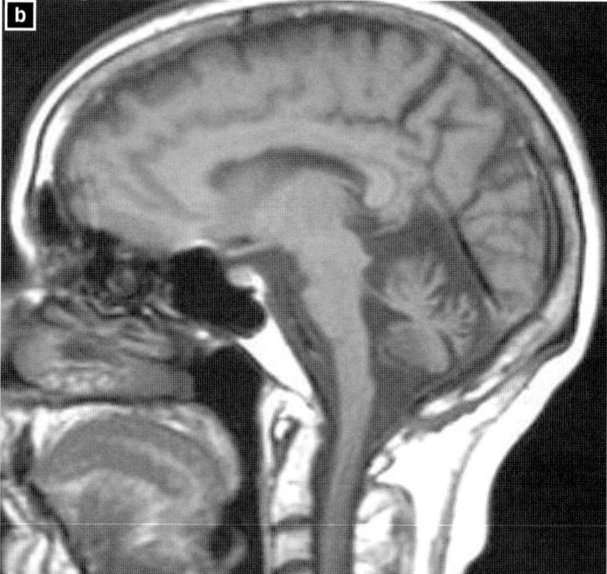

Fig. 5.18. **(a) T2 axial and (b) T1 sagittal 63-year-old male patient with a clinical diagnosis of MSA-C. There is marked atrophy of the pons and cerebellum. The T2 axial images show a typical "hot cross bun" sign in the belly of the pons. Case courtesy of Dr. Whitney Pope, UCLA Department of Radiology.**

cerebellar signs. Hence, the Movement Disorders Society Scientific Issues Committee Report of 2003 suggested that MSA be further subdivided into MSA-P (P for parkinsonian), where parkinsonian features predominate, and MSA-C (C for cerebellar), where cerebellar features predominate. The term MSA-P would thus replace SND, while the designation MSA-C would replace sporadic OPCA/OPCD. Both groups of patients tend to have a high preponderance of autonomic features, and hence SDS is no longer a particularly useful addition. It is estimated that about 80 percent of patients with MSA are in the MSA-P category, while 20 percent are in the MSA-C category.

Discuss the MR imaging features of MSA.

The imaging features tend to reflect the underlying pathologic changes. In patients with MSA-P, the concentration of GCIs and associated neuronal degeneration is relatively high in the putamen. Also, the putamen has been shown to have a significant increase in iron deposition, up to five times normal. Hence, on imaging, there is atrophy of the putamen as well as abnormal T2-weighted hypointensity of the putamen on 1.5 tesla MR systems due to the susceptibility effect of iron. This is most pronounced along the posterolateral putaminal margins, and often progresses to the point that the putamen becomes darker than the globus pallidus on T2. This is known as "signal inversion" between the putamen and the globus pallidus, and has been considered a characteristic imaging finding in MSA-P (see Fig. 5.16 above). It has been hypothesized that the excess iron deposition may play a role in catalyzing oxidation reactions which cause neuronal damage, as discussed with Parkinson's disease. The resultant gliosis and neuronal degeneration is felt to cause the T2 hyperintensity seen along the lateral margins of the dark putamen. This combination of darkening of the posterolateral putamen on T2, with thin slits of T2 hyperintensity along the lateral-most margin of the dark putamen, has in our experience been the most reliable MR imaging sign of MSA-P.

Some clinicians have taken to using gradient echo T2-axial images in an effort to "bring out" the T2 hypointensity along the lateral putaminal margins, since gradient echo sequences are more sensitive to the susceptibility effects of iron than the spin-echo or fast spin-echo sequences conventionally used in brain imaging. This is illustrated in the patient (Fig. 5.17).

Imaging, however, is at this point just an adjunct to the diagnosis, and there is no definitive data to assess the sensitivity and specificity of MRI compared to pathological diagnosis at autopsy. One study, however, states that MRI helped classify only 50 percent of MSA-P patients (Schrag et al., 2000).

The situation is a bit better when dealing with MSA-C (or what used to be called the sporadic form of OPCA/OPCD). In these cases, the neuronal degeneration is more pronounced in the pons, cerebellum, and inferior olives, and this is reflected both clinically and on imaging, where MRI scans have been estimated to help classify patients 70 percent of the time (Schrag et al, 2000). MRI scans tend to show significant atrophy of both the pons and the cerebellum. Also, an interesting imaging appearance of the atrophic pons has been noted in some cases. This consists of cruciform hyperintensities on T2 in the belly of the pons, leading to the so-called "hot cross bun" sign (see Fig. 5.18).

Some interesting new forays into the uses of imaging in the diagnosis of Parkinson-plus syndromes include PET imaging with ligands for dopamine receptors to try to distinguish Parkinson's disease (decreased D1 but upregulated D2 receptor profile) from MSA and PSP (decreased D1 and D2 receptor profile). This was briefly discussed in Case 5.1 – Parkinson's disease.

References

Schrag, A., Good, C. D., Miszkiel, K. et al. Differentiation of atypical parkinsonian syndromes with routine MRI. *Neurology* 2000; **54**: 697–702.

Stacy, M., and Jankovic, J. Differential diagnosis of Parkinson's disease and the Parkinsonism Plus syndromes. E-article – http://www.parkinsons-information-exchange-network-online.com/archive/091.html.

Case 5.4

64-year-old male presents with a 3-year history of progressive gait difficulties, with axial instability, loss of balance and frequent falls for 2 years. In the last year, he has also been complaining of progressive visual difficulties, with difficulty walking down stairs and difficulty reading, as well as dysarthria. Physical examination reveals some bradykinesia, as well as increased tone and pronounced axial rigidity. Strength was normal. The patient exhibits a significant vertical gaze palsy and attempts to compensate using a doll's eye maneuver.

MRI images are presented (Fig. 5.19), with a normal control for comparison. What are the findings? What is your diagnosis?

Diagnosis

The clinical history, as well as the imaging findings, strongly suggest the diagnosis of progressive supranuclear palsy (PSP).

Briefly discuss the clinical findings and pathogenesis of PSP.

PSP is an idiopathic neurodegenerative disease first characterized as a distinct entity in the 1960s. It is also known by the eponym "Steele–Richardson–Olszewski syndrome," for short (just kidding – but that is really its eponym). It is the most common of the atypical parkinsonisms, estimated to affect about 5 percent of parkinsonian patients. Disease onset is usually in the seventh decade. Early in the course of the disease, the most common clinical features are postural instability with frequent falls (usually occurring within the first year), axial rigidity, dysarthria, and bradykinesia. The most characteristic feature – a supranuclear vertical gaze palsy affecting down-gaze more than up-gaze – usually manifests about 3 years after disease onset. PSP also has cognitive manifestations with frontal lobe dysfunction, often manifest as apathy and frontal release signs. Pseudobulbar palsy is also often part of the clinical picture.

In the early stages of the disease, it may be difficult to differentiate PSP from PD or the other atypical parkinsonian syndromes. The presence of a levodopa unresponsive parkinsonism with early postural instability and frequent falls should suggest the diagnosis, as this is a relatively late feature in PD. Likewise, dysarthria as a prominent early feature should suggest PSP. Although a frank vertical gaze palsy usually occurs later, there is often a pronounced slowing of vertical saccades at a relatively early phase. In PD, there is no slowing of saccades, while in CDB, there is reportedly increased latency but normal speed of saccades, without distinction between horizontal and vertical direction. Therefore, careful testing of ocular motility is important. It is useful to recall that the vertical gaze palsy is supranuclear, i.e., occurring above the level of the ocular motor nuclei. With a supranuclear palsy, there will often be an improvement in the vertical gaze excursion with activation of the vestibular ocular reflex, or with attempting to elicit the Bell phenomenon (the involuntarily rolling upward of the eyes as the lids close). In a patient unable to voluntarily perform up-gaze, the eyes can be held half open by the examiner. When the patient is asked to try to close his eyes, if the eyes roll upward, this suggests that the palsy is supranuclear.

As mentioned earlier, PSP is considered a *tauopathy*, with abnormal tau protein aggregates causing neurofibrillary tangles within neurons and glial cells. In the glial cells, the tau aggregates of PSP form a so-called "astrocytic tuft." The neuronal degeneration of PSP is most pronounced in the midbrain, as well as in the ocular motor nuclei, the pedunculopontine nucleus, the striatum, and the GPi.

Briefly discuss the imaging findings and the utility of imaging in PSP.

The main imaging findings are well illustrated by our patient. They consist of significant atrophy of the midbrain, including the tectal plate. One reference suggests using an axial midbrain diameter of 17 mm as a cutoff point (Schrag et al., 2000). However, we have found the sagittal images to be more characteristic, showing a very atrophic midbrain above the belly of the pons.

Other additional findings include *ex vacuo* dilatation of the third ventricle, signal increase in the midbrain, frontotemporal atrophy, and atrophy of the red nucleus.

The reference (Schrag et al., 2000) found that, in attempting to differentiate between patients with PSP, MSA, CBD, and

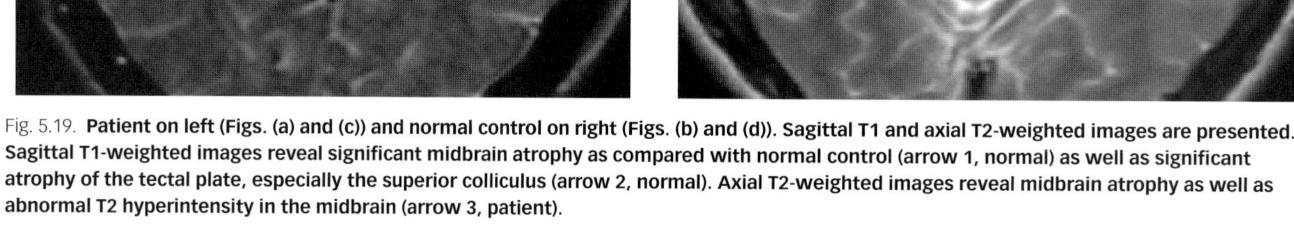

Fig. 5.19. **Patient on left (Figs. (a) and (c)) and normal control on right (Figs. (b) and (d)). Sagittal T1 and axial T2-weighted images are presented. Sagittal T1-weighted images reveal significant midbrain atrophy as compared with normal control (arrow 1, normal) as well as significant atrophy of the tectal plate, especially the superior colliculus (arrow 2, normal). Axial T2-weighted images reveal midbrain atrophy as well as abnormal T2 hyperintensity in the midbrain (arrow 3, patient).**

control subjects, MRI correctly classified the PSP patients more than 70 percent of the time, and was judged as a useful adjunct to the diagnosis.

More recent work has focused on assessing DWI imaging in the discrimination of MSA-P and PSP from PD and from each other. Seppi *et al.* (2003) have found that diffusion-weighted imaging shows a higher regional apparent diffusion coefficient (rADC) in the basal ganglia in patients with PSP and MSA as compared with PD. Using rADC values in the putamen, the authors could discriminate PSP from PD with a sensitivity of 90 percent and a positive predictive value of 100 percent. However, it is not possible to reliably distinguish PSP from

MSA-P, as both have increased apparent diffusion coefficients compared to patients with PD.

References

Schrag, A., Good, C. D., Miszkiel, K. *et al.* Differentiation of atypical parkinsonian syndromes with routine MRI. *Neurology* 2000; **54**: 697–702.

Seppi, K., Schocke, M. F. H., Esterhammer, R. *et al.* Diffusion-weighted imaging discriminates progressive supranuclear palsy from PD, but not from the parkinson variant of multiple system atrophy. *Neurology* 2003; **60**: 922–927.

Case 5.5

61-year-old female patient who presents with a 3-year history of progressive difficulty dressing and using her left arm. She complains that lately, her left arm "seems to have a mind of its own," and that she is often unaware of its position. Examination reveals bradykinesia and rigidity of the left arm. There is also relative left hemisensory neglect and a left-sided agraphesthesia (i.e., the patient cannot recognize words scratched on her left palm). There was no significant ideomotor apraxia, but when asked to draw a cube, the patient showed a significant construction apraxia. Also, there was evidence of some left-sided magnetic apraxia, with groping by the left hand and clutching of objects placed in it with difficulty releasing them. MRI examination showed no lesions of the corpus callosum.

MRI image presented (Fig. 5.20). What are the findings, and what is your leading differential diagnostic possibility?

The patient's history and examination findings are remarkable for an asymmetric parkinsonism of the left arm, construction apraxia, left-sided sensory findings, and a left-sided "alien limb" syndrome. The MRI examination, by report, shows no evidence of lesions of the corpus callosum. The provided images, however, show right frontoparietal cortical atrophy.

Diagnosis

Corticobasal ganglionic degeneration (CBD).

CBD, known as either corticobasal or cortical basal ganglionic degeneration, is a fairly rare atypical parkinsonian syndrome, and one which is difficult to diagnose. It typically presents in the sixth or seventh decade, and is not diagnosed below age 45.

The MRI imaging findings are limited, with the typical descriptions in the literature focusing mainly on focal unilateral frontoparietal atrophy usually in the region of the central sulcus. Some investigators have also reported relative T2 hypointensity in the putamen and globus pallidus (see, for example, Hauser *et al.*, 1996). The findings, though, are typically quite subtle, and one has to really look carefully at the scans, and correlate them with the clinical findings.

Like PSP, CBD is also a tauopathy, and both share the same tau haplotype. Thus, some investigators consider CBD to be integrally related to PSP. However, unlike PSP, CBD often presents with a *unilateral* levodopa unresponsive parkinsonism, as well as limb apraxia on the affected side, which may progress to a frank "alien limb" syndrome. Apraxia, by the way, can be defined as a "motor agnosia," i.e., the inability to perform learned skilled movements in the absence of motor weakness or sensory deficits. Such unilateral motor, sensory and cognitive deficits are highly unusual in PSP. The presence of an "alien limb" syndrome, in the absence of a lesion of the corpus callosum, is suggestive of the diagnosis of CBD. Other important differences between CBD and PSP are the lack of postural instability and early falls with CBD, the occasional presence of myoclonus in CBD (an unusual feature in PSP) and the lack of a characteristic vertical gaze palsy in CBD. However, it is noted that CBD patients may present with non-specific visual difficulties and show latency of saccades on examination. As stated previously, though, there is no gross slowing of saccades or preferential involvement of the vertical gaze direction.

In this case, since the right cortex was involved, the diagnosis was perhaps a bit more challenging, since the apraxia displayed is a right brain apraxia, consisting of deficits in 3-D visuospatial and construction deficits. A more typical suspected case of CBD is shown above (Fig. 5.21), where the patient presented with gradually progressive right-sided parkinsonism (remember, Parkinson's disease usually begins unilaterally, so this is not so helpful) as well as an ideomotor apraxia (this is quite helpful, as it is usually not seen in

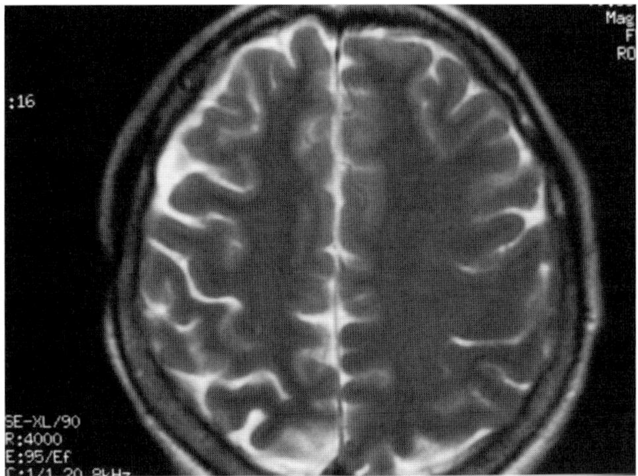

Fig. 5.20. **T2-weighted axial MRI image shows asymmetric cortical atrophy involving the right frontoparietal convexity.**

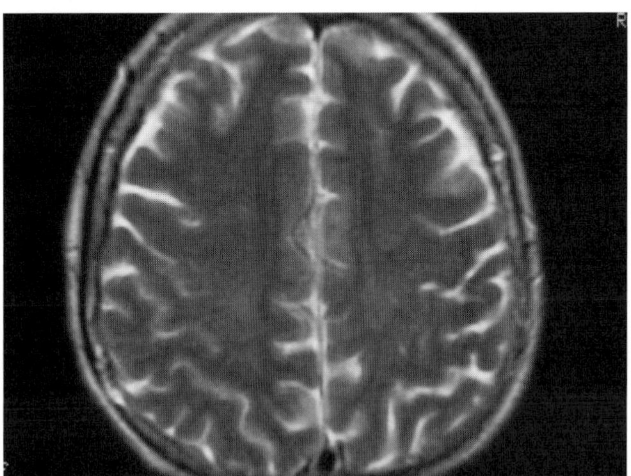

Fig. 5.21. **T2-weighted MRI scan shows left frontoparietal cortical atrophy in a patient who presented with right-sided parkinsonism and ideomotor apraxia. The patient is suspected to have CBD.**

Parkinson's disease). This can be tested by asking the patient such things as "show me how you would cut a piece of paper with scissors," or "show me how you would hammer a nail," i.e., asking the patient to pantomime movements that would require them to understand the use of tools and to formulate an action plan. This sort of apraxia is what is seen with lesions in the left brain, and may affect both limbs. The patient above, it is noted, did not have an "alien hand" syndrome.

Less commonly, CBD may present as a frontal lobe dementia, with progressive aphasia and attention disorder.

Pathologically, CBD is characterized by swollen neurons with poor cytoplasmic staining (achromasia) in the frontoparietal cortex, basal ganglia, and substantia nigra. Also, abnormal tau aggregates are found in the neurons and glial cells, where they form so-called astrocytic plaques (as compared to the astrocytic tufts seen in PSP).

Reference

Hauser, R. A., Murtaugh, F. R., Akhter, K. *et al.* Magnetic resonance imaging of corticobasal degeneration. *Journal of Neuroimaging* 1996; **6**(4): 222–226.

Case 5.6

41-year-old male presents with a 2-year history of difficulty concentrating and increasing irritability. On examination, he has mild generalized chorea. He has a broad-based gait, and when asked to protrude his tongue, he could not sustain the protrusion, and his tongue quickly darted back into his mouth. The patient's mother was alive and well in her late 60s. His father had died of suicide while the patient was still a young child.

What is chorea and what are some of its possible causes? Chorea is defined as spontaneous, random, fidgeting movements, which may begin as subtle movements of the fingers as if one was playing the piano, or as facial grimaces, and may progress to large amplitude violent flinging movements. When it combines with writhing dystonic movements, it is called choreoathetosis. Chorea, of course, automatically calls to mind Huntington's disease (sometimes called Huntington's chorea). However, it actually has a large number of causes. In a recent series of consecutive patients seen for chorea, a vascular etiology such as a deep infarct or bleed was the most common (40 percent). Other common etiologies included drug-induced chorea (14 percent), Huntington's disease (10 percent), and AIDS (10 percent) (for a more complete discussion, see Piccolo *et al.*, 2003). Numerous other less common causes have also been described, and a useful (but incomplete) classification is presented below:

I. Neurodegenerative diseases
   - Huntington's disease
   - Huntington's disease-like syndromes
   - Fahr's disease
   - Neuroacanthocytosis
   - Wilson's disease
II. Vascular lesions
   - Infarct
   - Hemorrhage
   - Moyamoya
   - Anoxia
III. Drug induced
   - Cocaine
   - Amphetamines
   - Anticonvulsants
   - Tricyclic antidepressants
IV. Infections
   - AIDS (primary HIV infection)
   - AIDS (secondary infections)
   - Creutzfeldt–Jakob disease
V. Metabolic
   - Acquired hepatocerebral degeneration
   - Hyponatremia
   - Hyperglycemia
VI. Toxic
   - Carbon monoxide
   - Manganese
   - Thallium
VII. Immune mediated
   - Antiphospholipid antibody syndrome
   - Sydenham's chorea
   - Postinfectious chorea
   - Paraneoplastic chorea (small cell lung cancer, lymphoma, thymoma, renal cell)

Our patient's images are presented (Figs. 5.22 and 5.23). What are the findings and what is your diagnosis?

On the MRI scan our patient shows significant atrophy of the caudate and putamen compared to a normal age-matched control, with ballooning of the frontal horns of the lateral ventricles. The PET scans of our patient show absent fluorodeoxyglucose uptake in the striatum. The normal control shows uptake in the caudate (arrow 1) and putamen (arrow 2), not present in our patient. Both patients show uptake in the thalami (arrow 3).

Diagnosis

Huntington's disease.

Please discuss Huntington's disease, including clinical manifestations, genetics, and a putative neuropathology in terms of the basal ganglia circuits discussed thus far.

Huntington's disease is an autosomal dominant progressive neurodegenerative disorder which affects the motor, cognitive, and emotional–psychiatric domains. In the early 1990s, the underlying neurogenetics of Huntington's disease were elucidated with the isolation of a distinct genetic anomaly on a section of the short arm of chromosome 4 known as the Huntington gene or the huntingtin gene. This region codes for an essential protein called huntingtin, found normally in all cells, but appearing to be essential to the function of neurons. Under normal circumstances, this gene has several CAG nucleotide triplets near the beginning of its DNA sequence (less than 30). Huntington's disease is caused by having too many of these CAG trinucleotide repeats (greater than 40). The CAG triplet codes for the amino acid

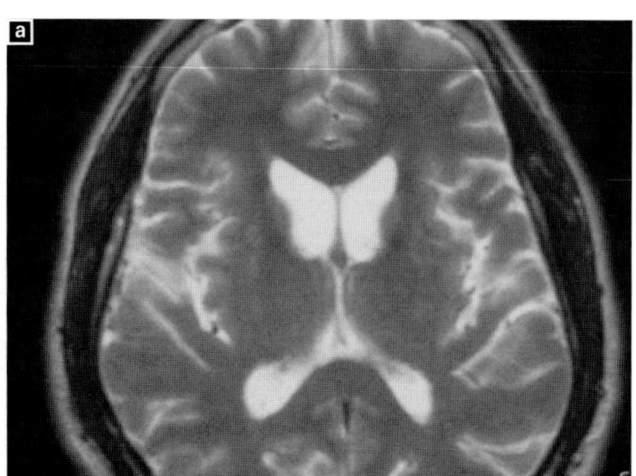

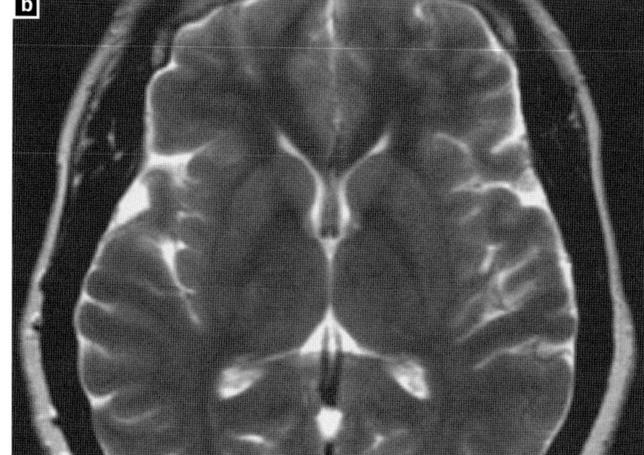

Fig. 5.22. **T2-weighted axial MRI scans at the level of the striatum. Our patient on left (a), with normal control on right (b). See text for findings.**

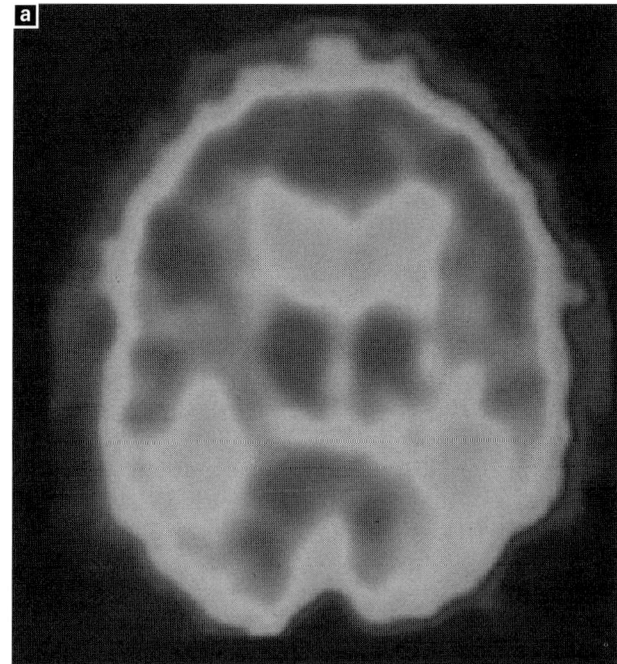

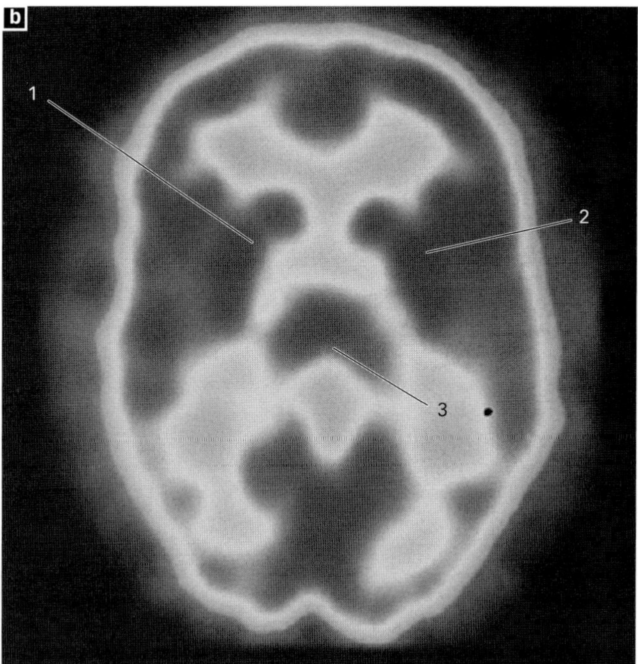

Fig. 5.23. **Fluorodeoxyglucose PET scans at the level of the striatum. Our patient on left (a), with normal control on right (b) (see plate section for color image).**

glutamine. Therefore, in Huntington's disease, an abnormal huntingtin protein is formed with too many glutamine residues. The precise mechanism by which the presence of this abnormal huntingtin protein leads to neuronal death is now a matter of active research. It seems that this protein folds abnormally and forms aggregates which cannot be properly degraded by the cell's protein cleanup machine known as the ubiquitin–proteasome degradation pathway. These protein clumps may then "tie up" other essential regulatory proteins and hence cause cell death. The age of disease onset and rapidity of progression are linked to the number of CAG repeats. Therefore, patients with greater than 60 CAG repeats almost always manifest early, with a disorder termed juvenile Huntington's. In older textbooks, this was referred to as the Westphal variant of Huntington's disease, but this term is essentially no longer used.

There is a definite preferential susceptibility of certain neuron populations to the presence of abnormal huntingtin. Patients with Huntington's disease, it turns out, show significant degeneration of the striatum, with volume loss in the caudate and putamen. Cytologic examination shows that the volume loss appears to preferentially affect the medium spiny neurons of the striatum.

The degeneration of the striatum is felt to preferentially affect the neurons involved in the indirect dopaminergic pathway. Under normal circumstances, the indirect pathway is inhibitory to the motor cortex. Degeneration of this pathway thus leads to a disinhibition of the excitatory thalamocortical motor input, and thus causes a disorder of increased motion, manifest by the choreiform movements typical of Huntington's disease (see Fig. 5.24).

As the disease progresses into its later stages, there is also degeneration of the direct pathway, leading to bradykinesia, and rigidity. In fact, in the terminal stages of disease, choreoathetosis gives way to akinesia. It is noted that, in juvenile Huntington's patients, the predominant presentation may be one of bradykinesia or akinesia, rather than the classic choreiform movements.

The disease onset typically begins at middle age, with subtle choreiform movements, which progress to more violent, random excess motions which may combine with athetosis to produce choreoathetosis. There is also a characteristic motor impersistence, where motor tasks cannot be completed. Clinically, this may manifest as a "darting tongue" sign, where the patient is unable to sustain protrusion of his or her tongue. Later in the disease, it manifests with buckling of the knees while walking, thus severely impairing gait. In combination with choreiform movements of the arms and torso, the gait takes on a marionette-like quality.

The prevalence of Huntington's disease is approximately 4–8 per 100 000 in the population. Accurate incidence estimates are difficult to obtain, but there are probably somewhere in the vicinity of 30 000 patients currently diagnosed with Huntington's disease, with an additional 150 000 "at-risk" patients.

In the setting of a positive family history, the diagnosis is usually made by the patient's clinical presentation, and further genetic or imaging testing is not usually necessary. However, approximately 6 percent of patients with Huntington's disease have a genuinely negative family history. Much of this may be secondary to instability of the CAG repeats, with a tendency to expand over generations, especially when inherited from the paternal side. Hence, patients may present with Huntington's disease confirmed by genetic testing, but with a negative family history. Study of the parents will often reveal abnormal increased CAG repeats in the 30–35 range in one of the parents, indicating a premutation. Instability and expansion of the CAG repeats will take the number above 40, and manifest as frank Huntington's disease in the affected children. It is for this reason that juvenile Huntington's disease is felt to be usually secondary to paternal transmission, as CAG repeat instability and expansion occurs significantly more during spermatogenesis, and is therefore more likely to be transmitted through the father's DNA.

As described above, the most obvious clinical manifestations of Huntington's are in the motor domain. However, previous discussions have elucidated that there are multiple cortical-basal ganglia loops, which also impact cognitive and emotional functions. For example, the frontal lobe–caudate loop is involved in cognitive activity, and hence degeneration of the striatum would also be expected to produce cognitive deficits. In fact, a significant proportion of Huntington's disease patients exhibit cognitive abnormalities, with dysexecutive disorders and loss of impulse control, which is often expressed as irritability. In addition to cognitive abnormalities, a large number of Huntington's disease patients also experience major affective disorders, most significantly depression. It has been noted that there is an exaggerated rate of suicide among Huntington's disease patients. This is, in fact, one of the causes of a negative family history as well (the affected parent may have disappeared, or committed suicide, and not have been identified as a Huntington's disease patient).

In approximately 1 percent of patients who present with a clinical picture of Huntington's disease, there is no definite family history, and genetic testing does not show the abnormal Huntington's gene. Under these circumstances, it may be reasonable to consider a group of genetic diseases called Huntington's disease-like (HDL) disorders. Several of these have been described in the last decade, which involve various genetic mutations. For example, HDL-2 is caused by CAG/CTG repeat expansions in a gene on chromosome 16 (for an excellent overview of the material in this case discussion, as well as some more discussion of HDL disorders, see Shannon, K. M., Huntington's disease and other choreas. *Continuum*, 2004, **10**(3): 65–83).

Thus far, there is no cure or available treatment which seems to delay the onset of symptoms or slow the progression of neuronal degeneration. However, the motor and psychiatric manifestations may be partially ameliorated. The psychiatric manifestations may be treated with antidepressants. The motor manifestations may be treated with atypical neuroleptics, and with some dopamine and catecholamine depletion agents. The most successful of these is tetrabenazine, which, while not currently available in the United States, may be obtained in Europe or Canada.

Imaging does not play a significant role in the diagnosis of Huntington's disease due to the availability of a direct genetic test (available since 1993). Older literature stressed that such measurements as the bicaudate diameter on MRI scans can show the characteristic caudate and putaminal atrophy. In patients with juvenile Huntington's, there is also often abnormal T2-weighted hyperintensity in the striatum. As seen above, PET scans show decreased fluorodeoxyglucose uptake in the striatum in a pronounced fashion. Prior to genetic testing, these were some of the methods for assessing at risk patients.

Finally, it is interesting to note that the genetic defect responsible for Huntington's disease (excess CAG trinucleotide repeats) also underlies several other diseases of the CNS. Thus, with advances in neurogenetics, Huntington's is now known to be part of a larger family of "polyglutamine" diseases, each with excess CAG repeats in distinct loci in the human genome. Currently, there are seven other such polyglutamine syndromes, among which are dentatorubropallidoluysian atrophy (DRPLA), and spinocerebellar ataxia types 1,2,3,6 and 7 (SCA1, SCA2, SCA3, SCA6, SCA 7).

Reference

Piccolo, I., Defanti, C. A., Soliveri, P. *et al*. Cause and course in a series of patients with spontaneous chorea. *Journal of Neurology* 2003; **250**: 429–435.

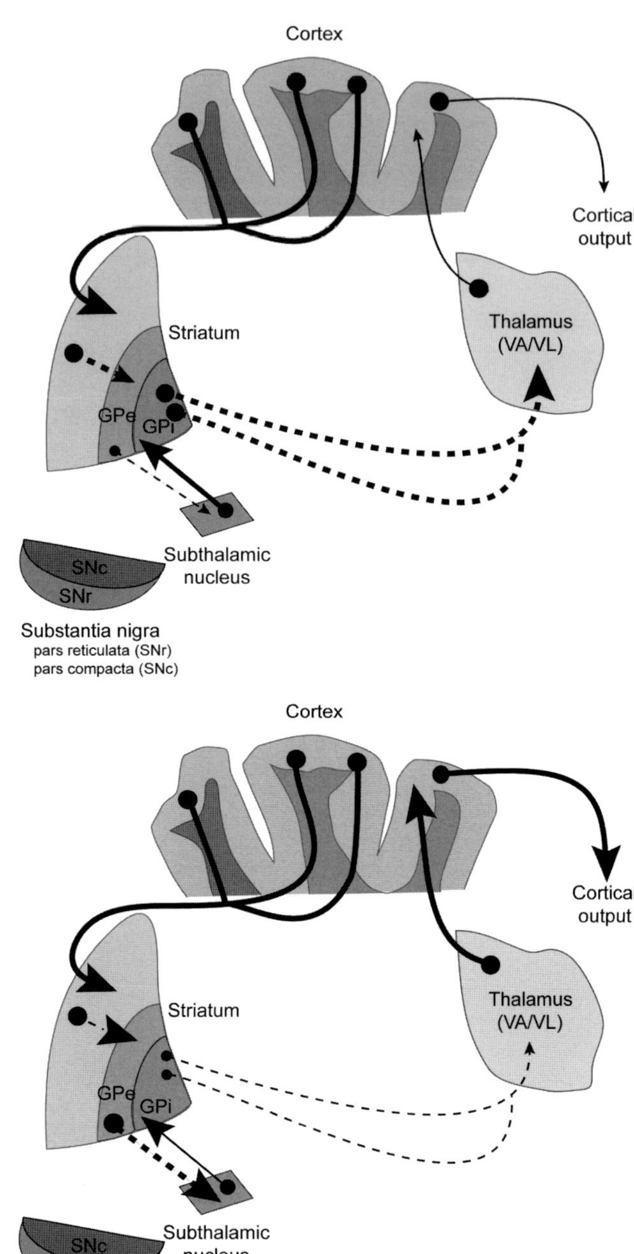

Fig. 5.24. **Top: Normal indirect pathway. Bottom: Degeneration of the indirect pathway, leading to disinhibition of the excitatory thalamocortical pathway. Less inhibitory output from the putamen to the GPe causes the GPe to increase its inhibitory output to the subthalamic nucleus. The STN sends less excitatory impulses to the GPi, thus lessening its inhibition of the thalamic motor areas, leading to a net excitation of the thalamocortical circuit compared to baseline. Excitatory pathways are solid while inhibitory pathways are dashed. The thickness of the lines indicates the strength of the output.**

Case 5.7

58-year-old male with a 5-week history of flinging movements of his right arm. Clinical examination quickly confirmed the history provided by the patient; intermittent involuntary large-amplitude violent flinging of the right arm was indeed observed. The medical student on the team had recently finished a psychiatry rotation, and thought that the patient was exhibiting a hysterical reaction.

The patient's MRI scan is shown (Fig. 5.25). What are the findings? What is your diagnosis?

The scans show a small cystic area consistent in appearance with a chronic lacunar infarct in the region of the left subthalamic nucleus (Fig. 5.25 (a) and (b)). Figure 5.25 (c) and (d) show deep brain stimulator electrodes in the subthalamic nuclei of a different patient, hence marking the location of the STN. Notice that, on axial images, the subthalamic nucleus projects over the zona compacta. However, the diagnosis of an old lacunar infarct in this location should be made with extreme caution, as the midbrain is a frequent location for Virchow–Robin (perivascular) spaces,

which would have an identical appearance and are much more frequent (see, for example, Saeki *et al.*, 2005). The diagnosis was made in this patient due to a typical clinical presentation, lack of other lesions, as well as absence of a perivascular space in this location on an MRI from 14 months prior.

Diagnosis

Hemiballismus secondary to lacunar infarct of the subthalamic nucleus.

Briefly discuss hemiballismus, including the functional neuroanatomy of the basal ganglia in this disorder.

Ballismus refers to involuntary, sudden, large-amplitude flinging movements of a limb. It is almost always unilateral, and has been classically considered secondary to lesions of the contralateral subthalamic nucleus, usually infarcts or bleeds. Given what we have reviewed thus far about the indirect pathway, it is relatively straightforward to come up with a putative explanation for this, as shown in Figure 5.26. Damage to the

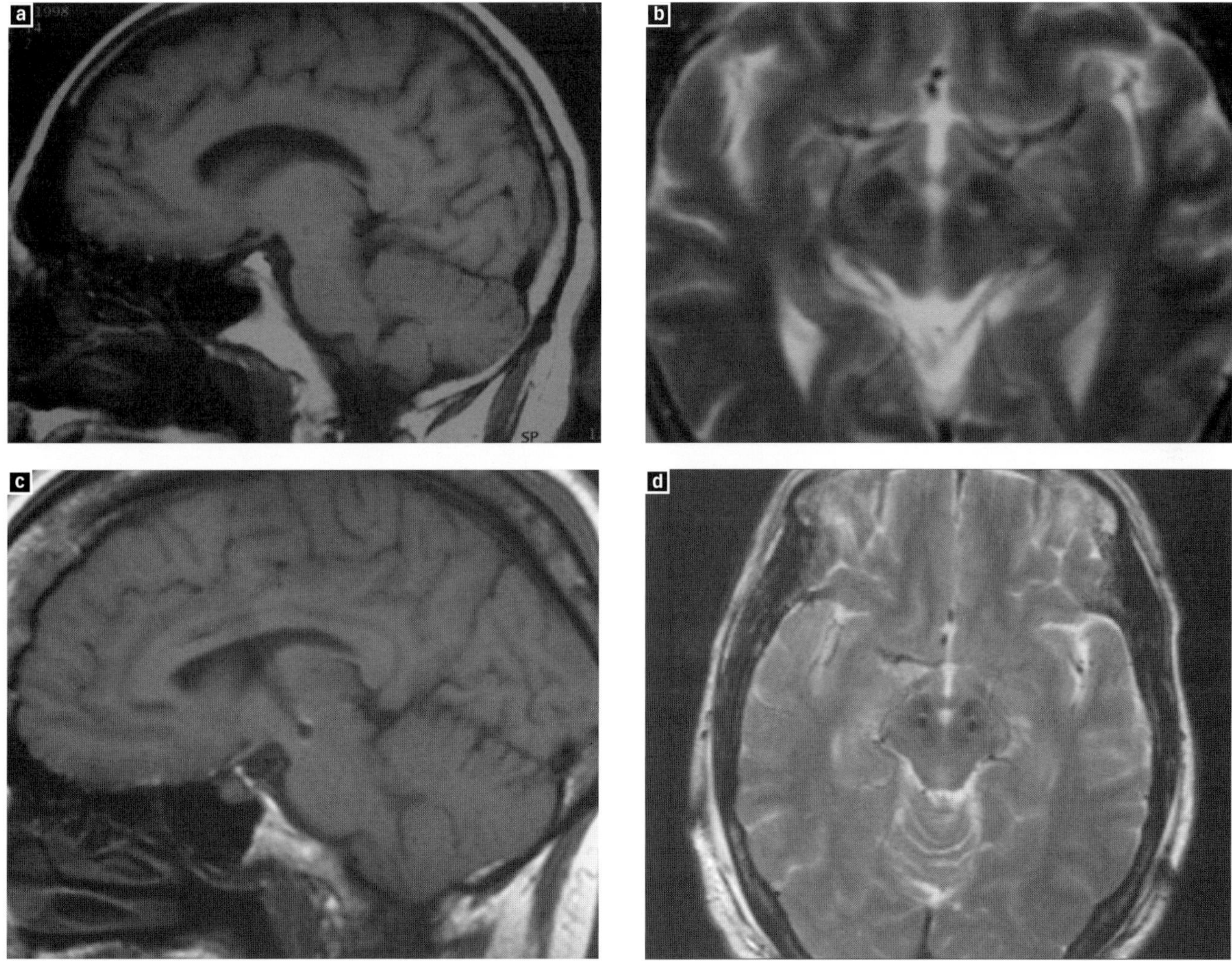

Fig. 5.25. **(a) Sagittal T1 and (b) axial T2-weighted MRI images of our patient. (c) Sagittal T1 and (d) axial T2-weighted images in a different patient with subthalamic nucleus (STN) deep brain stimulators to mark the location of the STN.**

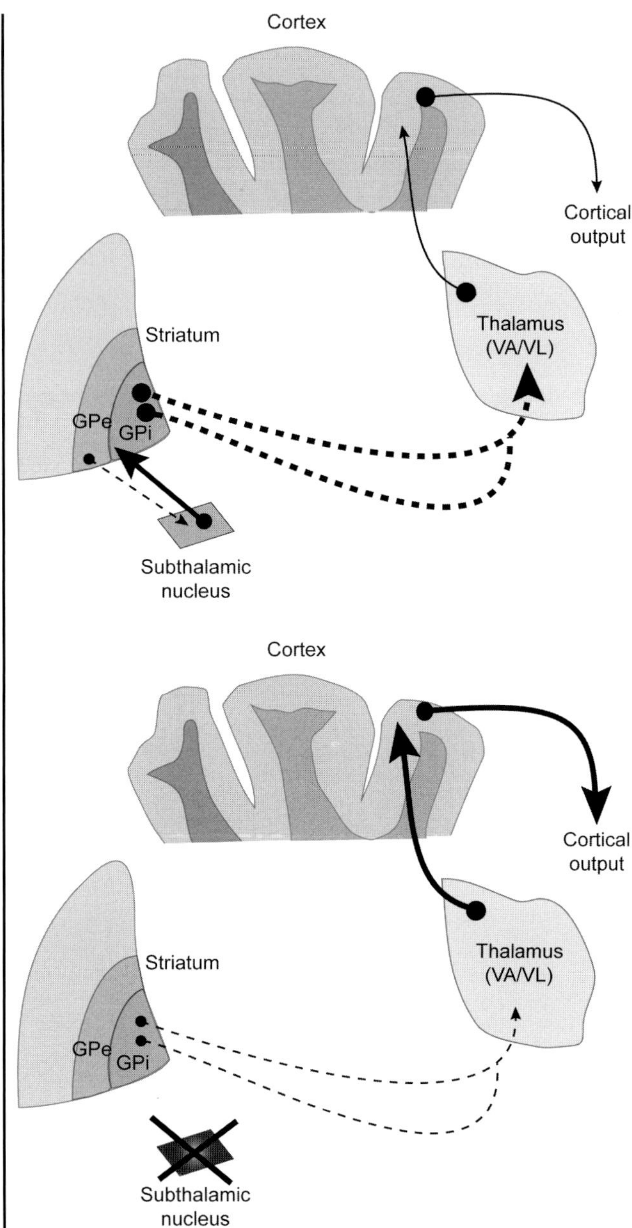

Fig. 5.26. **Top: Normally, the subthalamic nucleus sends excitatory impulses to the globus pallidus interna (GPi), stimulating it to exert an inhibitory effect on the motor areas of the thalamus, which excite the motor cortex. Bottom: With damage to the subthalamic nucleus, it no longer stimulates the GPi. Thus, the normal inhibitory tone maintained by the GPi over the thalamus is lost, leading to disinhibition of the excitatory thalamocortical pathway, and a disorder of excess motion – in this case, hemiballismus. Excitatory pathways are solid, while inhibitory pathways are dashed. The thickness of the lines indicates the strength of the output.**

subthalamic nucleus leads to disinhibition of the excitatory thalamocortical pathway. For those who do not know the neuroanatomy, the disorder is sometimes mistaken for a hysterical reaction.

This functional neuroanatomic explanation suggests that there should be a close relationship between hemiballismus and chorea – both represent a disruption of the indirect pathway, which normally exerts an inhibitory tone on the thalamus. In the case of chorea, the dysfunction is at the level of the putamen, while in the case of hemiballismus, the dysfunction is at the level of the subthalamic nucleus. It turns out that there is, indeed, a close relationship between the two disorders of movement, with many neurologists considering them to be parts of the same spectrum, with hemiballismus representing a choreic movement of proximal limb muscles. Others have noted that some patients who initially present with hemiballismus gradually show a decrease in the flinging movements of the proximal limb muscles, and evolve into a choreoathetosis of the hand and fingers. This is felt to represent a partial recovery.

Hemiballismus sometimes responds to treatment with haloperidol or phenothiazine. If not, we can once again look to the neuroanatomy for a surgical treatment. Since the motor nuclei of the thalamus (VA and VL) have become disinhibited and are sending too many excitatory impulses to the motor cortex, it stands to reason that stereotactic lesions of the ventrolateral thalamus might prove beneficial. Neuroanatomy does not lie, and such surgery is a possible, and usually effective, option for severe cases (see Krauss and Mundinger, 1996).

Finally, it is noted that, although hemiballismus has been classically linked to lesions of the subthalamic nucleus, recent studies suggest that we need to broaden our differential list. One study, in fact, found that only 26 percent of patients with hemiballismus have lesions in the subthalamic nucleus, while 53 percent had lesions elsewhere, including the caudate, globus pallidus, thalamus, and cortex. Moreover, 20 percent of patients had no demonstrable lesion at all (Postuma and Lang, 2003).

References

Krauss, J. K., and Mundinger, F. Functional stereotactic surgery for hemiballism. *Journal of Neurosurgery* 1996; **85**(2): 278–286.

Postuma, R. B., and Lang, A. E. Hemiballism: revisiting a classic disorder. *Lancet Neurology* 2003; **2**: 661–668.

Saeki, N., Sato, M., Kubota, M. *et al.* MR imaging of normal perivascular space expansion at midbrain. *American Journal of Neuroradiology* 2005; **26**: 566–571.

Case 5.8

12-year-old male with a 6-year history of progressive difficulty walking, such that the patient now spends most of the time in a wheelchair. The symptoms began with cramping and inversion of the left foot when walking, which progressed to spasms and inversion with any attempted movement. Symptoms progressed to involve both legs and the trunk. It was noted that the patient was significantly less symptomatic in the morning, when he could do some walking, but progressively worsened throughout the day. Examination showed a cognitively intact young male with flexion of the left leg at the hip and knee and inversion of the left foot. A vague family history of a similarly afflicted uncle was provided.

What is dystonia? What are the differential diagnostic possibilities in this case?

Dystonia is defined as sustained abnormal muscle contractions which lead to either repetitive movements or abnormal postures.

The salient features in this case are:

(1) A progressive childhood-onset dystonia which began in a single lower extremity leading to a marked gait disturbance, and then generalized over time.

(2) A diurnal variation of symptoms.

(3) A possible familial component.

The differential diagnosis of dystonia is vast, as it can be secondary to a large number of basal ganglia disorders, including tumor, infarct, toxic, and inherited and non-inherited metabolic disorders, or it can occur as a primary dystonia syndrome or a dystonia-plus syndrome. A much fuller discussion than will be presented here can be found in the excellent article "Dystonia and related diseases," by Cynthia Comella, *Continuum,* 2004; **10**(3): 89–112.

The progressive nature of the disease, its childhood onset, and possible familial component suggest a genetic dystonia syndrome. Thus far, 13 such syndromes have been described (DYT1–DYT13). The most important of these is DYT1, an autosomal dominant early onset dystonia. It is secondary to a GAG deletion in a gene on chromosome 9, and causes an abnormal form of a ubiquitous protein known as torsin A. This disease is important to know because it is the only one of the DYT syndromes which has a direct genetic test, and because it alone accounts for 40–65 percent of limb early-onset dystonia.

It is important to note the following clinical pearl: childhood dystonias often begin in the foot and then generalize over time; adult-onset dystonias, by contrast, begin in the cervical region, upper body or face, and typically remain focal. Therefore, an adult who presents with a generalized dystonia or a hemibody dystonia should not be considered to have a primary dystonia syndrome. Likewise, an adult who presents with a leg dystonia should be investigated for other etiologies (which may include Parkinson's disease).

Our particular patient displayed a suggestive clinical feature – diurnal variation, with worsening of symptoms in the evening.

What diagnosis does this suggest? What diagnostic maneuver would you like to try?

The diurnal variation of symptoms along with the early onset of a lower limb dystonia and prominent gait disturbance raises the possibility of what used to be called Segawa's syndrome, and is now referred to as dopamine-responsive dystonia, or DRD. As the name implies, the dystonia here is markedly improved by dopamine administration, to which patients show a profound and sustained response. Thus, we would like to try a course of levodopa. It was tried, and the patient showed significant improvement.

Diagnosis

Dopamine-responsive dystonia (DRD).

DRD is also classified as DYT5. There are two main variants, a more frequent autosomal dominant type and a less frequent autosomal recessive type. The genetics here is interesting, and so we'll take a brief excursion. Autosomal dominant DRD is now known to be secondary to a mutation on chromosome 14, on the gene for guanosine triphosphate (GTP) cyclohydrolase I. This, in turn, contributes to the synthesis of tetrahydrobiopterin, which is a cofactor for the enzyme tyrosine hydroxylase, key in the synthesis of dopamine. The autosomal recessive variety is from a mutation on chromosome 11, in the tyrosine hydroxylase gene itself! Thus, DRD is, in essence, a dopamine deficiency, but without neuronal damage. Thus, it is responsive to levodopa. This pathophysiology also correlates with the well-known clinical observation that dopamine antagonsists can sometimes produce dystonia. Along this vein, it is interesting to note that DRD often presents with superimposed parkinsonian features.

What about the imaging?

Since this is a neuroimaging book, we need to include some images, which were indeed obtained in the course of the workup (Fig. 5.27).

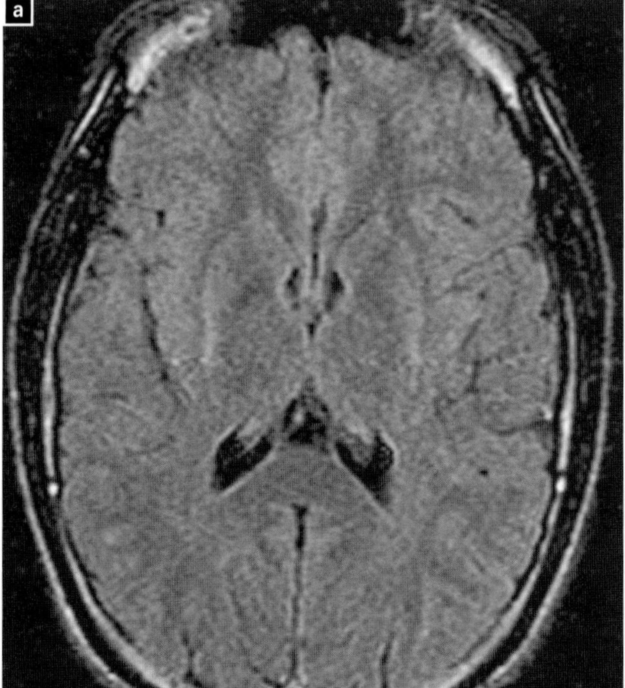
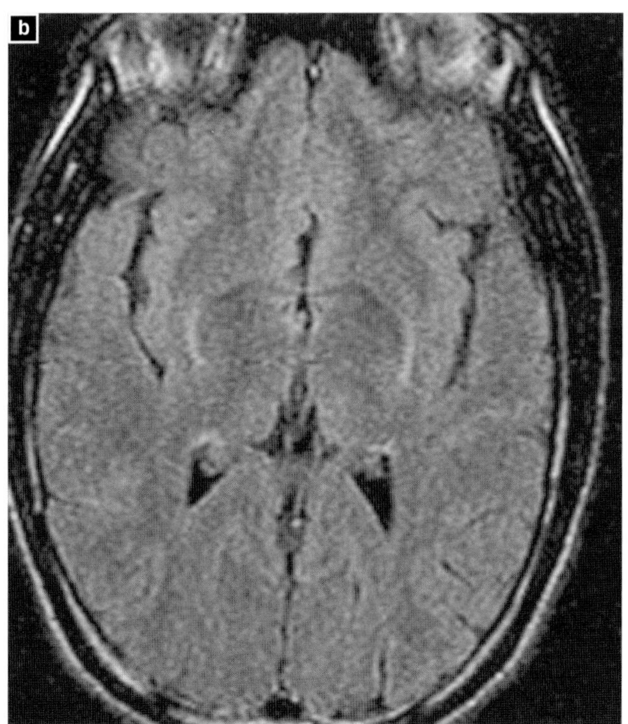

Fig. 5.27. **(a), (b) FLAIR axial images through the basal ganglia are obtained. The images are remarkable only for very thin strips of subtle hyperintensity along the lateral putaminal margins. Other than this very subtle finding, the images are normal. (Case courtesy of Dr. Suzie Bash, UCLA Department of Radiology.)**

In DRD (as well as primary dystonias in general) MRI imaging is usually normal, or with non-specific subtle abnormalities such as seen above. This is consistent with the notion that dystonias result from defective cell function rather than from a well-defined pathological lesion in a given cell population. However, MRI helps to exclude other entities which may present with childhood dystonia, such as Wilson's disease, juvenile Huntington's disease, Hallervorden–Spatz syndrome, mitochondrial encephalopathies, certain aminoacidopathies, and vascular, infectious, or neoplastic lesions involving the basal ganglia. All of these entities should show MRI abnormalities.

We show this case for the intrinsic interest of the DRD syndrome, as well as to underscore that, for effective clinical practice, it is important to know when imaging is *not* going to make a significant contribution to a case workup or diagnosis.

Case 5.9

22-year-old female patient presents with 2-year history of tremor and increasing irritability and depression. Examination reveals symmetric bradykinesia, rigidity, as well as a proximal appendicular tremor that increased when the arms were outstretched. The patient was notably dysarthric.

MRI images are provided (Fig. 5.28). What are the findings? What differential diagnostic possibilities are you entertaining?

The images through the basal ganglia reveal symmetric abnormal T2 hyperintensity in the bilateral caudates, putamina, and thalami. In the putamen, there is an inner zone of slight hyperintensity with a more lateral "strip" of marked hyperintensity at the lateral putaminal margins. In the midbrain, there is abnormal T2-weighted hyperintensity in the midbrain tegmentum with some sparing of the cerebral peduncles.

Among the differential diagnostic possibilities for a young person with an extrapyramidal movement disorder would be young-onset Parkinson's disease, familial parkinsonian syndromes, hereditary dystonias, secondary parkinsonisms, and juvenile Huntington's disease.

What additional tests would you like to order?

In evaluating young people with movement disorders, we should always remember to test for one other disease which we have not yet mentioned. To give you a hint, let's order a serum ceruloplasmin level. The result of the test is 15 mg/dL.

Diagnosis

Wilson's disease. This is an extremely important diagnosis to make, because it is a treatable disease. With proper therapy, progression of symptoms may be halted, while if left untreated, the disease is lethal.

Discuss Wilson's disease, including the genetics, pathophysiology, and radiologic findings.

Wilson's disease is an autosomal recessive genetic disorder of copper metabolism. The signs and symptoms are secondary to an excess of copper deposition predominantly in the liver and brain, with increased deposition also seen in the eyes and kidneys. The excess copper deposition appears to lead to accelerated cell death due to increased oxidative stress. The underlying genetic defect is a mutation in a copper-transporting adenosine triphosphate (ATPase) gene known as ATP7B, located on chromosome 13. Over 200 mutations of this gene have been identified, and hence any significant defect in the copper-transporting ATPase can lead to Wilson's disease. Because there are so many different genetic mutations, there is as yet no clinically useful genetic test for Wilson's disease. It is interesting to note that about 1 in 100 people has a "Wilson's disease" gene. These individuals are heterozygotes, and hence do not have Wilson's disease. The odds that a man and woman chosen at random will each carry the gene is thus 1 in 10 000. Of their children, 1 in 4 will be homozygous, and so a crude incidence of 1 in 40 000 births for Wilson's disease may be arrived at.

Normally, copper is absorbed by the intestine, and excess copper is excreted by the liver into the bile. In Wilson's disease, this hepatic excretion process is impaired (since ATP7B functions in the vesicular transport of copper into bile) and so there is a

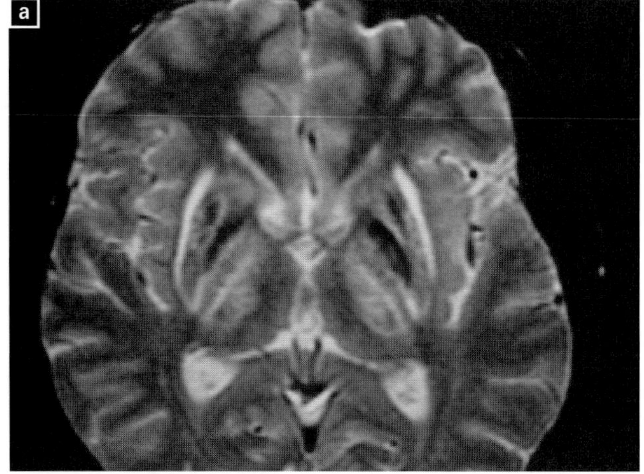

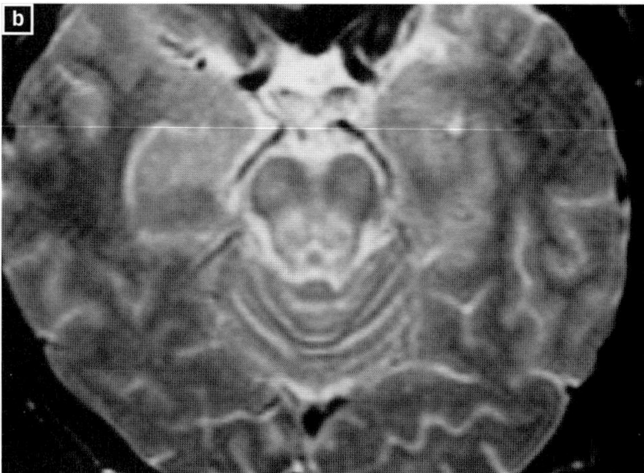

Fig. 5.28. **(a). T2-weighted axial images through the basal ganglia and (b) the midbrain. See text for findings. (Case courtesy of Dr. Suzie El-Saden, UCLA Department of Radiology.)**

buildup of copper in the liver. Eventually, the copper will "spill over" into the blood stream, and deposit in the brain, leading to damage in the striatum, brainstem tegmentum, and multiple white matter pathways, including the dentatorubrothalamic tract.

Wilson's disease has two main clinical manifestations. When it presents in childhood, the manifestation is usually hepatic, with cirrhosis, hepatitis, or liver failure. When the disease presents in adulthood, the manifestations are more often neurologic and neuropsychiatric, although there is usually underlying liver damage as well. The neurologic manifestations run the range of the extrapyramidal disorders. The most frequent of these is tremor, which is often an appendicular tremor which increases as the arms are outstretched, known as a "wing-beating tremor" as was found in our patient. Other patients may present with superimposed parkinsonism, dystonia, or chorea. The dystonia may be in the limbs, but there is also a peculiar orofacial dystonia, which has been likened to a sardonic grimace. A fairly characteristic feature of Wilson's disease is that the extrapyramidal features often focus on the corticobulbar pathways, and then spread caudally. Hence, patients often present with prominent dysarthria, dysphagia, and drooling. The neurospsychiatric symptoms often involve poor impulse control, irritability, and cognitive decline.

The diagnosis is usually made on clinical grounds, plus a variety of highly suggestive biochemical tests. The initial non-invasive tests consist of the following:

Ophthalmologic examination for Kayser–Fleischer rings

These are brownish rings around the limbus of the cornea secondary to deposition of copper in Descemet's membrane. These are best seen on slit-lamp examination. Kayser–Fleischer rings are present in nearly all patients with neurologic manifestations, although they may be absent in younger patients with hepatic manifestations. For test purposes and roundsmanship (as well as sometimes in real life) it is good to know that Kayser–Fleischer rings, while highly suggestive in the right clinical setting, are not pathognomonic for Wilson's disease as was once thought. They are sometimes seen in severe cholestatic disorders, such as partial biliary atresia or primary sclerosing cholangitis.

Serum ceruloplasmin levels

Ceruloplasmin is the most important serum protein for copper transport. Levels are usually low in Wilson's – less than 20 mg/dL in 80–90 percent of patients – with normal ranges being >25 mg/dL. However, not all patients will have low ceruloplasmin levels. Also, asymptomatic heterozygotes may have reduced ceruloplasmin. Many textbooks do not link the low ceruloplasmin levels to the ATP7B genetic defect responsible for Wilson's, and hence the student is unclear on why ceruloplasmin would be low if copper excretion into bile is impaired. It turns out that the ATP7B is also responsible for incorporating copper into apoceruloplasmin, and for posttranslational changes in this protein. Therefore, defects in ATPB7 also lead to low ceruloplasmin.

Total serum copper

Because most serum copper is bound to ceruloplasmin, total serum copper is also usually low or normal (not high as we might intuitively expect). However, knowing total serum copper and ceruloplasmin, we can calculate free copper, which is usally elevated.

Urinary copper excretion

Because free copper is high, there is an increased urinary excretion of copper over a 24-hour collection period (greater than 100 mg/24 h versus a normal of less than 40 mg).

Liver copper concentration

If, after the above battery of tests, there is still some question as to the diagnosis, a liver biopsy may be performed to quantitate the copper in the liver. A concentration of 250 micrograms copper per gram of liver is considered diagnostic (normal 15–55 mcg/g) in the right clinical setting.

Given the above diagnostic algorithm, what then is the role of imaging? One role is to exclude other disease processes. When it comes to positively making the diagnosis (rather than excluding other diseases), even MRI is not terribly sensitive or specific. However, there are three or four findings that you should be aware of:

- Abnormal T2 hyperintensity in the striatum and the bilateral thalami. The hyperintensity in the putamen can actually be fairly suggestive if it has a lamellated pattern, with modest hyperintensity medially in the putamen and an outer strip of marked hyperintensity (as was present in our patient). This probably corresponds to gliosis from copper-mediated damage.
- Sometimes, especially later in the disease, there is deposition of iron in the zones of gliosis, and the putamen and caudate become quite hypointense on T2. However, the lateral putaminal margins will typically remain markedly hyperintense, again reflecting the lamellated pattern described above. These findings are shown in the case below of a 30-year-old male patient with Wilson's disease (Fig. 5.29), but are seen in only a minority of cases.
- There is abnormal T2-weighted hyperintensity in the tegmentum of the midbrain and sometimes in the belly of the pons (this was also clearly present in our patient). It has been noted in the literature that the T2-weighted hyperintensity in the midbrain tegmentum often spares the red nuclei and the medial margins of the pars reticulata as well as the superior colliculi. All of these structures appear dark against

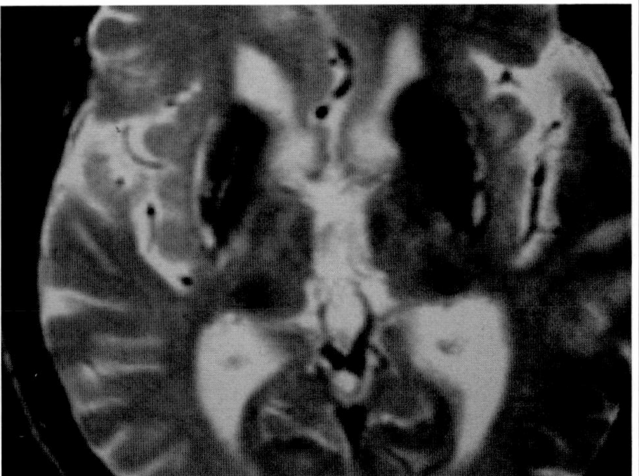

Fig. 5.29. **30-year-old male with Wilson's disease. A T2-weighted axial image shows marked hypointensity of the lentiform nucleus, with a strip of hyperintensity at the lateral putaminal margins.**

the bright midbrain tegmentum, and produce a fairly characteristic pattern called the "face of the giant panda" sign. This is illustrated in Fig. 5.30.

What treatments are available for Wilson's disease?

Very briefly, copper-chelating agents such as Penicillamine and Trientine can arrest disease progression by chelating excess copper. Also, oral zinc salts can reduce intestinal copper absorption. If proper therapy is instituted, there is an excellent prognosis for halting disease progression. It has even been noted that the radiologic abnormalities may be reversible with treatment (Zagami and Boers, 2001). Therefore, while imaging may not play a central role in diagnosis, it is a useful adjunct, and may also be useful in treatment follow up. Lastly, there is also some interesting work with MR spectroscopy showing that there may be a role for spectroscopy in assessing the degree of neurologic involvement. Wilson's disease patients with neurologic manifestations had lower levels of N-acetylaspartate and N-acetylaspartylglutamate on ^{1}H spectroscopy as compared with normal controls, while those with hepatic manifestations only did not (Page *et al.*, 2004). Thus, in the future, spectroscopy may also have a role in following treatment.

References

Page, R. A., Davie, C. A., MacManus, D. *et al.* Clinical correlations of brain MRI and MRS abnormalities in patients with Wilson disease. *Neurology* 2004; **63**(4): 638–643.

Zagami, A. S., and Boers, P.M. Disappearing "face of the giant panda." *Neurology* 2001; **56**(5): 665.

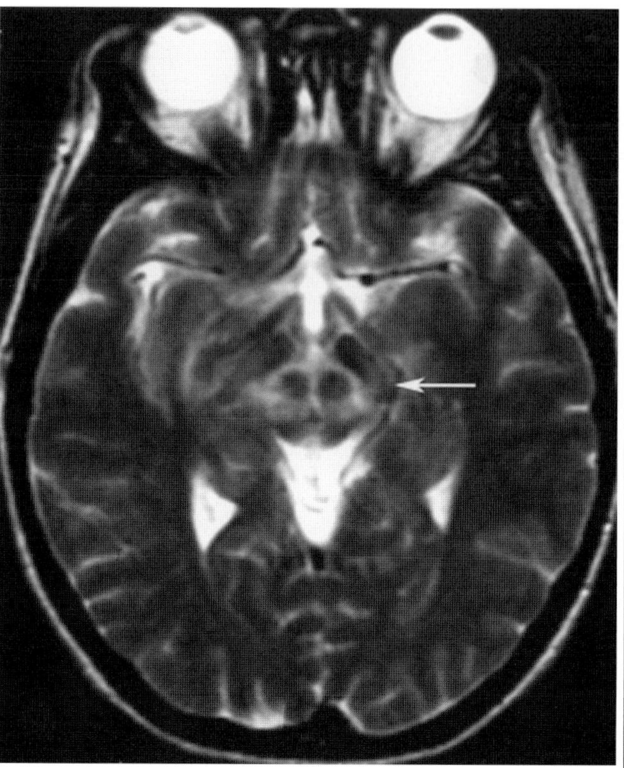

Fig. 5.30. **T2-weighted axial image in a patient with Wilson's disease, showing the classic "face of the giant Panda" sign in the midbrain as described above. This is said to be quite characteristic of Wilson's disease. (Image from Jacobs, D. A. Markowitz, C. E. Liebeskind, D. S. and Galetta, S. L. The "double panda sign" in Wilson's disease. *Neurology* 2003; 61(7):969. Used with permission.)**

Case 5.10

14-year-old male presents with a 2-year history of abnormal posturing, with difficulty walking and cognitive decline, as well as progressive visual impairment. On examination, there was rigidity of the upper and lower extremities with dystonia. There was some generalized bradykinesia, and mild spasticity in the lower extremities. The patient was noted to be dysarthric. There was no history of encephalitis, head trauma, or birth asphyxia.

What is your differential based on the history thus far?

This is a difficult question. As we have seen, there is a vast range of primary dystonia syndromes (including dystonia-plus syndromes), which may present with dystonia, possibly with additional parkinsonian features, in childhood and adolescence. However, it is important to recall that primary dystonia syndromes do not usually present with cognitive impairment or spasticity. Prominent among the remaining differential diagnostic possibilities would be Wilson's disease, which may present in this fashion, as well as juvenile Huntington's. As mentioned briefly, juvenile Huntington's tends to present with rigidity-akinesia rather than choreoathetosis, and so is in the differential list for this patient. Both disorders may also have neuropsychiatric and cognitive findings.

MRI images are provided (Fig. 5.31). What are the findings? What is your provisional diagnosis?

The spin echo T2-weighted images show central hyperintensity in the globi pallidi, surrounded by prominent T2 hypointensity.

In the literature, this pattern has been referred to as the "eye of the tiger" sign. On the T2 GRE sequence, which is more sensitive to magnetic susceptibility effects, such as from iron, there is marked blooming of the T2-weighted hypointensity in the globi pallidi. These findings, along with the patient's age and clinical presentation, are highly suggestive of a diagnosis.

Diagnosis

Hallervorden–Spatz syndrome.

Please discuss Hallervorden–Spatz syndrome.

This disease, described in the 1920s, is characterized by progressive extrapyramidal dysfunction and dementia, coupled with abnormal iron deposition in the brain, most prominently in the globus pallidus. The most classic form is an autosomal recessive disorder with a genetic defect on chromosome 20, involving the pantothenate kinase 2 gene (PANK2).

Pathologically, there is excess iron deposition most prominent in the globus pallidus and its analog, the pars reticulata of the substantia nigra. The iron is found both intracellularly and extracellularly. There is associated neuronal loss, gliosis, and demyelination. There are also swollen axons with vacuolated cytoplasm, known as spheroid bodies. The precise role of the excess iron in the production of these changes is unknown. In fact, it is unclear whether the excess iron deposition is a cause or effect of the neuronal degeneration. Likewise, the precise role of

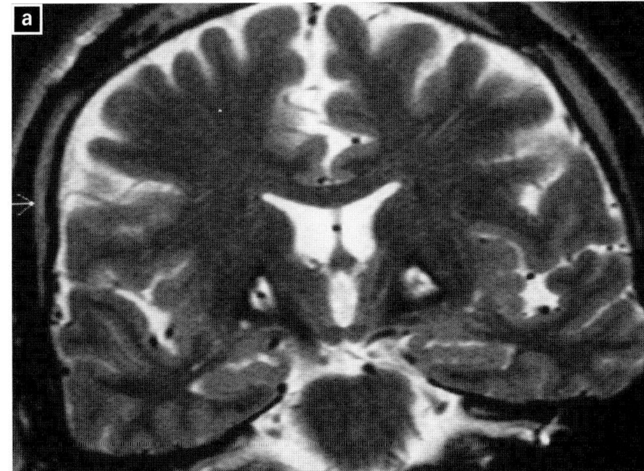
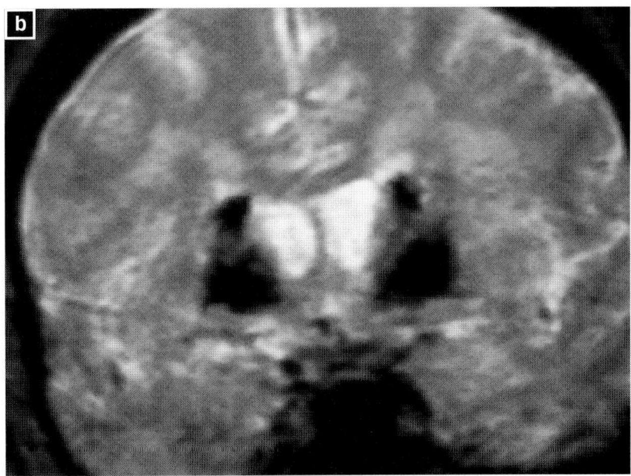

Fig. 5.31. **(a) Coronal spin echo T2 and (b) coronal gradient echo T2-weighted images through the basal ganglia. (Case courtesy of Dr. Noriko Salomon, UCLA Department of Radiology, and Dr. Ashok Panigrahy, Los Angeles Children's Hospital.)**

the PANK2 mutation in the pathogenesis of this disease is unclear. PANK2 appears to play a key role in the production of coenzyme A, which in turn is needed for proper metabolism of carbohydrates, fats, and some amino acids. It is speculated that deficient or abnormal PANK2 may lead to an accumulation of cysteine in the basal ganglia. Cysteine, in turn, chelates iron, which may accelerate free radical formation due to auto-oxidation of cysteine in the presence of iron. However, this all remains quite provisional.

Clinically, the disease typically presents in childhood or early adolescence with extrapyramidal movement disorders and cognitive decline. The disease is progressive, usually leading to death in about 10 years. While the clinical presentation is somewhat variable, dystonia and rigidity are usually prominent features. There may also be parkinsonism, tremor, or choreoathatosis. Dysarthria and dysphagia often appear as the disease progresses. Visual problems, either from optic atrophy or retinitis pigmentosa, may also occur.

As mentioned above, the differential diagnosis for Hallervorden–Spatz disease will include juvenile Huntington's and Wilson's disease, both of which may overlap with Hallervorden–Spatz clinically. Also on the clinical differential would be juvenile ceroid lipofuscinosis, which is a genetic storage disease that presents with visual loss, dementia, rigidity, and dystonia. Since there is no genetic or biochemical test for Hallervorden–Spatz, MRI imaging is quite useful as an adjunct to diagnosis. The typical features are as above, with abnormal T2-weighted hypointensity in the globus pallidus due to excess iron deposition. The resultant neuronal death and gliosis may produce a central zone of T2 hyperintensity within the hypointensity – the "eye of the tiger" sign, as seen in our patient. However, the "eye of the tiger" may not be present, and the images may just show prominent T2-weighted hypointensity in

the basal ganglia, especially in the globi pallidi. In the right clinical setting, these MRI findings are highly suggestive.

Once again, Hallervorden–Spatz underscores a theme which we have tried to make prominent in this chapter: diseases of the basal ganglia involve more than just extrapyramidal movement disorders, and often have cognitive and affective components as well.

Also, this disease introduces one of the important differential diagnostic gamuts in the imaging of the basal ganglia: prominent T2 hypointensity. The differential diagnostic possibilities here are limited, with the commonest entities being:

Hallervorden–Spatz
Ferrocalcinosis of the basal ganglia (such as Fahr's disease)
Exaggerated physiologic iron deposition
Parkinson-plus (MSA) syndromes

Lastly, it is probably important to mention that there seems to be some effort to rename this syndrome. This is in large measure due to the Nazi affiliation of Dr. Julius Hallervorden (see Shevell, 2003). Some names by which it is now referred to are "neurodegeneration with brain iron accumulation type I" (NBIA-1), or "pantothenate kinase-associated neurodegeneration" (PKAN).

An excellent overall review of this syndrome, including possible pathophysiology, can be found in the emedicine article by Garg and Hanna, 2005.

References

Garg, N. and Hanna, P. Hallervorden-Spatz disease. Emedicine, http://www.emedicien.com/neuro/topic151.htm; last modified 3/3/05; accessed 4/5/05.

Shevell, M. Hallervorden and history. *New England Journal of Medicine* 2003; **348**: 3–4.

Case 5.11

56-year-old male patient with 2-year history of progressive bradykinesia, gait difficulties, and postural instability. Examination confirmed a symmetric bradykinesia with rigidity and cogwheeling. The patient showed a postural tremor of the extremities, and episodic dystonia of the extremities as well as the neck.

What differential diagnostic possibilities are you considering?

Parkinsonian features would suggest Parkinson's disease as the most likely diagnosis. Somewhat atypical, however, is the early postural instability. Parkinson-plus syndromes, such as multiple system atrophy, would certainly be a differential diagnostic possibility, as well as possibly drug-induced extrapyramidal symptoms from neuroleptics or other dopamine depleting agents.

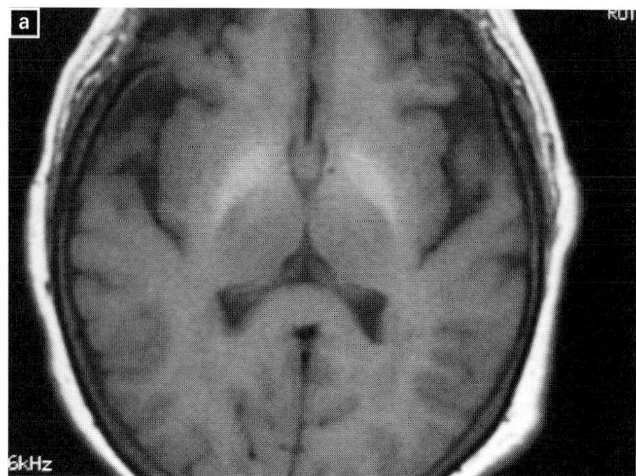
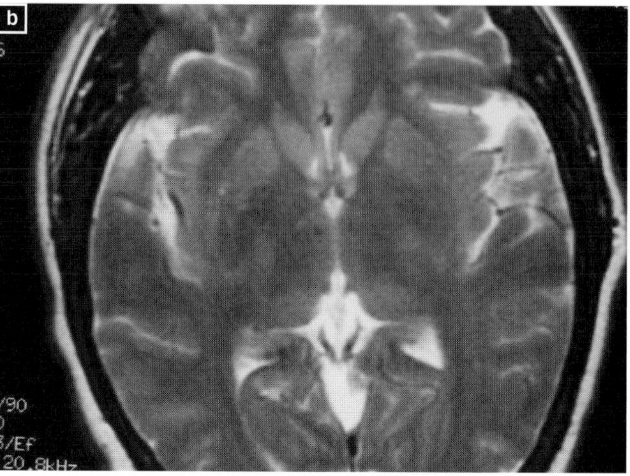

Fig. 5.32. **(a) Axial T1- and (b) T2-weighted images of the brain are obtained without contrast. See text for findings.**

MRI images are presented (Fig. 5.32). What are the findings? What is your differential? Is there any other specific history that you would like to know?

The T1-weighted image shows marked abnormal symmetric T1 hyperintensity in the globus pallidus bilaterally. The T2-weighted images do not show any corresponding signal abnormality.

The finding of T1-weighted hyperintensity in the lentiform nuclei, especially in the globi pallidi, suggests a rather limited differential diagnostic set. By far the most common cause is liver cirrhosis or serious chronic liver disease. Two other less common possibilities are manganese toxicity and total parenteral nutrition. Rarely, T1-weighted hyperintensity in the globi pallidi may be due to portosystemic shunting in the liver in the absence of liver disease.

To complete the differential, we note that other reported causes of patchy T1-weighted hyperintensity in the globi pallidi include rare cases of Wilson's disease, where the copper acts as a paramagnetic substance and shortens T1, petechial hemorrhage after bilateral globus pallidus ischemic infarcts, hamartomas in the basal ganglia such as with neurofibromatosis, rare instances of Japanese encephalitis, treated toxoplasmosis, and sometimes basal ganglia calcification (calcium may sometimes shorten the T1 time of adjacent hydrogen protons in water, and cause T1-weighted hyperintensity on MRI).

T1 hyperintensity in the basal ganglia

(1) Chronic liver disease
(2) Total parenteral nutrition
(3) Petechial hemorrhage after ischemic injury
(4) Hamartomas (such as with neurofibromatosis)
(5) Manganese toxicity
(6) Portosystemic shunts
(7) Basal ganglia calcifications
(8) Treated toxoplasmosis
(9) Rare cases of Japanese encephalitis
(10) Rare cases of Wilson's disease

For those interested in this particular pattern, the article by Lai *et al.* (1999) may be helpful.

Now, to get back to our case. The prominent globus pallidus T1-weighted hyperintensity clearly distinguishes this case from Parkinson's disease or Parkinson-plus syndromes. Therefore, the key question you would like to ask is: does the patient have chronic liver disease? The answer, in this case, is yes! The patient has cirrhosis secondary to hepatitis C.

Diagnosis

Acquired hepatocerebral degeneration.

This syndrome is difficult to pin down precisely. Some use the term to describe the classic MRI findings shown above, regardless of whether the patient has neurologic symptoms. This probably is not a good idea, since even the very early descriptions of T1 hyperintensity in the basal ganglia in association with chronic liver disease pointed out that this finding did not necessarily correlate with neurologic status, but merely served as a marker for the presence of significant chronic hepatic dysfunction (for example, Brunberg *et al.*, 1998). Furthermore, it is found in a high percentage of cirrhotic patients (up to 75 percent). Others use the term to refer to the fairly acute shifts in sensorium as well as tremor and asterixis which may accompany liver disease. Still others confine the usage to chronic motor abnormalities which do not change with sensorium alterations and which are present when the patients are relatively "clear." We prefer the last of these options, separating acquired hepatocerebral degeneration both from neurologically asymptomatic cirrhosis and from episodes of acute hepatic encephalopathy.

When the patients do have motor abnormalities, they may range from parkinsonian-type presentations, as in our patient, to dystonia, tremor, or choreiform movements. The most well-defined presentation seems to be that of a parkinsonian syndrome with early onset postural instability and a postural (but not resting) tremor, along with episodic dystonia. However, it is noted that this represents only a subset of patients with acquired hepatocerebral degeneration, no matter which definition is used. One paper, looking at all cirrhotic patients who were candidates for liver transplantation for over 1 year, found that this subset accounted for 21 percent of those with advanced liver disease (Burkhard *et al.*, 2003).

Pathologically, it has been found that there is microcavitation and neuronal degeneration in the lentiform nuclei, especially the globus pallidus. The precise pathophysiology of this degeneration is unclear. However, the most popular hypothesis, by far, is that the effects are secondary to excess manganese deposition in the globi pallidi, which is felt to be neurotoxic. Manganese, being paramagnetic, shortens the T1 time of adjacent protons and leads to the observed T1 hyperintensity. The evidence in support of this hypothesis is several-fold:
– there is a significant increase in serum and CSF manganese levels in patients who have abnormal T1 hyperintensity in the globus pallidus in the setting of chronic liver disease.

- autopsy series in this same subset of patients reveal a signifi-cant increase in elemental manganese concentration in the globi pallidi compared to normal controls. There is a concomi-tant loss of D2 dopamine receptors. This is an extremely inter-esting correlate to the extrapyramidal signs exhibited by these patients.
- liver transplantation has been shown to lead to reversal of the T1 hyperintensity in the basal ganglia along with a normaliza-tion of serum manganese levels.
- the T1 hyperintensity in the globus pallidus in acquired hepa-tocerebral degeneration is identical to that seen in the rare reported cases of occupational manganese intoxication.

For further reading on this topic, the articles by Butterworth *et al.* (1995) and Maeda *et al.* (1997) are suggested.

Please briefly discuss manganese toxicity.

This diagnosis would be entertained in a patient presenting with extrapyramidal (usually parkinsonian) signs and symptoms who displays the charactersistic T1 hyperintensity in the basal ganglia illustrated above, but without liver disease. Manganese toxicity was initially described at the turn of the century in mine workers who inhaled significant amounts of manganese dust. In the acute phase, this caused emotional lability, nervousness and hallucinations, and became known as "manganese madness."

Currently, toxicity is usually seen in steel alloy workers who do welding involving manganese. The high temperatures cause vaporization of the manganese which is then inhaled, absorbed in the pulmonary circulation, and deposited in the brain. The cause for the selective sensitivity of the globus pallidus remains unclear.

In the chronic phase, a bradykinetic syndrome with rigidity, resembling Parkinson's disease, is seen. This probably correlates with the dopaminergic dysfunction in the striatum noted above. However, it has been noted that the gait of patients with manga-nese toxicity is distinct from that in Parkinson's disease, with a characteristic "cock walking" on the tips of the toes.

In normal patients, manganese, like copper, is absorbed in the intestine and then the excess is excreted by the liver. With hepatic dysfunction, there may be limited excretion. Also, the portosystemic shunting which accompanies cirrhosis may "dump" manganese into the systemic circulation, bypassing the portal circulation. Thus, it is interesting to note that patients on total parenteral nutrition also exhibit the same T1 hyperintensity in the globus pallidus as patients with acquired hepatocerebral degeneration and manganese toxicity; this is probably because the manganese in the TPN bypasses the portal circulation as well. More interestingly still (trying to hold your interest here!) is that a similar imaging appearance of basal ganglia T1 hyperintensity has been described in a case of portosystemic shunting without liver disease due to a hepatic vascular malformation. This cor-rected once the vascular malformation was repaired and the portosystemic shunt ablated (da Rocha *et al.*, 2004).

References

Brunberg, J., Kanal, E., Hirsch, W. *et al.* Chronic acquired hepatic failure: MR imaging of the brain at 1.5 T. *American Journal of Neuroradiology* 1998; **19**: 485–487.

Burkhard, P. R., Delavelle, J., Du Pasquier, R., *et al.* Chronic parkinsonism associated with cirrhosis; a distinct subset of acquired hepatocerebral degeneration. *Archives of Neurology* 2003; **60**: 521–528.

Butterworth, R. F., Spahr, L., Fontaine, S. *et al.* Manganese toxicity, dopa-minergic dysfunction and hepatic encephalopathy. *Metabolic Brain Disease* 1995; **10**(4): 259–267.

da Rocha, A. J., Braga, F. T., da Silva, C. J., *et al.* Reversal of Parkinsonism and portosystemic encephalopathy following embolization of a congenital intrahepatic venous shunt: brain MR imaging and ^{1}H spectroscopic find-ings. *American Journal of Neuroradiology* 2004; **25**: 1247–1250.

Lai, P. H., Chen, C., Liang, H. L., and Pan, H. B. Hyperintense basal ganglia on T1-weighted MR imaging. *American Journal of Neuroradiology* 1999; **172**: 1109–1115.

Maeda, H., Soto, M., Yoshikawa, A. *et al.* Brain MR imaging in patients with hepatic cirrhosis: relationship between high intensity signal in basal gang-lia on T1-weighted images and elemental concentrations in brain. *Neuroradiology* 1997; **39**: 546–550.

Case 5.12

55-year-old male patient who presented with 3 months' history of difficulty walking and frequent falls. Clinical examination revealed axial and proximal bradykinesia, freezing gait, and pos-tural instability. There was no tremor, significant rigidity, or distal akinesia.

The remainder of the history is withheld. For those who do imaging, this is the natural state of affairs. When our depart-ment started requiring that clinical histories be put in before a brain MRI or head CT would be done, our clinical colleagues were quick to defeat this initiative, with the typical one- or two-word histories they entered being: "sick," "ER visit," and "298.8." This last history seems to be a psychiatry code number of some sort.

Please look at the MR image (Fig. 5.33). What are the findings? What is your differential?

There is bilateral, abnormal T2-weighted hyperintensity in the globus pallidus bilaterally. T1-weighted images (not shown) revealed only subtle associated hypointensity.

The pattern of T2-weighted hyperintensity in the basal ganglia (with or without associated T1-weighted hypointensity) is one of the most interesting in neuroradiology. The following category-based diagnostic paradigm is suggested in analyzing these cases:

I. Primary hypoxic or anoxic injury, i.e., low oxygen delivery. This probably represents the majority of cases showing this pattern.

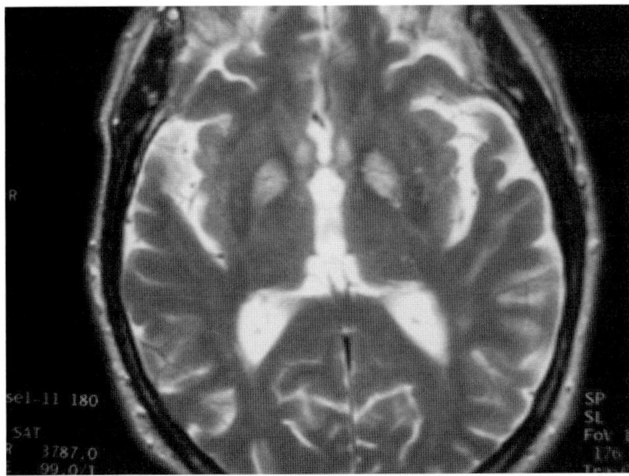

Fig. 5.33. **Axial T2-weighted image of the brain.**

II. Functional hypoxia (i.e., lack of efficient ATP synthesis) – in other words, oxygen is being delivered, but cannot be efficiently utilized. We usually view oxygen as the bottom line: no oxygen and we're dead. Thus, we seldom stop to ask why oxygen is necessary.

It is needed to make ATP via oxidative phosphorylation, predominantly in the mitochondria. Thus, enzymatic defects or genetic disorders which hamper oxidative metabolism or cause mitochondrial dysfunction may produce a hypoxic injury pattern in the basal ganglia. Among these are:
- Leigh's syndrome.
- Mitochondrial disorders, such as MELAS (mitochondrial encephalopathy with lactic acidosis and stroke).
- Certain aminoacidopathies. It turns out that not only glucose, but certain amino acids as well as fatty acids enter the Krebs cycle and produce ATP. If there is a disruption of the metabolism of these substrates in the Krebs cycle, a pattern of injury results similar to that seen in hypoxia. The main aminoacidopathies in this category are methylmalonic acidemia, propionic acidemia, glutaric aciduria and maple syrup urine disease.

III. Profound hypoglycemia. Why? Oxygen doesn't make ATP by itself! It needs glucose to go through the Krebs cycle first (actually glucose is broken down to pyruvate which goes through the Krebs cycle to yield a small amount of ATP, and NADH and FADH2, which are then oxidized by oxygen in the cytochrome chain to make much more ATP – and you thought you'd never use this stuff again!).

After finishing everything to do with hypoxia/ATP synthesis, we now need to turn to other categories of disease.

IV. Degenerative disorders
- Wilson's disease (i.e., hepato *lenticular* degeneration; we've seen this before).
- Juvenile Huntington's disease.
- Dysmyelinating disorders. The basal ganglia may be involved in certain disorders of myelin maintenance, including Krabbe's disease and Canavan's disease. Also, osmotic myelinolysis, such as extrapontine myelinolysis can affect the basal ganglia.

V. Toxic exposure
- Methanol; this is fairly toxic to the striatum, and tends to preferentially involve the putamen and caudate.
- Various "zebras": there are rare reports of basal ganglia necrosis after hydrogen sulfide or carbon disulfide exposure, wasp stings or exposure to certain Eastern herbal supplements.

VI. Encephalitis – various viral encephalitidies may involve the basal ganglia in an inconstant fashion, and these include West Nile virus, Japanese encephalitis, and Epstein–Barr encephalitis.

Diagnosis

Hypoxic injury to the basal ganglia status post respiratory arrest (this is the history which was withheld).

Please discuss further the category of hypoxic injury to the basal ganglia.

The basal ganglia, particularly the globus pallidus, seem to have a high metabolic rate, and hence suffer early in the setting of hypoxia. Inciting causes may be respiratory arrest or near drowning, for example. While there are differences in brain injury patterns between hypoxia and hypotension, the end-artery supply pattern of the basal ganglia also makes them sensitive to combined hypotensive-hypoxic insults such as cardiac arrest. In adults, the globus pallidus may be more commonly injured than the striatum, but caudate and putamen hypoxic injuries also occur. In children, hypoxic injury seems to injure the striatum more than the globus pallidus (this is noted in tabular form in Dr. Barkovich's outstanding textbook, *Pediatric Neuroimaging*, 1995 edition).

The difference in injury distribution contributes to significant differences in clinical presentation. It has been noted by several authors that hypoxic lesions of the globus pallidus tend to present with a parkinsonian akinetic-mutism type of syndrome. Conversely, lesions of the striatum tend to present with dystonia. Thus, after hypoxic injury, children are more likely to present with dystonia, while adults are more likely to present with parkinsonism. Some interesting references which make these points are Nagarajan *et al.* (1995), Kuoppamaki *et al.* (2005), and Hawker and Lang (1990).

Another interesting observation is that the parkinsonism in hypoxic injury of the globus pallidus tends to show some differences from that seen in Parkinson's disease and Parkinson-plus syndromes. Hypoxic lesions of the globus pallidus have been described as producing more pronounced axial bradykinesia, freezing gait, speech difficulties, and postural disturbances, and relatively less peripheral bradykinesia, rigidity, or appendicular tremor. This constellation has led some to hypothesize that the globus pallidus functions mainly in axial motor control (see Feve *et al.*, 1993)

It is important to realize that the extrapyramidal movement disorders manifested in hypoxic injury to the basal ganglia usually have a delayed onset of weeks to months, and may rarely be progressive over a period of years (Bhatt *et al.*, 1993).

There are some additional interesting mechanisms of hypoxic-type injury to the basal ganglia, which we would like to note, as they may not come immediately to mind:

Carbon monoxide poisoning

Carbon monoxide (CO) is a colorless, odorless, poisonous gas which binds to hemoglobin with an affinity approximately 250 times greater than oxygen. Thus, it easily displaces oxygen from hemoglobin. It also causes a leftward shift of the oxyhemoglobin dissociation curve. Thus, it results in oxygen deprivation, with the brain and heart being especially sensitive. With serious exposure, neurologic sequelae may be present in up to 40 percent of cases. The globi pallidi are especially sensitive to CO intoxication, and often show infarction, which may be hemorrhagic. The striatum is less sensitive, and less likely to show imaging abnormalities (see Fig. 5.34).

Like other hypoxic injury to the globus pallidus, patients are often left with parkinsonism. However, they may also have chorea or dystonia. Some investigators have hypothesized that the neurologic sequelae are related not only to hypoxia, but to a direct toxicity of CO to neurons, since the severity of the sequelae does not seem to correlate with the COHb levels. The take home point from the perspective of neuroimaging: carbon monoxide tends to damage the globus pallidus.

From an epidemiologic angle, it is good to know that carbon monoxide is the leading cause of accidental poisoning death in the US, claiming about 2000 lives per year. Some interesting references for those who wish to read further are Cobb and Etzel (1991), Hardy and Thom (1994), Sokal and Kralkowska (1985), and Hsiao *et al.* (2004).

Cyanide poisoning

Cyanide is a highly lethal poison which inactivates the enzyme cytochrome oxidase (cytochrome oxidase aa3), a terminal enzyme in the electron transport chain. Cyanide may enter the body through inhalation, ingestion as a sodium or potassium salt, or by dermal absorption, or may be produced from the

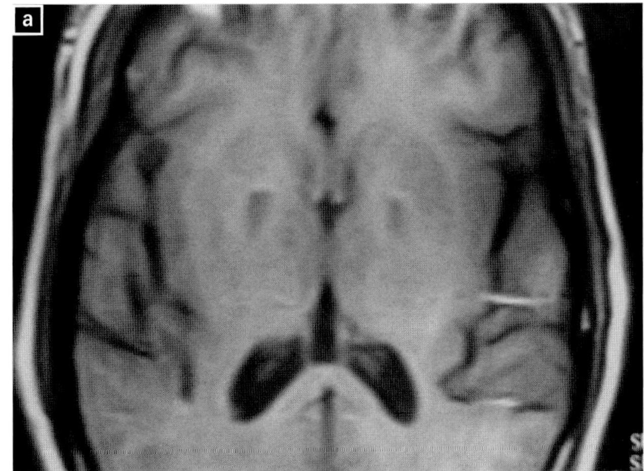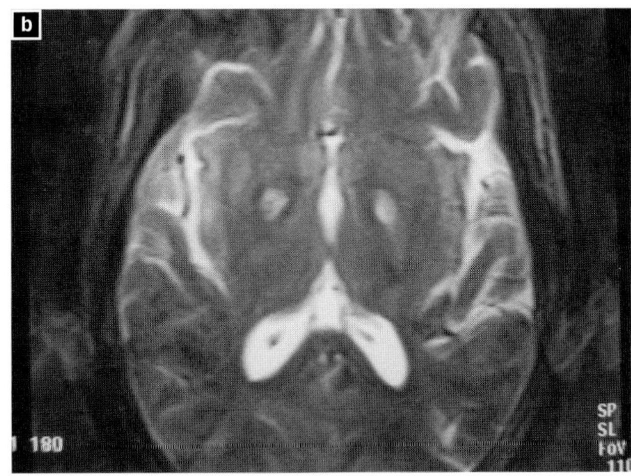

Fig. 5.34. **(a) Axial T1 and (b) T2-weighted images of the brain show bilateral necrosis of the globus pallidus in this 32-year-old male patient who attempted to commit suicide by carbon monoxide and was found in his garage. The patient showed axial bradykinesia, slowed speech, memory difficulty, and sphincter control problems.**

metabolism of certain compounds. Cyanide intoxication occurs in two main forms:

Intentional ingestion in a suicide attempt

This is lethal 95 percent of the time. In the survivors, the basal ganglia are once again preferentially affected.

Exposure

By far the most common cause here is smoke inhalation in a fire. Plastic compounds, as well as wool and silk, may produce hydrogen cyanide gas when they burn. Also, the metal plating and jewelry-making industries have a risk for cyanide exposure. Esoteric causes include prolonged therapy with sodium nitroprusside (with cyanide as a metabolic product) and eating foods high in cyanide, such as cassava. If you ever decide to play Jeopardy, you may want to know that cassava, also known as manioc, is a tropical, starchy staple of South American origin. It can be made into tapioca, or ground into flour. If its roots are properly disposed of, there should be little risk of cyanide poisoning.

In cases of prolonged low dose exposure, there is usually ataxia and optic neuropathy rather than profound ischemic insults.

Please look at the case (Fig. 5.35) of a 35-year-old laboratory worker who ingested cyanide in a failed suicide attempt. The patient initially had akinetic mutism, which slowly resolved. The patient was left with choreoathetosis in the limbs after sensory stimulation.

High altitude sickness

The hypoxia encountered at high altitudes may damage the basal ganglia, and there are case reports of mountain climbing leading to a subcortical dementia associated with imaging evidence of damage to the basal ganglia (Usui *et al.*, 2004; Jeong *et al.*, 2002). Interestingly, the patients did not present with a significant movement disorder.

AIDS and cocaine use

This is an odd heading. However, there have been reports of acute onset ischemic-type lesions in the basal ganglia in AIDS patients using cocaine. AIDS and a high incidence of renal failure was thought to potentiate the ischemic effects of cocaine and produce ischemic damage to the basal ganglia (Meltzer *et al.*, 1998).

Hemolytic–uremic syndrome

This syndrome, characterized by renal failure and microangiopathic hemolytic anemia, usually occurs after an *E. coli* diarrheal illness in children due to a toxin produced by the *E. coli*. It causes microthrombotic changes in the lenticulostriate perforators of the basal ganglia, and may result in abnormal T2 hyperintensity in the bilateral basal ganglia.

Lastly, we have been "lumping" the basal ganglia as one large unit. However, as we alluded to in our discussion of carbon monoxide poisoning, there are tendencies for certain disease processes that lead to T2 hyperintensity in the basal ganglia to involve preferentially the globus pallidus and for others to involve the striatum. This information is summarized below, and is taken from Dr. Barkovich's textbook, *Pediatric Neuroimaging*.

Globus pallidus

Hypoxic injury
Carbon monoxide poisoning
Methylmalonic and propionic acidemia
Kearns–Sayre syndrome
Canavan's disease
Maple syrup urine disease

Striatum

Hypoxic–ischemic injury or asphyxia in a child
Leigh's disease
MELAS
Hypoglycemic injury
Juvenile Huntington's disease
Wilson's disease
Cyanide
Methanol toxicity
Glutaric aciduria

References

Barkovich, J. A. *Pediatric Neuroimaging*. New York: Raven Press, 1995.

Bhatt, M. H., Obeso, J. A., and Marsden, C. D. Time course of postanoxic akinetic-rigid and dystonic syndromes. *Neurology* 1993; **43**: 314–317.

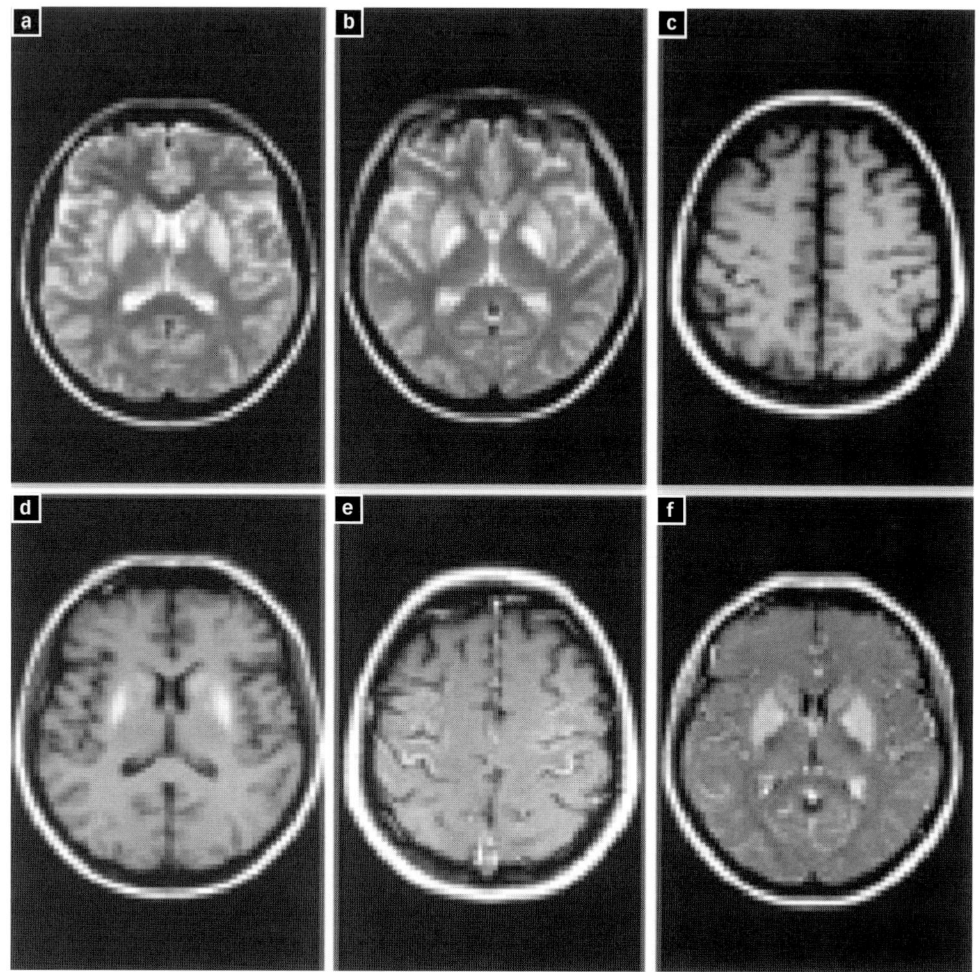

Fig. 5.35. **(a), (b) Axial T2-weighted images, (c), (d) axial T1 images and (e), (f) axial post-contrast T1 images are provided. There is marked T1 and T2 hyperintensity in the bilateral basal ganglia involving the caudate, putamen, and globus pallidus, consistent with hemorrhagic infarction. There is enhancement of the basal ganglia and the motor and premotor cortical ribbons, again consistent with subacute infarct. (Case used with the kind permission of the American Society of Neuroradiology, from Rachinger, J., Fellner, F., Stieglbauer, K. *et al*. M.R. Changes after acute cyanide intoxication. *American Journal of Neuroradiology* 2002; 23: 1398–1401, Fig. 2.**

Cobb, N. and Etzel, R. A. Unintentional carbon monoxide-related deaths in the United States, 1979 through 1988. *Journal of the American Medical Association* 1991; **266**(5): 659–663.

Feve, A. P., Fenelon, G., Wallays, C. *et al*. Axial motor disturbances after hypoxic lesions of the globus pallidus. *Movement Disorders* 1993; **8**(3): 321–326.

Hardy, K. R. and Thom, S. R. Pathophysiology and treatment of carbon monoxide poisoning. *Journal of Clinical Toxicology* 1994; **32**(6): 613–629.

Hawker, K. & Lang, A. E. Hypoxic-ischemic damage of the basal ganglia. Case reports and a review of the literature. *Movement Disorder* 1990; **5**: 219–224.

Hsiao, C. L., Kuo, H. C., and Huang, C. C. Delayed encephalopathy after carbon monoxide intoxication – long-term prognosis and correlation of clinical manifestations and neuroimages. *Acta Neurologica Taiwan* 2004; **13**(2): 64–70.

Jeong, J. H., Kwon, J. C., Chin, J. *et al*. Globus pallidus lesions associated with high mountain climbing. *Journal of Korean Medical Science* 2002; **17**(6): 861–863.

Kuoppamaki, M., Bhatia, K. P., and Quinn, N. Progressive delayed-onset dystonia after cerebral anoxic insult in adults. *Movement Disorder* 2002;**17**(6):1345–1349.

Kuoppamaki, M., Rothwell, J. C., Brown, R. G. *et al*. Parkinsonism following bilateral lesions of the globus pallidus: performance on a variety of motor tasks shows similarities with Parkinson's disease. *Journal of Neurology, Neurosurgery, and Psychiatry* 2005; **76**(4): 482–490.

Meltzer, C. C., Wells, S. W., Becher, M. W. *et al*. AIDS-related MR hyperintensity of the basal ganglia. *American Journal of Neuroradiology* 1998; **19**: 83–89.

Nagarajan, L., Appleton, D. B., and Earwaker, J. S. Case report: MRI in post-hypoxic parkinsonism. *Journal of Child Neurology* 1995; **10**: 63–65.

Sokal, J. A., & Kralkowska, E. The relationship between exposure duration, carboxyhemoglobin, blood glucose, pyruvate and lactate and the severity of intoxication in 39 cases of acute carbon monoxide poisoning in man. *Archives of Toxicology* 1985; **57**(3): 196–199.

Usui, C., Inoue, Y., Kimura, M. *et al*. Irreversible subcortical dementia following high altitude illness. *High Altitude Medicine and Biology* 2004; **5**(1): 77–81.

Case 5.13

52-year-old male patient with 3-year history of progressive generalized dystonia and choreiform movements. The patient's family also related that the patient now suffered from memory deficits, cognitive impairments, and depression.

What do you think so far?

As discussed in previous cases, the differential diagnosis for chorea and dystonia is very broad, and may reflect any number of primary or secondary disorders of the basal ganglia. Certainly, the history, including the dementia and the depression, would be consistent with Huntington's disease, but the age of onset is a bit old. We need some extra information. Imaging is a great way to look at the basal ganglia for obvious pathology.

Imaging is provided (Fig. 5.36). What are the findings? What is your differential? Would you like to order any other tests?

The differential diagnostic list for basal ganglia calcifications is quite long, and includes the following:

Physiologic basal ganglia calcifications
Disorders of calcium metabolism
– hypoparathyroidism
– pseudo- and pseudopseudohypoparathyroidsim
– hyperparathyroidism
ToRCH congenital infections (toxoplasmosis, rubella, cytomegalovirus, and herpes)
Pediatric HIV infection
Fahr's disease
Cockayne syndrome
Aicardi–Goutières syndrome
Down's syndrome

For those interested in further reading on basal ganglia calcifications, the article by Cohen *et al.* (1980) may be helpful.

While many entities may cause basal ganglia calcifications, the characteristic distribution of the calcifications in this case (basal ganglia, subcortical white matter, dentate nuclei of the cerebellum) make Fahr's disease and hypoparathyroidism the two most likely differential diagnostic possibilities. Therefore, the key question we would like to ask is about the patient's calcium level, to distinguish these two possibilities. The calcium level was normal, excluding hypoparathyroidism.

Diagnosis

Fahr's disease.

Not much is known about this disease. It is characterized by abnormal deposits of calcium in the brain, most prominently in the basal ganglia, but also in the thalami, white matter, and cerebellum. The pathophysiology of the calcium deposition and the accompanying neuronal degeneration remain unclear. Thus, the disease goes by many names: idiopathic basal ganglia calcification (IBGC), striatopallidodentate calcinosis, and cerebrovascular ferrocalcinosis, in addition to Fahr's disease. Older books referred to it as a genetic disease with instances of autosomal recessive and autosomal dominant inheritance, and also as an oftentimes sporadic occurrence.

Recently, however, genetic analysis in a family with autosomal dominant transmission identified the first chromosomal locus for the disease on chromosome 14q. This locus is now known as IBGC1 (Geschwind *et al.*, 1999). With this discovery, the trend seems to be shifting to consider Fahr's disease as an autosomal dominant disorder of idiopathic calcium deposition, primarily in the basal ganglia.

A precise clinical presentation also remains elusive. Like other basal ganglia disorders, it has motor, cognitive, and psychiatric manifestations. The most common psychiatric manifestation is depression. Attention deficit, mood swings, anxiety, and irritability are also described. The cognitive impairment is predominantly a frontal subcortical dementia. The movement disorders range from chorea and dystonia to parkinsonism, and may include dysarthria and spasticity.

Some sources suggest that the parkinsonian features occur late in the disease. However, a recent survey of Fahr's disease patient's found that parkinsonism is the most common movement disorder, seen in 57 percent of patients, with chorea found in 19 percent (Manyam *et al.*, 2001).

Surprisingly, the degree of calcification does not appear to correlate with the neurological presentation. Finally, it has been reported that Fahr's disease may have purely behavioral–neuropsychological manifestations. PET scanning in one such case report showed significant hypometabolism of the basal ganglia and the frontal lobes, suggesting a disruption of the frontostriatal circuits (Benke *et al.*, 2004).

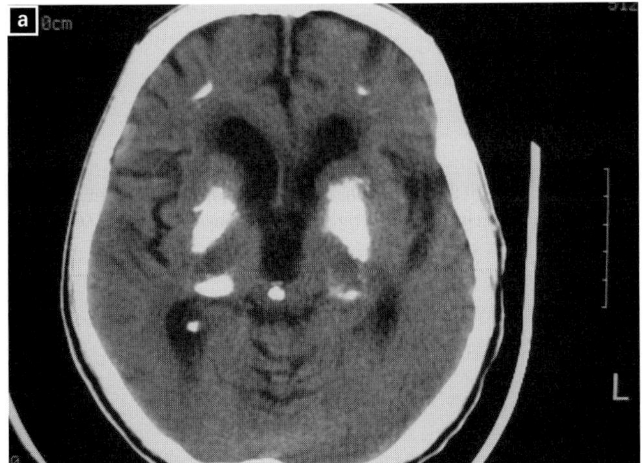

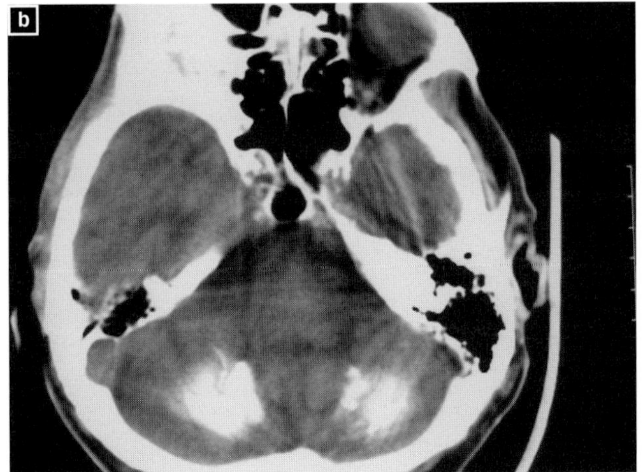

Fig. 5.36. **(a), (b) Selected axial non-contrast CT images of the brain. The axial CT images show extensive calcifications of the bilateral basal ganglia, bilateral thalami, and extensive calcification of the dentate nuclei and white matter of the cerebellum. Higher slices (not shown) revealed some calcifications of the subcortical white matter as well. (Case courtesy of Dr. Suzie El-Saden, UCLA Department of Radiology.)**

Please take a look at the CT scan of a 48-year-old patient, who presented with progressive dementia and parkinsonism over 4 years (Fig. 5.37). What are the findings? What is your differential? Are there other laboratory tests which you would like?

Once again, with this characteristic pattern, Fahr's disease and hypoparathyroidism should come to mind. The calcium level in this patient was 6 mg/dL, and the diagnosis was hypoparathyroidism. Paradoxically, in these patients with hypocalcemia, there is often dystrophic calcification of the basal ganglia. The neurological manifestations in the chronic setting may be identical to Fahr's disease, but the parkinsonian symptoms are sometimes reversible with the administration of parathyroid hormone (Tambyah *et al.*, 1993).

Pseudohypoparathyroidism is a condition where there is hypocalcemia, but with elevated levels of parathyroid hormone, and a biological resistance to its activity. This condition may be due to a variety of genetic defects. In terms of neuroimaging, its appearance can be identical to hypoparathyroidism. The reason it was not included with Fahr's and hypoparathyroidism in the differential of the above cases is because it is quite rare. However, for your viewing pleasure, is a case of pseudohypoparathyroidism (Fig. 5.38).

Finally, in the imaging workup of movement disorder patients, we often go directly to MRI, bypassing the CT. Therefore, it is good to see the appearance of such dense calcifications on MRI (Fig. 5.39). They often give a characteristic mix of T1 and T2 hypointensity with a hyperintense halo, as in the case below. We have previously noted that calcifications may sometimes present with T1 hyperintensity, and this sometimes fools junior residents, until they have seen a few such cases. If you see such an appearance, order the non-contrast CT to look for calcifications.

References

Benke, T., Karner, E., Seppi, K. *et al*. Subacute dementia and imaging correlates in a case of Fahr's disease. *Journal of Neurology Neurosurgery, and Psychiatry* 2004; **75**(8): 1163–1165.

Cohen, C. R., Duchesneau, P. M., & Weinstein, M. A. Calcification of the basal ganglia as visualized by computed tomography. *Radiology* 1980; **134**: 97–99.

Geschwind, D. H., Loginov, M., and Stern, J. M. Identification of a locus on chromosome 14q for idiopathic basal ganglia calcification [Fahr disease]. *The American Journal of Human Genetics* 1999; **65**: 794.

Manyam, B. V., Walters, A. S., and Narla, K. R. Bilateral striopallidodentate calcinosis: clinical characteristics of patients seen in a registry. *Movement Disorder* 2001; **16**(2): 258–264.

Tambyah, P. A., Ong, B. K., and Lee, K.O. Reversible parkinsonism and asymptomatic hypocalcemia with basal ganglia calcification from hypoparathyroidism 26 years after thyroid surgery. *American Journal Medicine* 1993; **94**(4): 444–445.

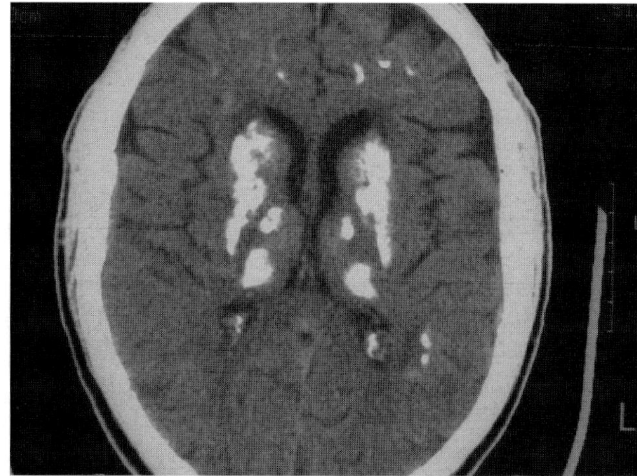

Fig. 5.37. **Axial non-contrast CT scan demonstrates heavy calcifications in the bilateral basal ganglia, thalami, and subcortical white matter. Lower images (not shown) illustrated some calcifications in the cerebellum as well. The pattern is essentially identical to our last case.**

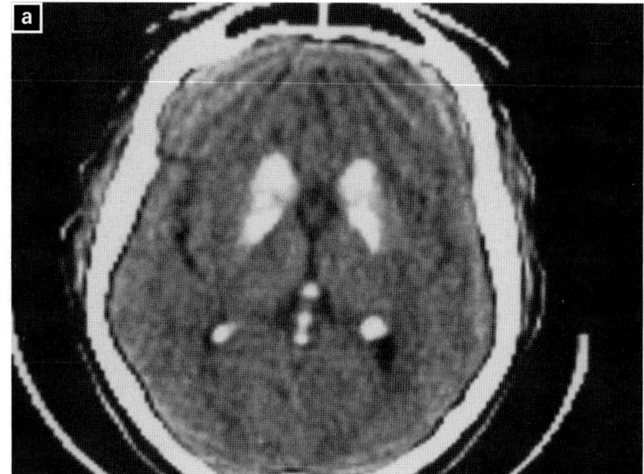
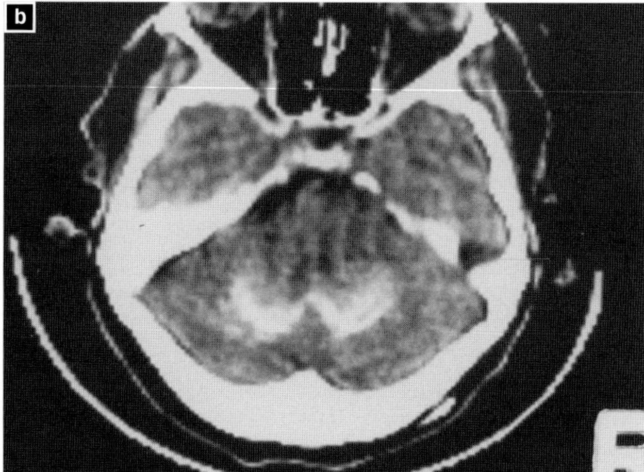

Fig. 5.38. **(a), (b) Patient with pseudohypoparathyroidism showing dense basal ganglia and cerebellar calcifications on a very old set of CT images. (Case courtesy of Dr. Suzie El-Saden, UCLA Department of Radiology.)**

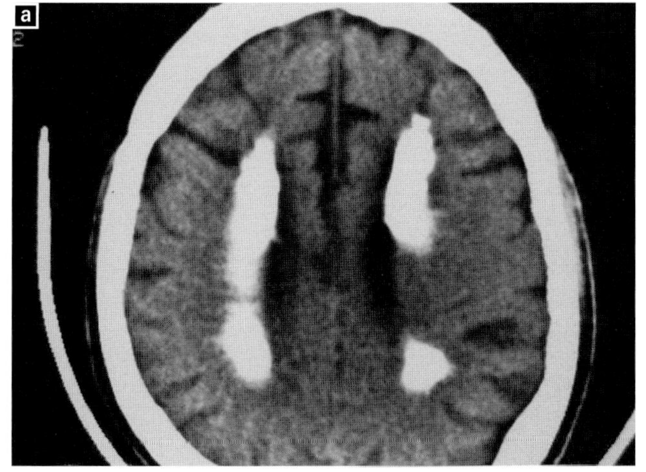

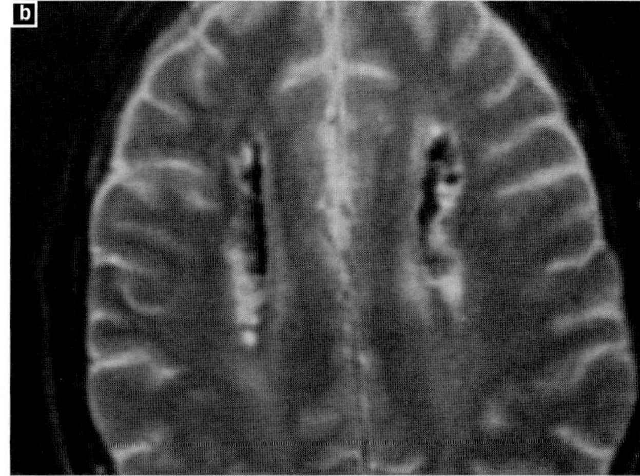

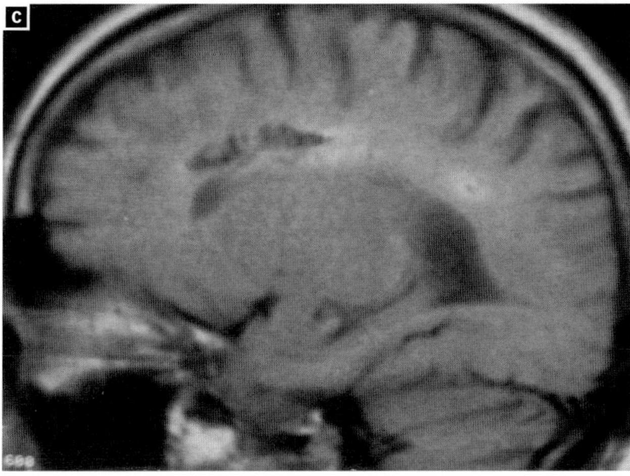

Fig. 5.39. (a) Axial non-contrast CT showing dense periventricular calcifications. (b), (c) T2 axial and T1-weighted sagittal MRI images, respectively, showing T1 and T2 hypointensity with halos of hyperintensity on both T1 and T2. This bizarre appearance should suggest heavy calcification and prompt a CT.

Case 5.14

4-year-old male patient with ataxia, nystagmus, and dysarthria, progressive for 1 year. On examination, the patient showed diminished muscle mass, incoordination, dysarthria, slowed saccades with irregular eye movements, and horizontal nystagmus.

MRI images are shown (Fig. 5.40). What are the findings? What is your differential?

The MRI images show abnormal symmetric T2-weighted hyperintensity in the inferior aspect of the lentiform nuclei, medial thalami, dorsal midbrain, pontine tegmentum, and dorsal medulla.

The bilaterally symmetric distribution suggests a metabolic disorder. The involvement of the basal ganglia, thalami, and upper and lower brainstem in the locations shown above suggests Leigh's syndrome. Some have likened the distribution of abnormalities to Wernicke's encephalopathy, while others have likened it to Wilson's syndrome.

Diagnosis

Leigh's syndrome.

Leigh's syndrome, or subacute necrotizing encephalomyelopathy, is a progressive neurodegenerative disorder characterized by enzymatic defects, which affect ATP production and mitochondrial function. It is, in fact, any of a wide constellation of individual genetic defects which lead to a characteristic neuropathology of vacuolization and spongiform degeneration in the basal ganglia, thalami, brainstem, and possibly the cerebellum or cerebral white matter. It turns out that the molecular genetics of Leigh's syndrome are thus an exceedingly complex subject. However, we try to note a few useful points.

- A very large number of individual genetic defects can produce Leigh's syndrome.
- The defects tend to be of two major types: those involving the citric acid cycle, such as pyruvate dehydrogenase or pyruvate decarboxylase deficiency, and those involving the cytochrome chain.
- The cytochrome chain is composed of five complexes (I–V), which are elaborated by mitochondrial DNA (the mitochondria, like the nucleus, contain DNA. In the human, mitochondrial DNA is composed of 37 genes). Defects in any of these complexes may produce Leigh's syndrome. An excellent overall review of mitochondrial respiratory

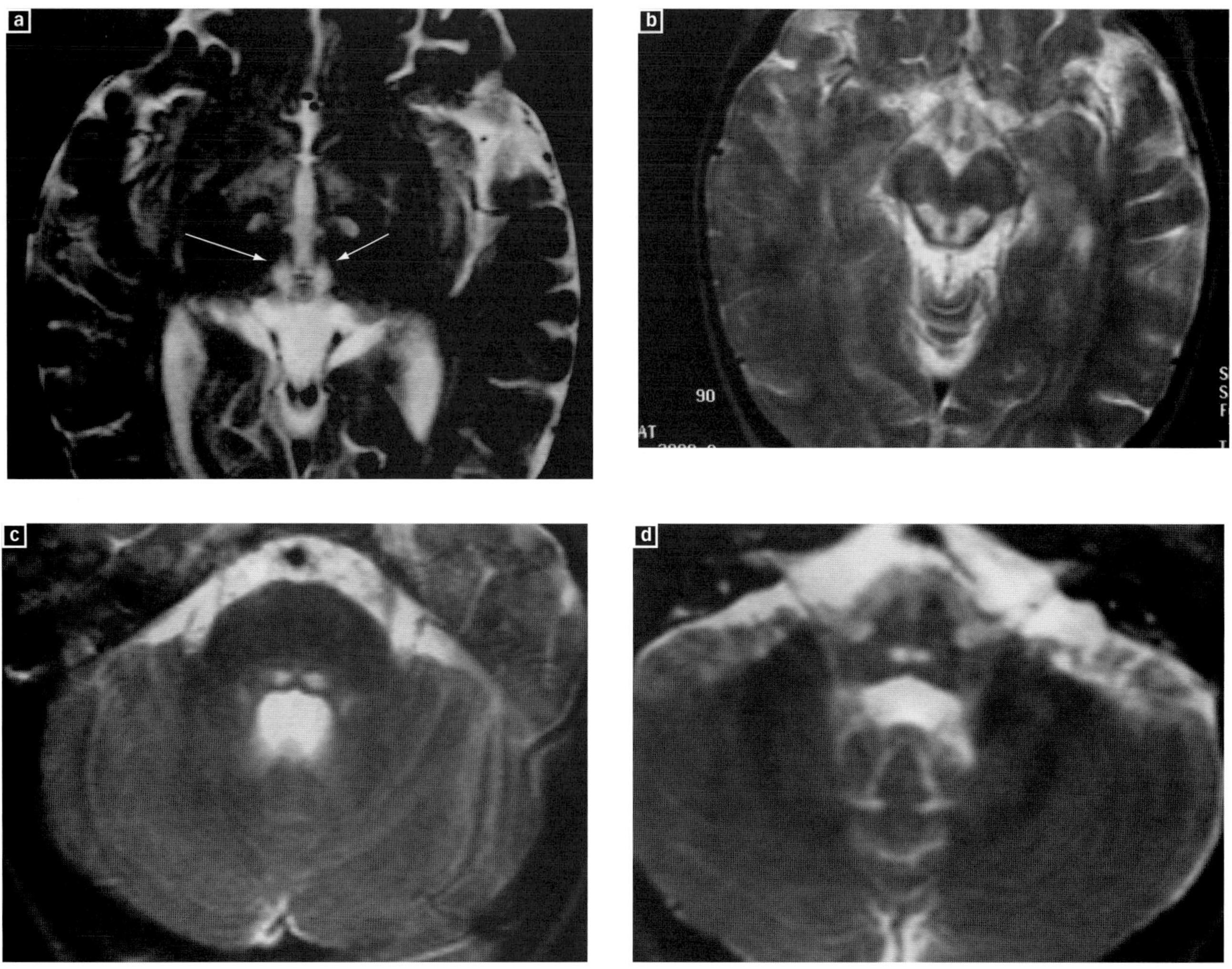

Fig. 5.40. **(a)–(d) T2-weighted axial MRI images at the levels of the inferior basal ganglia, midbrain, pons and medulla. (Case courtesy of Dr. Ashok Panigrahy, Los Angeles Children's Hospital.) The hyperintensities in the medial thalami are indicated by the arrow, since they are subtle, and may blend with the signal of the third ventricle.**

chain genetics and diseases by DiMauro and Schon (2003) is referenced.

– The most common defect seems to be in the cytochrome c oxidase system, also known as complex IV. Within complex IV, mutations in Leigh's syndrome have been found in the surfeit-1 gene (SURF1), and in genes known as COX10 and COX15. There is also a French-Canadian (Saguenay–Lac Saint Jean) variant of Leigh's with a different COX deficiency.

– In those with cytochrome c oxidase deficiencies, there are differences in imaging, based on whether the SURF 1 gene is involved. In that subset of patients, the brainstem and cerebellum tend to be heavily involved. Those without SURF 1 mutations are more likely to show abnormalities of the basal ganglia, particularly the putamen. For those interested in parsing out the imaging correlates, the articles by Farina *et al.* (2002) and Rossi *et al.* (2003) may be useful.

– Clinically, the syndrome consists of a variety of presentations. However, it is usually seen in infancy or early childhood, presenting with hypotonia, muscle wasting, ataxia, nystagmus, deafness, ocular motility disorders, dysphagia, pyramidal, and extrapyramidal movement disorders, and

respiratory insufficiency with periods of apnea. Death is often secondary to respiratory failure. An interesting imaging correlate is that near fatal respiratory failure tends to be strongly associated with the presence of lower brainstem lesions (such as in our patient) on MRI (see Arii and Tanabe, 2001).

– Because of the heterogeneity of the defects, there are three types of inheritance patterns associated with Leigh's syndrome: X-linked recessive (some pyruvate dehydrogenase deficiencies), mitochondrial (disease may be inherited directly through mitochondrial DNA, which is essentially always passed maternally), and autosomal recessive.

– The disorder was originally described by Denis Leigh, a British neuropathologist, in 1951. It turns out he pronounced his name "Lee", and not "Lay." This may be the most useful piece of information in this case presentation. Somewhere along your training, one of your attendings is bound to mention "Lay's" syndrome. That's when you jump in and say, "Don't you mean 'Lee's' syndrome, Professor? That is, after all, the correct pronounication." You will be a favorite of that attending forever after, guaranteed!

References

Arii, J. and Tanabe, Y. Leigh syndrome: serial MR imaging and clinical follow-up. *American Journal of Neuroradiology* 2000; **21**: 1502–1509.

DiMauro, S., & Schon, E. A. Mitochondrial respiratory-chain diseases. *New England Journal of Medicine* 2003; **348**: 2656–2668.

Farina, L., Chiapparini, L., Uziel, G. *et al*. MR findings in Leigh syndrome with COX deficiency and SURF1 mutations. *American Journal of Neuroradiology* 2002; **23**(7): 1095–1100.

Rossi, A., Biancheri, R., Bruno, C. *et al*. Leigh syndrome with COX deficiency and SURF1 gene mutations: MR findings. *American Journal of Neuroradiology* 2003; **24**(6): 188–191.

Case 5.15

6-year-old patient with subacute onset of generalized chorea over the last week. Two weeks ago, the patient had been diagnosed with infectious mononucleosis.

MRI images are provided adjacent (Fig. 5.41). What are the findings? What is your diagnosis?

The MRI image shows diffuse abnormal hyperintensity in the bilateral putamen and caudate nuclei.

Diagnosis

Epstein–Barr virus (EBV) encephalitis involving the basal ganglia.

The diagnosis here is extremely difficult, and not something which you are expected to get *a priori*. However, we thought this would be a useful case to see, so that if you encounter it again, you would think of this rare entity.

As we have previously discussed, the differential of T2-weighted hyperintensity in the basal ganglia is broad, with infectious etiologies a possible but not common cause.

Of the possible infections without mass lesions, confluent gelatinous pseudocysts in dilated perivascular spaces from cryptococcal infection may simulate diffuse smooth symmetric hyperintensity. Also, several viral encephalitidies may involve the basal ganglia in an inconstant fashion. Among these are Eastern equine encephalitis, rabies, and West Nile encephalitis. It is difficult to be more specific, as cases of these encephalitides will also be present without basal ganglia involvement. Japanese encephalitis may involve the basal ganglia, but much more commonly involves the thalami. Murray Valley encephalitis tends to involve the thalami and spare the basal ganglia. Nipah valley encephalitis, meanwhile, is distinctly different, with lesions at the gray–white matter junctions and little involvement of the deep gray structures.

Finally, post-infectious acute disseminated encephalomyelitis (ADEM) may involve the basal ganglia and has been reported post streptococcal infection, post-mycoplasma infection and even post-Hepatitis B vaccination.

If you scan the literature on EBV encephalitis, you will find that basal ganglia involvement may occur, but once again is not a particularly common manifestation. Various lesions involving cortical gray matter, white matter, the brainstem, the cerebellum, the basal ganglia, and the thalami have been reported. Moreover, CNS involvement with EBV infection is uncommon (less than 10 percent of cases) and most of the cases where it is clinically felt that there is some CNS involvement are negative on imaging. For those who are interested in a good case series on this topic, please see Shian and Chi (1996).

However, if you have a patient who has recently been diagnosed with infectious mononucleosis and presents with extrapyramidal

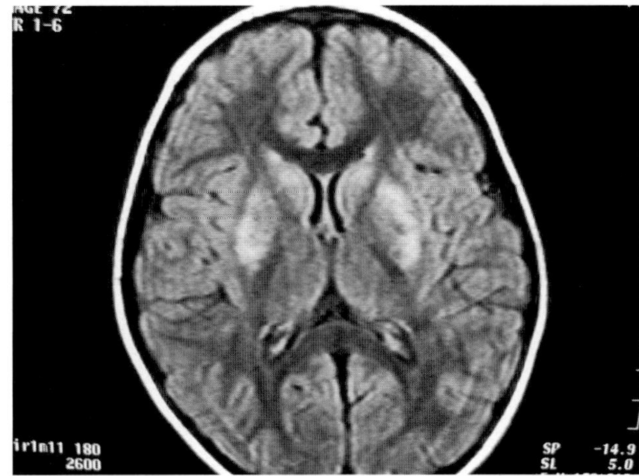

Fig. 5.41. **Axial FLAIR MRI image.**

findings and has abnormal T2 hyperintensity of the basal ganglia, think of this unusual entity: EBV encephalitis involving the basal ganglia. This bilaterally symmetric basal ganglia involvement secondary to EBV encephalitis has been well documented in two prior case reports (Cecil *et al.*, 2000 and Donovan and Zimmerman, 1996).

It is also useful to remember that ADEM as a response to chronic EBV infection is reported in the brain, and should be included in your differential if the patient has known EBV infection.

In their 29 patient case series of EBV encephalitis cited above, Shian and Chi noted that the clinical presentation is variable, with the most common findings being an alteration in the level of consciousness, seizures and visual hallucinations. Cranial nerve palsies have also been reported.

Thus, while EBV encephalitis involving the basal ganglia is a rare entity, you are now in a position to suggest it in the right clinical setting.

References

Cecil, K. M., Jones, B. V., Williams, S. *et al*. CT, MRI and MRS of Epstein–Barr virus infection: case report. *Neuroradiology* 2000; **42**: 619–622.

Donovan, W. D., and Zimmerman, R. D. MR findings of severe Epstein–Barr virus encephalomyelitis. *Journal of Computer Assisted Tomography* 1996; **20**: 1027–1029.

Shian, W. and Chi, C. Epstein–Barr virus encephalitis and encephalomyelitis: MR findings. *Pediatric Radiology* 1996; **26**: 690–693.

Case 5.16

63-year-old patient presents with 2-day onset of right arm hemichorea and hemiballismus. Clinical examination confirms the history. The patient denies a family history of Huntington's disease and denies HIV infection.

The CT and MRI images are presented (Fig. 5.42). What are the findings? What other piece of clinical history would you like to know now that you have seen the scans? What is your diagnosis?

The CT scan shows subtle hyperdensity in the left putamen and left caudate head. The non-contrast MRI scans show subtle

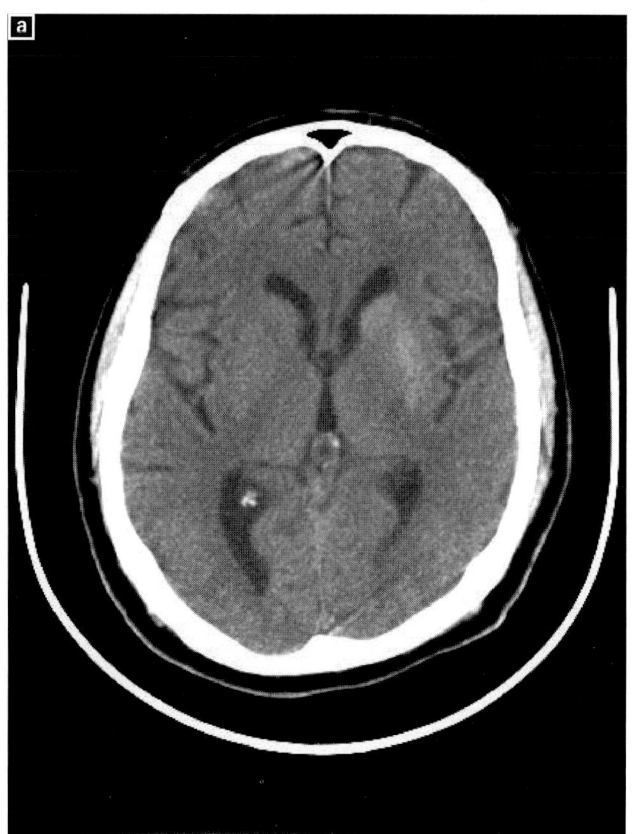 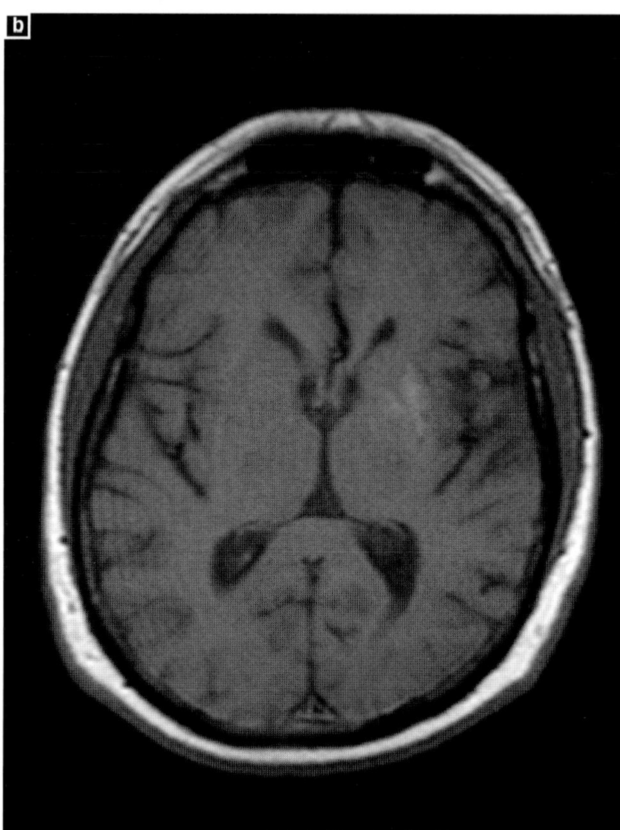

Fig. 5.42. **(a) Axial non-contrast CT and (b) axial T1-weighted MRI scans of the brain are obtained.**

T1-weighted hyperintensity. T2-weighted and FLAIR images (not shown) were normal in appearance.

This appearance of hyperdensity on non-contrast CT and T1-weighted hyperintensity on non-contrast MRI in the putamen in the setting of recent onset contralateral hemichorea–hemiballismus has been described in the literature in a very specific clinical setting.

Is there any other clinical data that you wish? *Hint*: Ask for a blood glucose. In our patient, it was 540 mg/dL, and he had a history of primary diabetes.

Diagnosis

Hemichorea–hemiballismus in association with non-ketotic hyperglycemia.

One of the unusual causes of hemichorea–hemiballismus is non-ketotic hyperglycemia (see, for example, Lai *et al.*, 1996 and Wintermark *et al.*, 2004).

Once you have seen a case (such as this one), you will never forget it. That is lucky, because there is little else we can say about it. The pathophysiology of this disorder is unclear. Some authors have hypothesized that hyperglycemia causes decreased blood flow to the basal ganglia and disturbs normal GABA concentrations. Others have implicated osmotic disturbances, while others suggest ischemia due to hyperviscosity. The truth remains elusive, but the association seems definite. It is an important association to recognize, because the condition is quite treatable. The movement disorder responds extremely well to normalization of the blood glucose levels. Our patient's findings, for example, resolved in 48 hours. It is also important not to mistake the

imaging findings and clinical presentation for an ischemic stroke. Thus, be aware that subtle diffusion-weighted hyperintensity and ADC map hypointensity may be present.

Not only is the pathophysiology of this disorder unclear, but so is the cause of the hyperdensity on CT and the T1-weighted hyperintensity on MRI. The leading hypotheses are either an influx of calcium associated with hyperglycemia (recall that calcium may sometimes be hyperintense on T1-weighted MRI), or petechial hemorrhage in the basal ganglia. The imaging findings seem slowly reversible with normalization of the blood glucose, but definitely lag behind the usually dramatic clinical improvement.

The putamen is usually involved, but the caudate may also be abnormal. The involvement may be unilateral (that seems slightly more common), in which case the hemiballismus–hemichorea is on the contralateral side, or the involvement may be bilateral.

References

Lai, P. H., Tien, R. D., Chang, M. H., *et al.* Chorea-ballismus with nonketotic hyperglycemia in primary diabetes mellitus. *American Journal of Neuroradiology* 1996; **17**: 1057 –1064.

Wintermark, M., Fischbein, N. J., Mukherjee, P., Yuh, E. L., and Dillon, W. P. Unilateral putaminal CT, MR, and diffusion abnormalities secondary to nonketotic hyperglycemia in the setting of acute neurologic symptoms mimicking stroke. *American Journal of Neuroradiology* 2004; **25**(6): 975–976.

Case 5.17

33-year-old male patient with several weeks of progressive left-sided chorea. Patient denies family history of movement disorders.

An MRI image is presented (Fig. 5.43). What are the findings? After seeing the scan, is there other clinical history which you would like? What is your diagnosis?

The image shows a large lobulated rim-enhancing mass in the right basal ganglia, with a large amount of surrounding edema. A similar but smaller mass is seen in the left basal ganglia.

The lobulated appearance of the right basal ganglia lesion (as well as a location in the basal ganglia) make metastatic disease less likely, although it is, of course, a possibility. The appearance and multiplicity of the lesions make primary CNS tumor less likely, although that is also a possibility. However, the location of the lesions in the basal ganglia, and the large amount of surrounding edema suggest the possibility of a particular infection: toxoplasmosis. Given that, the relevant piece of missing clinical data we are after is the patient's HIV status. After the MRI scan, the patient was tested, and found to be HIV positive.

Diagnosis

AIDS-related chorea.

This is not a specific disease entity, but rather another interesting association. Of course, there is nothing specific about AIDS and chorea. Any basal ganglia lesion could potentially lead to extrapyramidal movement disorders. However, it has been noted that about 3 percent of AIDS patients have clinically significant movement disorders, and that with prospective follow-up, up to 50 percent may develop some degree of extrapyramidal movement disorder (see Cardoso, 2002).

The AIDS-associated extrapyramidal movement disorders can be thought of as two broad groups, the hyperkinesias and the hypokinesias (parkinsonism). The most common hyperkinetic extrapyramidal disorder is hemiballismus–hemichorea, with the vast majority of cases being secondary to AIDS-related opportunistic infections, especially toxoplasmosis, as in our patient. Other hyperkinetic disorders include dystonia or myoclonus. AIDS patients may, instead, show features of parkinsonism. As

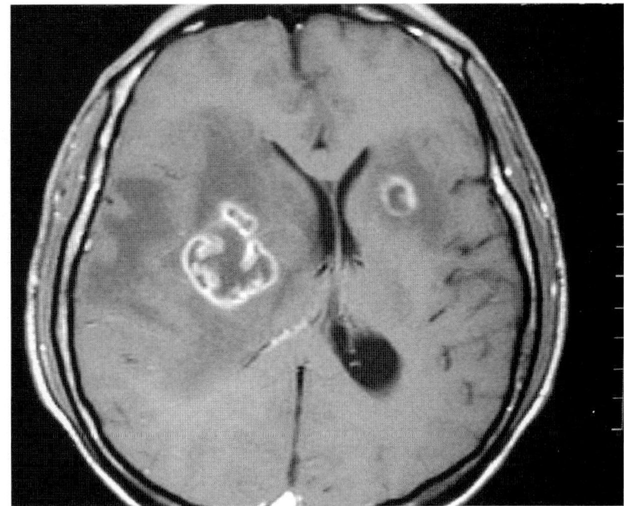

Fig. 5.43. **Axial post-contrast T1-weighted MRI scan of the brain is provided.**

opposed to the hyperkinetic disorders, parkinsonism or tremor is usually not secondary to opportunistic infections, but to dopaminergic dysfunction associated with primary HIV infection of the CNS. Some other interesting references on this topic are Piccolo *et al.* (1999) and Tse *et al.* (2004).

References

Cardoso, F. HIV-related movement disorders: epidemiology, pathogenesis and management. *CNS Drugs* 2002; **16**(10): 663–668.

Piccolo, I., Causarano, R., Sterzi, R. *et al.* Chorea in patients with AIDS. *Acta Neurologica Scandinavia* 1999; **100**(5): 332–336.

Tse, W., Cersosimo, M. G., Gracies, J. M., Morgello, S., Olanow, C. W. and Koller, W. Movement disorders and AIDS: a review. *Parkinsonism and Related Disorder* 2004; **10**(6): 323–334.

Case 5.18

10-year-old girl presents with several months of slowly worsening left arm dystonia. On taking a more careful history, we find out that the dystonia has remained only in the arm, and has not spread further.

What are your initial thoughts?

As you recall, primary dystonia syndromes which begin in childhood often (but, of course, not always) begin in the foot and then generalize. Thus, this is not the typical pattern, and should raise the possibility of a focal lesion.

An MRI is shown (Fig. 5.44). What is your diagnosis?

The MRI image shows multiple serpiginous tangled flow voids involving primarily the right lentiform nucleus. The appearance is consistent with a tangle of vessels, and is diagnostic of an arteriovenous malformation (AVM). The AVM has deep venous drainage into a large subependymal vein.

Diagnosis

Focal left-sided dystonia secondary to a right basal ganglia AVM.

There is no particular association between AVM and dystonia. As we have seen, a myriad of basal ganglia disease processes may lead to dystonia. It is but another example of such a disease process – not terribly common, but definitely previously reported (Friedman *et al.*, 1986; Kurita *et al.*, 1998).

Please discuss briefly the management of AVMs.

As you know, AVMs are congenital vascular malformations. Although they are present at birth, they tend to become symptomatic later in life, usually in the third or fourth decades. They consist of one or more large arterial feeders supplying a complex vascular tangle known as the nidus, which then drains into one or more large draining veins. AVMs have an estimated annual risk of hemorrhage of about 2–4 percent per year, with an estimated mortality rate of 10 percent when a bleed occurs.

In an attempt to guide therapy, neurosurgeons usually grade AVMs based on the Spetzler–Martin grading scheme, a five-point system which grades the AVM based on the size of the nidus at angiography, whether the AVM is located in eloquent brain, and whether or not it has deep venous drainage (or drains only to superficial cortical veins).

Size		Location		Venous drainage	
< 3 cm	1	Non-eloquent brain	0	Superficial	0
3–6 cm	2	Eloquent brain	1	Deep	1
> 6 cm	3				

AVMs may thus range from grade 1 to 5, with higher grades heralding a poorer prognosis. In general, neurosurgeons will attempt to manage grades 1–3 and sometimes grade 4 operatively. Grade 5, and sometimes grade 4 are generally felt to be poor operative candidates, who may be managed by endovascular techniques such as embolization. A third possible option, and one often favored for the management of deep AVMs, is stereotactic radiosurgery. Data regarding the effectiveness of radiosurgery for AVMs in the deep gray matter is mixed. One recent study showed an overall obliteration rate of 60 percent. However, post-radiation complications occurred in 19 percent of cases, while post-treatment hemorrhage occurred in 10 percent (Andrade-Souza *et al.*, 2005). Another study showed slightly less favorable outcomes, with 48 percent of the patients obtaining an excellent outcome (defined as obliteration of the lesion without any new deficits) after one or more radiosurgical procedures, and 39 percent of the patients obtaining an excellent outcome after one radiosurgical procedure (Pollock *et al.*, 2004). This, of course, means that just over half the patients could not obtain an excellent outcome. Thus, care must be taken in choosing which patients are referred for stereotactic radiosurgery. It turns out that outcome is very closely linked to what the neurosurgeons term "the AVM score." Patients with an AVM score of <1.5 do much better than those with an AVM score of >1.5. The AVM score is calculated as follows (see Pollock and Flickinger, 2002):

AVM score = (0.1)(AVM volume in cm^3) + (0.02)(patient age in years) + (0.3)(location of lesion). To obtain a numerical value for the location, the following criteria are used: frontal or temporal = 0; parietal, occipital, intraventricular, corpus callosum, cerebellar = 1; basal ganglia, thalamic, or brainstem = 2.

With that, you should be ready to converse with your neurosurgeon friends, and hopefully help manage your patients with this difficult problem.

References

Andrade-Souza, Y. M., Zadeh, G., Scora, D. *et al.* Radiosurgery for basal ganglia, internal capsule, and thalamus arteriovenous malformation: clinical outcome. *Neurosurgery* 2005; **56**(1): 56–63.

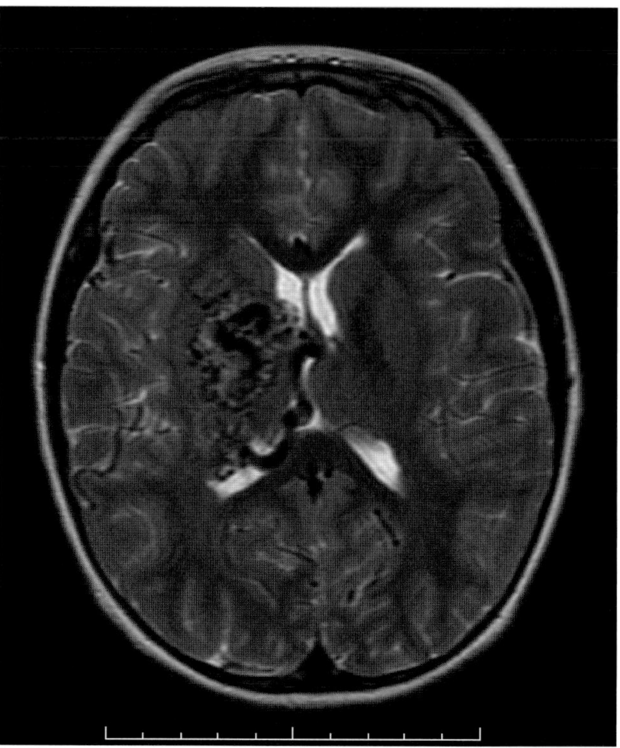

Fig. 5.44. **Axial T2-weighted MRI. (Case courtesy of Dr. Ashok Panigrahy, Department of Radiology, Los Angeles Children's Hospital.)**

Friedman, D. I., Jankovic, J., and Rolak, L. A. Arteriovenous malformation presenting as hemidystonia. *Neurology* 1986; **36**(12): 1590–1593.

Kurita, H., Sasaki, T., Suzuki, I., and Kirino, T. Basal ganglia arteriovenous malformation presenting as "writer's cramp." *Childs Nervous System* 1998; **14**(6): 285–287.

Pollock, B. E. and Flickinger, J. C. A proposed radiosurgery-based grading system for arteriovenous malformations. *Journal of Neurosurgery* 2002; **96**(1): 79–85.

Pollock, B. E., Gorman, D. A., and Brown, P. D. Radiosurgery for arteriovenous malformations of the basal ganglia, thalamus, and brainstem. *Journal of Neurosurgery* 2004; **100**(2): 210–214.

Case 5.19

72-year-old male patient who 1 year ago developed an acute confusional epsiode. Head CT at that time was negative. The patient has since shown a decline in mental status with a component of abulia, lack of initiative, and mild left-sided hemineglect.

MRI examination is shown (Fig. 5.45). What are the findings? What is your diagnosis?

The MRI shows a large old infarct of the right caudate head.

Diagnosis

Abulia and cognitive decline secondary to caudate infarct.

This short case is intended to introduce the reader to the association between caudate infarcts and both acute and chronic behavioral abnormalities. As discussed in the introduction, the caudate nucleus participates in a frontal cortex – basal ganglia loop. Therefore, it is not unreasonable to assume that caudate lesions may be associated with some degree of behavioral and cognitive abnormalities.

There are, indeed, several papers which have investigated and corroborated this notion. Caplan *et al.* (1990) found that in patients with caudate infarcts, there was a high incidence of cognitive and behavioral abnormalities. Of 18 patients with caudate infarcts, abulia was noted in 10, agitation and hyperactivity were noted in 7, and contralateral hemineglect was noted in 3. The contralateral hemineglect was noted exclusively in those with right caudate infarcts.

Mendez *et al.* (1989) studied 12 patients with caudate infarcts, 11 of whom had unilateral infarcts, and found that dorsolateral caudate infarcts tended to cause apathy and decreased verbal and motor output, while small ventromedial infarcts tended to cause disinhibition and poor impulse control. The laterality of the lesion did not affect the presentation. This particular study also showed that caudate infarcts tended to be associated with acute behavioral changes.

Another study by Kumral and Evyapan (1999) involving 31 patients with caudate infarct also found a high percentage of neurospychiatric abnormalities. The most frequent abnormalities were abulia and psychic akinesia in 48 percent, frontal system abnormalities in 26 percent, speech deficits in patients with left-sided lesions (23 percent), and neglect syndromes in those with right-sided lesions (10 percent).

Lastly, there is some evidence to suggest that along with the behavioral changes noted above, patients with caudate infarcts often suffer long-term cognitive decline as a chronic sequela of these infarcts (Bokura and Robinson, 1997).

References

Bokura, H. and Robinson, R. G. Long-term cognitive impairment associated with caudate stroke. *Stroke* 1997; **28**: 970–975.

Caplan, L. R., Schmahmann, J. D., Kase, C. S. *et al.* Caudate infarcts. *Archives of Neurology* 1990; **47**: 133–143.

Kumral, E., Evyapan, D., and Balkir, K. Acute caudate vascular lesions. *Stroke* 1999; **30**: 100–108.

Mendez, M. F., Adams, N. L., and Lewandowski, K. S. Neurobehavioral changes associated with caudate lesions. *Neurology* 1989; **39**(3): 349–354.

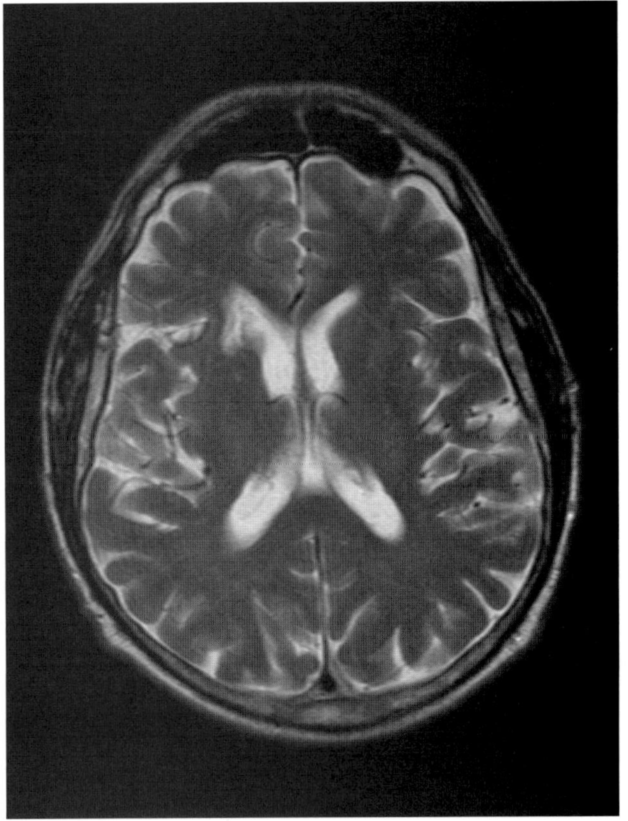

Fig. 5.45. **T2 axial MRI examination.**

Conclusion

At the end of this long journey, we would briefly like to reiterate a few of the points made in the introduction. After examining a variety of diseases of the basal ganglia, it is clear that there is neither a specific relationship between disease process and imaging appearance, nor between basal ganglia lesions and clinical symptoms and signs.

If the disease of the basal ganglia is not an infarct, mass (either tumor or infection), bleed, or vascular lesion, then it is probably a metabolic or degenerative process. The imaging abnormalities for these metabolic and degenerative disease categories are likely to involve only signal changes of the basal ganglia. There are three main categories of signal abnormalities.

Abnormal T2-weighted hyperintensity

This is by far the most frequent pattern of signal abnormality, and the differential for this pattern was covered in Case 5.12.

Abnormal T1-weighted hyperintensity

This is much less frequent. The differential for this pattern was covered in Case 5.11.

Abnormal T2-weighted hypointensity

This is the rarest of all, and its differential was covered in Case 5.10.

Another important point is that two patients with the same disease process (e.g., anoxic damage of the basal ganglia) may present with different symptoms, e.g., dystonia and choreoathtosis versus parkinsonism and bradykinesia. An interesting paper by Bhatia and Mardsen (1994) examining the clinical correlates of basal ganglia lesions illustrates this lack of specificity, while allowing us to identify some general patterns. In this excellent paper, the authors review 240 cases of basal ganglia lesions (caudate, putamen, and globus pallidus). Of the motor disorders present, dystonia was the most frequent (36 percent), especially when the putamen was involved. Less common movement disorders occurring with the same types of lesions were chorea (8 percent) and parkinsonism (6 percent), with dystonia–parkinsonism occurring least frequently (3 percent).

Finally, we have tried to stress that, while extrapyramidal motor disorders may be the most obvious (or most frequently thought of) manifestation of disease of the basal ganglia, the basal ganglia serve other important functions, subtended by multiple cortex–basal ganglia loops. Some of these involve the frontal lobes and the caudates, while others involve the limbic cortex and the ventral striatum. Thus diseases of the basal ganglia have cognitive, emotional, and behavioral aspects, as well as motor manifestations. We have tried to stress the ubiquity of cognitive and neuropsychiatric findings in such entities as Parkinson's disease or Huntington's disease, but the principle holds across the board. In the paper mentioned above (Bhatia and Mardsen, 1994), behavioral consequences of basal ganglia lesions were also detailed. The most common behavioral abnormality was abulia, i.e., apathy with loss of spontaneous verbal output and initiative. This was present in 13 percent. Disinhibition was less common (4 percent). Interestingly, isolated lesions of the caudates rarely caused motor disturbances, but commonly caused behavioral problems, especially abulia.

In fact, there is probably a significant role for the basal ganglia in some purely psychiatric disorders, such as obsessive–compulsive disorder and depression, which do not have significant extrapyramidal motor manifestations. We did not discuss these due to the lack of imaging correlates. However, we would like to leave you with an excellent review of the neuropsychiatric aspects of diseases of the basal ganglia, including many of the processes discussed in this chapter, to help stress the point we have been making (Ring and Serra-Mestres, 2002).

References

Bhatia, K.P., and Mardsen, C.D. The behavioral and motor consequences of focal lesions of the basal ganglia in man. *Brain* 1994; **117**: 859–876.

Ring, H.A., and Serra-Mestres, J. Neuropsychiatry of the basal ganglia. *Journal of Neurology, Neurosurgery, and Psychiatry* 2002; **72**: 12–21.

"Excellence is in the details. Give attention to the details and excellence will come."

Perry Paxton

The diencephalon, which sits between the cerebral hemispheres, has extremely widespread neuronal connections. Although it is only about 2 percent of the CNS by weight, its components are of tremendous functional significance. These components are:

(1) The thalamus, which makes up about 80 percent of the diencephalon.
(2) The epithalamus, comprised mainly of the pineal gland and the habenula.
(3) The subthalamus, whose main functional components include the superior aspects of the substantia nigra and red nucleus, as well as the subthalamic nucleus and the zona incerta. The zona incerta is a collection of neurons which sits in a slit-like fashion between the subthalamic nucleus and the thalamus, and appears to be continuous with the midbrain reticular formation. However, in terms of clinical–pathologic correlation, we are, as of yet, not certain of its function. The subthalamic nucleus and the substantia nigra have largely been discussed in the chapter on the basal ganglia, and so the subthalamus will not be discussed further here.
(4) The hypothalamus.

This chapter will first discuss the thalamus, then briefly discuss the hypothalamus and the pituitary gland, which is largely under hypothalamic control.

The thalamus

Anatomically, the thalami are paired structures that sit close to the midline of the brain, above the brainstem (although some anatomists are adamant that there is only one thalamus, with right and left hemithalami). The thalamus is an egg-shaped structure which is located just medial to the posterior limb of the internal capsule. It extends anteriorly to the foramen of Monro and medially to the walls of the third ventricle (Fig. 6.1).

Functionally, the thalamus is part of a very large number of neuroanatomic loops. It acts as a relay station for all sensory modalities (with the exception of olfaction, which projects directly to the cortex), as well as for numerous motor pathways from the cerebellum and basal ganglia on their way to the cortex. The thalamus also has important connections with the limbic and memory systems, giving it an important role in affective function and memory.

These various neuronal circuits project on distinct areas of the thalamus, which is anatomically subdivided into multiple separate nuclei. It is probably simplest to first study this internal anatomy and then return to reclassify the nuclei into different functional groups based on the loops in which they participate as well as on their pattern of input–output connections. Before delving into these tasks, it is worth noting that, despite the multiple distinct loops and functional zones, the basic schema of thalamic connections is relatively uniform at the "big picture" level. The thalamus receives inputs from various subcortical structures, and outputs to various areas of the cerebral cortex. The thalamic outputs, though, are modulated by numerous feedback connections from the cortex to the thalamus, as well as by some interthalamic relays.

Internal anatomy of the thalamus (Fig. 6.2)

The thalamus is divided along most of its long axis into medial and lateral portions by a thin sheet of myelinated fibers called the *internal medullary lamina*. At the anterior pole of the thalamus, though, this lamina divides to enclose the *anterior nucleus* of the thalamus.

The medial portion of the thalamus is fairly easy to describe. It is conventionally considered to contain only one nucleus, the *dorsomedial* (DM) nucleus. However, inferior to the dorsomedial nucleus, there is a thin layer of neurons which covers the medial surface of the thalamus along the wall of the third ventricle. This sheet makes up the *midline* nuclei of the thalamus. These are a continuation of the periaqueductal gray matter. These nuclei occasionally fuse across the midline to form

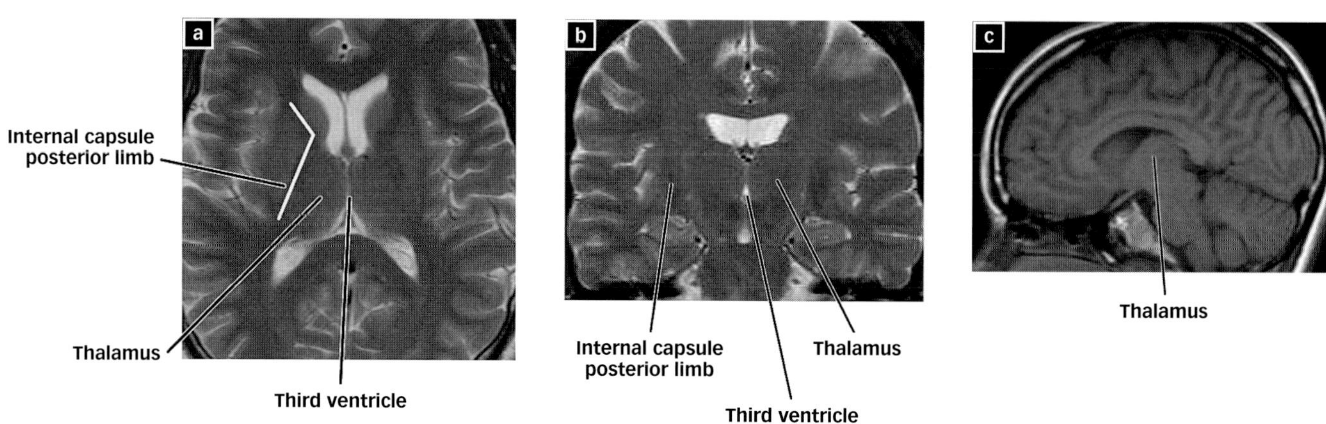

Fig. 6.1 (a) T2 axial and (b) coronal, and (c) T1 sagittal images show the thalamus in relation to the posterior limb of the internal capsule and third ventricle.

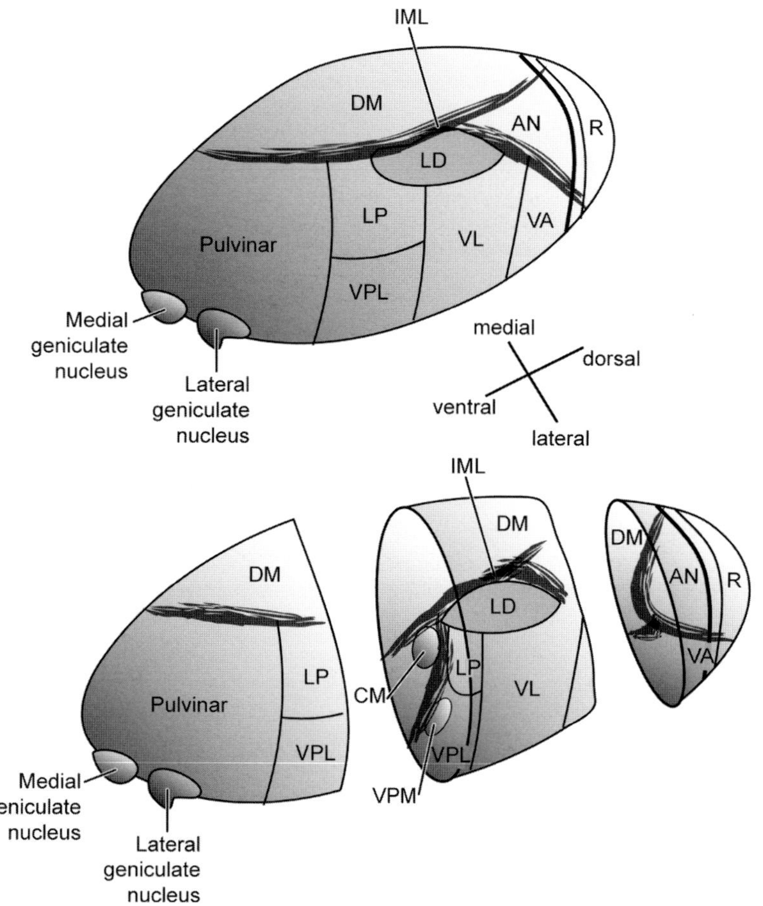

Fig. 6.2. **A slightly rotated image of the thalamus showing the location of the various nuclei and the internal medullary lamina. (a) Whole thalamus on one side. (b) Thalamus that has been divided into three parts to demonstrate the internal medullary lamina and how it divides the thalamus into various nuclei, as well as illustrating nuclei contained within the thalamus. Anterior nucleus (AN), reticular nucleus (R), ventral anterior nucleus (VA), ventral lateral nucleus (VL), lateral dorsal nucleus (LD), dorsal medial nucleus (DM), lateral posterior nucleus (LP), ventral posterolateral nucleus (VPL), ventral posteromedial nucleus (VPM), centromedian nucleus (CM).**

the interthalamic adhesion in the 70 percent of people in which it is present.

The lateral portion of the thalamus is more complex. It is divided into ventral and dorsal nuclear groups. The dorsal nuclei include the large *pulvinar* which forms the posterior border of the thalamus, as well as the *lateral posterior* nucleus (which is continuous with the pulvinar) and the *lateral dorsal* nucleus. The ventral tier of nuclei, going from anterior to posterior, is composed of:

Table 6.1. Thalamic nuclei and their connections

Type	Name of nucleus	Major subcortical input	Major output
Specific relay	Lateral geniculate	Optic tract (retinal ganglion cells)	Viscual cortex
	Medial geniculate	Inferior brachium (inferior colliculus)	Auditory cortex
	Ventral posterolateral	Medial lemniscus, spinothalamic tract	Somatosensory cortex
	Ventral posteromedial	Trigeminothalamic tracts (chief sensory/spinal nucleus)	Somatosensory cortex
	Ventral lateral, ventral anterior (VL/VA)	Cerebellum, basal ganglia	Motor/premotor cortex
	Anterior	Mammillothalamic tract (mammillary body)	Cingulate gyrus
Association	Pulvinar	Retinal ganglion cells, superior colliculus	Parietal-occipital-temporal
	Lateral posterior	Superior colliculus	Association cortices
	Lateral dorsal	Mixed	Parietal association cortex
	Dorsomedial	Amygdala, septal area, olfactory cortex	Cingulate gyrus Prefrontal cortex
Non-specific	Part of VA	Various thalamic nuclei	Prefrontal cortex
	Intralaminar	Reticular formation, basal ganglia, cerebellum, somatosensory systems	Collaterals to widespread cortical areas
Subcortical	Reticular	Thalamus	Thalamus

(1) the *ventral anterior* (VA) nucleus,

(2) the *ventral lateral* (VL) nucleus,

(3) the *ventral posterior* nucleus. This is further subdivided into medial and lateral parts, the *ventral posteromedial* (VPM) and the *ventral posterolateral* (VPL) nuclei respectively.

(4) the *medial* and *lateral geniculate* nuclei. These are located posterior and ventral to the VPM/VPL, along the undersurface of the pulvinar. They function as relay stations for the auditory (medial geniculate) and visual (lateral geniculate) pathways.

Between the medial and lateral portions of the thalamus, sitting within the internal medullary lamina, sits a group of nuclei known as the *intralaminar* nuclei. The most prominent of these is the *centromedian* (CM) nucleus. The centromedian nucleus is directly medial to the VPM, and invaginates it, giving the VPM a concave or semilunar shape.

Finally, there is a thalamic nucleus which defies this anatomic classification scheme, the *reticular* nucleus. This is actually a thin sheet of neurons which sits along the lateral surface of the thalamus, between the lateral nuclear group and the posterior limb of the internal capsule.

Functional categorization of thalamic nuclei

The type of input and output connections of the various thalamic nuclei described above allows them to be grouped into two broad functional categories: *relay* nuclei and *association* nuclei (Table 6.1). Not all nuclei fit into this categorization, and there are also *non-specific* thalamic nuclei, which include the intralaminar and midline nuclei and the reticular nucleus.

The input and output connections are also illustrated diagrammatically in Figs. 6.3 and 6.4. Figure 6.3 shows subcortical inputs to various thalamic nuclei, while Fig. 6.4 shows outputs of the various thalamic nuclei to the cortex. It must be recalled that there are almost always feedback loops from the cortex to the thalamus, i.e., if a thalamic nucleus outputs to a specific region of the cerebral cortex, it also receives input from that region as well.

Relay nuclei

Relay nuclei are characterized by having a specific well-defined input bundle, and by projecting to a specific functional area of the cerebral cortex. The sensory, motor, and limbic systems all have thalamic relay nuclei. The input–output connections of the relay nuclei are shown in Figs. 6.3 and 6.4.

Sensory system

Somatic sensation utilizes the VPM and VPL nuclei, with the body represented in the VPL and the face represented in the VPM. The medial lemniscus body fibers, carrying light touch, vibration, and proprioception information from the arms, legs, and trunk project onto the VPL. The spinothalamic tract, carrying light touch, pain, and temperature sensation from the body also projects to the VPL. The facial portion of the medial lemniscus, as well as the trigeminothalamic tract (equivalent of the spinothalamic tract for the head), project to the VPM.

Special sensory systems

The medial geniculate nucleus receives auditory inputs from the brachium of the inferior colliculus and outputs to the auditory cortex in the superior temporal lobe. The lateral geniculate nucleus receives inputs from the optic tract, and outputs to the visual cortex in the occipital lobe.

The motor system

The VA and VL nuclei comprise the motor areas of the thalamus. They receive inputs from the cerebellum via the dentatothalamic tract (predominantly the VL nucleus) and from the basal ganglia via the thalamic fasciculus (predominantly the VA nucleus). The VA and VL project to the motor and premotor cortex. The VA projects more to the premotor cortical regions while the VL projects more prominently to the motor cortex.

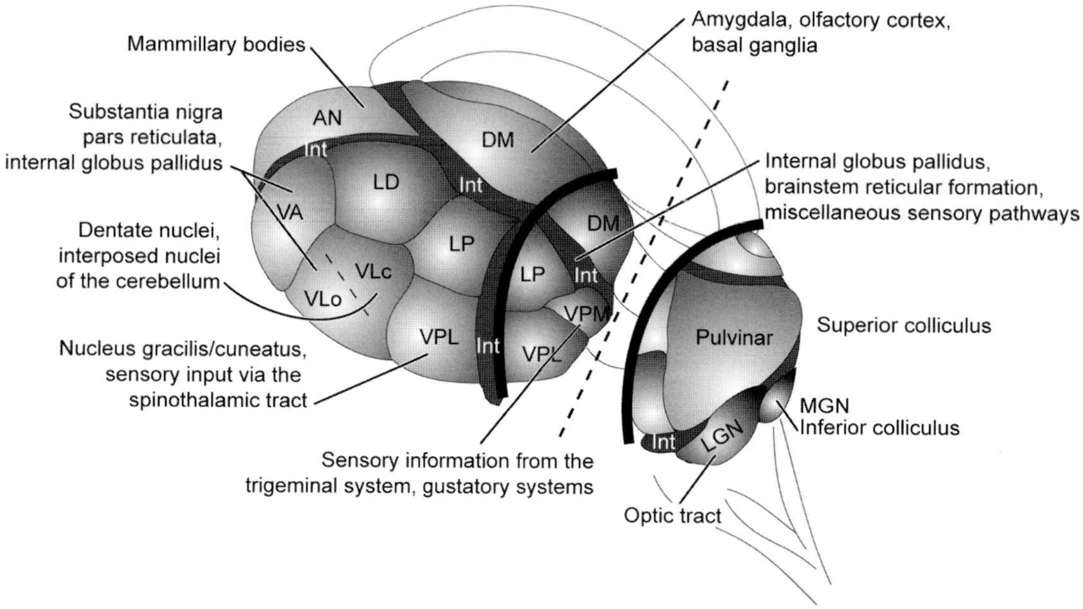

Fig. 6.3. **Non-cortical inputs into the thalamic nuclei. Anterior nucleus (AN), reticular nucleus (R), ventral anterior nucleus (VA), ventral lateral nucleus (VLo/VLc), lateral dorsal nucleus (LD), dorsal medial nucleus (DM), lateral posterior nucleus (LP), ventral posterolateral nucleus (VPL), ventral posteromedial nucleus (VPM), centromedian nucleus (CM), intralaminar nuclei (Int).**

The limbic system

The relay nuclei for the limbic system are the anterior nucleus and the lateral dorsal nucleus. The anterior nucleus receives inputs from the mammillothalamic tract (coming from the hippocampus), and outputs to the cingulate gyrus. The lateral dorsal nucleus does not receive a well-defined input bundle, but also outputs to the cingulate gyrus, and is considered part of the limbic thalamus. These nuclei are thus involved in emotional behavior and memory and new learning.

Association nuclei

There are two main association nuclei in the thalamus, the dorsomedial (DM) nucleus, and the pulvinar. The lateral posterior nucleus is connected to the pulvinar, and appears functionally linked to it, and so these two nuclei are often referred to as the pulvinar/LT complex. The main subcortical inputs are shown in Fig. 6.3 and the main cortical connections are shown in Fig. 6.4.

In contrast to relay nuclei, association nuclei do not receive input bundles from modality-specific long tracts. Rather, they receive inputs from broad regions of cortex, some subcortical structures and other thalamic nuclei. Likewise, they do not output to a specific functional cortical area, such as the motor cortex or visual cortex, but rather to the broad regions of cortex known as the association cortex.

The two main regions of association cortex in the human brain are the prefrontal cortex, located in the frontal lobes anterior to the motor regions, and the parietal–occipital–temporal association cortex, adjacent to the sensory, visual, and auditory cortices. Each of these association areas is connected with a thalamic association nucleus.

The dorsomedial nucleus is connected with the prefrontal association cortex. It receives inputs both from the prefrontal cortex itself, as well as from the limbic system, including the amygdala. It is involved in high-level cognitive function, emotional behavior and memory. As a side note, the surgical operation called prefrontal lobotomy interrupted the pathway from the frontal association cortex to the dorsomedial nucleus.

The pulvinar/LP complex is connected with the parietal–occipital–temporal association cortex and receives reciprocal inputs from it. It also receives inputs from the lateral geniculate and the superior colliculus. Thus, it is involved in visuospatial processing. Interestingly, and not immediately clear from its pattern of neuronal connections, the pulvinar also seems to have a role in speech. Lesions in the dominant pulvinar have been associated with anomia.

Non-specific nuclei

The intralaminar and midline nuclei seem to be important in the functioning of the basal ganglia and the limbic system, but the details here are far from known. They have a very broad range of inputs, including the reticular activating system, the limbic system, and the basal ganglia, and they project back to these same areas as well as to the cerebral cortex. These broad, non-specific connections suggest that the intralaminar and midline nuclei may help regulate the level of cortical excitability. The centromedian nucleus, though, probably functions a little more specifically with the basal ganglia and the motor system.

The reticular nucleus covers the outer surface of the thalamus. Inputs and outputs connecting the thalamus to various areas of cortex give off collaterals to the overlying portion of the reticular nucleus. The reticular nucleus, in turn, projects back to those areas of the thalamus. For example, the area of the reticular nucleus overlying the VPL receives collaterals from the VPL and the sensory cortex, and projects back to the VPL. Thus, the reticular nucleus is the one thalamic nucleus

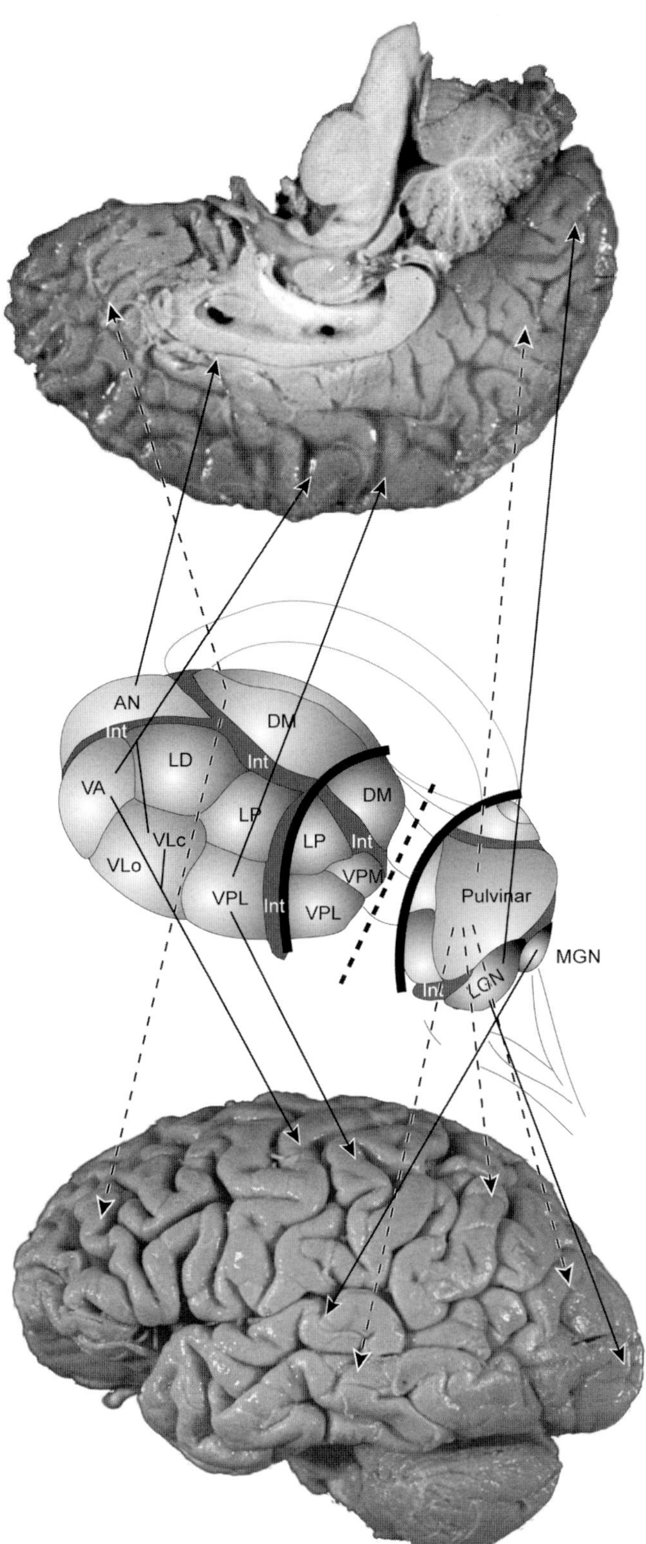

Fig. 6.4. **Major outputs of the thalamic nuclei. Specific relay nuclei are denoted by a solid line; association nuclei are denoted by a dashed line.**

which has no outputs going to the cortex. It probably helps to control thalamic output, and seems important in regulating and modulating the output of the thalamus to the cortex during different phases of sleep.

Internal circuitry of the thalamus

A key question that is sometimes lost in the scuffle of attempting to learn the various nuclei and their connections is: what does the thalamus actually do? Derivative questions are: why do the various sensory and motor pathways pass through the thalamus? Is it just a relay station, where these fibers synapse on their way to the cortex, or does it somehow process, alter, augment, etc., the information flowing through it? We are much less adept at answering these questions than in describing the anatomic connections. The thalamus seems to function in several ways: as a gateway to the cortex, deciding which and how much sensory information arrives at the cortex; integrating motor information before delivering it to the cortex; affecting cortical arousal and excitability in the face of these impulses which will be delivered to it; impacting the affective response of the cortex; and facilitating memory and learning of the information it gates to the cortex. How the thalamus accomplishes these functions is not clear. However, we can describe in slightly more detail the path of neural impulses in the thalamus and the circuitry behind the integrative functions (Fig. 6.5).

Within the thalamus are two types of neurons: projection neurons (so named because they carry impulses out of the thalamus, such as to the cortex) and local-circuit interneurons, which synapse with the projection neurons. Both the projection neurons and the local-circuit interneurons receive inputs from subcortical structures (e.g., the spinothalamic tract, basal ganglia, etc.) as well as from the cerebral cortex. Most of these are excitatory neurons using glutamate or aspartate as their

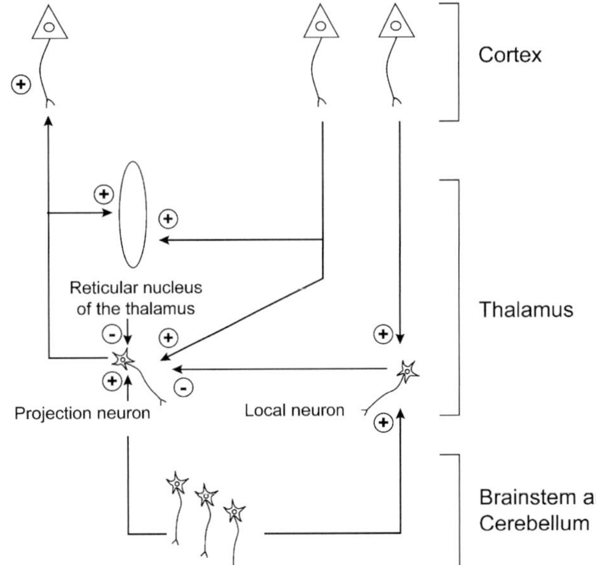

Fig. 6.5. **Internal circuitry of the thalamus.**

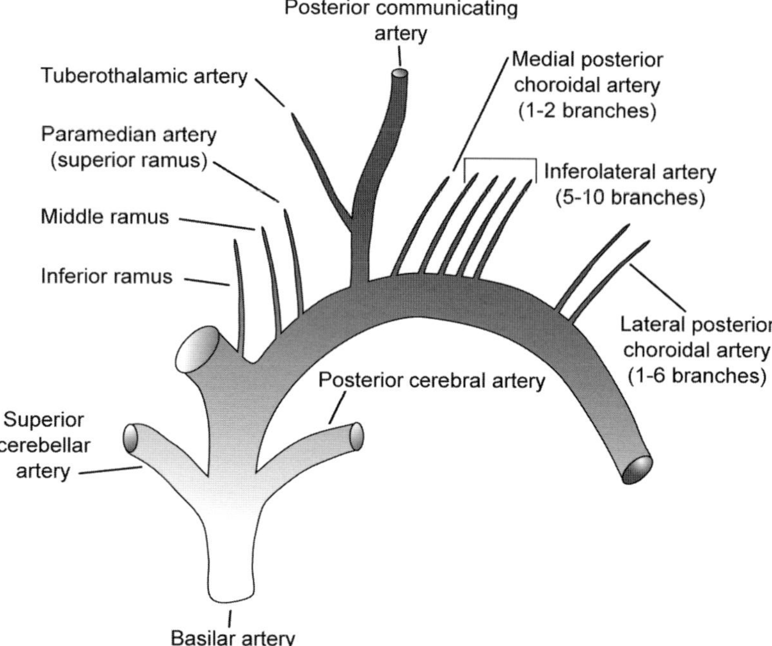

Fig. 6.6. **The thalamus is supplied by four main arteries, which divide it into four vascular territories. These are the tuberothalamic artery, the paramedian artery, the inferolateral arterial group, and the lateral posterior choroidal arterial group. (Figure adapted from Schmahmann, J. D. Vascular syndromes of the thalamus. *Stroke* 2003; 34(9):2264–2291.**

neurotransmitter. One exception to this, as you recall, is that neurons coming from the globus pallidus interna (GPi) are inhibitory, using gamma-aminobutyric acid (GABA) as their neurotransmitter. The local-circuit interneurons, in turn, send out inhibitory GABAergic fibers to the projection neurons. The reticular nucleus functions as a zone of local-circuit interneurons, receiving excitatory inputs from the cortex, and sending inhibitory GABAergic fibers to the projection neurons. Thus, the projection neurons receive excitatory inputs from the subcortical structures (except the GPi) and from the cortex, and inhibitory inputs from the local-circuit interneurons and the reticular nucleus. They then balance and integrate all of this information, and then pass it to the cortex in the form of excitatory impulses.

Thalamic vascular territories

To study clinicopathologic correlations of thalamic lesions, it is generally agreed upon that patients with thalamic infarcts provide the most precise information. Other lesions, such as bleeds, gliomas, or encephalitis, tend to be more diffuse. Therefore, the study of thalamic strokes provides the best structure–function correlation available and is probably the most useful approach for the clinician, since thalamic infarcts represent the most common pathology encountered.

Although a precise functional correlation for each thalamic nucleus is not possible, as infarcts usually involve multiple nuclei, and since arterial territories have both variability and overlap, it is possible to delineate in broad terms several thalamic stroke syndromes. This delineation is based on the different vascular territories of the thalamus. Therefore, in an attempt

to be interactive, we pose the question: what are the vascular territories of the thalamus?

Anatomists such as Foix and Hillemand, and later Percheron (among others) have delineated four main arterial territories in the thalamus based on the arteries that supply it (see Fig. 6.6). A simplified description of them is provided, giving the main areas supplied in each territory (see Fig. 6.7).

(1) The territory of the tuberothalamic artery (also known as the polar artery of Percheron and the premammillary pedicle of Foix and Hillemand). The tuberothalamic artery originates from the posterior communicating artery. It follows the course of the mammillothalamic tracts and supplies predominantly the anterior portion of the thalamus, including the anterior nucleus, the ventral anterior (VA) nucleus, part of the ventrolateral (VL) nucleus, the ventral part of the dorsomedial (DM) nucleus, the mammillothalamic tract, and the ventral amygdalofugal pathway. This vascular territory is known as the anterior territory.

(2) The territory of the paramedian artery (also known as the paramedian pedicle, the retromammillary pedicle of Foix and Hillemand, or the posterior thalamosubthalamic paramedian artery of Percheron). Now you see why we will just refer to it as the paramedian artery. This artery arises from the P1 portion of the posterior cerebral artery, as part of a group of so-called interpeduncular branches or rami. The inferior and middle rami supply the midbrain, while the superior ramus is the paramedian artery. The paramedian artery runs from the ventromedial aspect of the thalamus to its dorsolateral portion. It supplies most of the dorsomedial nucleus, and portions of the internal medullary lamina, and most of the intralaminar

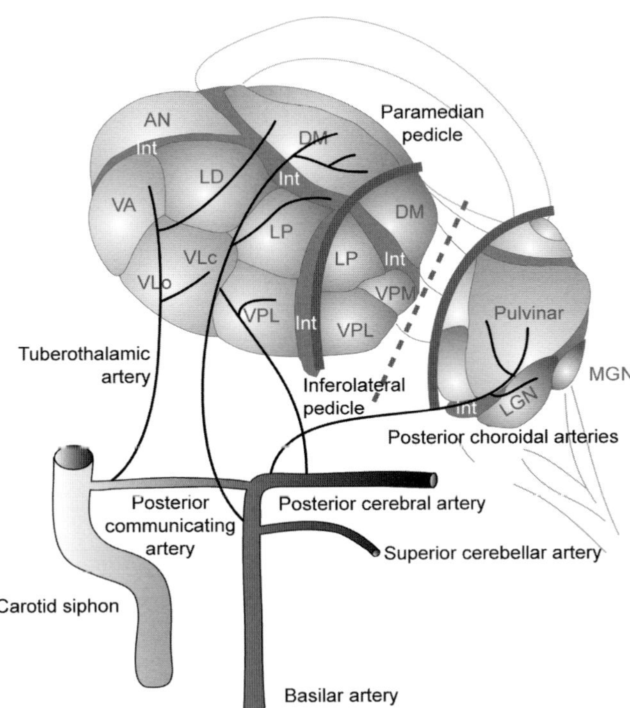

Fig. 6.7. **The arterial supply of the thalamus. Anterior nucleus (AN), reticular nucleus (R), ventral anterior nucleus (VA), ventral lateral nucleus (VLo/VLc), lateral dorsal nucleus (LD), dorsal medial nucleus (DM), lateral posterior nucleus (LP), ventral posterolateral nucleus (VPL), ventral posteromedial nucleus (VPM), centromedian nucleus (CM), intralaminar nuclei (Int).**

nuclei. This vascular territory is known as the paramedian territory.

It is noted that in about one-third of patients, the tuberothalamic artery is absent, and its territory is also supplied by the paramedian artery.

(3) The territory of the inferolateral arteries (also known as the thalamogeniculate pedicle of Foix and Hillemand, or simply the thalamogeniculate perforators). These are multiple arteries arising from the P2 portion of the posterior cerebral artery (i.e., the portion distal to the posterior communicating artery). The inferolateral arteries mainly supply the ventral posterior nuclear group (VPM and VPL), and also contribute to the supply of the medial geniculate nucleus and to the rostral and lateral portions of the pulvinar. This vascular territory is known as the inferolateral territory.

(4) The territory of the posterior choroidal arteries. The posterior choroidal arteries also arise from the P2 portion of the posterior cerebral artery, and are comprised of a number of branches. These supply predominantly the lateral geniculate nucleus, the inferolateral portion of the pulvinar and the lateral posterior (LP) nucleus and the lateral dorsal nucleus. Other branches may supply a portion of the medial geniculate and the posterior portions of the intralaminar nuclei. This vascular territory is known as the posterior territory.

Variant territories

As if having to remember the four classical territories and names of the supplying arteries were not enough, there has been a recent addition to these in the form of variant territories (see Carrere *et al.*, 2004). The authors, in a major review of the Lausanne Stroke Registry, found that 30 percent of all thalamic stroke patients apparently do not know their vascular anatomy. These patients presented with thalamic strokes that could not be easily classified into one of the four classical categories. An analysis of those patients led to a description of three variant vascular territories, hypothesized to be based either on variations in vascular supply or a watershed ischemia pattern:

(1) *Anteromedian territory*: infarcts here overlap the classical anterior and paramedian territories, usually combining the posterior part of the anterior territory with the anterior part of the paramedian territory.

(2) *Central territory*: infarcts here are in the center of the thalamus, and thus in involve the adjacent parts of all four classical territories.

(3) *Posterolateral territory*: infarcts here overlap the classical inferolateral and posterior territories, usually involving the posterior part of the inferolateral territory with the anterior part of the posterior territory.

Summary

In summary, then, the thalamic nuclei seem to function in five domains: processing sensory information; participating in general motor functions and speech; affecting general arousal (the reticular and intralaminar nuclei are important here); participating in high-level cognitive functions, such as judgment, reasoning, memory and visuospatial processing (the association nuclei are important here); interacting with the limbic system to impact mood, affect, and motivation (the anterior thalamic nuclei are most important here). Various nuclei participate in each of these functions, and thalamic lesions, including infarcts, destroy these nuclei in varied combinations. Thus, clinicopathologic correlations can be difficult. However, using the neuroanatomic approach we have described, at least a measure of order may be imposed on the chaos.

Probably the most important "take home" point of this chapter is that the thalamus is a complex structure with involvement in multiple brain systems. Most physicians outside the realm of neurology/neuroradiology associate only one sort of clinical presentation with thalamic lesions: contralateral sensory deficits. Hopefully, this chapter will illustrate that thalamic pathology provides a much richer and more complex spectrum of clinical abnormalities and clinicopathologic correlations.

With that, let's take some cases!

Reference

Carrere, E., Michel, P., and Bogousslavsky, J. Anteromedian, central, and posterolateral infarcts of the thalamus: three variant types. *Stroke* 2004; **35**: 2826.

Case 6.1

48-year-old female patient, who presented initially with "altered mental status" 7 days ago. Notable on the patient's neurologic evaluation was abulia with diminished verbal output and hypophonia, mild left-sided weakness, a suggestion of left-sided hemineglect, and word-finding difficulties with perseveration during speech. Comprehension and repetition were intact. No sensory deficit was elicited. Memory testing revealed decreased word recall as well as visual memory impairment. The patient also had constructional apraxia. The patient seemed disoriented in time, unable to sequence events properly during her hospital stay, overlapping events from last week onto events of today.

For non-neurologists, the above history may be a bit daunting. For example, what is abulia? What is hemineglect and how can we test for it? How can we test for visual, or visuospatial, memory impairment?

Gradually gaining familiarity with terms typically used by neurologists in describing patient findings is important for neuroradiologists. The author has found that this knowledge accrues in bits and pieces. Therefore, here are a few bits. Abulia refers to apathy or lack of spontaneous action not accounted for by a decreased level of consciousness. Hemineglect is failure to respond to stimuli coming from one side of space, not accounted for by a motor or sensory deficit. Therefore, not responding to visual stimuli in the right visual field after a left occipital infarct does not count as hemineglect, because it is caused by a homonymous hemianopsia secondary to the stroke. The neglected side is opposite to the side of the responsible brain lesion. Briefly, hemineglect may be sensory (i.e., ignoring sensory stimuli to one side of the body or coming from one side of space), motor (lack of motor response in the affected half of space), or representational (being unable to properly generate mental images; half of the image is ignored). Hemineglect may also be personal (ignoring half of one's body, such as not combing the hair on one side of the head) or spatial (ignoring half of the outside space, such as not eating the food on one half of a plate). Typical tests for hemineglect include the line bisection test and cancellation tests. The line bisection test consists of drawing a line and asking the patient to divide it in half. If the patient ignores one-half of the line and proceeds to bisect only the half which he perceives, the mark will be off midline. Therefore, a patient with a right-sided brain lesion will have left hemineglect. He will ignore the left half of a horizontal line, and his bisection mark will be off midline toward the right. Cancellation tests involve such things as using a variety of figures scattered across a piece of paper and asking the patient to cross out one particular type, such as "stars." The patient with left hemineglect will only cross out stars on the right half of the paper. Another test for representational hemineglect is to ask the patient to draw a clockface. If the patient neglects one half of the clock, or tries to bunch up all of the numbers on one semicircular arc, then this suggests hemineglect. An excellent reference on the topic of hemineglect is Plummer *et al.*, 2003. Three common tests of memory are (a) the 15-word test, where the patient tries to recall 15 words read by the examiner, and may have multiple tries in which he learns the words; (b) Hebb's audioverbal span test, where the patient repeats longer and longer series of numbers read by the examiner; and (c) Corsi blocks visuospatial memory test, where the patient must mimic the examiner by touching an increasing number of blocks in the right order. The well-known game Simon, with the flashing lights, is the commercial version of this test.

Speaking of memory impairment, it may appear that we have forgotten about our patient. Figure 6.8 shows an image from her MRI scan. What are the findings? What is your diagnosis?

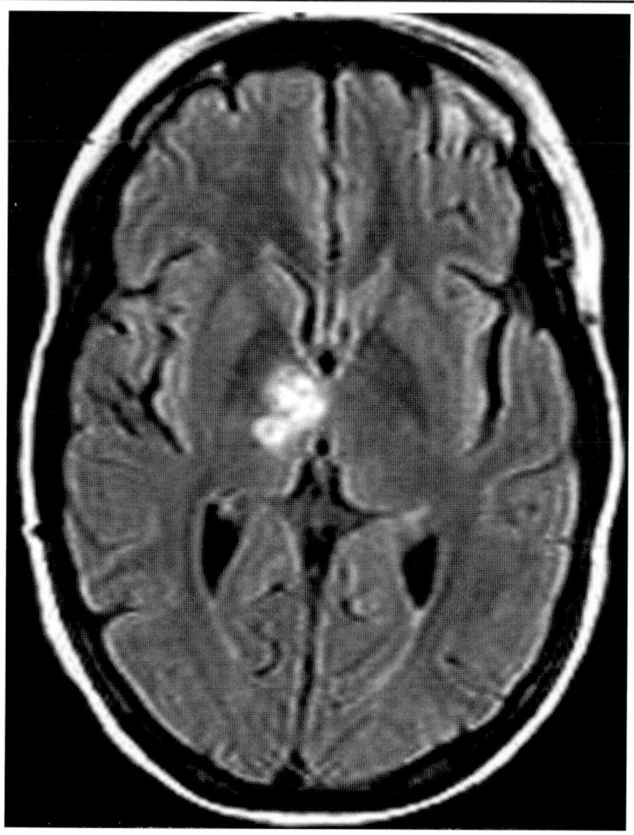

Fig. 6.8. **Axial FLAIR image.**

Diagnosis

The scan shows abnormal hyperintensity in the anterior aspect of the right thalamus. The most likely diagnosis is an infarct, which this turned out to be.

In what thalamic vascular territory does the infarct lie? What structures are typically involved by infarcts in this territory? What is the typical clinical presentation for such infarcts?

This infarct is in the tuberothalamic artery territory, which supplies the anterior thalamus. A common synonym for this artery is the polar artery. This artery, once again, originates from the posterior communicating artery, whereas the remainder of the thalamic supply is from the posterior cerebral artery. The structures typically involved by infarcts in this territory are the anterior nucleus (ANT), the ventral anterior nucleus (VA), the rostral part of the ventral lateral nucleus (VL), the ventral part of the dorsomedial nucleus (DM), the mammillothalamic tract, and the anterior portion of the internal medullary lamina. The typical clinical findings are termed "neuropsychological" and consist of:

(a) *Abulia.* The patient may show apathy and lack of spontaneity.
(b) *Impairment of recent memory and new learning.* This is thought to result from infarction of the mammillothalamic tracts, which connect the hippocampal formations to the anterior thalamic nuclei, as well as infarction of the anterior thalamic nuclei themselves. Various reports suggest that visual memory is more involved in right-sided tuberothalamic strokes, whereas verbal memory is more affected in left-sided tuberothalamic strokes.
(c) *Hemineglect and visuospatial impairment.* This is thought to be more common in right tuberothalamic strokes.
(d) *Dysphasia.* According to some, this is a milder form of aphasia. According to others, it is the same as aphasia, the difference

being that Americans say "aphasia" whereas Europeans say "dysphasia." Anterior thalamic infarcts lead to a particular form of dysphasia, typified by word-finding difficulties, hypophonia, paraphasias and perseveration. Paraphasia is the production of unintended syllables or words during speech. It may involve saying only part of a word instead of the whole word or inverting part of a word (i.e., tevilision instead of television) – this is literal paraphasia. It may also involve word substitutions, such as saying one word when you mean your mother … er, when you mean another. This is verbal paraphasia. Typically, the dysphasia associated with anterior thalamic infarcts shows relatively preserved comprehension and preserved repetition.

The conventional wisdom is that dysphasia is more common with left-sided tuberothalamic infarcts whereas visuospatial deficits are more common with right-sided infarcts. However, a nice paper on anterior thalamic infarcts, representing a fairly large series, failed to find this lateralization (see Ghika-Schmid and Bogousslavsky, 2000).

(e) *Disorientation to time and place.* These infarcts may actually show a most interesting feature, in which patients superimpose events that are unrelated in time upon each other, as if they had happened within the same temporal frame. This leads to a state of parallel expression of mental activities, each proceeding separately with the patient thinking that they all belong to the same time frame. This has been termed palipsychism by Ghika-Schmid and Bogousslavsky, from the Greek palin [again] and psyche [soul].

(f) *Facial aprosody.* Here, there is a hemifacial paresis only for emotional responses. In other words, the patient has decreased spontaneous facial expressions over one-half of the face in response to emotional stimuli, but no motor deficit if the patient intentionally tries to smile or frown.

References

Ghika-Schmid, F., and Bogousslavsky, J. The acute behavioral syndrome of anterior thalamic infarction: a prospective study of 12 cases. *Annals of Neurology* 2000, **48**. 220–227.

Plummer, P., Morris, M. E., and Dunai, J Assessment of unilateral neglect. *Physical Therapy* 2003; **83**(8): 732–740.

Case 6.2

63-year-old patient who initially presented with sudden onset altered mental status, characterized by decreased consciousness and confusion. The patient's sensorium cleared the day post-ictus but the patient remained confused and became agitated. Clinical examination showed astrexis of the right arm as well as upward gaze palsy. The patient had some antegrade memory deficit and confabulation. The patient's speech was hypophonic with reduced fluency but intact repetition.

Presented in Fig. 6.9 is an image from the patient's MRI scan. What are the findings? What is your diagnosis?

Diagnosis

There is a subacute infarct in the left paramedian thalamus, hyperintense on DWI. Paramedian infarcts are the second most common thalamic infarcts, following inferolateral territory infarcts.

What structures are typically involved in paramedian thalamic infarction? What are the signs and symptoms of infarcts in this territory?

The paramedian artery, once again, arises from the P1 portion of the posterior cerebral artery and courses within the thalamus from ventromedial to dorsolateral. It supplies predominantly the dorsomedial nucleus, the intralaminar nuclei including the centromedian nucleus, the midline nuclei, and variable portions of the internal medullary lamina.

Paramedian infarcts of the thalamus typically present with alterations in arousal and memory. There is decreased consciousness, which may last from minutes to days. After clearing of the sensorium, the presentation is similar to anterior (tuberothalamic) territory infarcts. There is often confusion, and sometimes apathy, while at other times there is aggressiveness and poor impulse control. There are memory deficits, with anterograde amnesia being the most prominent feature. This is often accompanied by confabulation. An interesting case has been reported where the memory deficit was predominantly autobiographical, with relative preservation of memory for famous events and people. This was thought to be secondary to disconnection of frontal and temporal memory circuits. A dysphasia typified by decreased verbal fluency, hypophonia, and paraphasias with intact repetition is also often present. This has been called by some the "adynamic aphasia

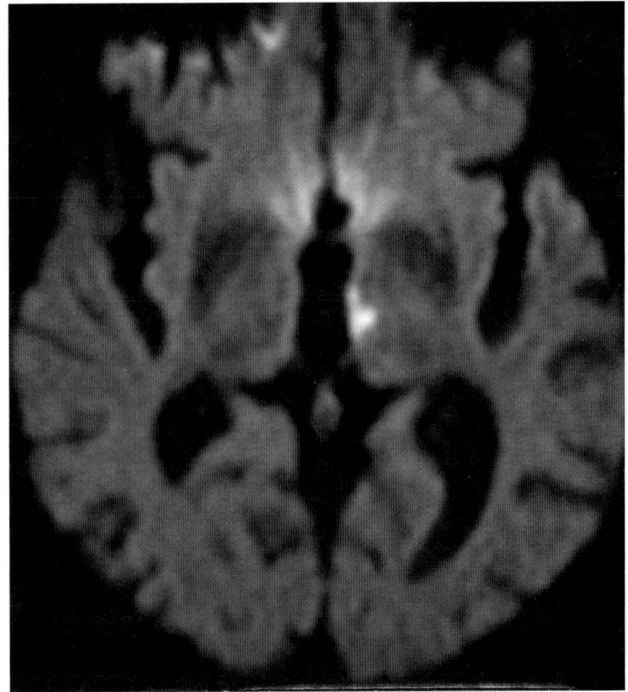

Fig. 6.9. **Axial DWI image.**

of Guberman and Stuss," based on their description of the findings (see Guberman and Stuss, 1983).

Interestingly, most patients also have oculomotor abnormalities, with the most common being upward gaze palsy. Other reported abnormalities include a vertical "one-and-a-half," as well as internuclear ophthalmoplegia and defects in lateral gaze which have been termed "pseudo-sixth nerve palsies."

Motor abnormalities are typically not pronounced, but mild hemiparesis as well as asterixis of the contralateral arm have been reported. Classically and importantly, there is typically no sensory deficit in these infarcts.

With paramedian infarcts, there does seem to be a left–right discrepancy in terms of dysphasia versus visuospatial deficits and hemineglect, with dysphasia more common in left-sided thalamic infarcts and decreased visual memory and hemineglect more common with right-sided infarcts. This is illustrated by the case of a 53-year-old male who showed left-sided hemineglect following a right paramedian thalamic infarct (Fig. 6.10). The patient had no evidence of dysphasia and no sensory deficits.

In summary, then, the salient features of paramedian thalamic infarcts are: (1) decreased arousal; (2) memory deficits, particularly anterograde amnesia, along with confabulation; (3) neuropsychological dysfunction characterized by confusion, apathy, and sometimes poor impulse control, agitation, and aggression; (4) thalamic dysphasia, more prominent in left-sided lesions; (5) decreased visuospatial processing and possibly contralateral hemineglect, more common in right-sided lesions; (6) oculomotor abnormalities, with upward gaze palsy being the most frequent feature.

It must be noted that these associations are mostly phenomenological: they come from carefully examining patients with paramedian thalamic infarcts and cataloguing their clinical findings. However, some putative links between symptoms and what we have discussed so far in regard to thalamic anatomy can be made. For example, there are two fiber systems key to learning and memory: the mammillothalamic tract and the amygdalofugal pathway. As already mentioned in the previous case discussion, the mammillothalamic tract connects the anterior nuclei of the thalamus with the hippocampal formations, at least partially explaining memory deficits with tuberothalamic infarcts. The amygdalofugal pathway links the medial portions of the dorsomedial thalamic nuclei with the limbic system and the frontal cortex. In particular, it connects the magnocellular portion of the dorsomedial nuclei with the basal forebrain, the amygadala and the orbitofrontal cortices. It is postulated that damage here leads both to memory deficits and emotional disturbances. This circuit may thus explain why, although both tuberothalamic and paramedian infarcts manifest with memory deficits, paramedian infarcts seem to have a higher predilection for deficits in judgment and emotional control.

The alterations in consciousness typical of paramedian infarcts may be due to involvement of the midline nuclei as well as the rostral portions of the intralaminar nuclei. These structures receive significant inputs from the midbrain reticular activating system, which are then widely distributed to the cerebral cortex (see Fig. 6.3).

There is also a plausible neuroanatomic explanation for the oculomotor abnormalities seen in paramedian infarcts. The medial thalamus contains fibers from the premotor cortex on their way to the interstitial nucleus of Cajal, the nucleus of Darkschewitsch

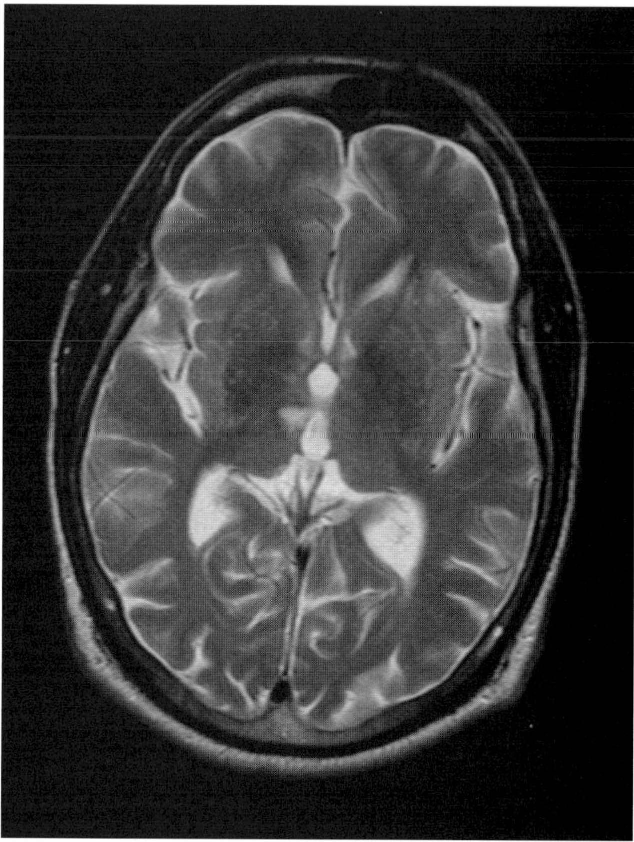

Fig. 6.10. **T2-weighted axial image shows a right paramedian thalamic infarct in a patient with left-sided hemineglect. The patient had no sensory deficits.**

and the rostral interstitial nucleus of the MLF in the midbrain. These nuclei are responsible for modulating vertical gaze, and disturbances of the pathways from the cortex to them probably underlie the observed oculomotor abnormalities.

Reference

Guberman, A. and Stuss, D. The syndrome of bilateral paramedian thalamic infarction. *Neurology*, 1983; **33**: 540–546.

Case 6.3

57-year-old male patient who abruptly lost consciousness. The patient's consciousness waxed and waned over the next 2 weeks. As the patient's sensorium cleared, he was noted to have severe memory impairment with perseveration and confabulation. The patient had a pronounced aphasia with marked decrease in verbal fluency and generalized apathy. Oculomotor testing revealed a vertical "one-and-a-half" syndrome (vertical gaze palsy in one eye and upward gaze palsy in the other).

The MRI images are provided in Fig. 6.11. What are the findings? How can the findings be explained?

The images show early subacute bilateral paramedian thalamic infarcts, with symmetric foci of T2 and DWI hyperintensity.

Diagnosis

Bilateral paramedian thalamic (a.k.a. artery of Percheron) infarcts.

This finding of bilateral paramedian thalamic infarcts is an important one to become familiar with. These infarcts, when isolated to the thalamus, are typically referred to as artery of Percheron infarcts (see, for example, Matheus and Castillo, 2003). Of course, either unilateral or bilateral paramedian infarcts can rightly be called artery of Percheron infarcts, since this is a synonym for the paramedian artery. However, Dr. Percheron's name has become most famously associated with the vascular variant (which he also described) leading to

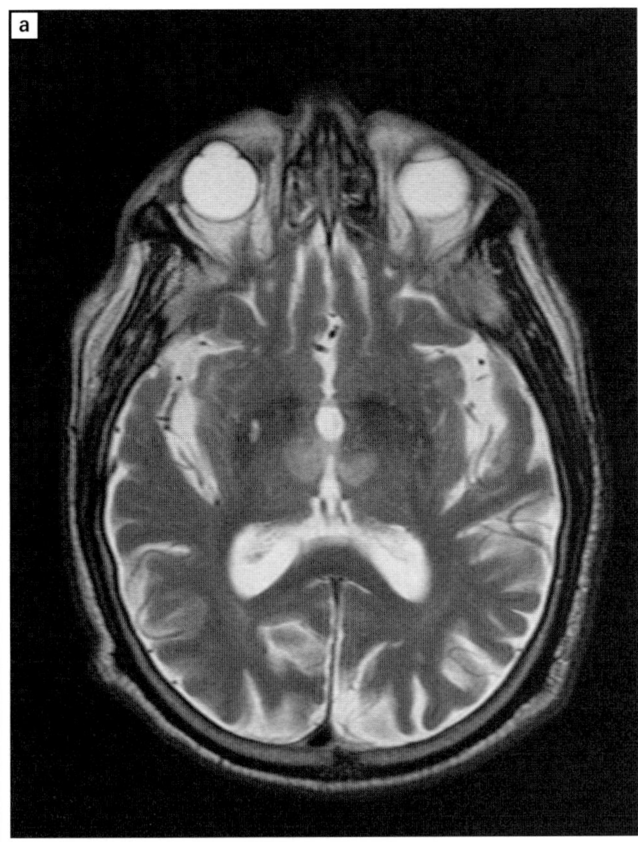

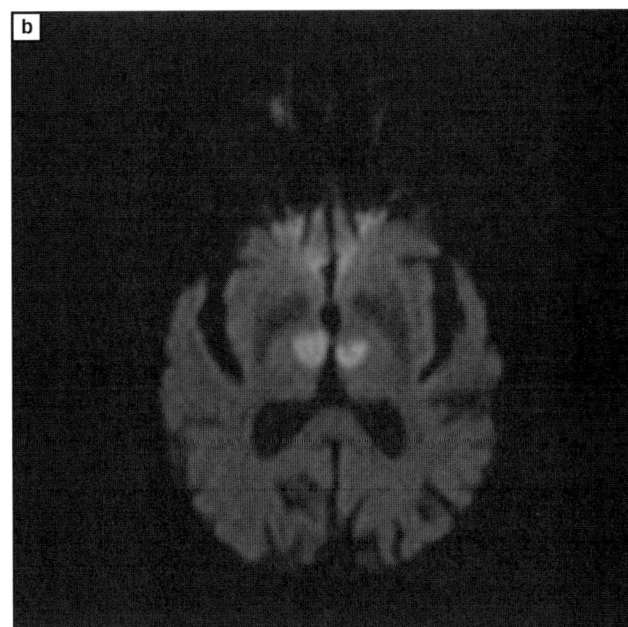

Fig. 6.11. **(a) T2 and (b) DWI axial MRI images.**

bilateral paramedian infarcts. In this variant, a single paramedian trunk, referred to as the artery of Percheron, arises from one or the other P1 portion, and then supplies both medial thalami. Thus, if this artery becomes compromised, the result is bilateral paramedian thalamic infarcts.

In the series of Bogousslavsky *et al.*, out of 14 patients with paramedian thalamic infarcts, 5 were bilateral. The same sort of infarct may be seen with "top of the basilar" syndrome, where there is thrombus in the distal basilar artery. In that situation, though, the paramedian thalamic infarcts tend to be part of a more extensive infarct pattern which typically includes the midbrain and the PCA territories.

Describe the clinical findings in bilateral paramedian thalamic infarcts.

The findings are of the same type as unilateral infarcts but tend to be more severe. In some cases, the alterations in consciousness are very profound, with the patients presenting with coma. Another possible sequela is a persistent vegetative state where the patient is awake but unresponsive. This is known as akinetic mutism (this can also occur with massive pontine infarcts). Such a case is presented adjacent (Fig. 6.12).

This patient was a 58-year-old who presented with decorticate coma. Over several weeks, the patient's the coma gave way to akinetic mutism. FLAIR images reveal extensive bilateral paramedian infarcts. On the left, the infarct also extends into the tuberothalamic (anterior) territory. This occurs because, as mentioned previously, the tuberothalamic artery is sometimes absent and its supply is taken over by the paramedian artery. For historical interest, the association between thalamic lesions and a

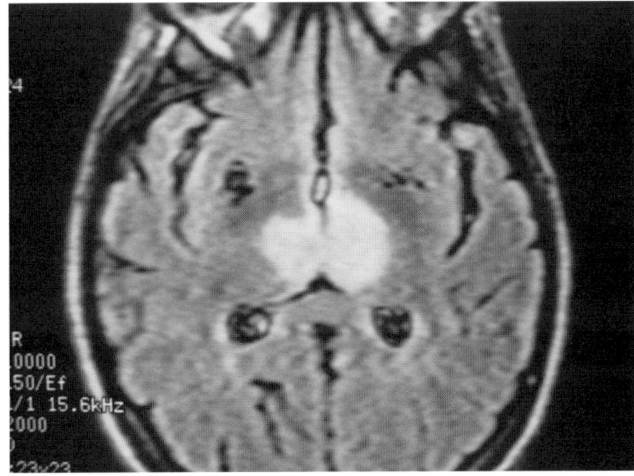

Fig. 6.12. **FLAIR image shows large bilateral paramedian thalamic infarcts.**

persistent vegetative state was highlighted by the autopsy findings of Karen Ann Quinlan, who lived in a persistent vegetative state for 10 years following a cardiac arrest, and whose condition galvanized the debate about life-sustaining measures for such patients. In her case, the most severe damage was in the bilateral thalami (see Kinney *et al.*, 1994).

Finally, to end this case with a bit of esoterica, it is noted that medial thalamic infarcts have also been reported to cause hypersomnia, where the patients may sleep excessively, up to 20 hours per day (Bassetti *et al.*, 1996). This suggests a role for the medial thalamus in regulating sleep–wake cycles. This association is corroborated by studies involving a rare condition known as the Kleine–Levin syndrome, or alternatively, the hypersomnia–hyperphagia syndrome. This is a bizarre disease which affects adolescent males, and is characterized by recurrent bouts, usually lasting a few days, of hypersomnia and excessive compulsive eating. The findings are sometimes accompanied by memory deficits and hypersexual behavior. The bouts may recur as frequently as every few months, but in-between bouts, the patients are typically normal. Clinicopathologic correlation suggests a role for the medial thalamus in this disorder (Carpenter *et al.*, 1982). For example, recent studies with SPECT scanning have shown hypoperfusion of the thalami during the symptomatic periods (Huang *et al.*, 2005).

References

Bassetti, C., Mathis, J., Gugger, M., *et al.* Hypersomnia following paramedian thalamic stroke: a report of 12 patients. *Annals of Neurology* 1996; **39**: 471–480.

Bogousslavsky, S., Regli, F., Uske, A. Thalamic infarcts: clinical syndromes, etiology and prognosis. *Neurology* 1988; **38**(6): 837–48.

Carpenter, S., Yassa, R., and Ochs, R. A pathologic basis for Kleine–Levin syndrome. *Archives of Neurology* 1982; **39**(1): 25–28.

Huang, Y. S., Guilleminault, C., Kao, P. F. *et al.* SPECT findings in the Kleine–Levin syndrome. *Sleep* 2005; **28**(8): 955–960.

Kinney, H. C., Korein, J., Panigrahy, A. *et al.* Neuropathological findings in the brain of Karen Ann Quinlan: the role of the thalamus in the persistent vegetative state. *New England Journal of Medicine* 1994; **330**(21): 1469–1475.

Matheus, M. G., and Castillo, M. Imaging of acute bilateral paramedian thalamic and mesencephalic infarcts. *American Journal of Neuroradiology* 2003; **24**: 2005–2008.

Case 6.4

60-year-old male patient who presented with a few minutes of right body tingling followed by a sensation of right-sided weakness and clumsiness. Clinical examination revealed a right-sided hemihypesthesia involving the face and body to pain and temperature as well as vibration and proprioception. The patient had mild right-sided weakness as well as right extremity ataxia with hypermetria and dysdiadochokinesis.

Do the clinical findings suggest a particular anatomic location for this lesion?

The patient presents with a hemisensory deficit combined with an ataxic hemiparesis. This combination is highly suggestive of a lesion in the thalamus contralateral to the side of symptoms, and more specifically, a lesion in the ventrolateral portion of the contralateral thalamus.

The patient's MRI is shown (Fig. 6.13). What are the findings? What is the diagnosis?

Diagnosis

MRI shows a subacute infarct involving the left ventrolateral thalamus, with T2 and DWI hyperintensity. The infarct is in the territory of the inferolateral or thalamogeniculate arteries. This is the territory most commonly involved in thalamic infarcts (followed by the paramedian artery territory).

Describe the structures involved in, and clinical presentation of, inferolateral thalamic infarcts.

The thalamogeniculate or inferolateral arteries are a group of perforators which arise from the P2 portion of the posterior cerebral

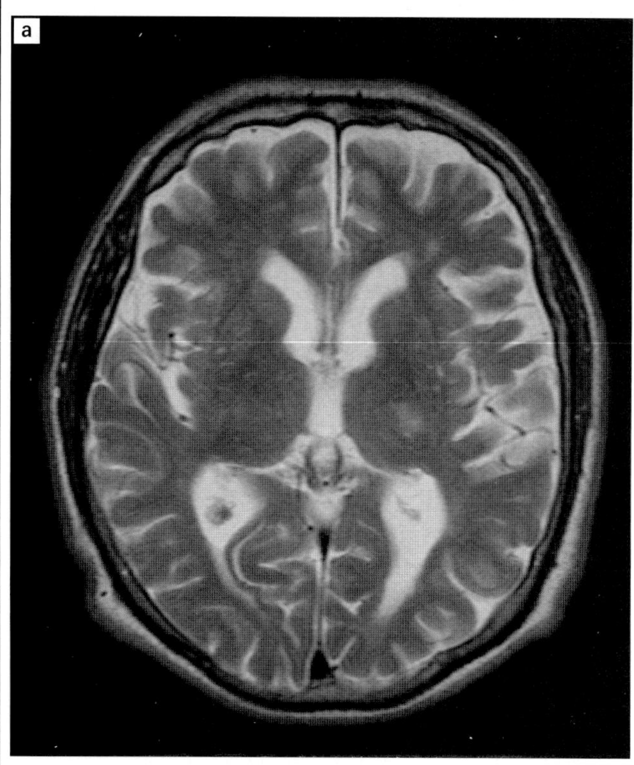

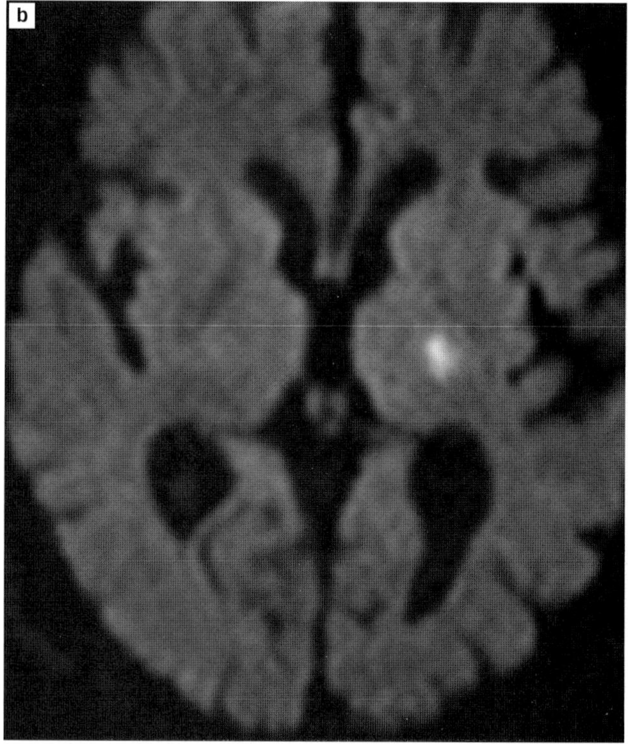

Fig. 6.13. **(a) T2 and (b) DWI axial MRI images.**

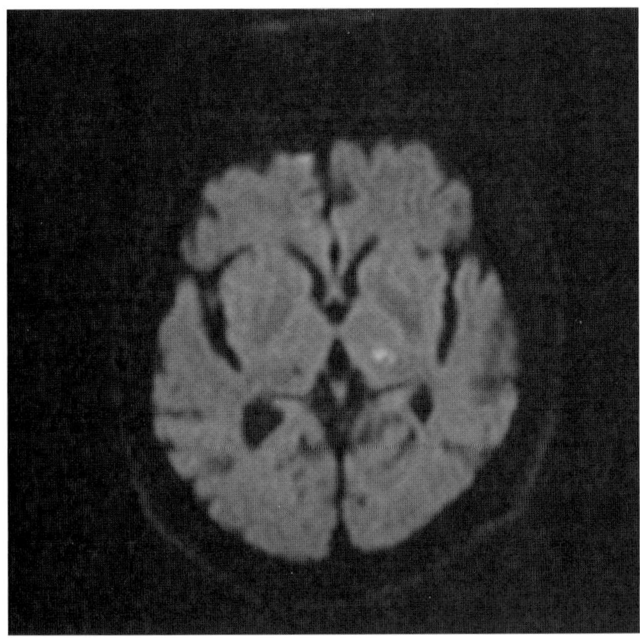

Fig. 6.14. **Axial DWI images show a small subacute infarct in the left ventrolateral thalamus. Patient is a 57-year-old male with a pure cheiro-oral syndrome.**

artery. They supply principally the VPM and VPL nuclei of the thalamus, as well as the ventral and lateral portions of the VL nucleus, with variable supply as well to portions of the pulvinar.

Therefore, the principal manifestations of infarcts in this region are hemisensory deficits, which may be across all modalities, or may affect only touch, pain and temperature. An interesting sensory manifestation, known as the cheiro-oral syndrome, may sometimes be observed with inferolateral thalamic infarcts. It consists of numbness of the corner of the mouth and of the hand. This may occur because of the somatotopic organization of the VPM and VPL nuclei, with the hand area putatively being medial in the VPL (which, as you recall, handles sensation in the body), adjacent to the mouth area, presumably lateral in the VPM (which handles sensation in the face). Thus, a small infarct may involve the medial VPL and lateral VPM, producing the cheiro-oral syndrome. A pure cheiro-oral syndrome was found in the patient adjacent (Fig. 6.14).

Sometimes, the corner of the mouth, the hand, and the foot on the same side are all involved, with sparing of the rest of the body. Naturally, this is called the cheiro-oral-pedal syndrome, and has also been described with ventrolateral thalamic infarcts (Yasuda *et al.*, 1993). However, we hasten to add that the literature is replete with case reports of the cheiro-oral or cheiro-oral-pedal syndrome also occurring with parietal cortical lesions, midbrain infarcts, and pontine hemorrhages. In fact, one source states, after a review of the literature, that pontine lesions are the most common cause of pure cheiro-oral syndrome (see Huang and Chu, 1994). Therefore, if a patient presents with cheiro-oral manifestations, wait to see the MRI scans.

Also, with ventrolateral thalamic infarcts, one occasionally encounters combinations which have not been specifically described in the literature, but make anatomic sense. For example, a patient (Fig. 6.15) presented with a right-sided

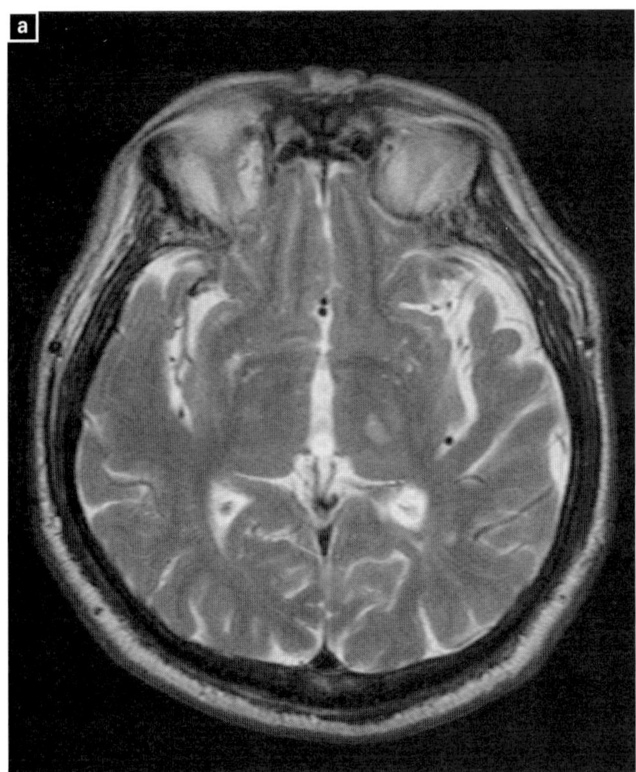

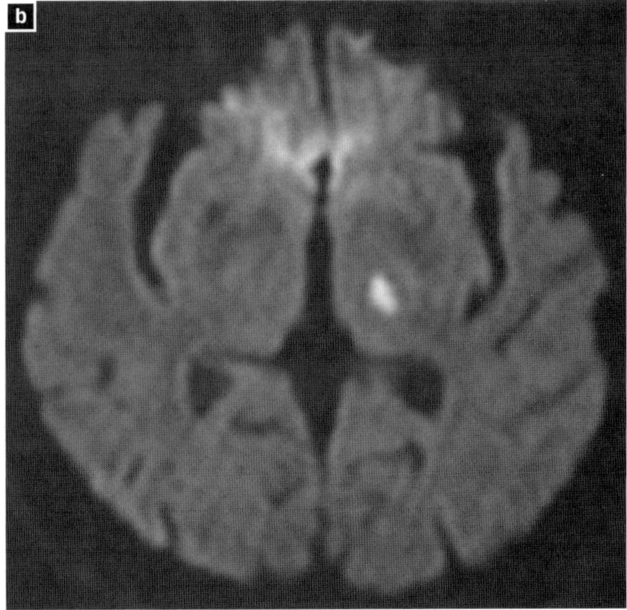

Fig. 6.15. **(a) Axial T2 and (b) DWI images show a subacute infarct in the left ventrolateral thalamus. Patient is a 61-year-old male with a cheiro-oral syndrome as well as ataxic hemiparesis of the right hand.**

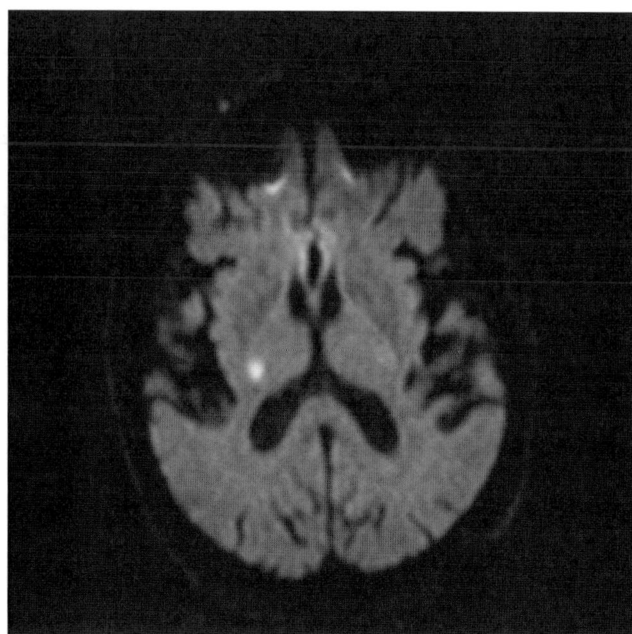

Fig. 6.16. **Axial DWI images of a 68-year-old male who presented with left hemisensory deficits. Four weeks later, the patient developed severe burning paroxysmal left body and face pain, consistent with a Dejerine–Roussy syndrome secondary to a right ventrolateral thalamic infarct.**

Several weeks after an inferolateral thalamic infarct, the contralateral hand may assume an athetoid posture, with wrist pronation and thumb adduction beneath the extended fingers. This is known as "thalamic hand."

It is important to note that cognitive and psychiatric manifestations (such as memory deficits or behavioral changes) and alterations of consciousness are essentially absent in inferolateral thalamic infarcts. Also, the thalamic dysphasia which occurs with tuberothalamic and paramedian infarcts is quite unusual in inferolateral infarcts.

In the aftermath of inferolateral thalamic infarcts, a distinct pain syndrome has been described. Please discuss it. Hint: it has a French eponym.

Weeks to months after an inferolateral thalamic infarct, the patient may develop severe paroxysmal pain in the contralateral body, often triggered by light touch. This "thalamic pain" is often poorly responsive to analgesia. The combination of the typical findings for an inferolateral infarct, such as hemihypesthesia and ataxic hemiparesis, followed by the paroxysmal pain syndrome just described, is known as the thalamic syndrome of Dejerine and Roussy. Interestingly, thalamic pain occurs more commonly with right-sided infarcts, suggesting that the right cerebral cortex is more involved in nociception (nociception is the recognition of painful stimuli). Other manifestations of the infarct, though, such as sensory deficits, weakness or ataxia do not show a propensity to lateralize. Another interesting bit of trivia is that, for thalamic pain syndrome, the right-sided predominance was more pronounced in men than women. A typical clinical example is shown in Fig. 6.16. A nice reference in this regard is Nasreddine and Saver (1997).

cheiro-oral syndrome, as well as ataxia of the right hand and mild right hand weakness.

This combination of sensory, motor and cerebellar findings, once again, is highly suggestive of ventrolateral thalamic infarcts. The cause of the sensory findings has been discussed. Because of involvement of the VL nucleus, the patients may also have contralateral weakness as well as ataxia (recall that cerebellar fibers coursing through the dentatothalamic tract on their way to the motor cortex synapse in the VL).

References

Huang, M. H., and Chu, N. S. Pure cheiro-oral syndrome due to a small pontine hematoma: report of a case and review of the literature. *Journal of the Formosa Medical Association* 1994; **93**(7): 636–639.

Nasreddine, Z. S., and Saver, J. L. Pain after thalamic stroke: right diencephalic predominance and clinical features in 180 patients. *Neurology* 1997; **48**(5): 1196–1199.

Yasuda, Y., Matsuda, I., Akiguchi, I. *et al.* Cheiro-oral-pedal syndrome in thalamic infarction. *Clinical Neurology and Neurosurgery* 1993; **95**(4): 311–314.

Case 6.5

58-year-old male complaining of "a few weeks of not seeing right." On examination, he is noted to have a left homonymous sectoranopia. He is otherwise neurologically intact.

What are your thoughts on the possible location of the lesion?

As will be covered more fully later, homonymous visual field deficits indicate a post-chiasmatic lesion contralateral to the side of the visual field defect. Possible locations would be a lesion involving the right-sided optic radiations, or possibly one lip of the right calcarine cortex.

The patient's CT examination is shown in Fig. 6.17. Other than the images shown, the CT was unremarkable. What you see?

Diagnosis

Hemorrhagic infarct of the right thalamus.

In which vascular territory is this infarct located? What structures are usually involved in such infarcts? What is the typical clinical presentation of these infarcts?

The infarct is in the posterior thalamus, in the territory of the posterior choroidal arteries. The posterior choroidal arteries arise from the P2 portion of the posterior cerebral artery. There are two groups: medial and lateral. The medial branches supply predominantly the midbrain and the subthalamic nucleus. The lateral posterior choroidal arteries supply the lateral geniculate nucleus, the inferolateral portion of the pulvinar, and the lateral dorsal nucleus and lateral posterior nucleus of the thalamus.

These infarcts are relatively infrequent, and they involve predominantly association areas of the thalamus, and therefore they are less well characterized in their clinical presentation. The most prominent clinical findings as reported by the Lausanne group (see Bogousslavsky *et al.*, 1988, as well as Neau and Bogousslavsky, 1996) is a contralateral homonymous quadrantanopia or sectoranopia (where a given sector of vision is homonymously absent). The quadrantanopia may be in the upper or lower part of the visual field, and the visual field deficits are thought to probably be secondary to infarction of, or adjacent to, the lateral geniculate nucleus.

An interesting concomitant of the homonymous quadrantanopia, also reported by the Lausanne group, is an impaired quick

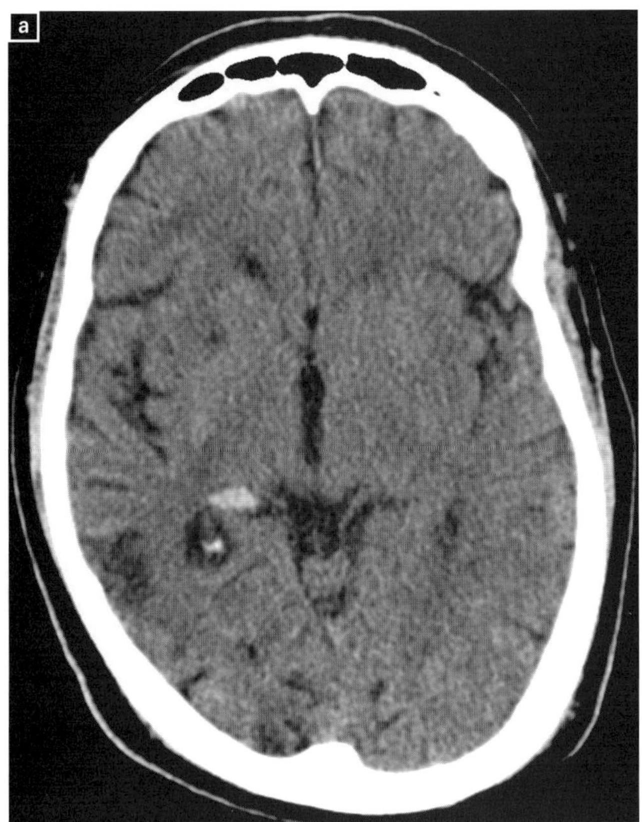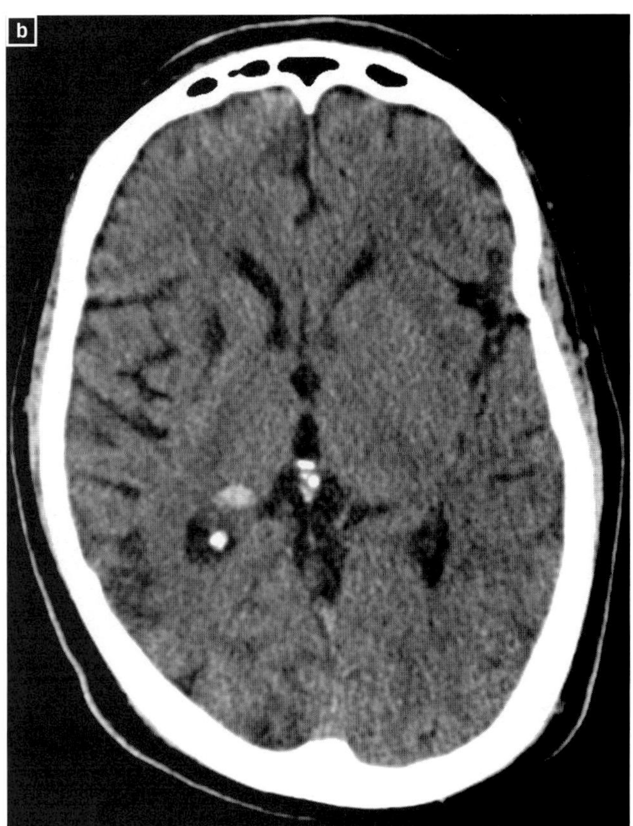

Fig. 6.17. **(a), (b) Contiguous non-contrast CT images show a bleed in the posterior right thalamus in this patient with a homonymous left-sided visual field defect.**

phase of the optokinetic response opposite to the lesion. What does this mean? Most of us are familiar with the vestibulo-ocular reflex (VOR). Another well-described reflex eye movement is the optokinetic reflex or optokinetic nystagmus. This is the sort of eye movement which occurs as we are riding a train and looking out at the scenery as it passes by. Our eyes track the moving scenery as we go by it. This is called the slow phase or smooth pursuit phase of optokinetic nystagmus. Then, as the objects leave our visual field, our eyes dart back to capture another scene and begin tracking it. This darting back is the fast or saccadic phase of optokinetic nystagmus. The smooth pursuit phase is mediated by interactions of the visual cortex and visual association areas with the vestibular nuclei and flocculonodular lobe of the cerebellum, ultimately projecting to the PPRF. The fast or saccadic phase is mediated by the frontal eye field projecting to the contralateral PPRF. Thus, lesions of the frontal eye fields, for instance, can cause disruption of the fast phase of optokinetic nystagmus. Apparently, so can lesions in the posterior thalamus.

Other possible manifestations of posterior choroidal infarcts which have been reported include:

(1) Spatial hemineglect opposite the side of an infarct or bleed in the pulvinar. Such is the case of the patient below. He is a 74-year-old male who had some left-sided hemineglect and mild constructional apraxia (Fig. 6.18). Non-contrast CT reveals a moderately large old infarct of the right pulvinar.

  Usually, visuospatial hemineglect occurs with right-sided thalamic lesions (see Karnath *et al.*, 2002 and Motomura *et al.*, 1986). This finding is probably due to the role of the pulvinar

in visuospatial processing and its connections with the temporal–occipital–parietal association cortex.

(2) There are sporadic reports of transcortical aphasia in patients with lateral posterior choroidal artery infarcts (see Neau and Bogousslavsky, 1996). This is consistent with some reports which assert that the pulvinar has a role in language processing and that intraoperative stimulation of the pulvinar can result in anomia (Ojemann *et al.*, 1968).

(3) Rarely, patients with infarcts in the posterior choroidal territory may develop an unusual movement disorder in a delayed fashion. This consists of ataxia, tremor, myoclonus, and chorea. It has been described by the Lausanne Stroke Group and termed the "jerky dystonic unsteady hand syndrome" (Ghika *et al.*, 1994).

(4) Rarely, patients with posterior thalamic strokes may develop scotoma. This is a very rare manifestation, but scotomas in association with posterior thalamic lesions have been previously reported (Wada *et al.*, 1999).

References

Bogousslavsky, J., Regli, F., Uske, A. Thalamic infarcts: clinical syndromes, etiology, and prognosis. *Neurology* 1988; **38**(6): 837–848.

Ghika, J., Bogousslavsky, J., Henderson, J. *et al.* The " jerky dystonic unsteady hand" : a delayed motor syndrome in posterior thalamic infarctions. *Journal of Neurology* 1994; **241**: 537–542.

Karnath, H. O., Himmelbach, M., Rorden, C.. The subcortical anatomy of human spatial neglect: putamen, caudate nucleus and pulvinar. *Brain* 2002; **125**(2): 350–360.

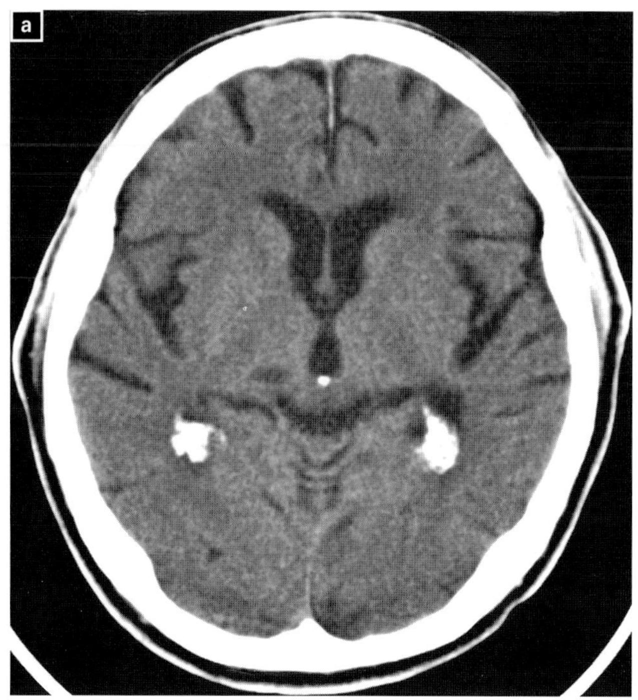
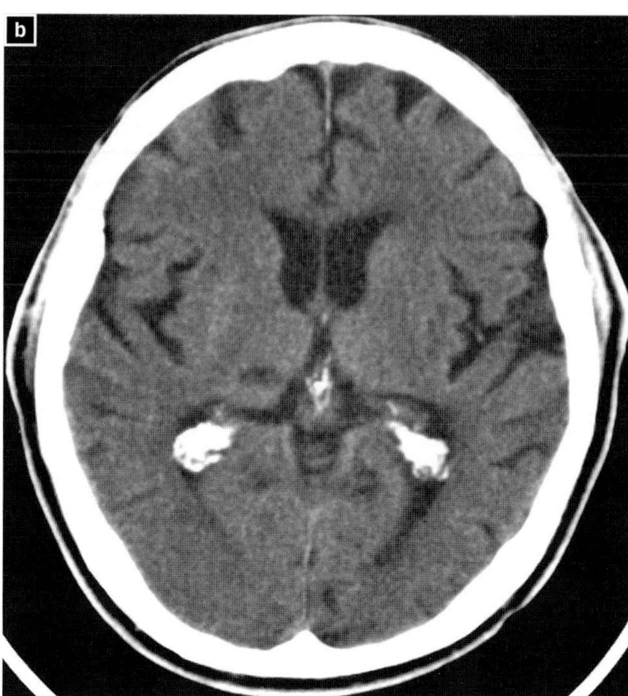

Fig. 6.18. **(a), (b) CT images show a moderately large, old infarct involving the right pulvinar.**

Motomura, N., Yamadori, A., Mori, E. *et al*. Unilateral spatial neglect due to hemorrhage in the thalamic region. *Acta Neurologica Scandinavia* 1986; **74**: 190–194.

Neau, J. P., and Bogousslavsky, J. The syndrome of posterior choroidal artery territory infarction. *Annales of Neurology* 1996; **39**: 779–788.

Ojemann, G. A., Fedio, P., and Van Buren, J. M. Anomia from pulvinar and subcortical parietal stimulation. *Brain* 1968; **91**: 99–116.

Wada, K., Kimura, K., Minematsu, K. *et al*. Incongruous homonymous hemianopic scotoma. *Journal of Neurological Science* 1999; **163**(2): 179–182.

Case 6.6

34-year-old female patient found unconscious. The patient was comatose with posturing and bilateral positive Babinski's sign. Her family stated that, 3 days ago, she had been complaining of headaches, nausea, and vomiting.

MRI examination is provided in Fig. 6.19. What are the findings? What is your differential? What test would you order at this point?

There is marked abnormal FLAIR hyperintensity in the bilateral thalami, as well as diffuse swelling. No discrete mass lesion is seen, and the appearance is fairly symmetric. The differential diagnosis for this appearance is quite limited, and includes as leading possibilities:

(1) Bilateral thalamic infarcts, such as in "artery of Percheron" infarcts or "top of the basilar" syndrome.

(2) Deep cerebral vein thrombosis, such as involving the internal cerebral veins or vein of Galen.

(3) Viral encephalitis.

(4) Infiltrative glioma crossing through the massa intermedia.

Such an appearance of the thalami should therefore immediately prompt us to look closely at the vein of Galen. Did you notice this structure in the above images? The fact is, we hardly ever notice it as we read routine MRIs. Look again at our patient's sagittal image with a normal control for comparison (Fig. 6.20). What do you notice now?

A closer examination of our patient's MRI images suggests thrombus in the vein of Galen. The next step in the workup should then be an MR venogram.

The MR venogram is shown (Fig. 6.21), with a normal control. What are the findings? What is the diagnosis?

The phase-contrast MR venogram of our patient shows a robust superior sagittal sinus. However, comparison with the normal control shows complete absence of flow signal in the internal cerebral veins, vein of Galen and the straight sinus.

Diagnosis

Deep cerebral vein thrombosis (DCVT) and thrombosis of the straight sinus. DCVT is defined as thrombosis of the internal cerebral veins and/or the vein of Galen.

The relevant anatomy is as follows: the septal, anterior caudate, and thalamostriate veins join at the level of the foramen of Monro to form the paired internal cerebral veins (ICV). The ICVs run in a paramidline location in the cistern of the velum interpositum along the superior margins of the thalami. Just inferior to the spelnium of the corpus callosum, they join the basal veins of Rosenthal to form the vein of Galen, which then joins the inferior sagittal sinus (seen in only 50 percent of cases on MR venography) to form the straight sinus (see Fig. 6.22).

For those interested in a review of the venous anatomy and its variants with MRV, please refer to Ayanzen *et al.*, 2000.

DCVT is an unusual and highly dangerous clinical entity. It tends to have rather high mortality and morbidity rates, but may also be potentially treatable – therefore, it is important to think of it and diagnose it. It is necessary to distinguish DCVT

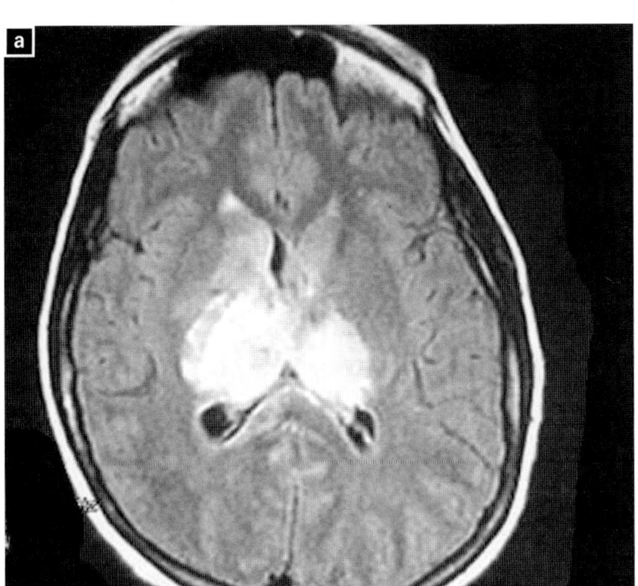
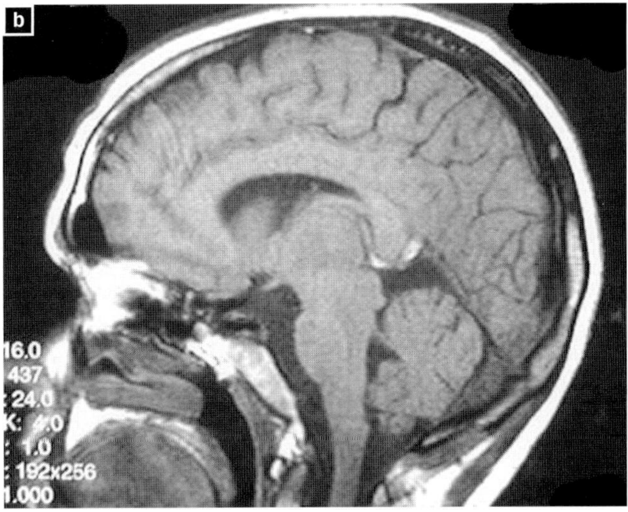

Fig. 6.19. **(a) FLAIR axial and (b) T1 sagittal images are provided. Case courtesy of Dr. Gavin Udstuen, Division of Neuroradiology, University of Cincinnati Medical Center.**

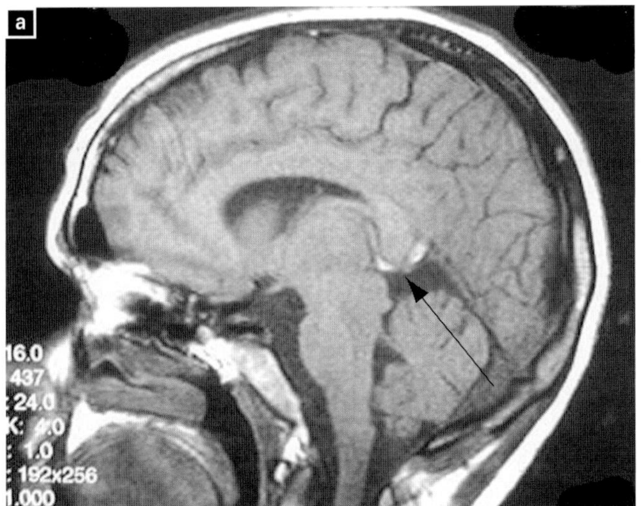
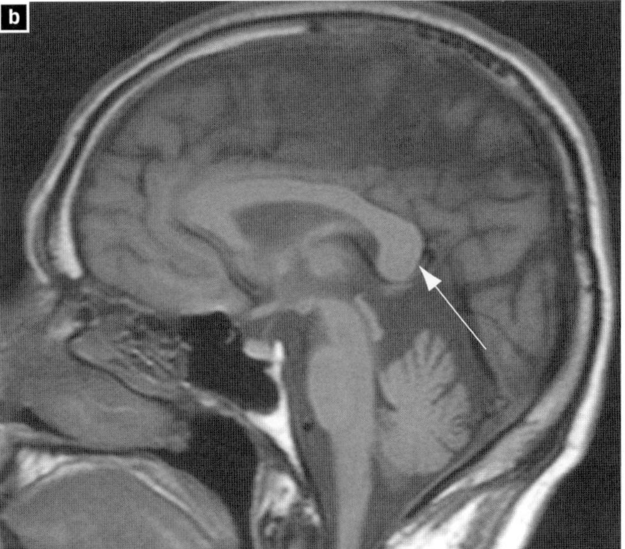

Fig. 6.20. **(a) Sagittal midline T1-weighted images of our patient, same as above. (b) Sagittal midline T1-weighted image of a normal control. Notice the subtle abnormal T1-weighted hyperintensity in the vein of Galen (arrow (a)). In the normal situation, the vein of Galen usually shows as a small curvilinear flow void beneath the splenium of the corpus callosum (arrow (b)) which we are not likely to notice unless we specifically look for it.**

from dural sinus thrombosis (such as thrombosis of the superior sagittal sinus). This distinction is not drawn in most papers or books, but is important because DCVT has a significantly higher mortality rate than dural sinus thrombosis. A nice discussion of DCVT is found in Crawford *et al.* (1995). In this paper, the authors review the clinical course of seven of their patients with DCVT. Three of these patients died and two remained severely disabled, illustrating the sort of mortality and morbidity characteristic of DCVT. Their case series and review of the literature demonstrated that in contrast to dural sinus thrombosis, patients with DCVT tended to have a more rapidly declining clinical course with altered consciousness and long tract signs. They were, though, less likely to present with the seizures, papilledema, and focal deficits, which are characteristic of dural sinus thrombosis. The absence of seizures in DCVT is probably due to a lack of the cortical irritation which occurs with dural sinus thrombosis.

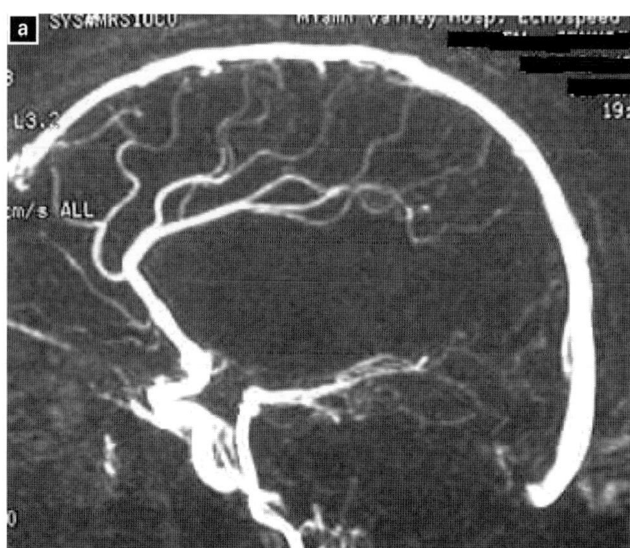

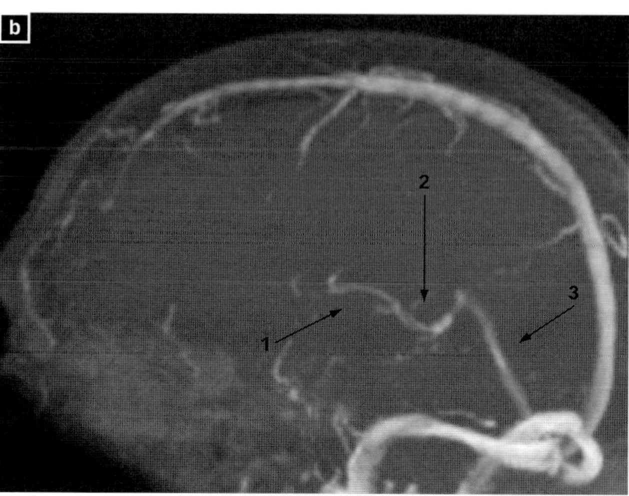

Fig. 6.21. **(a) Phase-contrast MR venogram of our patient, midline slab. Note the presence of the anterior cerebral artery, portions of the internal carotid, basilar and posterior cerebral arteries, which are present in this phase contrast acquisition. You are probably used to seeing time of flight acquisitions, where the arterial structures are absent. (b) Time-of-flight MR venogram of a normal control for comparison. Note the presence of the internal cerebral veins (arrow 1), vein of Galen (arrow 2) and the straight sinus (arrow 3), all absent in our patient.**

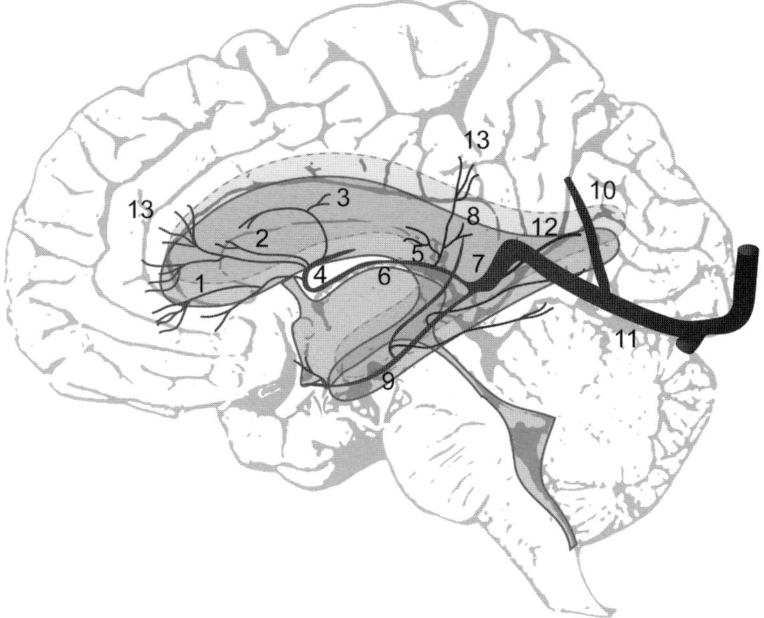

Fig. 6.22. **Anatomic diagram of deep venous anatomy. 1. Septal vein. 2. Anterior caudate vein. 3. Terminal vein. 4. Thalamostriate vein. 5. Direct lateral vein. 6. Internal cerebral vein. 7. Vein of Galen. 8. Inferior ventricular vein. 9. Basal vein of Rosenthal. 10. Inferior sagittal sinus. 11. Straight sinus. 12. Medial atrial vein. 13. Medullary veins.**

Conversely, dural sinus thrombosis may present with focal deficits secondary to isolated cortical venous infarcts; these are not seen in DCVT. Both DCVT and dural sinus thrombosis typically present with headache. Nausea and vomiting, though, seem more characteristic of DCVT. It is interesting to note that DCVT appears to show a strong female predominance (about 8:1 in the small series cited above). Also, most patients with DCVT seem to have a predisposing risk factor. These include polycythemia, oral contraceptives, malignancy, pregnancy, and puerperium, and inflammatory bowel disease. To sum up, then, DCVT is characterized by a high female predominance, the presence of a rapidly declining clinical course with headaches, nausea, vomiting, altered consciousness, and long tract signs, and absence of the papilledema, seizures, and focal deficits characteristic of dural sinus thrombosis.

The clinical presentation can, in part, be correlated to the diffuse thalamic involvement, as well as to hypoxia and increased venous pressure in the remainder of the territory drained by the deep venous system, which includes the basal ganglia, periventricular white matter, and portions of the cerebral peduncles.

The management of DCVT is not well defined, as there are relatively few cases. Because of the rapid clinical course and high mortality and morbidity rates, it is felt that some sort of treatment should be quickly instituted. There are reports of successful therapy with high dose heparin, even in the face of intracranial hemorrhage (Erbguth *et al.*, 1991). This seems to be the mainstay of therapy. There have also been reports of successful treatment by local infusion of thrombolytics delivered via a catheter introduced from the jugular veins into the straight sinus (Holder *et al.*, 1997). If you have a good neurointerventional service, consult them for their opinion on the matter!

As has become our wont, we end with some esoterica. The appearance of the thalami in DCVT is probably due to a mixture of increased hydrostatic pressure in the capillary beds as well as hypoxia, both due to lack of adequate venous outflow. Therefore, it stands to reason that elevation of venous pressures and impedance of venous outflow in the internal cerebral veins from any cause would produce similar imaging findings to our case above. Thus, it is not surprising to learn that there have been reports of arteriovenous malformations or fistulas draining into the deep venous system which present with bithalamic edema. These entities can be added toward the bottom of our differential. The findings seem reversible if the malformation or fistula is treated. For example, see Greenough *et al.*, 1999 and Ito *et al.*, 1995. Lastly, there are rare reports of unilateral internal cerebral vein thrombosis, leading to unilateral thalamic edema, but this is extremely rare (see Herrmann *et al.*, 2004).

References

Ayanzen, R. H., Bird, C. R., Keller, P. J. *et al.* Cerebral MR venography: normal anatomy and potential diagnostic pitfalls. *American Journal of Neuroradiology* 2000; **21**: 74–78.

Crawford, S. C., Digre, K. B., Palmer, C. A. *et al.* Thrombosis of the deep venous drainage of the brain in adults: analysis of seven cases with review of the literature. *Archives of Neurology* 1995; **52**: 1101–1108.

Erbguth, F., Brenner, P., Schuierer, G. *et al.* Diagnosis and treatment of deep cerebral vein thrombosis. *Neurosurgery Review* 1991; **14**(2): 145–148.

Greenough, G. P., Mamourian, A., and Harbaugh, R. E. Venous hypertension associated with a posterior fossa dural arteriovenous fistula: another cause of bithalamic lesions on MR images. *American Journal of Neuroradiology* 1999; **20**: 145–147.

Herrmann, K. A., Sporer, B., and Yousry, T. A. Thrombosis of the internal cerebral vein associated with transient unilateral thalamic edema: a case report and review of the literature. *American Journal of Neuroradiology* 2004; **25**: 1351–1355.

Holder, C. A., Bell, D. A., Lundell, A. L., Ulmer, J. L., and Glazier, S. S. Isolated straight sinus and deep cerebral venous thrombosis: successful treatment with local infusion of urokinase. *Journal of Neurosurgery* 1997; **86**: 704–707.

Ito, M., Sonokawa, T., Mishina, H. *et al.* Reversible dural arteriovenous malformation-induced venous ischemia as a cause of dementia: treatment by surgical occlusion of draining dural sinus: case report. *Neurosurgery* 1995; **37**: 1187–1192.

Case 6.7

44-year-old female patient presented with left-sided motor weakness, ataxia, and left-sided body and face numbness. Patient initially evaluated at an outside hospital, at which time she also displayed an altered level of consciousness with somnolence and decreased attention.

MRI is shown (Fig. 6.23). What are the findings? What is your diagnosis?

There is a region of mixed signal intensity, with a rim of T1-weighted hyperintensity and central isointensity, in the central and lateral portion of the right thalamus. The lesion displays the typical MR characteristics of a subacute hemorrhage.

Diagnosis

Right thalamic subacute hemorrhage.

Please discuss the presentation and prognosis of thalamic hemorrhages as compared with ischemic thalamic strokes.

Let us begin by providing two sources of further reading on this difficult to answer question: Steinke *et al.* (1992) and Saez de Ocariz *et al.* (1996).

Thalamic bleeds are usually hypertensive in etiology, but may also occur secondary to vascular malformations or hemorrhagic metastases. In general, it is very difficult to distinguish thalamic infarct from thalamic hemorrhage based on clinical presentation. Overall, in the series of Saez de Ocariz *et al.* (1996), out of 28 patients with MR confirmed thalamic lesions, 22 had thalamic infarcts while 6 had hemorrhage (thus, hemorrhage accounts for about 21 percent of the total). While hemorrhages are clinically difficult to distinguish from infarcts, they seem to have a significantly worse prognosis. To some extent, that is because thalamic bleeds sometimes rupture into the ventricular system, which heralds a high risk of death. Clinically, if a patient with thalamic

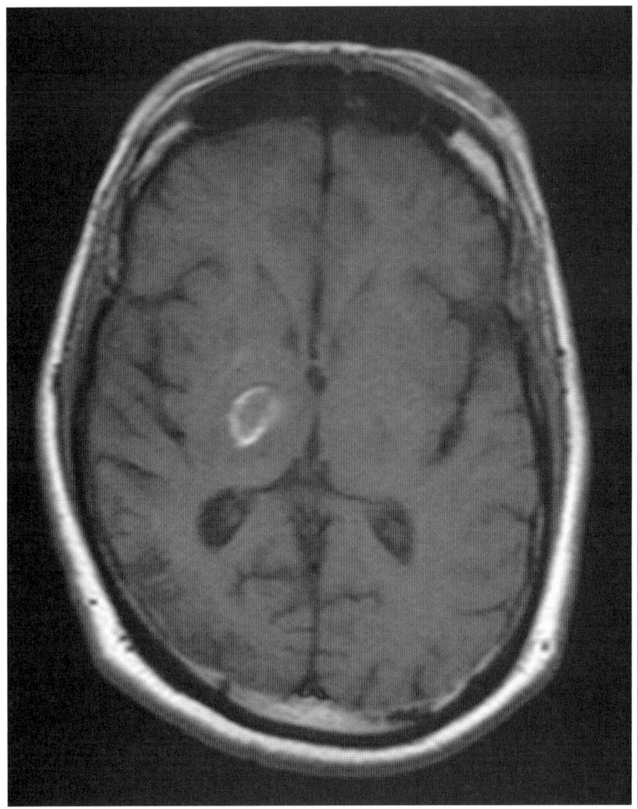

Fig. 6.23. **Axial T1-weighted MRI image.**

hemorrhage presents with stupor or coma, there is also a high risk of death. In terms of imaging, other than the presence of intraventricular blood, the size of the thalamic hemorrhage seems to be the next most important indicator of prognosis. Two series (Walshe *et al.*, 1977 and Weisberg, 1986) document that, if the thalamic hemorrhage exceeds about 3 cm in size, this is associated with an almost uniformly fatal outcome (see Fig. 6.24):

One interesting aside that emerges from a review of thalamic strokes is that in 56 percent of patients with ischemic thalamic infarcts, the neurologic deficit was present upon awakening, as compared with only 5 percent of patients with thalamic hemorrhage (see Steinke *et al.*, 1992, cited above). This probably reflects the circadian variation of infarct occurrence, with the highest likelihood being in the early morning hours (see Marler *et al.*, 1989).

References

Marler, J. R., Price, T. R., Clark, G. L. *et al.* Circadian rhythmicity of stroke onset. *Stroke* 1989; **20**: 473–476.

Saez de Ocariz, M., Nader, J. A., Santos, J. A. *et al.* Thalamic vascular lesions: risk factors and clinical course for infarcts and hemorrhages. *Stroke* 1996; **27**: 1530–1536.

Steinke, W., Sacco, R. L., Mohr, J. P. *et al.* Thalamic stroke: presentations and prognosis of infarcts and hemorrhages. *Archives of Neurology* 1992; **49**: 703–710.

Walshe, T. M., Davis, K. R., and Fisher, C. M. Thalamic hemorrhage: a computed tomographic-clinical correlation. *Neurology* 1977; **27**: 217–222.

Weisberg, L. A.. Thalamic hemorrhage. Clinical-CT correlations. *Neurology* 1986; **36**: 1382–1386.

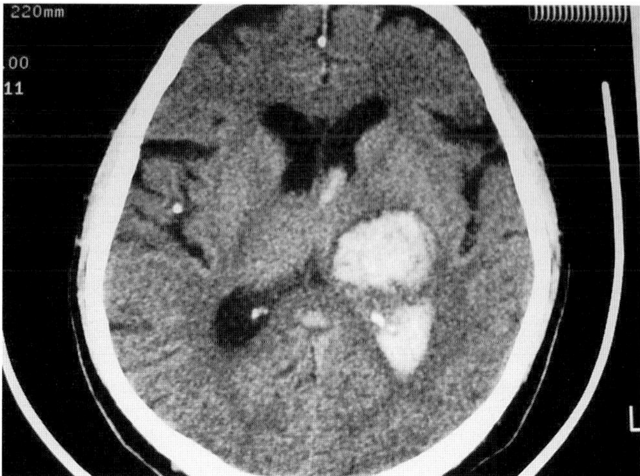

Fig. 6.24. **Non-contrast axial CT image showing large left thalamic hemorrhage (3.2 cm) with intraventricular extension.**

Case 6.8

50-year-old man presents with altered mental status progressive over 48 hours. He has horizontal nystagmus and is unable to fully abduct his eyes on lateral gaze. He is confused, being disoriented to time and place. He shows no focal motor weakness, but walks with a broad-based ataxic gait, and shows ataxia on both finger-nose and heel-shin testing. His biceps and knee-jerk reflexes are slightly decreased bilaterally.

What are the important elements of the history?

If we distill the history down, we have a 50-year-old male patient presenting with ophthalmoplegia (bilateral lateral rectus palsy), confusion and ataxia. Does this ring any bells?

Here is the patient's MRI scan (Fig. 6.25). What are the findings?

There is abnormal FLAIR hyperintensity in the periaqueductal gray matter, in the hypothalamus along the anterior walls of the third ventricle, along the columns of the fornix and in the bilateral medial thalami. Post-contrast, there is symmetric enhancement in the periaqueductal gray matter. Coupling the MRI scan with the clinical findings, there is one best differential diagnosis. What is it?

Diagnosis

Wernicke's encephalopathy.

Wernicke's encephalopathy is an acute or subacute illness characterized by a clinical triad of of ophthalmoplegia, ataxia and confusion. It is caused by a deficiency of thiamine (vitamin B1), which results in impaired cerebral glucose utilization. That is because thiamine (which is converted to its active form, thiamine pyrophosphate, in the liver) is a cofactor for key enzymes in the pentose-phosphate pathway (transketolase) and the tricarboxylic acid cycle (pyruvate dehydrogenase and alpha-ketoglutarate dehydrogenase). The lack of thiamine, therefore, disables glucose metabolism through these pathways and results in local lactic acidosis in the brain (because of its marked dependence on glucose metabolism), with subsequent cellular damage in highly susceptible areas. These turn out to be predominantly the periaqueductal gray matter, medial thalami, pontine tegmentum and mammillary bodies, as well as the cerebellar vermis and vestibular nuclei. In particularly severe cases, the cerebral cortex may also be involved. The ophthalmoplegia (most commonly abducens palsy and nystagmus) results from involvement of the brainstem tegmentum and the vestibular apparatus; the ataxia results from involvement of the cerebellum and the vestibular apparatus. The confusion (often manifest as apathy and decreased sensorium, sometimes to the point of coma) probably results from involvement of the medial thalami.

Wernicke's encephalopathy is often progressive, and confusion may progress to coma and death in 10–20 percent. Of those who survive, up to 80 percent end up with a Korsakoff psychosis, characterized by antegrade and retrograde amnesia and confabulation. That is why the disorder is commonly referred to as Wernicke–Korsakoff syndrome. The memory deficits are probably secondary to involvement of the mammillary bodies (impacting transmission of impulses from the hippocampal formations to the thalami through the mammillothalamic tracts) as well as the medial thalami.

Wernicke's encephalopathy is most commonly seen in alcoholics, both because their general malnutrition leads to thiamine deficiency and because the associated liver disease in the form of alcoholic hepatitis or cirrhosis leads to decreased activation of thiamine to thiamine pyrophosphate. However, Wernicke's encephalopathy can definitely occur in non-alcoholic conditions, where it may be harder to diagnose because of low clinical suspicion. Among the other causes noted are dialysis, AIDS, imposed starvation, prolonged vomiting and pancreatitis (see Zhong *et al.*,

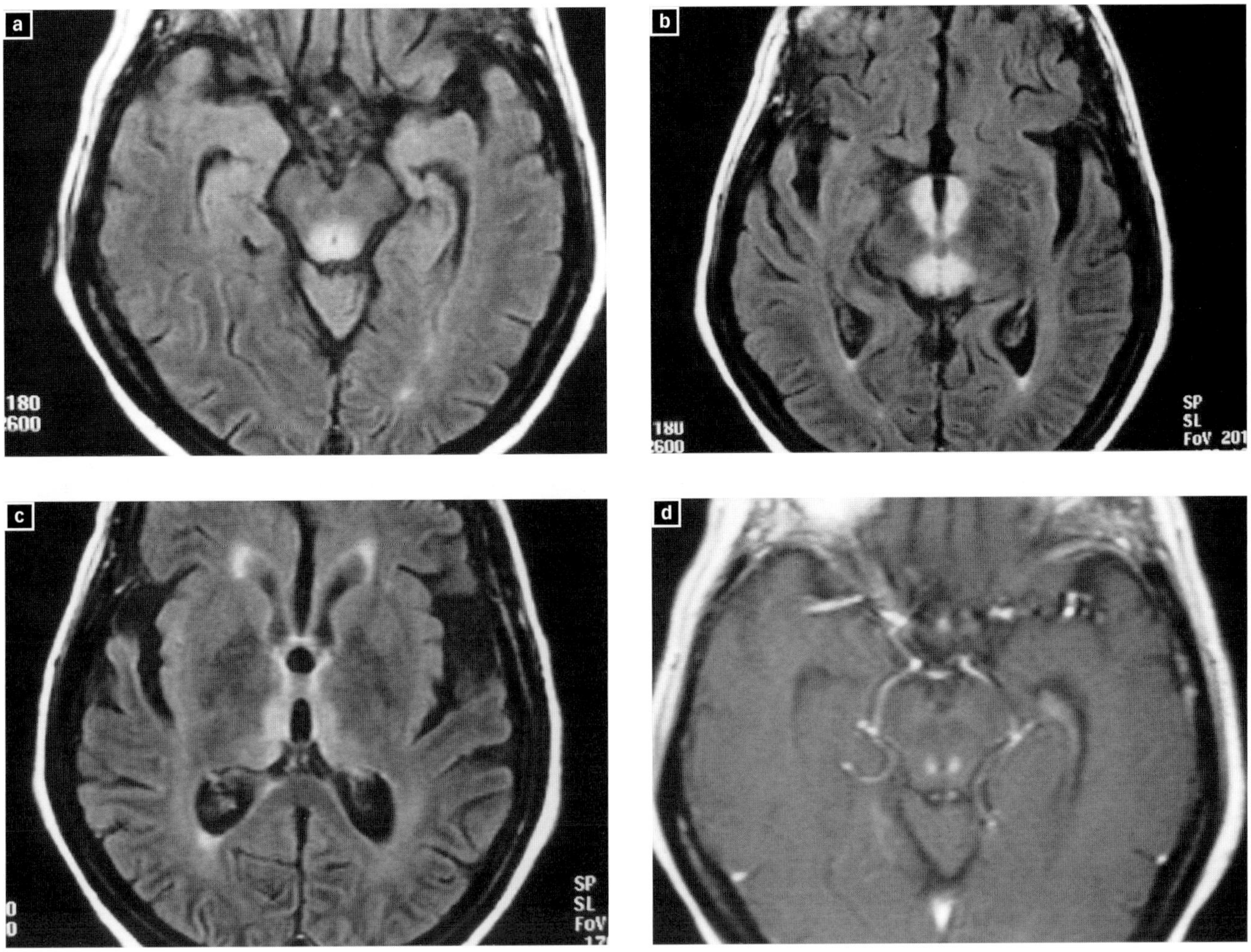

Fig. 6.25. **(a)–(c) Axial FLAIR images. (d) Axial T1 post-contrast image.**

2005). For example, look at the case of the patient adjacent (Fig. 6.26). This patient was a 49-year-old non-alcoholic male who had prolonged intractable vomiting and decreased oral intake secondary to a bout of gallstone pancreatitis. After being started on total parenteral nutrition, the patient developed nystagmus and confusion. MRI examination showed abnormal FLAIR hyperintensity in the paramedian thalami, and the diagnosis of Wernicke's encephalopathy was made.

It is important to note that in patients with borderline thiamine reserves, an acute Wernicke's encephalopathy may be precipitated by glucose administration, since the available thiamine stores are rapidly used up. The same thing may happen with the administration of TPN after prolonged fasting when thiamine is not included in the TPN regimen. This is why thiamine is always administered with glucose to alcoholic patients in the emergency room.

The treatment for Wernicke's, as expected, is thiamine administration, usually 100 mg i.v. in the immediate setting with daily supplementation thereafter. With treatment, the ophthalmoplegia component often responds quite rapidly, followed by improvements in ataxia, and then hopefully by improvement in the mental state. However, 25 percent of the patients who get Korsakoff's syndrome never recover full memory, and a sizeable minority of patients needs to be institutionalized.

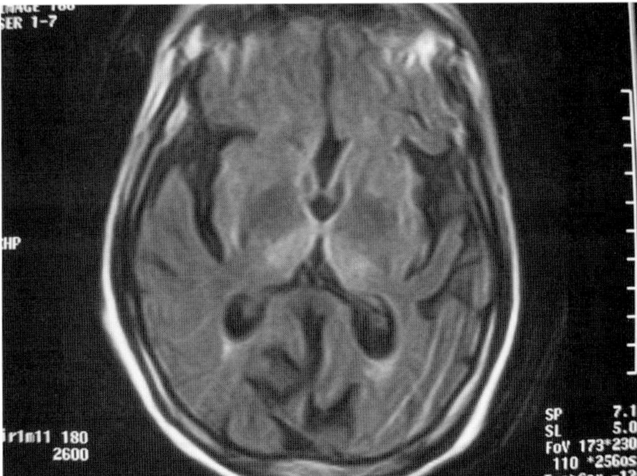

Fig. 6.26. **Axial FLAIR image, poor quality secondary to patient motion. There is abnormal hyperintensity in the bilateral medial thalami.**

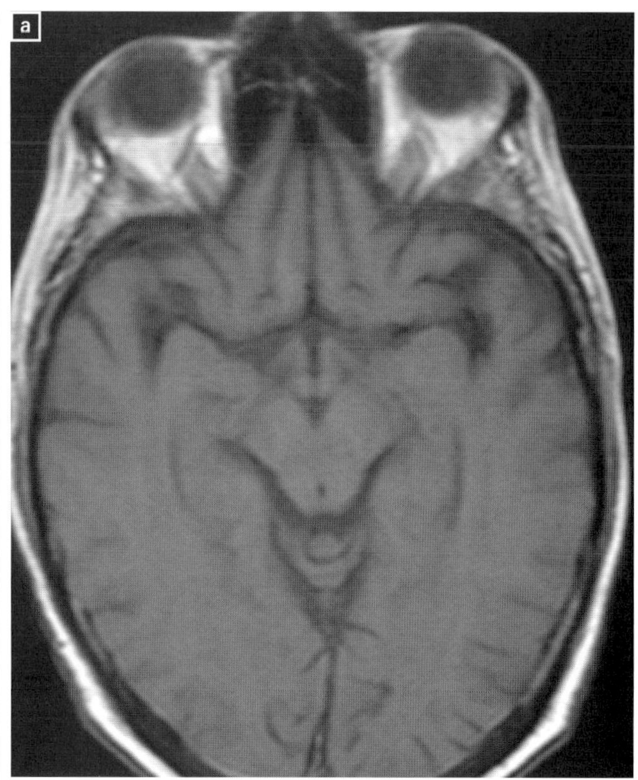
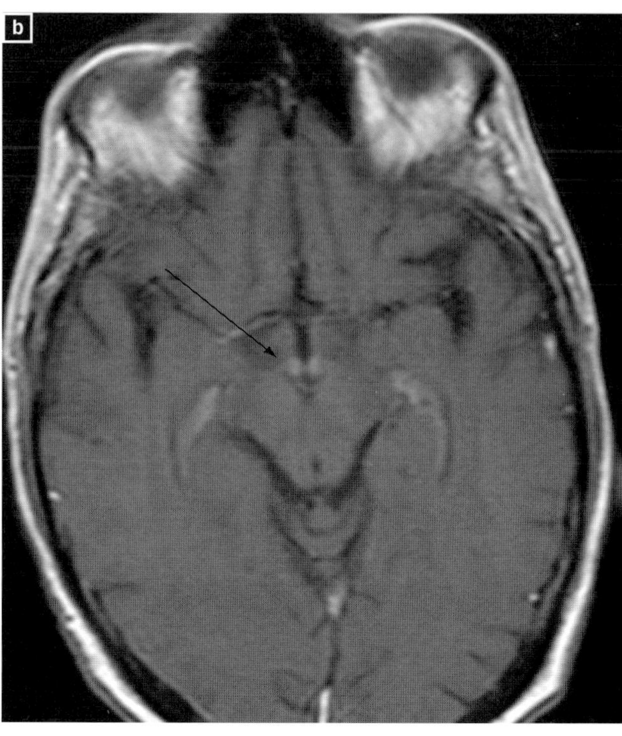

Fig. 6.27. **(a) Pre- and (b) post-contrast T1 axial images show abnormal enhancement of the mammillary bodies (arrow) in this patient with Wernicke's encephalopathy. No other abnormalities were present on this examination. Specifically, the mammillary bodies were not hyperintense on T2.**

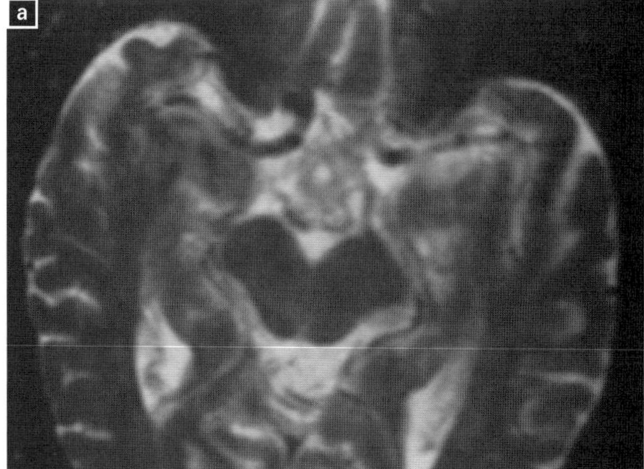
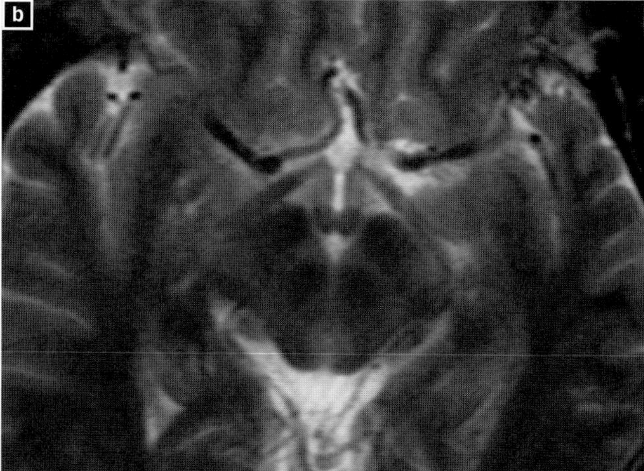

Fig. 6.28. **(a) Axial T2-weighted images of a patient with Korsakoff's syndrome. (b) Comparable image in a normal control. Our patient shows abnormal T2-weighted hyperintensity of the mammillary bodies.**

Describe the imaging findings of Wernicke's encephalopathy.

An easy way to remember the findings is that they tend to be midline. There may be abnormal FLAIR and T2 hyperintensity in the periaqueductal gray matter and midbrain tegmentum, along the walls of the third ventricle and in the paramedian thalami. Rarely, there may also be abnormal gyriform hyperintensity in the cerebral cortex.

It is interesting to note that imaging is not only helpful in making the diagnosis, but may also correlate with clinical presentation and prognosis. For example, patients with periaqueductal signal abnormality alone seem to have the mildest symptoms with less disturbance of the sensorium. Those with abnormal signal in the medial thalami tend to have a decreased sensorium, confusion and memory deficits. The rare patients with cortical ribbon signal abnormality appear to have a very bad prognosis with coma and death as highly likely outcomes (see Zhong *et al.*, 2005, also cited earlier). Another fairly suggestive finding is abnormal enhancement of the mammillary bodies (see Fig. 6.27), which may occur alone or with the other imaging manifestations of Wernicke's encephalopathy.

With time, the signal abnormalities seen on FLAIR and T2 sequences resolve, but this does not seem to correlate with the degree of residual clinical impairment on follow-up examinations. These tentative conclusions, though, are from a small patient series (White *et al.*, 2005).

Finally, we point out some of the findings which may be seen with a chronic Korsakoff's syndrome. In such cases, the acute Wernicke's encephalopathy clears, but the patient is left with significant antegrade and possibly also some retrograde amnesia, with prominent confabulation. Such a typical patient is presented (Fig. 6.28), showing T2-weighted hyperintensity in the mammillary bodies. On sagittal images, one may also see atrophy of the mammillary bodies.

References

White, M. L., Zhang, Y., Andrew, L. G. *et al.* MR imaging with diffusion weighted imaging in acute and chronic Wernicke encephalopathy. *American Joural of Neuroradiology* 2005; **26**: 2306–2310.

Zhong, C., Jin, L., and Fei, G. MR imaging of nonalcoholic Wernicke encephalopathy: a follow-up study. *American Journal of Neuroradiology* 2005; **26**: 2301–2305.

Case 6.9

12-year-old boy presents with an approximately 6-month history of gradual personality change, with increasing apathy, decreased mentation, diminished memory and confusion. No significant motor, sensory or cerebellar abnormalities were elicited on examination. The patient was referred for both psychiatric and neurologic consultation.

The patient's MRI is presented (Fig. 6.29). What are the findings?

There is marked abnormal enlargement with T2-weighted hyperintensity of the bilateral thalami, left greater than right. The appearance is consistent with an infiltrative mass involving the left thalamus and extending to the right.

Diagnosis

Bilateral thalamic glioma. Recall that low grade gliomas typically do not enhance, so do not let the lack of enhancement dissuade you from the diagnosis.

Thalamic gliomas constitute approximately 1 percent of all primary brain tumors. Bilateral thalamic gliomas, however, are quite a rare entity, with only a few descriptions in the literature. To get a feeling for how rare they are, we note that when the Montreal Neurological Institute and Hospital surveyed their records from 1963 to 1991, they found only 8 cases of bilateral thalamic gliomas, and this stands as one of the largest series in print (Partlow *et al.*, 1992).

The typical clinical presentation is that illustrated by our case and summarized in the title of the above review article. Patients usually present with neuropsychiatric manifestations, including apathy, confusion and diminished memory, rather than overt motor or sensory deficits. This may be due to the relatively slow rate of tumor growth, allowing accommodation by the motor and sensory systems.

Treatment usually consists of radiation therapy, but prognosis seems to be uniformly poor for these deep tumors.

Reference

Partlow, G. D., del Carpio-O'Donovan, R., Melanson, D. *et al.* Bilateral thalamic glioma: review of eight cases with personality change and mental deterioration. *American Journal of Neuroradiology* 1992; **13**(4): 1225–1230.

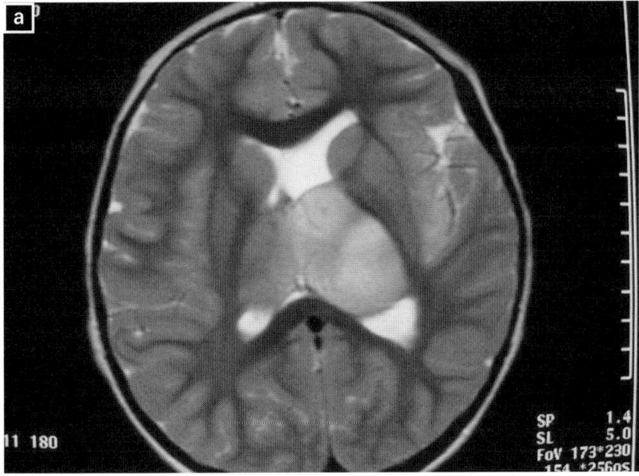
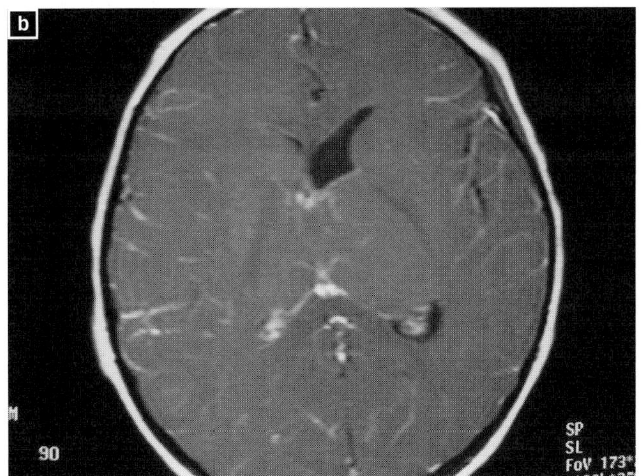

Fig. 6.29. **(a) Axial T2 and (b) post-contrast T1-weighted MRI images of the brain.**

Case 6.10

45-year-old male presents comatose with decorticate posturing. The family states that he had fever and mouth ulcerations for 3 days, then began having seizures.

An MRI image is presented (Fig. 6.30). What are the findings? What is your differential?

The FLAIR image shows symmetric bilateral hyperintensity involving the medial thalami, as well as the cortical opercular regions.

When we are able to confine a process to the gray matter, it makes our job much easier. The mantra which I give the residents is that for a gyriform pattern, think: infarct, infarct, infarct, encephalitis. Certainly, this is not an exhaustive list, as other pathology can affect the cortical gray matter, such as protoplasmic astrocytomas which like to infiltrate the cortex. However, it is a good starting point.

Diagnosis

Viral encephalitis.

The distribution of pathology on imaging and the provided clinical history make encephalitis the best choice. The presence of bilateral symmetry is also suggestive of encephalitis, since infarcts have no reason to be bilaterally symmetrical. Viruses, meanwhile, enter cells through protein gateways. Not all viruses infect all cells, and it stands to reason that the gateways which allow the viruses entry into specific cell populations are symmetrically distributed across the cerebral hemispheres.

A general discussion of viral encephalitis in the brain is beyond the scope of this case, as numerous etiologic agents may potentially infect the brain, from herpes virus (the most common cause of fatal endemic encephalitis) to the arboviruses, such as Eastern and Western Equine encephalitis, St. Louis encephalitis, Japanese encephalitis, and West Nile encephalitis.

The discussion of viral encephalitis is made more difficult by the fact that only a few viruses have a typical radiographic presentation which would allow that specific virus to be suggested on the basis of MRI findings. With regard to thalamic involvement in viral encephalitis, which is our topic here, a few observations are possible. If asked which viral encephalitis most typically affects the thalami, the best answer would probably be Japanese encephalitis,

where bilateral thalamic involvement is considered a typical finding. In one series of Japanese encephalitis patients, bilateral thalamic involvement was seen in 29 of 31 cases (Kalita and Misra, 2000). Involvement of the putamen is also very frequent. Japanese encephalitis is caused by a flavivirus belonging to what is known as the Japanese encephalitis antigenic complex. This is a group of closely related members of the flavivirus family which includes West Nile virus, St. Louis encephalitis virus, and Murray Valley encephalitis virus. These viruses seem to exhibit a neurotropism and hence have frequent CNS involvement. While St. Louis encephalitis has not been reported typically to involve the thalami, there is a small incidence of thalamic involvement in West Nile viral encephalitis. For example, in a recent case series, 8 of 16 cases of West Nile viral infection had brain findings suggestive of meningoencephalitis. Of these patients, 3 cases showed thalamic involvement, 2 as part of multifocal findings and 1 isolated to the thalami (Petropoulou *et al.*, 2005). Most interestingly, a case report of Murray Valley encephalitis, a disease seen almost exclusively in Australia, showed marked bilateral thalamic involvement. The imaging pattern was very similar to the reports of Japanese encephalitis, but with disease even more focused on the thalami in this particular case. The images below (Fig. 6.31) are those of a 49-year-old American woman who was living in Australia for over a year, and who presented with 3 days of fever, headache, vomiting, and confusion, as well as an expressive and mild receptive aphasia. A diagnosis of Murray Valley encephalitis was made with a positive CSF polymerase chain reaction (PCR) test for Murray Valley viral RNA.

There are very few reports in the literature regarding the imaging findings of Murray Valley encephalitis, but the bithalamic involvement, akin to Japanese encephalitis, suggests a similar neurotropism for these two closely related flaviviruses.

To further arouse your intellectual curiosity, we present the case of a patient who came to the emergency room obtunded. MRI, shown in Fig. 6.32, revealed bilaterally symmetric thalamic swelling and abnormal hyperintensity. A low white count and a CD4 of 8 led to HIV testing, and the patient was diagnosed with AIDS. HART therapy was instituted, and the bithalamic changes resolved over the course of about four weeks, leading to a presumptive diagnosis of HIV encephalitis involving the bilateral thalami. This manifestation, to the author's knowledge, has not been reported in the literature. The clinical service did not wish to pursue a brain biopsy just to help me write this book (and they call it a teaching hospital! Just kidding, folks). Therefore, the diagnosis remains presumptive and unreportable, but it certainly suggests that the thalami may be involved in a wide variety of encephalitides.

Now back to our original patient (Fig. 6.30). He was initially started on acyclovir as soon as he arrived in the ICU, based on the clinical history provided by the family. The MRI of Fig. 6.30, with bithalamic involvement, was highly atypical for herpes. After three negative PCR tests for HSV, the acyclovir was stopped. The CSF profile showed pleocytosis with a lymphocytic predominance, consistent with non-specific viral encephalitis. The clinical care team did not wish to pursue other viral serologic studies (and they call this a teaching hospital! This time, I'm not kidding, folks), so the specific etiologic agent in this case remains unknown. Within 2 weeks, the patient recovered from his coma, and eventually returned home with minimal deficits.

Thalamic involvement in viral encephalitis may also be unilateral, as in the case below of a 4-year-old girl with non-specific viral encephalitis, again based on CSF profile and clinical presentation (Fig. 6.33).

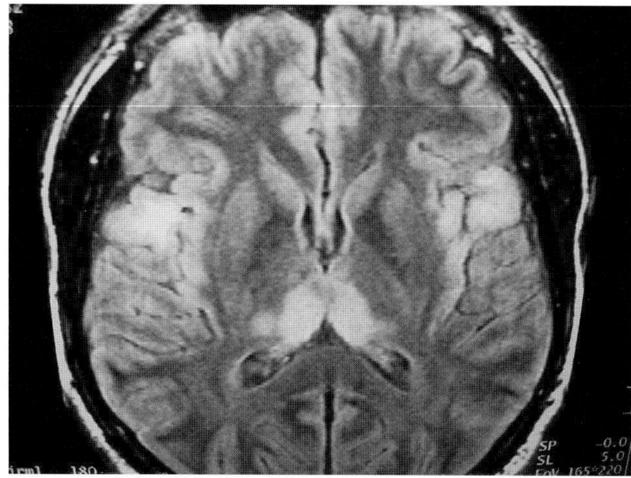

Fig. 6.30. **A single FLAIR axial MRI image.**

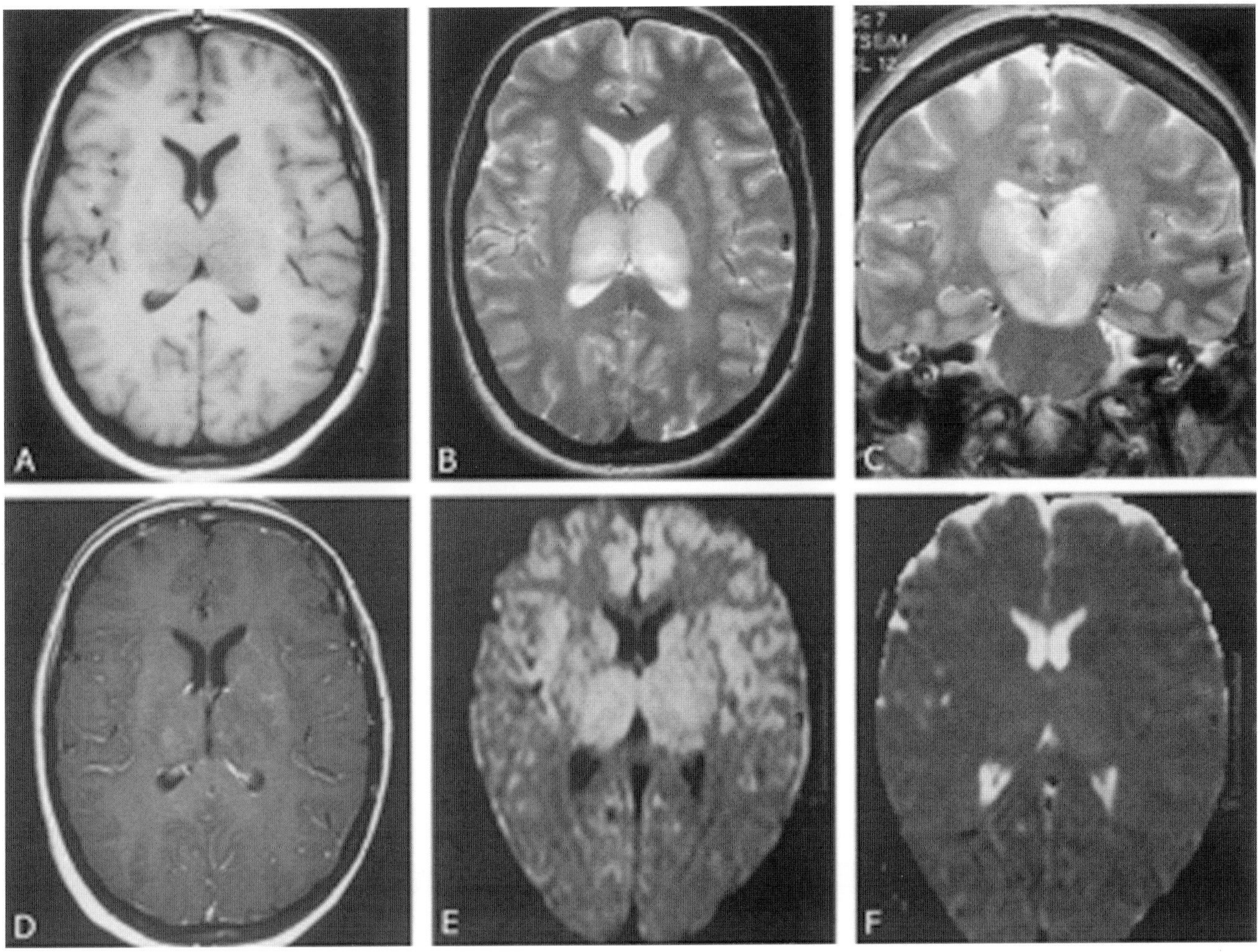

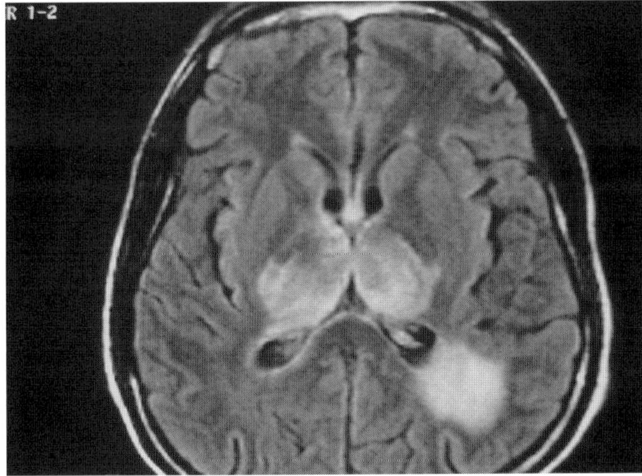

Fig. 6.31. **Top row, left to right – Axial T1, axial T2, coronal T2. Bottom row, left to right – post-contrast axial T1, DWI and ADC images. There is marked abnormal swelling and with T2 hyperintensity and T1 hypointensity of the bilateral thalami. There may be mild contrast enhancement. DWI and ADC images show some shine-through hyperintensity on the DWI images. Images are from figure 1 of Einsiedel, L., Kat, E., Ravindran, J.** *et al*. **MR findings in Murray Valley encephalitis.** *American Journal of Neuroradiology*. **Used with the kind permission of the ASNR.**

Fig. 6.32. **FLAIR axial MRI shows bilaterally symmetric thalamic hyperintensity and swelling in a case of possible HIV encephalitis of the thalami.**

Therefore, in "real life," we will have to reconcile ourselves to the fact that most cases of viral encephalitis involving the thalami will be non-specific and diagnosed by a combination of imaging, CSF profile and clinical presentation, without the isolation of a specific viral agent.

As a consolation, the cases above (as well as the preceding cases in this chapter), allow us to present the following differential for diffuse bilateral thalamic swelling with T2 hyperintensity:

(1) Deep cerebral vein thrombosis.
(2) Bilateral thalamic infarcts
   (a) Secondary to "top of the basilar" syndrome
   (b) Secondary to artery of Percheron infarcts
(3) Viral encephalitis
(4) Bilateral thalamic glioma

It would probably be reasonable to add anoxic–ischemic injury to this list, but the findings there are more likely to be in the basal ganglia than the thalamus.

Now, to end this discussion, here is a quiz case for you (Fig. 6.34). What do you think?

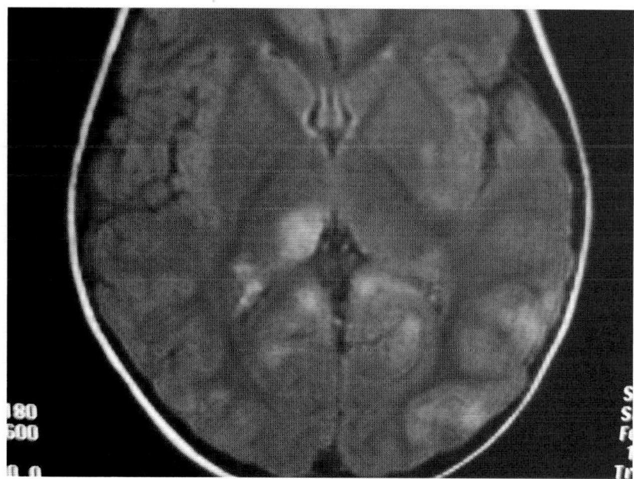

Fig. 6.33. **FLAIR axial image shows abnormal hyperintensity in the right thalamus, as well as multiple regions of gyriform cortical thickening and edema, consistent with viral encephalitis.**

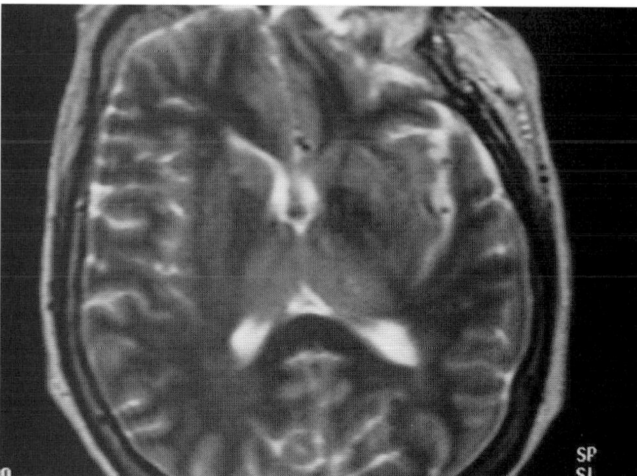

Fig. 6.34. **Axial T2-weighted image in a 35-year-old male, obtunded and confused. Image quality, once again, is degraded by patient motion. However, we see that there is subtle bilateral thalamic hyperintensity and swelling.**

Did you say viral encephalitis? If you did, I'm sorry to tell you that the patient had Wernicke's encephalopathy. Because you said non-specific viral encephalitis, the clinical team gave the patient supportive care, but did not think of administering thiamine. Unfortunately, the patient became acutely worse and died. In real life, the story played out differently and had a happy ending. But the moral of this frightening lesson is: please add Wernicke's to the above list!

References

Kalita, J. and Misra, U. K. Comparison of CT and MRI findings in the diagnosis of Japanese encephalitis. *Journal of Neurological Science* 2000; **174**: 3–8.

Petropoulou, K. A., Gordon, S. M., Prayson, R. A. *et al.* West Nile virus meningoencephalitis: MR imaging findings. *American Journal of Neuroradiology* 2005; **26**: 1986–1995.

Case 6.11

50-year-old male patient presents with headaches and vague visual complaints, including diplopia. Examination reveals no gross motor or sensory deficits. The patient, however, shows impairment of vertical gaze, more in the upgaze direction, as well as nystagmus with attempted convergence.

What are your thoughts on the possible location of the lesion?

The clinical description is consistent with Parinaud's syndrome, suggesting either a pineal lesion, or a lesion of the midbrain tectum.

Vertical gaze, as previously described in the midbrain chapter, is mediated through the rostral interstitial nuclei of the medial longitudinal fasciculus (riMLF), located above the oculomotor nuclei, as well as the interstitial nuclei of Cajal in the midbrain tectum. Therefore, pineal lesions pressing on the midbrain tectum frequently present with disturbances of vertical gaze, the main aspect of Parinaud's syndrome.

As a pointless historical aside (which most popular books seem to have), it is noted that Henri Parinaud was a French ophthalmologist who lived in the late 1800s. His name is also attached to another ophthalmologic syndrome, known as Parinaud's oculoglandular syndrome. This is a form of conjunctivitis caused by the bacteria *Bartonella henselae*, which is responsible for tularemia.

MRI examination of our patient, with a normal control for comparison, is presented (Fig. 6.35). What are the findings? What is your differential diagnosis?

Stereotactic biopsy revealed a pineocytoma. The pineal gland is the major component of the epithalamus, and hence part of the diencephalon. Therefore, this case provides a brief opportunity to review pineal region masses and make some observations about the physiologic role of the pineal gland.

Pineal region tumors account for approximately 1 percent of intracranial neoplasms, and are more common in children and young adults. Pineal region masses are most likely to be one of the following tumor categories, listed in descending order of frequency.

Germinomas

These arise from ectopic germ cell rests within the pineal gland, and are histologically identical to testicular seminomas. There is a significant male predilection (5–10: 1 male to female ratio). Germinomas are the most common pineal region tumor, accounting for approximately 50 percent of pineal masses. Making the diagnosis of germinoma is important as treatment with radiation therapy is very effective in tumor control.

Pineal parenchymal tumors

These account for 15–30 percent of pineal masses. There are two types of pineal parenchymal tumors.

Pineocytoma

This is usually a slow-growing tumor, considered to be a fairly benign neoplasm, originating from the pineocytes which make

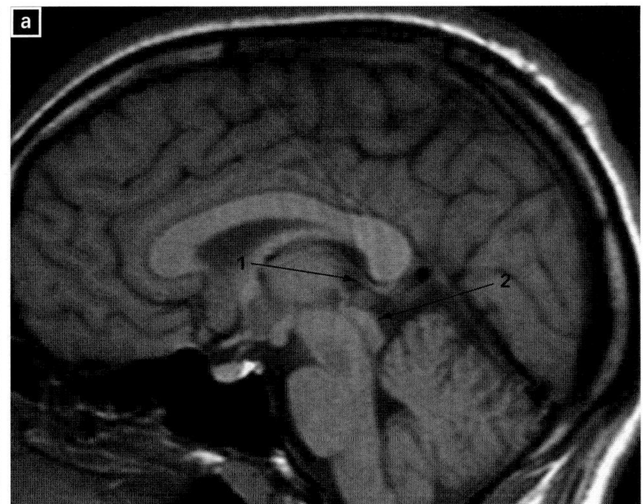

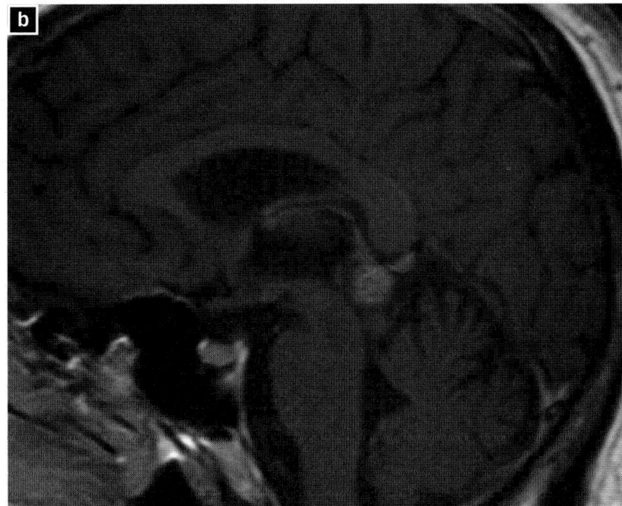

Fig. 6.35. **(a) Sagittal T1-weighted image of a normal control. The pineal gland is well seen (arrow 1) sitting above the tectal plate (arrow 2 shows the superior colliculus). (b) Sagittal post-contrast T1 weighted image of our patient. There is a small enhancing mass involving the pineal gland and impinging on the superior colliculus.**

up the pineal gland. Most pineocytomas have some degree of neuronal differentiation, hence making them fairly non-aggressive. However, the ones without neuronal differentiation are more aggressive and blend into the next tumor category.

Pineoblastoma

This is a malignant, poorly differentiated primitive neuroectodermal tumor, similar to medulloblastoma and neuroblastoma. Pineoblastoma tends to occur in younger patients, and has a very poor prognosis.

Pineal teratomas, another variety of germ cell tumor

This probably accounts for approximately 15 percent percent of pineal tumors.

Other germ cell tumors

These include choriocarcinoma, which may show an elevated beta human chorionic gonadotropin (hCG) in the blood and cerebrospinal fluid; endodermal sinus sinus or yolk sac tumor, which may show an elevated alpha-fetoprotein level; and embryonal cell carcinoma, a very rare intracranial tumor, often presenting with both elevated alpha-fetoprotein, and beta hCG.

Gliomas of the pineal gland, arising from glial cells within the pineal

The only one of these tumors which can be reliably differentiated from the others is pineal teratoma, due to the presence of the fat and cystic elements, as well as calcifications. The calcifications are usually not too helpful unless they are multiple and chunky, because the normal pineal gland is often calcified. It is important to note, though, that calcifications may normally be seen in 10 percent of 10-year-olds, and increase in frequency with age, but are not commonly seen in children under 10. Therefore, in a 7-year-old, pineal calcification would not usually be considered physiologic, and should raise concern for a teratoma.

The remaining tumors cannot be reliably differentiated from each other. Some general guidelines are that pineoblastomas tend to be more heterogeneous and poorly marginated than pineocytomas or germinomas. Also, some authors state that pineocytomas tend to "explode" the pineal calcifications because they are tumors of the pineal gland itself, whereas germinomas, which do not calcify, tend to displace the normal physiologic pineal calcification. Germinomas and pineoblastomas may show spread through the cerebrospinal fluid.

Discuss the physiologic function of the pineal gland.

The pineal gland can be considered an endocrine organ. Its main product is the hormone melatonin. Melatonin synthesis follows a circadian pattern, being secreted primarily during the dark portion of the day–night cycle. In lower vertebrates, the pineal gland is photosensitive, and melatonin secretion is directly suppressed by light. In higher mammals, including humans, the gland has lost direct photosensitivity, but responds to light through a complex set of neuronal relays.

As the nighttime becomes longer during the winter months, the period of secretion of melatonin during the dark cycle also increases. It is felt that this helps to regulate the estrus cycle in so-called photoperiodic mammals. Part of the regulation of the sexual cycle comes about because melatonin has antigonadotropic effects. With more melatonin, the estrus cycle is suppressed. With less melatonin, there is less antigonadotropic effect. Thus, many animals go "in heat" in the spring as the day begins to lengthen.

Along the same vein, there are sporadic case reports of pineal parenchymal tumors, with an excess secretion of melatonin, leading to hypogonadism and delayed puberty (see Walker *et al.*, 1996). Also, males with hypogonadotropic hypogonadism tend to have higher circulating melatonin levels than normal counterparts (Ozata *et al.*, 1996). These remain as general clinical observations about the antigonadotropic role of melatonin, without a fully detailed mechanism of the action and effect of melatonin known at present.

Conversely, pineal tumors are sometimes also associated with precocious puberty. One theory is that this occurs because tumors not of pineal parenchymal origin, such as germinomas, may destroy pineal cells and hence result in decreased melatonin levels, leading to an elimination of melatonin's antigonadotropic effect. It is more likely, however, that precocious puberty occurs secondary to ectopic production of hCG by choriocarcinomas, or possibly even by a small subgroup of germinomas with what are called syncytiotrophoblastic giant cells. Most germinomas, though, do not secrete beta hCG, and are not associated with precocious puberty. Choriocarcinomas, however, may be associated with precocious puberty in up to 5 percent of cases.

Lastly, it is becoming apparent that melatonin has multiple other roles in the human body. For example, it appears to be involved in immune function, with high levels promoting and low levels suppressing the immune response. Therefore, it may indeed be highly beneficial to get a good night's sleep when one is sick, or this may explain the propensity to get sick when traveling across time zones such that the melatonin circadian cycle is disrupted (and you thought it was the non-circulating air in the cockpit and the germ-laden airline pillows!). Melatonin receptors have, in fact, been detected in lymphoid tissue and on the surface of lymphocytes. Melatonin has even been shown to be a powerful antioxidant.

This case discussion would not be complete with at least a passing reference to Descartes' view regarding the pineal gland as the seat of the soul. This point is often quoted in neuroradioloy books for amusement. However, it was quite a serious matter to Descartes, who had a keen interest in anatomy and physiology, and linked his knowledge there to his philosophical theories. Descartes wrote most extensively about the pineal gland in his treatise, *The Passions of the Soul*. The following quote, however, in which he arrives at the function of the pineal gland using impeccable logic, is taken from some letters written a bit earlier:

> My view is that this gland is the principal seat of the soul, and the place in which all our thoughts are formed. The reason

I believe this is that I cannot find any part of the brain, except this, which is not double. Since we see only one thing with two eyes, and hear only one voice with two ears, and in short have never more than one thought at a time, it must necessarily be the case that the impressions which enter by the two eyes or by the two ears, and so on, unite with each other in some part of the body before being considered by the soul. Now it is impossible to find any such place in the whole head except this gland; moreover it is situated in the most suitable possible place for this purpose, in the middle of all the concavities; and it is supported and surrounded by the little branches of the carotid arteries which bring the spirits into the brain.

The interested reader may refer to Cottingham *et al.*, 1985/1991. This entire episode of the history of the pineal gland goes to show that impeccable logic can only get you so far. There needs to be clinical correlation! Thus far, there are no serious case reports of patients with pineal tumors having disruption of the soul, showing greater than average propensity to evil, or requiring exorcism. Therefore, on empirical grounds, the theory of Descartes must now be considered suspect.

References

Cottingham, J., Stoothoff, R., and Murdoch, D. *The Philosophical Writings of Descartes*, Cambridge University Press, 1985/1991.

Ozata, M., Bulur, M., Bingoi, N. *et al.* Daytime plasma melatonin levels in male hypogonadism. *Journal of Clinical Endocrinology and Metabolism* 1996; **81**(5): 1877–1881.

Walker, A. B., English, J., Arendt, J. *et al.* Hypogonadotrophic hypogonadism and primary amenorrhoea associated with increased melatonin secretion from a cystic pineal lesion. *Clinical Endocrinology* 1996; **45**: 353.

The hypothalamus and the pituitary

This section will briefly discuss the neuroanatomy of the hypothalamus, and to a lesser extent the pituitary gland. Since this is a book about neurology–neuroradiology correlations, the extent of this material is somewhat limited, as much of the clinical manifestations of hypothalamic and pituitary disorders are endocrine rather than neurologic. However, both the hypothalamus and the pituitary gland should be studied at least briefly, since the hypothalamus is part of the diencephalon and is, "pound for pound," one of the most important areas of the brain.

The hypothalamus is located along the anterior-inferior walls of the third ventricle, ventral to the thalamus. It is separated from the thalamus by a shallow groove in the walls of the third ventricle called the hypothalamic sulcus, which forms the dorsal boundary of the hypothalamus. Medially, the hypothalamus is delimited by the third ventricle, while its anterior border is the lamina terminalis. Along the ventral surface of the whole brain, the inferior margin of the hypothalamus can be seen directly behind the optic chiasm. An important landmark in the hypothalamus is the tuber cinerium, which literally means the "gray protuberance," a bulge located between the optic chiasm and the mammillary bodies. The infundibulum extends inferiorly from the region of the tuber cinerium down to the pituitary gland. The mammillary bodies are located along the posterior margin of the tuber cinerium and delineate its posterior extent (Fig. 6.36).

The hypothalamus, in general terms, is involved in the following sets of functions:

- *Autonomic*: it helps control brainstem and spinal cord autonomic centers.
- *Homeostatic*: it is involved in regulating appetite and eating, thirst and drinking, body temperature, sleep and circadian rhythms, and sexual behavior.
- *Endocrine*: it helps control the anterior and posterior pituitary.
- *Memory* and other limbic functions, including emotional behavior.

This global view of hypothalamic functions can be remembered using the clever mnemonic AHEM (autonomic, homeostatic, endocrine, memory), as in: "Ahem, ahem. Excuse me, but do you have a problem with your hypothalamus?"

This broad range of functions implies that the hypothalamus has a dizzying array of interconnections with the rest of the CNS, as well as multiple hypothalamic nuclei. Such is indeed the case, but we will try to limit detail to the minimum needed for clinical correlations. We will begin by first exploring some of the internal organization of the hypothalamus into different nuclei, and then explore some of the afferent and efferent network of connections that link the hypothalamus to the rest of the CNS. Finally, we will then discuss how the hypothalamus

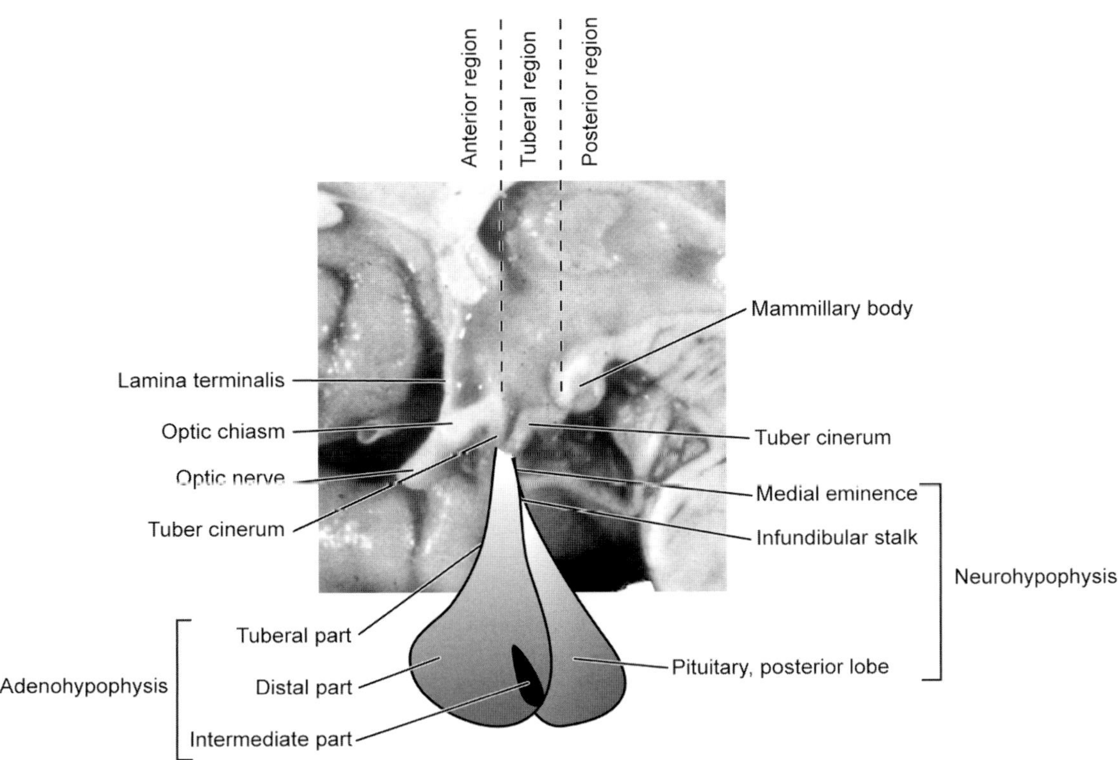

Fig. 6.36. **Midline brain section of the hypothalamus in relation to an anatomic diagram of the pituitary gland.**

participates in its AHEM functions and the clinical correlations to be expected with various hypothalamic lesions.

Internal organization of the hypothalamus

The hypothalamus is divided into medial and lateral portions by the fornix. The lateral region contains the lateral hypothalamic nucleus and a fiber tract known as the medial forebrain bundle, which links the basal forebrain, septal area and mibrain tegmentum to the hypothalamus. The medial portion of the hypothalamus contains multiple nuclei which are conventionally organized into four groups or regions (see Fig. 6.37).

Going from anterior to posterior, these are the:

Preoptic region
This contains the medial and lateral preoptic nuclei and the medial periventricular nucleus.

Anterior (or supraoptic) region
This contains the anterior hypothalamic nucleus, the paraventricular nucleus, the supraoptic nucleus and the suprachiasmatic nucleus.

Tuberal (or middle) region
This contains the ventromedial hypothalamic, dorsomedial hypothalamic, and arcuate nuclei.

Mammillary (or posterior) region
This contains the mammillary and posterior hypothalamic nuclei.

The hypothalamus is widely connected with the rest of the brain. Some of these connections are discussed briefly below:

Pituitary
The tubero-hypophysial (or tubero-infundibular) tract connects the hypothalamus to the anterior pituitary. The supraoptic-hypophysial tract connects the hypothalamus to the posterior pituitary. Both of these are one-way efferent tracts.

Hippocampal formation
Afferent and efferent fibers run in the fornix to connect the mammillary bodies to the hippocampal formations. The fornix is the major input to the mammillary bodies.

Amygdala
The amygdala is connected to the hypothalamus primarily through two pathways – the stria terminalis and the ventral amygdalofugal pathway. Some connections also run in the medial forebrain bundle. The stria terminalis connects the amygdala with the medial preoptic, anterior hypothalamic, ventromedial and arcuate nuclei of the hypothalamus. The amygdalofugal pathway connects the amygdala with the lateral hypothalamic nucleus. All of these tracts contain afferent and efferent fibers.

Thalamus
The major connection to the thalamus is the mammillothalamic tract, which contains afferent and efferent fibers linking the mammillary bodies with the anterior nucleus of the thalamus. For those who like eponyms, this is also known as the tract of Vicq d'Azyr. There is also an afferent tract called

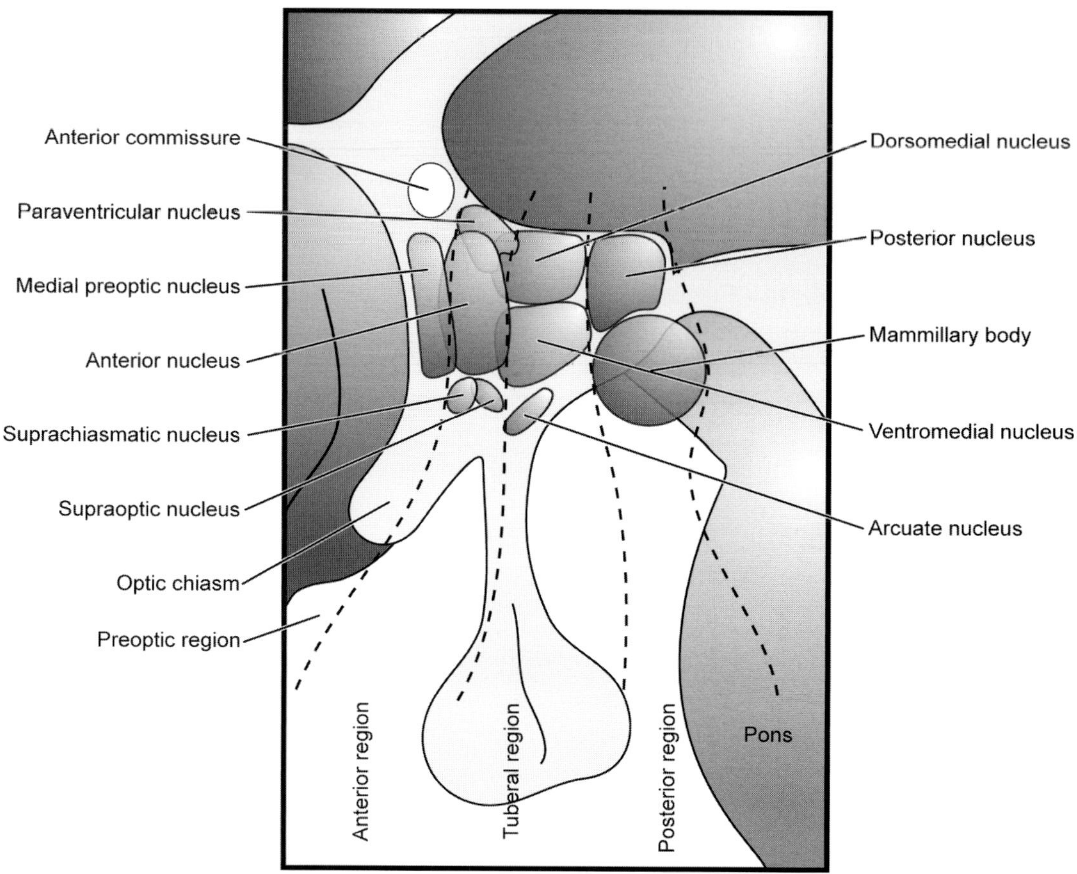

Fig. 6.37. **Medial hypothalamic nuclei divided into four zones from anterior to posterior: the preoptic area, the anterior (or supraoptic) region, the middle (or tuberal) region and the posterior (or mammillary) region. The specific hypothalamic nuclei are labeled.**

the thalamo-hypothalamic pathway which connects the dorsomedial and midline thalamic nuclei to the posterior and lateral portions of the hypothalamus.

Basal forebrain and prefrontal cortex

The medial forebrain bundle links the basal forebrain, including the olfactory cortex, the nucleus accumbens, the septal area, as well as areas of the prefrontal cortex, with the hypothalamus. The medial forebrain bundle also contains fibers back and forth to the hypothalamus from the brainstem reticular formation and the spinal cord.

Periaqueductal gray matter

The dorsal longitudinal fasciculus of Schutz carries afferent and efferent connections between the medial hypothalamus and the periaqueductal gray matter. Fibers linking the lateral hypothalamus to the periaqueductal gray matter run in the medial forebrain bundle.

Tegmental brainstem nuclei

Afferent fibers from the tegmental nuclei reach the mammillary bodies through a pathway called the inferior mammillary peduncle. Efferent fibers from the mammillary bodies to the brainstem tegmentum run in the mammillo-tegemental tract.

Autonomic nuclei

Efferent fibers leave the hypothalamus and connect with autonomic brainstem nuclei (dorsal motor nucleus of the vagus, nucleus solitarius, nucleus ambiguus). Also, preganglionic sympathetic fibers bound for sympathetic ganglia and the intermediolateral cell column of the spinal cord, and parasympathetic fibers bound for the sacral autonomic ganglia, run from the hypothalamus to the spinal cord. These pathways are collectively called descending autonomic fibers.

Retina

Afferent inputs come to the suprachiasmatic nucleus of the hypothalamus from the retina and optic chiasm via the retinohypothalamic pathway.

The complex internal structure of the hypothalamus and its vast network of connections function in the regulation of the four main areas as mentioned above. These will now be described in some more detail, along with some clinical correlates.

Endocrine

The hypothalamus is integral to the function of the anterior pituitary gland, and it synthesizes the hormones released

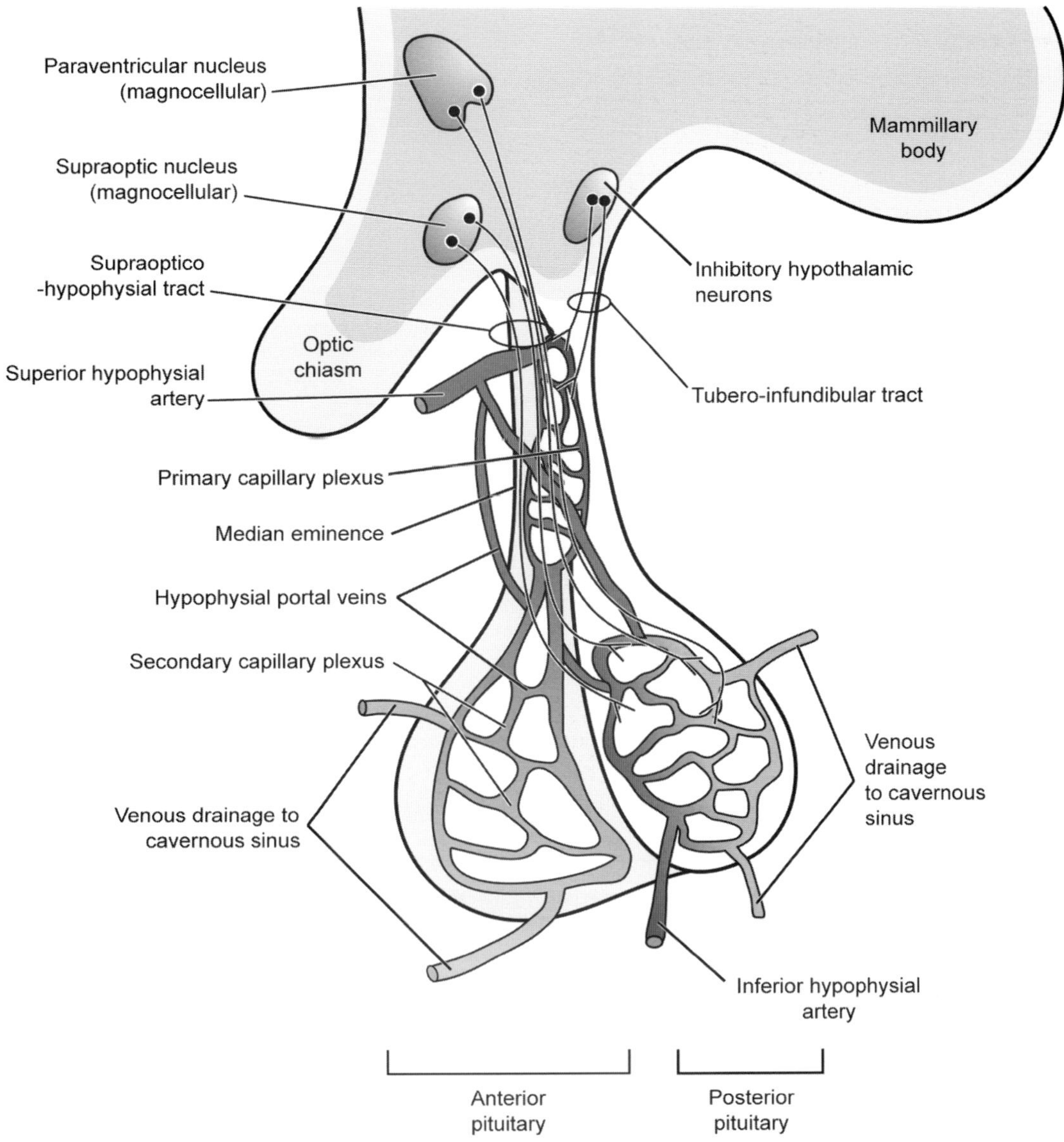

Fig. 6.38. **Hypothalamic regulation of the anterior and posterior pituitary. Hypothalamic neurons produce inhibitory and releasing factors into the median eminence (a capillary-rich zone). These factors are carried via the hypophysial portal veins to the anterior pituitary to modulate hormonal release. Hypothalamic neurons in the supraoptic and paraventricular nuclei release oxytocin and vasopressin into the posterior pituitary.**

by the posterior pituitary gland. The anterior and posterior portions of the pituitary gland have different embryological origins. The anterior pituitary, otherwise known as the adeno-hypophysis, arises from ectodermal cells along the roof of the embryologic pharynx which invaginate to form a structure called Rathke's pouch. The posterior pituitary, or neurohypophysis, extends inferiorly from the floor of the third ventricle, to meet Rathke's pouch. Together, the structures form the anterior and posterior lobes of the pituitary gland.

The hypothalamus is linked to the pituitary gland directly through the infundibulum, and indirectly through a regional set of vascular connections. The infundibulum has anterior and posterior portions, separated by the infundibular recess of the third ventricle. Along the anterior portion of the infundibulum, there is a slightly thickened area known as the median eminence.

The pituitary gland has a complex circulation pattern, which links it to the hypothalamus, and allows its endocrine products to enter the systemic circulation (Fig. 6.38).

The pituitary gland is supplied by the superior and inferior hypophyseal arteries, which are branches of the internal carotid artery. Internally, the pituitary gland has three main capillary plexi. The so-called primary capillary plexus is located in the median eminence, and is fed by the superior hypophyseal artery. It is in this location that the various hypothalamic neurons release their humoral factors to effect the release of pituitary hormones from the anterior pituitary gland (adenohypophysis). These humoral factors, usually known as the hypothalamic releasing factors (although some of them are inhibitory), are carried via hypophysial portal veins to the secondary capillary plexus in the anterior pituitary gland. In this location, most of these factors stimulate the cells of the pituitary gland to release various hormones, which are secreted into the secondary capillary plexus, and which go from there to the cavernous sinus, and then to the systemic circulation.

The anterior pituitary gland releases six hormones: adrenocorticotrophic hormone (ACTH), thyroid stimulating hormone (TSH), growth hormone (GH), prolactin, luteinizing hormone (LH) and follicle stimulating hormone (FSH). Each of these six hormones has a hypothalamic releasing factor to promote its release from the anterior pituitary. However, there are also three hormones which have hypothalamic inhibiting factors. TSH and GH are inhibited by a hypothalamic humoral factor called GIH (growth hormone inhibiting hormone). There is also a prolactin release-inhibiting factor, known as PIF, which turns out to be dopamine.

Thus, in summary, the hypothalamus exerts its control over the anterior pituitary as follows: hypopthalamic neurons project onto the median eminence, and release their humoral factors in the region of the primary capillary plexus. These are carried to the anterior pituitary via the hypophysial portal veins, and percolate through the secondary capillary plexus of the anterior pituitary gland, bathing the chromophil cells of the pituitary, and stimulating (or inhibiting) the release of pituitary hormones. The main hypothalamic nuclei projecting to the median eminence are the arcuate nucleus, the periventricular nucleus, the medial preoptic nucleus and portions of the paraventricular nucleus. Clinically, most of the problems related to the hormonal products of the anterior pituitary gland are not hypothalamic in origin. If there is an excess of hormonal activity, this is usually a result of pituitary microadenomas which secrete excess prolactin, ACTH, growth hormone, or rarely TSH, FSH and LH. Alternatively, pituitary insufficiency, or panhypopituitarism, occurs when the anterior pituitary cells are destroyed by tumors such as large non-functioning pituitary macroadenomas, or by hemorrhage or infection. However, hypothalamic tumors can also cause pituitary insufficiency by disruption of the hypothalamic releasing factors.

The posterior pituitary functions in a different fashion. It does not secrete hormones, but rather releases two hormones formed in the hypothalamus: oxytocin and vasopressin (also called antidiuretic hormone or ADH). The posterior pituitary gland contains a secondary capillary plexus similar to that of the anterior pituitary. Hypothalamic axons from the supraoptic and paraventricular nuclei travel through the posterior portion of the infundibular stalk (the supraoptic-hypophysial tract) and project directly onto the posterior pituitary. They then release oxytocin and vasopressin, which are stored in the cells of the posterior pituitary in the vicinity of the secondary capillary plexus. This plexus drains into the cavernous sinus, and thus carries these hormones into the systemic circulation as they are gradually released from the posterior pituitary. Some investigators state that the supraoptic nucleus secretes

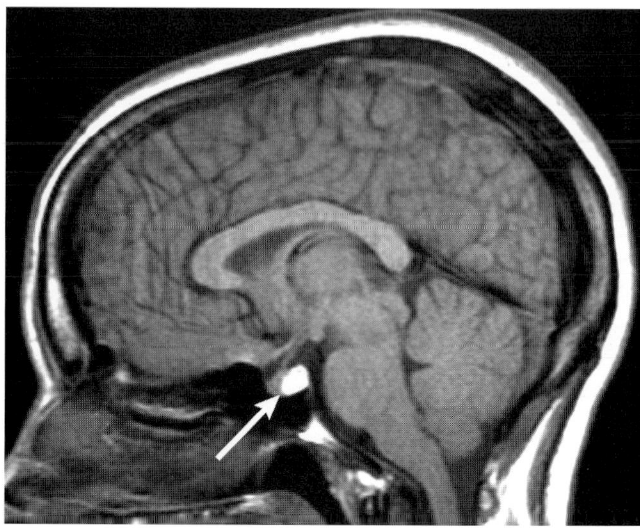

Fig. 6.39. **Sagittal T1-weighted non-contrast image showing the posterior pituitary bright spot (arrow). In this normal subject, it is more prominent than most.**

mainly ADH while the paraventricular nucleus secretes mainly oxytocin. An interesting imaging note is that while the normal anterior pituitary gland is isointense to brain on T1-weighted images, the posterior pituitary is normally hyperintense (see Fig. 6.39).

The cause of this T1-weighted hyperintensity remains a matter of some speculation. It may be secondary to carrier proteins called neurophysins located in neurosecretory granules in cells of the posterior pituitary. Alternatively, it may be secondary to intracellular lipids within pituicytes, or secondary to vasopressin itself. For those who would like to engage in this timeless debate, a couple of interesting sources are Arslan *et al.* (1999) and Lee *et al.* (2001).

In the paper by Lee *et al.* (2001) rabbits were deprived of water (for 7–9 days!) and the plasma concentration levels of vasopressin were assayed. With water deprivation and increases in plasma vasopressin (the vasopressin stored in the posterior pituitary presumably being released), there was a decrease in T1-weighted hyperintensity in the posterior pituitary. With water replenishment, there was a decrease in serum vasopressin (and presumably a build-up of stored vasopressin in the posterior pituitary), with a concomitant increase in T1 signal. Therefore, this paper suggests that the high T1 signal is due to the vasopressin secretory granules.

The important clinical correlate involving the hypothalamic-posterior pituitary axis is neurogenic (or central) diabetes insipidus, which results from a lack of vasopressin (ADH).

Autonomic

The hypothalamus, through its connections to the autonomic nervous system described above, is able to influence cardiovascular, gastrointestinal and respiratory functions. Once again, most of these autonomic influences are mediated by fibers carried in the dorsal longitudinal fasciculus and in the mammillotegmental tract. It is not possible to precisely delineate sympathetic and parasympathetic "centers" within the hypothalamus, as the integration of these functions appears to be too complex to be rigidly compartmentalized. However, in broad terms, the rostral and medial hypothalamus seems responsible for parasympathetic activation; stimulation of these regions, such as the preoptic and supraoptic areas, leads to a slowing of heart rate, decrease in blood pressure, increased GI motility and pupillary constriction. Conversely, the posterior and lateral portions of the hypothalamus (particularly the posterior) seem to be the source of sympathetic activation, causing the expected rise in heart rate, blood pressure, vasoconstriction, papillary dilation, etc. This autonomic regulation, of course, is integrated with the emotional functions of the hypothalamus and its links to the limbic system. Thus, when you are anxious, your heart pounds, you get "butterflies" in your stomach, and your palms begin to sweat. All of that is the hypothalamus!

Homeostasis

Appetite and eating

There appears to be a satiety center in the ventromedial nucleus of the hypothalamus. Therefore, bilateral lesions in this area lead to hyperphagia and obesity. How the hypothalamus regulates appetite is unclear. However, it is known that the hypothalamus contains receptors for the recently discovered hormone leptin. Leptin is considered to be a hormone with anti-obesity effects, helping to regulate food intake and metabolism. It binds to receptors in the arcuate nucleus of the hypothalamus. Recently, it has been shown that there are also important leptin binding sites in the ventromedial nucleus of the hypothalamus which, when blocked, lead to obesity in mice (Dhillon *et al.*, 2006). While these findings are in mice, they strongly support the notion that there is an important satiety center in the ventromedial hypothalamus, and are consistent with the fact that lesions in the ventromedial hypothalamic nuclei lead to hyperphagia and obesity. It is interesting to note that such lesions may also lead to rage reactions and aggressive behavior. This, of course, runs entirely counter to the "fat and jolly" stereotype.

An interesting clinical correlation to the role of the hypothalamus in feeding behavior and calorie balance is the Frohlich syndrome (also known as the Babinski–Frohlich syndrome). This results from damage to the tuberal regions of the hypothalamus, and is characterized by obesity, genital hypoplasia and growth retardation. The obesity is probably secondary to damage in the ventromedial nuclei, while the genital hypoplasia and growth retardation result from pituitary dysfunction secondary to interruption of the tuberohypophysial tract.

Whereas lesions in the ventromedial hypothalamus lead to hyperphagia and obesity, lesions in the lateral hypothalamus cause a decrease in appetite, with decreased food intake and weight loss. Some patients seem to entirely forget about eating, and have to be reminded to eat.

Calorie intake and weight regulation, though, are probably more complex than a simple balance between the satiety center in the ventromedial hypothalamus and the feeding center in the lateral hypothalamus. An example of this is a condition called the "diencephalic syndrome of infancy." This condition is characterized by progressive weight loss and emaciation during infancy, usually presenting as a failure to thrive. It is often caused by tumors of the anterior hypothalamus (usually low grade gliomas), and is sometimes accompanied by disorders of temperature regulation (for a nice series and discussion, see Poussaint *et al.*, 1997).

Thirst and drinking

Other than secretion of ADH, water regulation is influenced by the sensation of thirst and by drinking. Thirst seems to occur secondary to a rise in serum osmolality which stimulates osmoreceptors in the anterior and lateral hypothalamus. Animal studies show that drinking behavior occurs with stimulation of these regions despite overhydration. Conversely, lesions in this area abolish thirst and decrease water intake even in the face of dehydration.

Temperature regulation

This is a complex topic, as it involves such things as the metabolic rate, vasodilation or vasoconstriction of blood vessels near the skin, shivering, etc. The anterior hypothalamus appears to have thermoreceptors which respond to elevated body temperature and activate the various bodily mechanisms available for heat dissipation, such as sweating and vasodilation of surface vessels. Therefore, lesions of the anterior hypothalamus can cause hyperthermia. This sometimes occurs after surgery in this region or with head trauma. Some authors distinguish between sustained hyperthermia (associated with anterior hypothalamic lesions) and episodic hyperthermia which has been described with lesions of the ventromedial hypothalamus.

The posterior hypothalamus, by contrast, functions in heat conservation. Therefore, bilateral lesions in the posterior hypothalamus can cause either hypothermia or a condition called poikilothermia, where the body temperature fluctuates with the surroundings much like cold-blooded animals. An interesting clinical correlate in this regard is a condition called Shapiro's syndrome. This is a congenital condition characterized by episodic hypothermia along with episodic hyperhydrosis (excess sweating). These episodes can last from minutes to hours, and occur at various intervals. Shapiro's syndrome is often accompanied by agenesis of the corpus callosum, and may sometimes be associated with seizures. It is thought that the defect may be in the arcuate nucleus of the hypothalamus. Although this is an unusual syndrome, it has been reported several times in the literature and some authors suggest the possible use of clonidine as a treatment for the episodic hypothermia. There have also appeared in the literature reports of what is termed "reverse Shapiro's" syndrome, with agenesis of the corpus callosum, but episodic hyperthermia (see, for example, Hirayama *et al.*, 1994).

Circadian rhythms and sleep

The retinohypothalamic tract takes impulses from the retina to the suprachiasmatic nucleus of the hypothalamus, and this helps maintain the numerous circadian rhythms throughout the body. It has been known for some time that hypothalamic lesions can affect these circadian rhythms, and can also cause sleep disturbances. The precise etiology of the sleep disturbances is unclear, but it seems that there is a "waking center" in the posterior hypothalamus. Therefore, lesions of the posterior hypothalamus can cause hypersomnia. Interestingly, some authors state that anterior hypothalamic lesions may conversely cause insomnia. An interesting clinical correlate here is the Kleine–Levin syndrome. Patients with this rare syndrome, which typically affects teenage boys, display hyperphagia, hypersomnolence, and hypersexuality (according to some parents, this description would fit many of their teenage boys anyway!). This syndrome may occur with hypothalamic lesions as well as medial thalamic lesions.

Memory and other limbic functions

As we have described, the fornix represents the main input to the mamillary bodies in the posterior hypothalamus, carrying fibers from the hippocampal formations. Therefore, lesions of the hippocampi, fornices, or mammillary bodies can cause memory deficits, especially deficits in encoding new memories. Also, because of its connections with the limbic system, lesions of the hypothalamus may sometimes manifest with emotional disturbances. It is known, for example, that lesions of the ventromedial nucleus of the hypothalamus can produce a rage reaction, as mentioned above. Lesions of the posterior hypothalamus have been described to produce fear or apathy.

It is probably worthwhile to put these various clinical associations into tabular form to help with recall, and therefore the above material is summarized in Table 6.2.

In quickly referencing the table, we see for instance, that lesions of the posterior hypothalamus may make one sleepy, hypothermic, fearful and apathetic – a constellation sometimes found in junior residents.

Table 6.2. Hypothalamic anatomy: clinical correlates

Function	Disorder	Lesion location
Caloric intake	Hyperphagia (including Frohlich syndrome)	Satiety center, ventromedial nucleus
	Anorexia	Feeding center, lateral hypothalamus
	Diencephalic syndrome of infancy	Anterior hypothalamus
Thirst and drinking	Diabetes insipidus	Supraoptic and paraventricular nuclei, or infundibular stalk
Temperature regulation	Hypothermia	Posterior hypothalamus
	Hyperthermia	
	Sustained	Anterior hypothalamus
	Episodic	Ventromedial hypothalamus
Sleep	Hypersomnia	Waking center, posterior hypothalamus
	Insomnia	Anterior hypothalamus
Memory	Antegrade amnesia	Fornix, mammillary bodies
Limbic Functions	Rage	Ventromedial nucleus
	Fear and apathy	Posterior hypothalamus

References

Arslan, A., Karaarslan, E., and Dincer, A. High intensity signal of the posterior pituitary: a study with horizontal direction of frequency-encoding and fat suppression MR techniques. *Acta Radiologica* 1999; **40**(2): 142–145.

Dhillon, H., Zigman, J. M., Ye, C. *et al.* Leptin directly activates SF1 neurons in the VMH, and this action by leptin is required for normal body-weight homeostasis. *Neuron* 2006; **49**(2): 191–203.

Hirayama, K., Hoshino, Y., Kumashiro, H. *et al.* Reverse Shapiro's syndrome. A case of agenesis of corpus callosum associated with periodic hyperthermia. *Archives of Neurology* 1994; **51**(5): 494–496.

Lee, M. H., Choi, H. Y., Sung, Y. A., *et al.* High signal intensity of the posterior pituitary on T1-weighted images: correlation with plasma vasopressin concentration to water deprivation. *Acta Radiologica* 2001; **42**(2): 129–134.

Poussaint, T. Y., Barnes, P. D., Nichols, K. *et al.* Diencephalic syndrome: clinical findings and imaging features. *American Journal of Neuroradiology* 1997; **18**: 1499–1505.

Case 6.12

6-year-old boy presents with a 2-week history of increasing frequency of urination, as well as severe thirst. Over 24 hours, he urinated 5800 ml. His blood glucose was normal. His urine specific gravity was low at 1.008, urine osmolality was 111 mOsm/kg, and his serum osmolality was high at 292 mOsm/kg.

What do these findings suggest? What might be the cause?

The patient is presenting with polyuria and polydipsia, and is excreting a very dilute urine in the face of increased serum osmolality. These findings are consistent with diabetes insipidus.

Where you think the lesion could be? What are the different types of diabetes insipidus?

Diabetes insipidus is usually caused by a deficiency of vasopressin, otherwise known as antidiuretic hormone (ADH). ADH acts on the renal collecting tubules, causing them to resorb water. When it is absent or deficient, there is insufficient resorption of water, which is then excreted into the urine. The urine is therefore copious in amount (polyuria) and dilute. Because so much free water has been excreted, there is a rise in serum osmolality, leading to thirst and polydipsia.

As previously covered, ADH is formed in the supraoptic (and possibly paraventricular) nuclei of the hypothalamus, and transported via the supraoptic-hypophysial tract within the infundibulum to the posterior pituitary, where it is released. Therefore

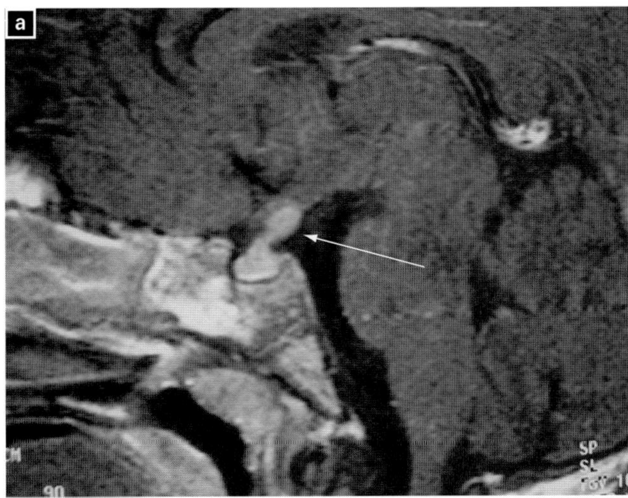
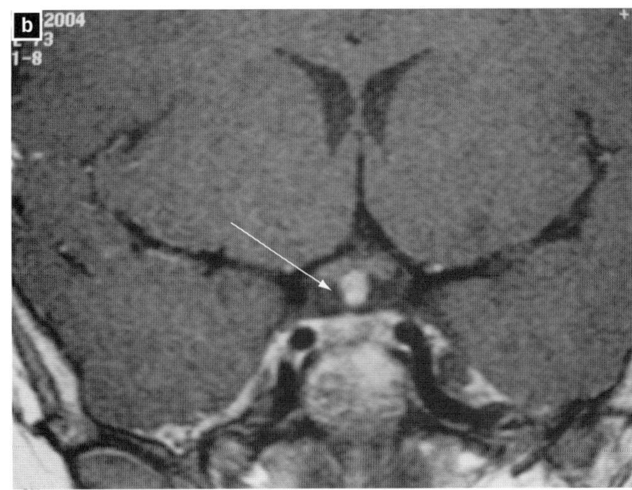

Fig. 6.40. **(a) Sagittal and (b) coronal post-contrast T1-weighted images of the pituitary gland.**

lesions of the ventral hypothalamus or of the infundibular stalk would interfere with this process, and produce diabetes insipidus. The scenario just described applies to what is called neurogenic (or central) diabetes insipidus, the most common type by far. It is also possible to have nephrogenic diabetes insipidus, where there is no deficiency of ADH, but there is development of insensitivity to ADH in the kidney. These two conditions can be distinguished from each other by subcutaneous administration of the synthetic vasopressin analogue, desmopressin or DDAVP. After such administration, patients with neurogenic diabetes insipidus show an increase in urine osmolality of greater than 50 percent in 1 hour, while those with nephrogenic diabetes insipidus do not show a siginificant rise.

Our patient showed a significant rise in urine osmolality to 380 mOsm/kg after administration of DDAVP, consistent with neurogenic diabetes insipidus.

MRI images are shown (Fig. 6.40). What are the findings? What is your differential?

The images show thickening and enhancement of the infundibular stalk (arrows) without a discrete mass. Differential diagnostic possibilities in children would be histiocytosis X (Langerhans cell histiocytosis) while in adults, sarcoid would be an excellent differential. In both age groups lymphocytic infiltration such as with lymphoma or leukemia are additional possibilities. Also, granulomatous diseases such as tuberculosis may cause this pattern, as may lymphocytic hypophysitis. Of course, neurogenic diabetes insipidus may also be caused by perisellar tumors such as germinoma, meningioma, glioma or metastatic disease, and by trauma which may lead to transection of the infundibular stalk.

Diagnosis

Langerhans cell histiocytosis. This disease has gone by many names, but they all refer to idiopathic infiltration of monocytes, macrophages and dendritic (Langerhans) cells in various areas of the body, causing damage through an inflammatory immune-mediated cascade. Originally, the disease was called histiocytosis X, and was subdivided into three separate entities based on severity of disease, with the mildest form called eosinophilic granuloma, a moderate form called Hand–Schuller–Christian disease and a severe early onset form called Letterer–Siwe disease. Recently, it has been found that these are all part of the same disease spectrum, now called Langerhans cell histiocytosis. The disease may be isolated to bones, such as the long bones or the skull, or may involve various organs, including skin, lymph nodes and the central nervous system. The CNS is involved in 15–25 percent of cases, and our patient's presentation is the typical one, with diabetes insipidus being the most common presentation of CNS Langerhans cell histiocytosis. Sometimes, hypothalamic involvement also leads to growth retardation and short stature.

The diagnosis may be presumptively made by imaging, and confirmed, if need be, by biopsy. To help you in conferring with the pathologists, it is good to know that Langerhans cells are moderately large homogeneous cells with a granular cytoplasm on H&E stains. The definitive diagnosis, however, rests on demonstrating so called Birbeck granules within the cytoplasm on electron microscopy, and demonstrating that the cells are positive for CD1 cell-surface markers (CD1 refers to a class of molecules that are found on the surface of dendritic cells and monocytes and function in the presentation of antigens to the immune system).

Case 6.13

41-year-old male who presents with a 1-year history of personality change and hyperphagia. The patient has shown gradually declining memory, and apathy with emotional lability manifest by bursts of anger. The patient lost his job 2 months prior to presentation. Also, the patient's eating habits have changed dramatically. He now eats voraciously, and has gained approximately 100 pounds in the last 10 months.

The constellation of findings, especially the development of aggressive hyperphagia, suggest the hypothalamus as a possible culprit for the patient's condition. As we have discussed, ventromedial hypothalamic lesions can cause both hyperphagia and rage reactions.

An MRI of the brain was obtained (Fig. 6.41). What are the findings? What is your differential diagnosis?

The MRI shows marked abnormal leptomeningeal and parenchymal enhancement along the ventral brain surface, especially along the hypothalamus. In the differential diagnosis would be sarcoidosis, basilar meningitis secondary to tuberculosis or fungal

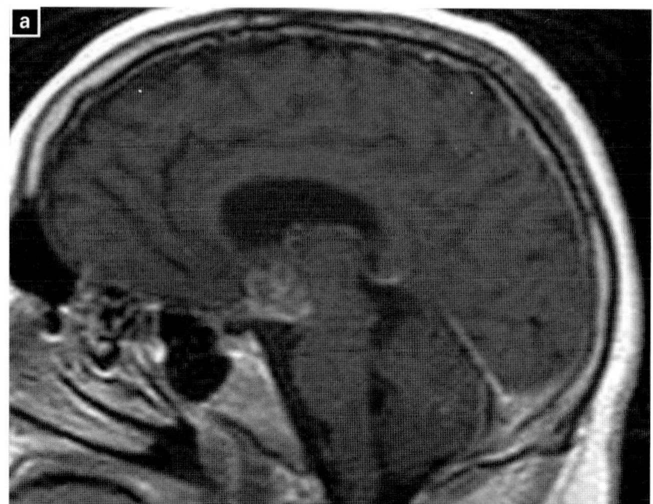
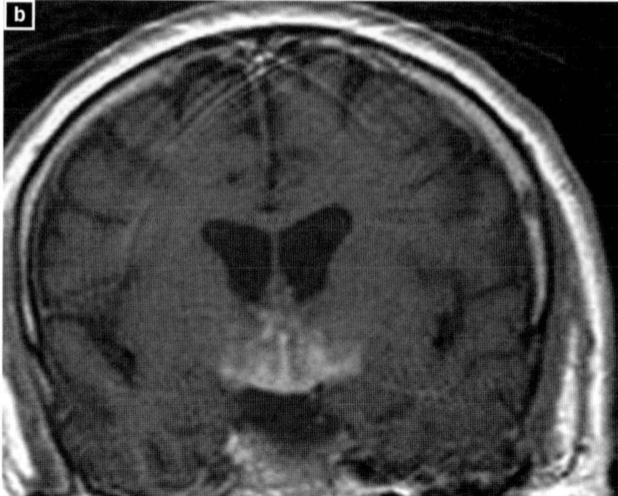

Fig. 6.41. **(a) T1-weighted sagittal and (b) coronal post-contrast MRI images.**

disease, lymphoma or acute lymphocytic leukemia, and leptomeningeal carcinomatosis. The patient had no relevant history of any of these diseases.

A thorough workup was undertaken, ending with the biopsy of a skin plaque which revealed non-caseating epithelioid granulomas.

Diagnosis

Neurosarcoidosis.

Sarcoidosis is an idiopathic disease characterized by the presence of non-caseating epithelioid granulomas. It may involve multiple organ systems, including the eyes, lungs, skin and lymph nodes. Clinical neurologic involvement occurs in about 5 percent of patients, with autopsy series showing involvement of the CNS in 14–27 percent of cases, suggesting a significant prevalence of subclinical disease. An interesting case series exploring the imaging and clinical findings in neurosarcoidosis is that of Christoforidis *et al.*, 1999. This series, using rigorous criteria to define neurosarcoidosis, found evidence of CNS involvement in 8.3 percent of 461 sarcoidosis patients. Of the population with neurosarcoidosis, 63 percent had neurologic symptoms as their first manifestation (this is about 5 percent of the total patient population in this study). Eleven percent of the neurosarcoidosis group (about 1 percent of the total patient population) had disease confined to the CNS.

The imaging manifestations of neurosarcoidosis are quite variable, and can be divided into six broad categories: (1) dural thickening or mass, (2) leptomeningeal involvement, (3) enhancing brain parenchymal lesions, (4) non-enhancing brain parenchymal lesions, (5) cranial nerve involvement, and (6) spinal cord and root involvement. All categories were well represented in the above case series, with cranial nerve involvement being a slightly more common finding. The most commonly involved cranial nerves are the optic nerves/optic chiasm and the seventh cranial nerves.

In our patient, marked involvement of the hypothalamus presented as hyperphagia, mood disturbances, personality changes and memory loss/dementia. This constellation of findings is quite consistent with the neuroanatomy of the hypothalamus, and has in fact been reported several times before in association with neurosarcoidosis (Vanhoof *et al.*, 1992; Sommer *et al.*, 1991; Martin and Riskind, 1992).

That hypothalamic lesions can cause hyperphagia and obesity is thus well-documented. Less clear is the mechanism by which they do so. Some data suggests that rats with ventromedial hypothalamic lesions show increased insulin secretion in response to glucose, promoting storage of the food energy in the form of adipose tissue. This occurs even during calorie restriction. The same mechanism seems to operate in humans, and there have been trials of treating patients with octreotide, a somatostatin agonist which suppresses insulin release at the beta cell level. These trials have shown some success in insulin suppression and weight loss (see Lustig, 2002). Thus, when people complain that they are getting fat despite dieting, they may be onto something!

It is interesting to note that nearly the opposite clinical presentation – cachexia – has also been associated with hypothalamic lesions, usually tumors. This was briefly mentioned above as the "diencephalic syndrome of infancy." This is also known as Russell's syndrome, after the doctor who initially described the association of cachexia with preserved linear growth, hyperactivity, and hypothalamic tumors. It has been described several times since. Two case series that offer a good discussion are Burr *et al.* (1976) and Fleischman *et al.* (2005).

References

Burr, I. M., Slonim, A. E., Danish, R. K., *et al.* Diencephalic syndrome revisited. *Journal of Pediatrics* 1976; **88**: 439–444.

Christoforidis, G. A., Spickler, E. M., Recio, M. V. *et al.* MR of CNS sarcoidosis: correlation of imaging features to clinical symptoms and response to treatment. *American Journal of Neuroradiology* 1999; **20**: 655–669.

Fleischman, A., Brue, C., Poussaint, T. Y., *et al.* Diencephalic syndrome: a cause of failure to thrive and a model of partial growth hormone resistance. *Pediatrics* 2005; **115**(6): e742–748.

Lustig, R. Hypothalamic obesity: the sixth cranial endocrinopathy. *Endocrinologist* 2002; **12**(3): 210–217.

Martin, J. B. and Riskind, P. N. Neurologic manifestations of hypothalamic disease. *Progress in Brain Research* 1992; **93**: 31–40.

Sommer, N., Weller, M., Petersen, D. *et al.* Neurosarcoidosis without systemic sarcoidosis. *European Archives of Psychiatry and Clinical Neuroscience* 1991; **240**(6): 334–338.

Vanhoof, J., Wilms, G., and Bouillon R. [Hypothalamic hypopituitarism with hyperphagia and subacute dementia due to neurosarcoidosis: case report and literature review.] *Acta Clinica Belgica* 1992; **47**(5): 319–328.

Case 6.14

6-year-old male presents with precocious puberty.

An MRI scan is presented (Fig. 6.42). What are the findings? What is your diagnosis?

The MRI examination shows a pedunculated mass (arrow) arising from the undersurface of the hypothalamus, in the region of the tuber cinerium. The mass is slightly hypointense on T1 and hyperintense on FLAIR. Post-contrast images (not shown) revealed no enhancement. Given its location, the diagnosis of hamartoma of the tuber cinerium was felt to be the most likely diagnostic possibility. However, biopsy revealed a low grade hypothalamic glioma.

Diagnosis

Hypothalamic glioma with precocious puberty.

The endocrinologic workup of precocious puberty is beyond our scope. However, in broad terms, it is divided into two major types: central precocious puberty and pseudoprecocious puberty. Central precocious puberty is secondary to premature activation (or failure of the normal prepubertal suppression) of the hypothalamic gonadotropin-releasing hormone (GnRH) pulse generator. This stimulates the pituitary gonadotropin-gonadal axis, and sets in motion the events of puberty at too early an age. It is identified by a pattern of response of LH to a GnRH stimulation challenge similar to that seen in normal puberty. This form of precocious puberty is also called GnRH-dependent precocious puberty. It may be idiopathic in etiology, or secondary to a variety of CNS processes. Most common among these are hypothalamic lesions, particularly hamartomas of the tuber cinerium. However, hypothalamic gliomas have been reported as a possible cause as well. Both boys and girls may develop precocious puberty secondary to such hypothalamic lesions. Head trauma and CNS infections, especially with basilar meningitis, are also reported causes. How precisely hypothalamic hamartomas or gliomas cause precocious puberty is unclear. In the opinion of some, these tumors actually secrete substances which stimulate the GnRH pulse generator, which should normally be dormant in the pre-pubertal phase (see Rivarola *et al.*, 2001).

Pseudoprecocious puberty, also called GnRH-independent precocious puberty, is due to sex hormone production outside the control of the GnRH pulse generator, and it may be due to gonadal or adrenal tumors. In boys, it may also be secondary to tumors which secrete hCG or LH. In our discussion of pineal germ cell tumors, we mentioned the syndrome of precocious puberty secondary to increased hCG production. This sort of precocious puberty is part of the pseudoprecocious puberty syndrome. Interestingly, girls do not typically get precocious puberty with pineal germ cell tumors that secrete hCG because the ovaries need a balance of both LH and FSH to be stimulated.

For our purposes, it is sufficient to note that children with central precocious puberty should be worked up with MRI, with special attention to the hypothalamus.

A last question to be asked before leaving this case is the frequency of endocrinologic abnormalities in patients similar to ours. While the mechanism of endocrine abnormalities with hypothalamic gliomas is somewhat understandable, the frequency of such abnormalities is a much more difficult question to answer. Surprisingly, it seems that only about 20 percent of patients with "opitco-hypothalamic" gliomas present with endocrine abnormalities. The majority present with visual disturbances and headache, without obvious endocrine dysfunction, even with pituitary stimulation testing (Martinez *et al.*, 2003). These statistics, it must be stressed, apply only to gliomas, and the authors of the above paper suggest in their conclusions that the relative paucity of endocrine deficiencies in optico-hypothalamic gliomas, despite their often large size, can be used to help distinguish gliomas from other suprasellar lesions.

In unusual cases, other somatic manifestations may occur, such as hypersomnolence. In the case in Fig. 6.43, a 48-year-old male presented with an aggressive optic chiasm glioma, which over time invaded the hypothalamus. The patient gradually developed hypersomnolence, such that at the time of this writing, he was sleeping approximately 20 hours per day.

Such sleep disturbances as a manifestation of hypothalamic tumors has been previously reported (Rosen *et al.*, 2002).

References

Martinez, R., Honegger, J., Fahlbusch, R. *et al.* Endocrine findings in patients with optico-hypothalamic gliomas. *Experimental Clinical Endocrinolology and Diabetes* 2003; **111**(3): 162–167.

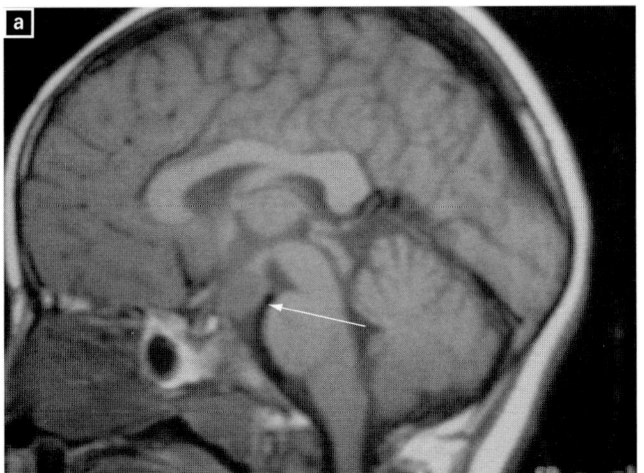
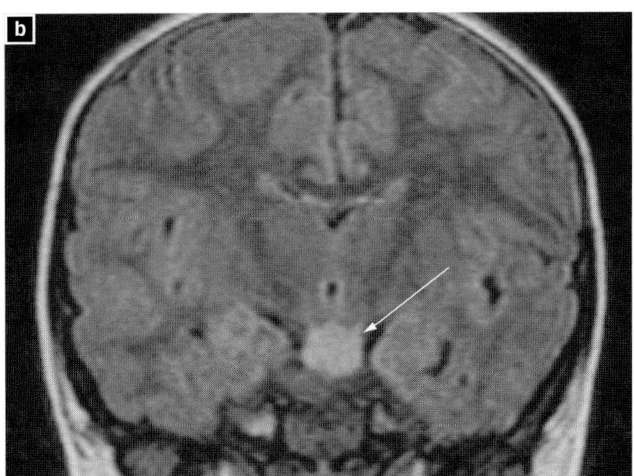

Fig. 6.42. **(a) Sagittal pre-contrast T1-weighted and (b) coronal FLAIR images are presented.**

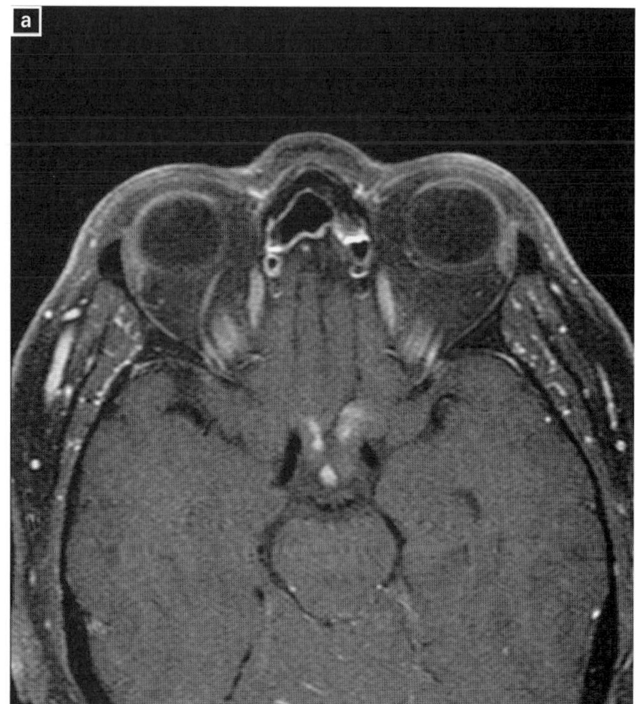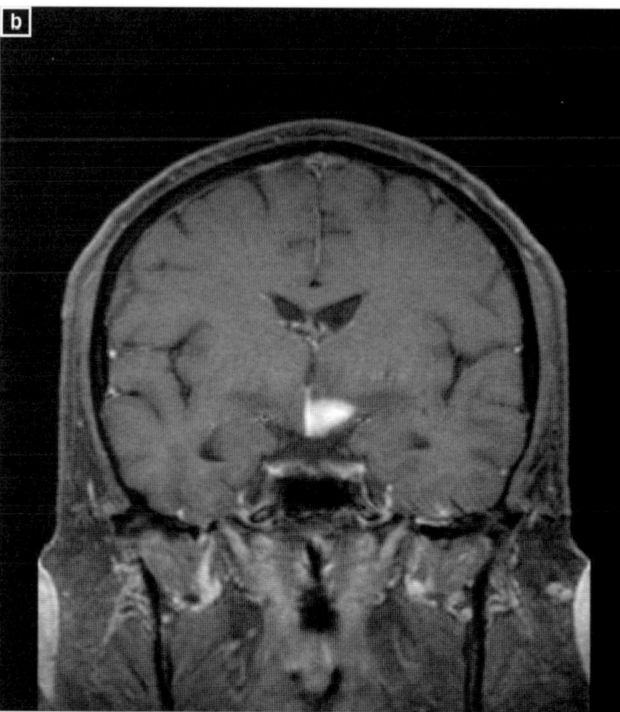

Fig. 6.43. **(a) Post-contrast fat-saturation T1-weighted axial images of the orbits at the time of presentation. There is thickening of the optic chiasm and both pre-chiasmatic optic nerves, left greater than right, with only mild enhancement. The patient had only visual symptoms at this time. (b) Coronal T1-weighted post-contrast image obtained 8 months later shows tumor invasion of the hypothalamus (more on the left) with marked enhancement. The patient now has profound hypersomnolence.**

Rivarola, M. A., Belgorosky, A., Mendilaharzu, H. *et al*. Precocious puberty in children with tumours of the suprasellar and pineal areas: organic central precocious puberty. *Acta Paediatrica* 2001; **90**(7): 751–6.

Rosen, G. M., Anne, E., Bendel, A. E. *et al*. Sleep in children with neoplasms of the central nervous system: case review of 14 children. *Pediatrics* 2002; **112**(1): e46–e54.

Case 6.15

33-year-old female patient presents with 6-month history of amenorrhea and galactorrhea. Upon further questioning, the patient also complains of weight gain and decreased libido. Neurologic testing was unremarkable.

What lab test would you like to order?

The combination of galactorrhea and amenorrhea should immediately make us think of elevated prolactin levels. Therefore, a prolactin level is ordered, and returns with a value of 160 ng/ml. It is important to have some idea of normal prolactin levels, which are either measured as ng/ml or as mg/L (these are equivalent units, the latter obtained from the former by multiplying numerator and denominator by 1000). Normal levels should roughly be less than 25 ng/ml. Once the levels have risen above 100–150 ng/ml, there is high suspicion for a prolactinoma. This is a functioning adenoma of the pituitary gland (usually a microadenoma, i.e., measuring less than 10 mm) which secretes excess prolactin. Before proceeding to an MRI of the pituitary gland, it is important to comment on mild elevations of prolactin. While these may still be secondary to a very small microadenoma (a micro microadenoma, if you will), they are often secondary to other causes. In fact, only about one-third of women with elevated prolactin levels have a prolactinoma, but the higher the prolactin level, the higher the odds. Once prolactin reaches the 150–200 ng/ml level, this is virtually diagnostic for a prolactinoma. For those of us who do neuroimaging, the following

scenario is all too common: an MR comes through, and the request states, "Elevated prolactin. Rule out prolactinoma." Naturally, the prolactin level is never given (radiologists have no business knowing such things). After struggling with the laboratory menu on the computer, we eventually unearth the prolactin level, and it is something like 32 ng/ml. At this point, we shake our heads and begin teaching the residents about what else may elevate prolactin levels. It turns out that there is quite a long list: food, chest wall lesions such as herpes zoster or trauma, sleep deprivation, stress, and medications. Therefore, the first thing to do with such mild hyperprolactinemia is to repeat the prolactin levels while the patient is fasting and to review the patient's medications. Among the medications which elevate prolactin are neuroleptic drugs such as antipsychotics or other psychotropic drugs, including monoamine oxidase inhibitors, amitriptyline, chlorpromazine, and haldol. Also, cimetidine and opiates may produce elevated prolactin.

Our review of the hypothalamus helps us to understand how at least some of these drugs elevate prolactin. As you recall, PIF, or prolactin inhibiting factor, is secreted by the hypothalamus to suppress release of prolactin from the pituitary. As you also recall, PIF is none other than dopamine. Therefore, dopamine antagonists will cause increased prolactin by disinhibiting the prolactin-secreting pituicytes. We are also in a position to understand how

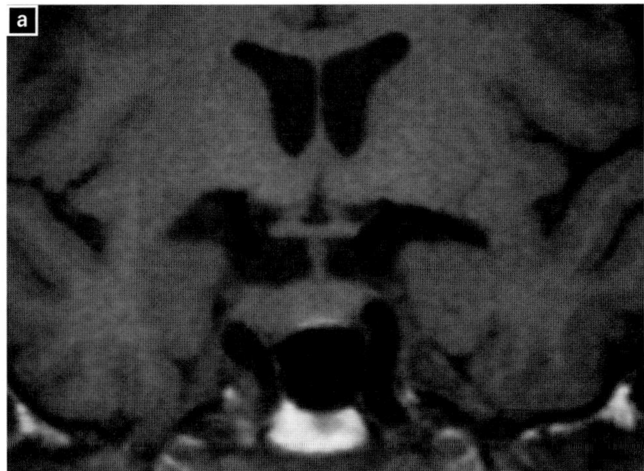
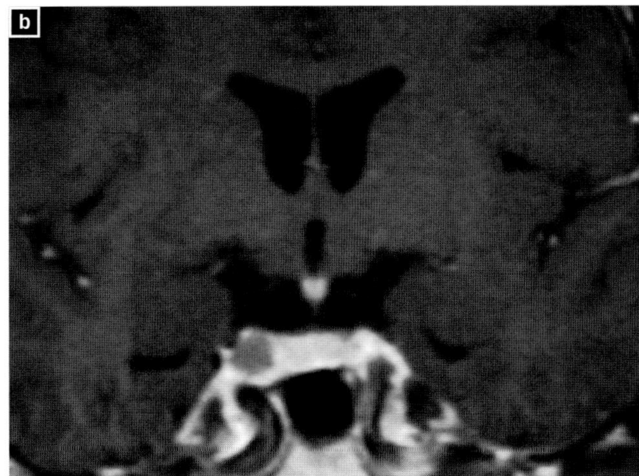

Fig. 6.44. **(a) Pre-contrast and (b) post-contrast T1-weighted thin slice coronal images through the pituitary gland.**

prolactinomas are treated. As opposed to other pituitary tumors, prolactinomas can often be successfully treated using medications rather than surgery. Based on the little bit of endocrinology above, we can now understand why the leading medications for treating prolactinomas are dopamine agonists, such as bromocriptine or cabergoline. These inhibit prolactin release and cause a shrinkage of the tumor. Also, we can understand a bit about how prolactinomas produce their symptoms. Prolactin, of course, directly stimulates lactation, producing galactorrhea. It seems that elevated prolactin levels, through a feedback loop, also decrease hypothalamic LHRH, which functions as the releasing hormone for LH and FSH. This produces amenorrhea. It is this same mechanism which delays the resumption of the menstrual cycle after childbirth during breast feeding. The decreased LH and FSH also lead to loss of libido.

Finally, a clinical pearl: in rare cases, patients may have markedly elevated prolactin levels without a prolactinoma or other contributory history such as medication-induced hyperprolactinemia. In such patients, it is important to know that there have been reports of other tumors outside the CNS leading to elevated prolactin. Such an association has sometimes been reported with cancer of the lung, kidney, thyroid, and breast, as well as multiple reports with colorectal cancer (see, for example, Bhatavdekar *et al.*, 2001). Therefore, such patients may benefit from a general cancer screening.

After this detour, we return to the evaluation of our patient. An MRI is provided (Fig. 6.44). What are the findings? What is your diagnosis?

There is a slightly hypointense lesion in the right lateral aspect of the pituitary gland, which stands out as an area of hypoenhancement after contrast. This appearance is consistent with a microadenoma, and in this case, highly consistent with a

prolactinoma. Usually, we give contrast to make tumors enhance against the background of the normal brain; not so with prolactinomas. Typically, the microadenoma will enhance less than the normal pituitary, and hence appear hypointense after contrast, opposite to the usual pattern we are used to. That is because the pituitary gland lacks a blood–brain barrier, and so enhances avidly (if it had a blood–brain barrier, it couldn't secrete its hormones into the bloodstream).

The definition of a microadenoma is an adenoma which is less than 10 mm in diameter. Anything bigger is called a macroadenoma. Overall, about 75 percent of pituitary adenomas are hormonally active. These tumors often come to attention as microadenomas, as the patient will have endocrine abnormalities that will force him or her to seek medical attention. Conversely, the non-functioning adenomas usually come to attention as macroadenomas, since they become symptomatic because of size and local mass effect rather than hormonal activities. Of the functioning pituitary adenomas, prolactinomas are by far the most common, accounting for about 50 percent of the total. In second place are growth hormone secreting adenomas, which can lead to gigantism or acromaegally, followed by ACTH secreting tumors, which lead to Cushing's disease. Adenomas which secrete TSH, LH or FSH have been reported as well, but these are quite rare.

Reference

Bhatavdekar, J. M., Patel, D. D., Chikhlikar, P. R., *et al.* Ectopic production of prolactin by colorectal adenocarcinoma. *Diseases of the Colon and Rectum* 2001; **44**(1): 119–127.

Case 6.16

63-year-old male presenting with several somatic complaints including a 2–3-week history of headaches, decreased libido, impotence, fatigue, and diminished appetite. The patient also reported blurring of vision, which he feels is now improved. No focal neurological signs were present on examination. Several laboratory studies were ordered, and some relevant abnormal values were: Testosterone 30 ng/dL (normal is greater than 300), Cortisol (AM) 2.2 ug/dL (normal 5–25 ug/dL), and Thyroxine 2.7 ug/dL (normal 4–12 ug/dL).

What are your thoughts on the patient's condition? What other tests would you like?

The patient has low testosterone, thyroxine and serum cortisol. These deficiencies point to the pituitary gland, and suggest the diagnosis of panhypopituitarism. Therefore, an MRI of the pituitary gland is warranted at this point.

MRI is presented below (Fig. 6.45). What are the findings? What is your diagnosis?

The pre-contrast MRI scan shows an enlarged pituitary gland with abnormal T1-weighted hyperintensity, with some mild expansion of the sella. The T1-weighted hyperintensity is consistent with subacute hemorrhage, with blood in the methemoglobin phase. Hemorrhage within an enlarged pituitary gland plus the signs and symptoms of pituitary insufficiency strongly suggest the diagnosis of pituitary apoplexy. Follow-up images obtained several weeks later (not shown) demonstrated resolution of hemorrhage and shrinkage of the pituitary gland.

The term pituitary apoplexy is somewhat vague, as it is used to refer to several different related conditions. The most comprehensive definition is that it represents either hemorrhage or infarction of the pituitary gland. The infarction may be bland, without a hemorrhagic component. Pituitary apoplexy, in the vast majority of cases, occurs in the setting of a pre-existing pituitary adenoma, which then either infarcts or bleeds into itself. However, it can also

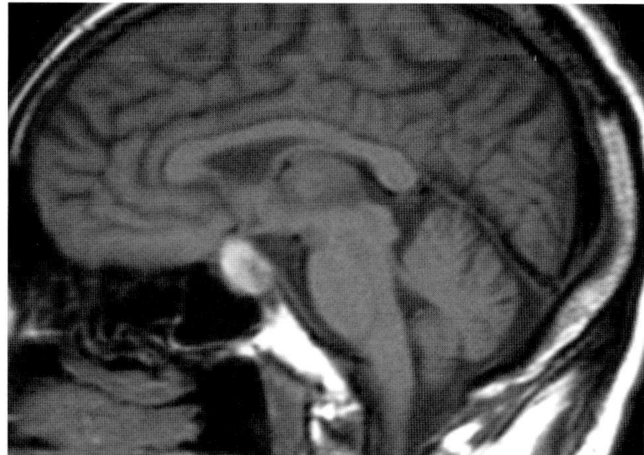

Fig. 6.45. **Sagittal T1-weighted pre-contrast MRI of the pituitary gland.**

occur without an adenoma being present, although this is much less common. There is some confusion as to whether to use the term "pituitary apoplexy" as a pathologic diagnosis or as a clinical one. Various series have revealed that necrosis or hemorrhage within a pituitary adenoma may occur 10–20 percent of the time. In most of these cases, the patients are asymptomatic with respect to the hemorrhage. However, in a small fraction of cases, probably under 1 percent, the patients manifest clinical symptoms. These symptoms may be abrupt, with headache, visual disturbances and altered mental status, or may be more gradual, as in our patient, manifesting with hypopituitarism. The imaging findings depend on whether there is pituitary infarction or hemorrhage. With hemorrhage, if it is imaged in the acute phase, there will be isointensity on T1 and hypointensity on T2. In the subacute phase (considered to be after about 3 days), the hemorrhage becomes hyperintense on T1-weighted images. With infarction, the enlarged gland is isointense on T1-weighted images, but post-contrast shows only rim enhancement. The finding of rim enhancement of an enlarged gland (without internal enhancement, as would be expected in a macroadenoma) has been suggested as a highly suggestive finding of pituitary infarct (Fig. 6.46).

Interestingly, diffusion weighted imaging may be quite useful in the diagnosis of pituitary apoplexy secondary to bland pituitary infarct, with the gland showing diffusion-weighted hyperintensity in cases of infarction (Rogg et al., 2002).

The hypopituitarism which may accompany pituitary apoplexy tends to manifest as a deficiency of the hormones of the anterior pituitary. While diabetes insipidus may occur, it is distinctly less common. The reason for the anterior pituitary's increased susceptibility to apoplexy is thought to be secondary to its unique blood supply (see Fig. 6.38). The posterior pituitary is supplied directly by the inferior hypophysial artery, a branch of the meningohypophysial trunk which arises from the cavernous portion of the internal carotid artery. Thus, with cerebral angiography, an immediate posterior pituitary "blush" is typically seen. The anterior pituitary gland, though, is supplied indirectly. As discussed previously, superior hypophysial arterial branches

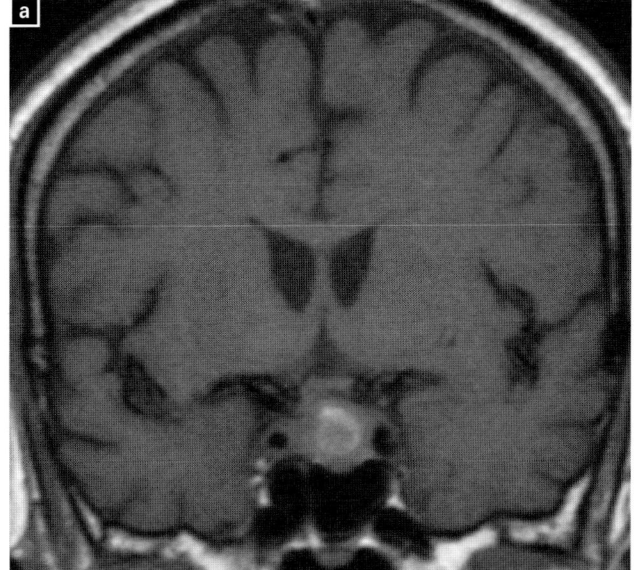
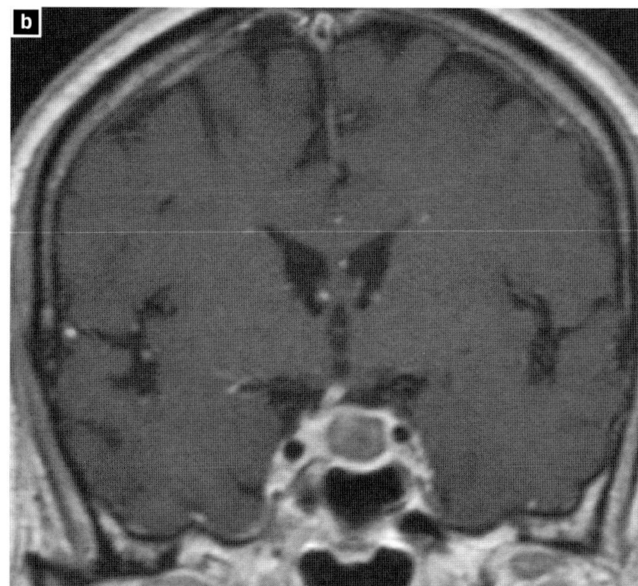

Fig. 6.46. **(a) Pre- and (b) post-contrast T1 coronal images show hemorrhagic infarction of the pituitary in a 51-year-old female who presented with panhypopituitarism. The blood products are hyperintense on the T1 pre-contrast images, but appear hypointense relative to the surrounding rim enhancement on the post-contrast images.**

(arising from the supraclinoid portion of the internal carotid artery or from the posterior communicating arteries) feed the pituitary portal system (primary capillary plexus and then the hypophysial portal veins), which then supplies the anterior pituitary. Therefore, at angiography, the anterior pituitary gland blush is delayed compared to the posterior pituitary, and typically less intense. This portal system probably results in decreased perfusion pressure to the anterior pituitary gland, and renders it more susceptible to ischemia in the setting of tumor or systemic hypotension.

A closely related disorder in the realm of pituitary infarction is Sheehan's syndrome, which is pituitary apoplexy in the postpartum setting, typically occurring in a normal gland. This uncommon syndrome almost always occurs in cases of complicated delivery with high blood loss, and was described by Dr. Sheehan in 1961. The infarcted gland is typically enlarged and shows rim enhancement. While Sheehan's syndrome may be a true emergency leading to pituitary insufficiency and rapid death, it is more often an indolent syndrome, manifesting with failure to lactate, failure of resumption of menses after delivery, and such secondary signs as failure of regrowth of shaved pubic hair.

Before leaving the topic of pituitary apoplexy and hemorrhage, it must be pointed out (for the lovers of esoterica) that Hantavirus infection has also been reported to produce apoplexy and hemorrhage of the anterior pituitary gland in the acute phase, and lead to hypopituitarism after recovery. This rare disease manifests with fever, hemorrhage, and renal failure, and has also been called hemorrhagic fever with renal syndrome (HFRS) and Korean hemorrhagic fever (see Suh *et al.*, 1995).

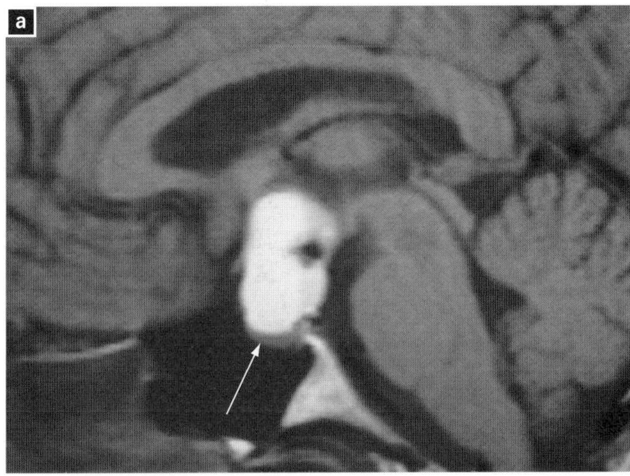
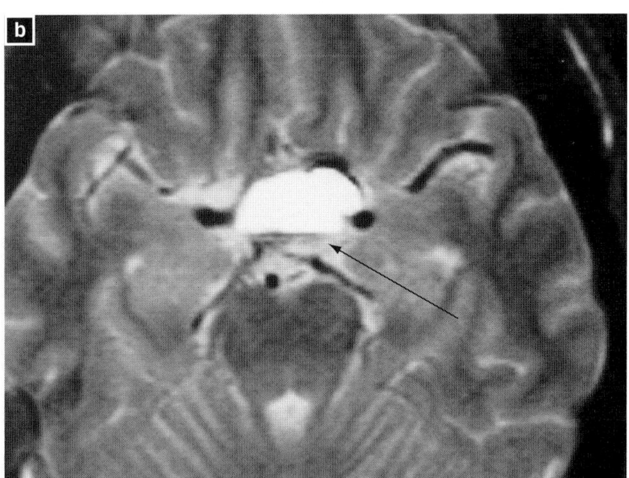

Fig. 6.47. **(a) Sagittal pre-contrast T1 and (b) axial T2 images of the pituitary are obtained. There is a large, lobulated intrasellar and suprasellar mass. The mass is hyperintense on T1 pre-contrast, due to hemorrhagic breakdown products, cholesterol crystals and proteinaceous fluid, and of mixed signal intensity on T2. Other than the typical mix of signal intensities, other clues to the diagnosis of craniopharyngioma are that the mass is separable from the pituitary gland (arrow in (a)), is cystic with a fluid–fluid level on T2 (arrow in (b)), and shows no significant enlargement of the sella for the size of the mass.**

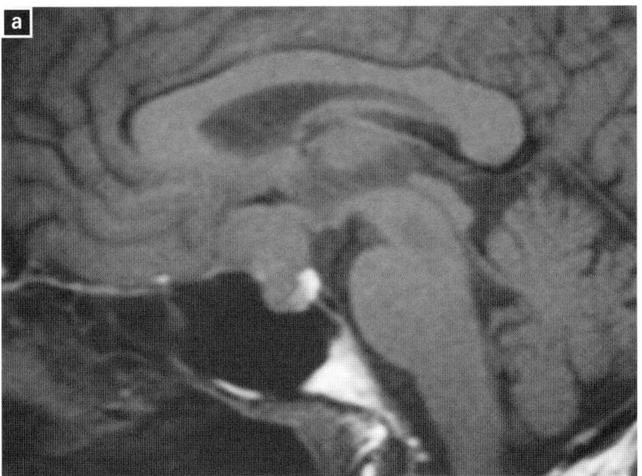
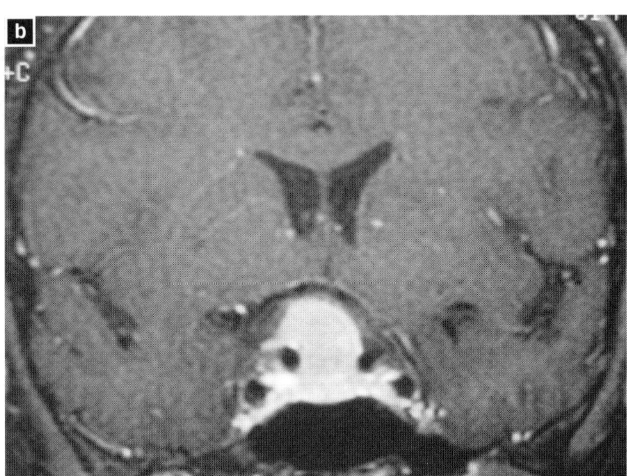

Fig. 6.48. **(a) Sagittal pre-contrast and (b) coronal post-contrast T1-weighted images of the pituitary show an isointense, homogenously enhancing intrasellar and suprasellar mass. Clues to the diagnosis of meningioma, other than isointense signal on pre-contrast T1 and homogenous enhancement post-contrast, include the forward leaning of the mass along the planum sphenoidale (macroadenomas tend to grow straight up) and the lack of significant enlargement of the sella for the size of the mass.**

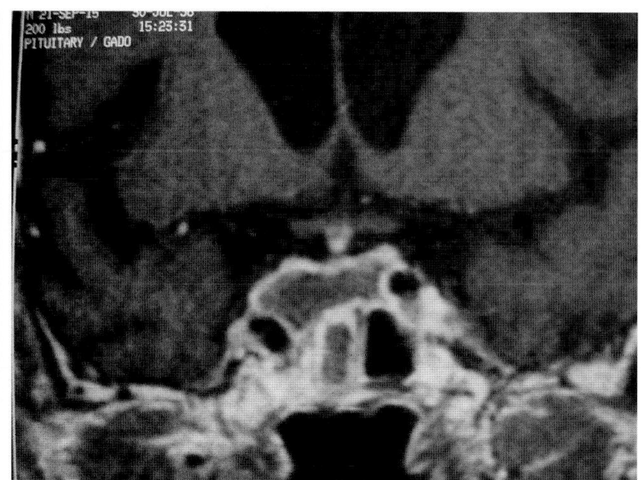

Fig. 6.49. **Post-contrast T1-weighted coronal images of the pituitary gland are obtained.**

Our two patients presented with panhypopituitarism, and turned out to have pituitary apoplexy. However, numerous other entities may cause panhypopituitarism, and these include other parasellar and intrasellar masses, such as metastases, meningioma, craniopharyngioma and large pituitary macroadenoma without hemorrhage or infarction, as well as trauma and hypothalamic lesions. Since craniopharyngiomas and meningiomas are both common lesions, they are shown in Figs. 6.47 and 6.48, respectively, just to familiarize you with their appearance. Neither of these patients, though, had hypopituitarism.

Finally, for your enjoyment, a very rare case is presented adjacent (Fig. 6.49) of a 66-year-old man who presented with headaches and hypopituitarism. Post-contrast T1-weighted images show a rim enhancing hypointense lesion filling the sella turcica.

As opposed to tumors, which typically extend superiorly, this mass seems to "flop" downward along the right aspect of the sella, depressing the right cavernous carotid artery. The appearance on post-contrast images suggests a rim-enhancing fluid collection. Beneath the mass, the right aspect of the sphenoid sinus is opacified and also shows rim enhancement. Do you have the diagnosis? This is a rare pituitary abscess. Pituitary abscess may be secondary to direct spread of infection from the sphenoid sinus, or may be secondary to hematogenous spread. The most common organisms are gram-positive cocci.

References

Rogg, J. M., Tung, G. A., Anderson, G. *et al*. Pituitary apoplexy: early detection with diffusion-weighted imaging. *American Journal of Neuroradiology* 2002; **23**: 1240–1245.

Suh, D. C., Park, J. S., Park, S. K. *et al*. Pituitary hemorrhage as a complication of hantaviral disease. *American Journal of Neuroradiology* 1995; **16**: 175–178.

7 | The cerebral cortex

The cerebral cortex, in the opinion of many, is what makes us who we are. The thin, highly convoluted layer of gray matter, which envelopes the white matter, contains an estimated 20 billion neurons. Although the cortex is the ultimate interpreter of sights and sounds and the initiator of motion, only a relatively small portion of the cortex is involved in the specific functions of receiving sensory input from the special senses or projecting motor outputs to the spinal cord. Over 80 percent of the cortex, the so-called association cortex, is involved in more general functions such as integrating information, cognition, language, and reasoning.

The most obvious way to study the cortex is based on the visible sulci and gyri along the cortical surface, as was done by the early anatomists. The cerebrum is divided into two hemispheres by the interhemispheric fissure, and each hemisphere is divided into four lobes (frontal, parietal, temporal, and occipital), and possibly a fifth "limbic" lobe if one wishes to consider it as such (Fig. 7.1). The Sylvian fissure (lateral sulcus) separates the temporal lobe inferiorly from the frontal and parietal lobes superiorly along the lateral cerebral convexity. The insula lies in the depth of the Sylvian fissure, and is covered by frontal, temporal and parietal opercula (lids). The central sulcus divides the frontal and parietal lobes along the lateral cerebral convexity. The parieto-occipital sulcus divides the parietal and occipital lobes along the medial brain surface. The occipital lobe is divided by the calcarine fissure, which runs nearly perpendicular to the parieto-occipital sulcus; its superior portion is called the cuneus, while the inferior portion is called the lingulus.

Other structures to take note of in Fig. 7.1 are the divisions of the frontal operculum into a pars frontalis, pars triangularis and pars opercularis, as well as the location of the supramarginal and angular gyri in the parietal lobe beneath the inferior parietal lobule. The supramarginal gyrus is found by following the Sylvian fissure posteriorly, while the angular gyrus is found by following the superior temporal sulcus posteriorly.

A more detailed way to study the cortex incorporates its microscopic anatomy. On the basis of detailed cytoarchitectural studies, neuroanatomists have thus classified the cortex into three types.

Neocortex

This cortex is a fairly recent evolutionary addition, characteristic of mammals, particularly humans. In the human being, neocortex accounts for about 90 percent of the cerebrum. Typically, it has six cellular layers, although in some portions of the cortex, such as in the motor cortex, some of the layers are so diminutive as to be nearly absent.

Allocortex

This sort of cortex is evolutionarily much older. It is composed of only three layers, and forms a significant portion of the limbic system, including the hippocampal formations and such areas as the primary olfactory cortex and piriform cortex.

Mesocortex

This sort of cortex can be thought of as a transition between neocortex and more primitive cortex, and has a variable number of layers between three and six. It comprises portions of the cingulate gyrus, entorhinal cortex, and parahippocampal gyrus.

The study of the microscopic structure of the cortex is fascinating, but is too specialized for the sorts of clinical correlations in which we are involved, so we will make only a few notes in passing:

- It is noted that the six cellular layers in typical neocortex migrate in reverse order, with layer six, the deepest layer, representing the first wave of migration of neuroblasts. The remaining layers continue migrating in reverse order, such that layer five represents the second wave of neuroblast

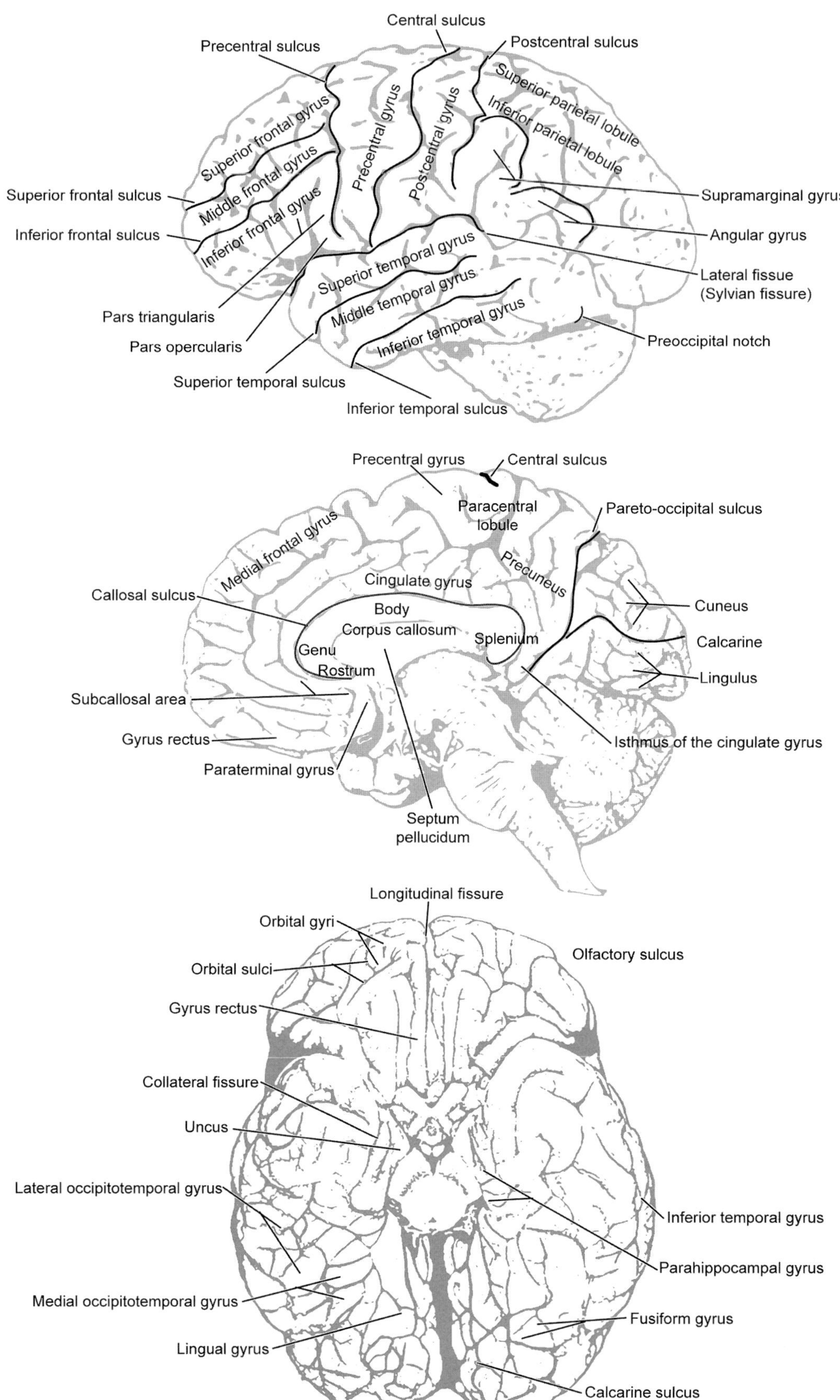

Fig. 7.1. **Anatomic diagram of cerebral sulci and gyri. Top: lateral surface of the brain. Middle: medial surface of the brain. Bottom: ventral surface of the brain.**

migration, and so on. Thus, neurons in the more superficial layers must migrate past the ones already layed down in the deeper layers. Disorders of this complex migrational scheme lead to so-called migrational disorders such as polymicrogyria, pachygyria, and gray matter heterotopia – all of which may be associated with seizures.

- Layers one, five, and six (the molecular, ganglionic, and multiform layers) are present in all three types of cortex, while layers two, three, and four (external granular, pyramidal, and internal granular layers) are the more recent additions found only in the neocortex. Various types of neuronal connections are more specific to some layers than others. For example, neurons in layers five and six are efferent: neurons in layer six give rise to corticothalamic fibers, and neurons in layer five give rise to fibers that project to the brainstem and spinal cord. Layers one through four have a more afferent and receptive function, and give rise to complex intracortical connections. For example, layer four is the major afferent connection for modality-specific inputs from the thalamus.

- Although the cortex can be thought of as functionally divided in a horizontal fashion according to its layers, the true functional units of cortex are probably vertically organized in a columnar fashion, with each vertical column containing all of the cortical layers. Various neuroanatomic studies have shown that such small vertical columns of cells in the cortex form functionally separate modules within the brain, with each module being selectively activated by specific peripheral stimuli. It is estimated that there are approximately 3 million such modules within the cerebral cortex.

- These modules can be thought of as the microstructural units of the cortex. However, there are regional variations within the cortex in such things as the width of each of the cellular layers and the cellular density within each layer. Neuroanatomists have used these variations to draw up regional cytoarchitectural maps of the cortex. The most famous of these is that drafted by the German neuroanatomist Brodmann nearly a century ago. He divided the cortex into 52 areas (see Fig. 7.2). This division, along with the typical anatomy of sulci and gyri, is probably the best way to talk about the functional anatomy of the cortex.

There are some interesting facts that you may (or, more likely, may not) have wondered about regarding Brodmann's areas. First, Brodmann's cytoarchitectural maps only loosely correspond to sulcal/gyral anatomy, with some areas being only part of a gyrus and others crossing over sulci to include portions of different gyri. Secondly, the areas seem to be numbered in a rather haphazard fashion. What is the etiology of the bizarre numbering? The numbering actually simply corresponds to the temporal order in which Brodmann studied the different areas of cortex (somewhat anticlimactic, huh?). Lastly, just for fun, ask your professors about Brodmann's areas 13–16. You will notice that these are absent from most textbook diagrams of Brodmann's areas, and correspond to deep insular regions not typically illustrated or discussed.

An equally fascinating area of study, again beyond the scope of this book, is the neurochemical organization of the cortex. Until recently, it was believed that inputs to cortical neurons came only from the thalamus (from both modality-specific thalamic nuclei and non-specific thalamic nuclei), and from other areas of cortex, in the form of short and long association fibers (which connect to neurons in the same cerebral hemisphere) and commissural fibers (which connect neurons in one hemisphere to others in the contralateral hemisphere). More recent advances, however, have revealed that there are significant subcortical extra thalamic sources of input to the cerebral cortex, which can best be considered in terms of separate chemical neurotransmitter systems. For example, serotonergic input to the cortex originates from the raphe nuclei in the brainstem, while cholinergic inputs originate from the nucleus basalis of Meynert in the basal forebrain, just beneath the anterior commissure. Certainly, these systems are important in neurobehavior. As we know, disorders of serotonin are now well implicated in affective disorder such as depression, while disturbances in cholinergic inputs to the cortex are involved in the genesis or progression of Alzheimer's disease.

With these introductory notes, it is time to begin looking at the functional anatomy of the cortex. For this purpose, the cortex can be thought of in terms of four broad categories (see Fig. 7.3):

Primary cortical areas

These are, by and large, the sensory areas of the cortex which receive inputs from modality-specific thalamic nuclei, as well as the motor cortex. There are six primary sensory cortical areas: somesthetic (or somatosensory), visual, auditory, vestibular, gustatory, and olfactory.

Unimodal association areas

The primary motor cortex, as well as the somatosensory, visual, and auditory primary sensory cortical areas, have associated unimodal association areas. That means regions of cortex which are located next to, and deal mainly with, their associated primary cortical areas. In the case of somatosensory, visual and auditory cortex, the unimodal association areas interpret the sensations which are perceived in a more raw form in the primary sensory cortex.

Multimodal association areas

Unlike the unimodal association cortex, multimodal association areas are not linked to a single primary cortical area. Rather, they integrate broadly across multiple sensory modalities, or serve broader cognitive functions. The largest multimodal association cortex is the prefrontal region of the frontal lobes, and the next largest is the parieto-temporo-occipital association cortex at the junction of the named lobes.

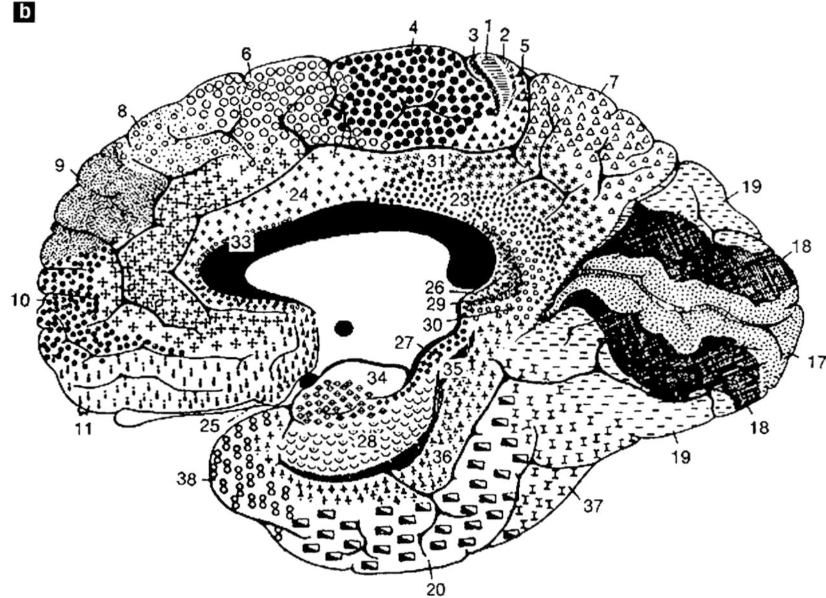

Fig. 7.2. **(a) Lateral view of the left hemisphere and (b) medial view of the right hemisphere showing Brodmann's areas.**

The limbic cortex

The term, "limbic cortex," is somewhat inaccurate, and is meant to denote the limbic system. For the purposes of clinical correlation, the limbic system is being considered as a separate brain system, although it functions in concert with a broad range of other cortical and subcortical structures to perform its main tasks: regulating drive and affective behavior, and playing a central role in learning and memory. The main components of the limbic system are the hippocampal formations, the parahippocampal gyri (particularly the portions known as the entorhinal cortex), the columns of the fornix, the mammillary bodies, the cingulate gyri, and portions of the amygdalas. Most of these structures are connected via a feedback neuronal circuit known as the Papez circuit. The term "limbic," by the way, comes from the Latin "limbus," or ring, denoting that many of the structures and interconnections of the Papez circuit wrap around the brainstem in a C-shaped loop or ring.

And now let us take some cases!

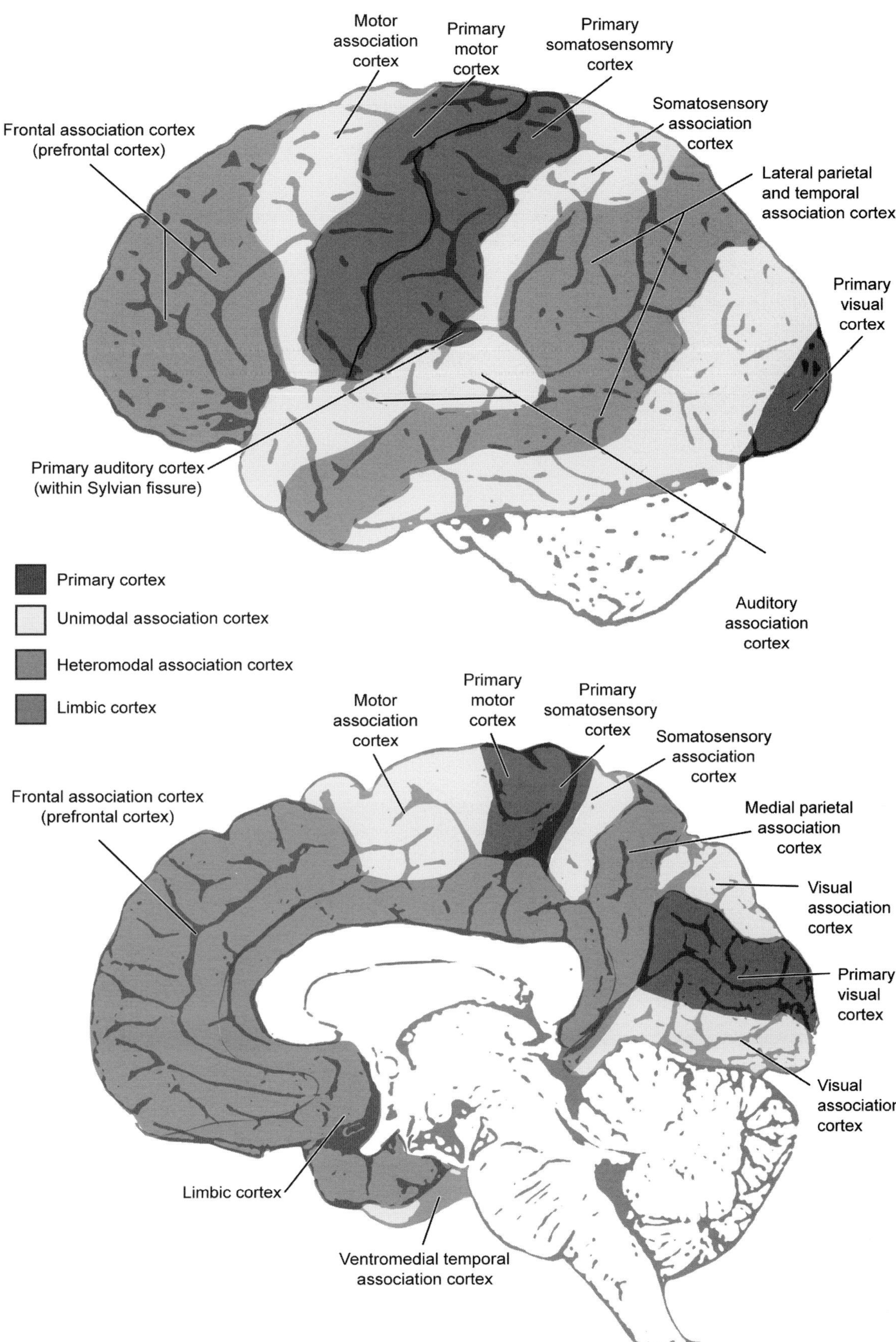

Fig. 7.3. **Illustration of the different categories of cerebral cortex. See text for details.**

Case 7.1

65-year-old patient presents with a gradual onset of worsening right upper extremity weakness and loss of hand dexterity.

MRI examination is presented (Fig. 7.4). Where is the lesion? What is your diagnosis?

There is hypointensity, consistent in appearance with vasogenic edema, involving the left motor strip (later post-contrast images showed an underlying metastatic lesion). That the motor strip is involved can be ascertained by finding the central sulcus (arrow in Fig. 7.4). Immediately anterior to it is the precentral gyrus, which houses the motor cortex. This corresponds to Brodmann's area 4. A lesion of the motor cortex produces contralateral hemiparesis. The location of the lesion in the motor cortex, along the high lateral convexity, corresponds to the arm and hand regions (see below).

Discuss the somatotopic organization of the motor cortex and some of its clinically relevant features.

The localization of the motor cortex is fairly easy along the superolateral surface of the cerebral hemisphere, as shown here. On the medial side of the hemisphere, localization is more difficult, and the motor cortex corresponds to the anterior aspect of the paracentral lobule.

The motor cortex is somatotopically organized with the contralateral half of the body represented in an orderly but disproportionate fashion along the motor strip, as depicted by the familiar figure of the motor homunculus (see Fig. 7.5). Notable in the homunculus are the disproportionately large

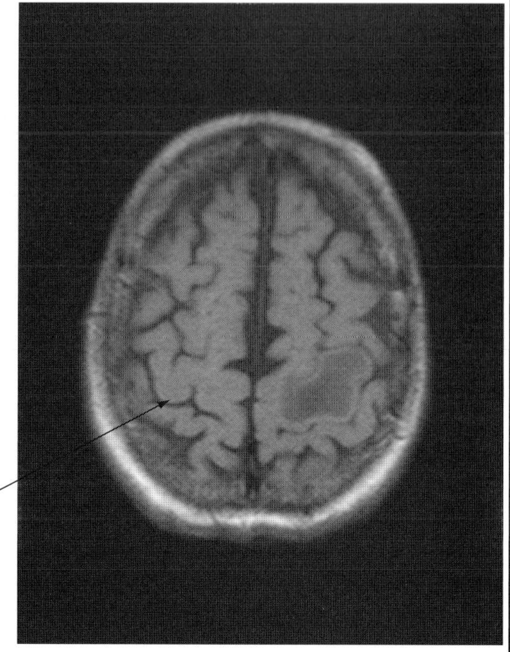

Fig. 7.4. **T1-weighted axial non-contrast MRI.**

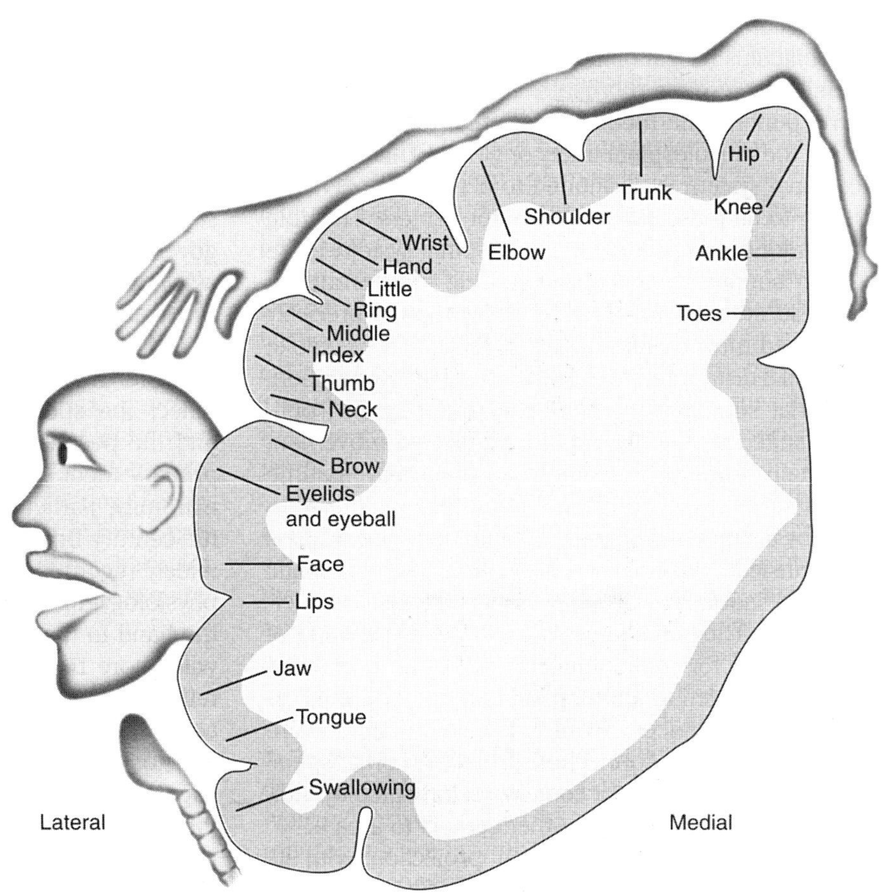

Fig. 7.5. **Representation of the motor homunculus along the motor strip.**

areas of representation for the tongue and the thumb, because of the importance of these regions in skilled hand movements and in speech.

The motor cortex receives projections from the motor areas of the thalamus (where impulses from the cerebellum and basal ganglia are transmitted), from the somesthetic sensory cortex and sensory association areas, and from the supplementary motor cortex (see Fig. 7.3). The motor cortex reciprocally outputs to these areas, as well as, of course, to the pyramidal tracts to exert motor control over the contralateral half of the body.

Important clinical points to note are as follows.

- Electrical stimulation of the motor cortex gives rise to discrete movements in isolated contralateral muscles or movements across a single joint in the contralateral body. However, there are bilateral responses in the extraocular muscles, upper face, tongue, larynx, and pharynx. Thus, ipsilateral cortical infarcts do not typically manifest with gross tongue deviation, contralateral vocal cord paralysis, or significant dysphagia, because corticobulbar innervation to the upper face, tongue, and larynx/pharynx is bilateral. The innervation, however, seems to have a contralateral predominance, so some mild component of dysphagia or tongue deviation, for example, may be present.
- Lesions isolated to the motor cortex usually lead to a loss in highly skilled, intricate movements of the distal muscles (writing, or performing surgery), whereas gross motor movements may be retained or recovered.
- Typically, a tumor or infarct of the motor cortex leads to initial contralateral weakness or flaccid paralysis, which is later followed by hypertonia and hyperreflexia, as well as a positive Babinski sign – the characteristics of upper motor neuron lesions. According to some authors, though, hyperreflexia and spasticity occur secondary to involvement of the subcortical/extrapyramidal pathways, and lesions isolated to the cortical ribbon of the motor cortex may produce only flaccid paralysis (see Fig. 7.6).

The putative pathophysiology of the spasticity which typically accompanies lesions of the motor pathways is that there is loss of descending inhibitory fibers to the gamma motor neurons of the anterior horn cells of the spinal cord. These gamma motor neurons innervate the intrafusal fibers of the muscle spindles. Loss of cortical inhibition stretches the mid-portion of the muscle spindle, lowering the threshold for activation. This, in turn, leads to hypertonia and hyperreflexia. It is interesting to note that this disinhibition is most pronounced in the flexors of the upper extremity and the extensors of the lower extremity, leading to the classic post-stroke posturing of a flexed arm and an outstretched leg with spasticity. However, it is important to stress that this is only one proposed mechanism, and that the etiology of prolonged flaccidity after cerebral infarct is not at all well understood, and remains a matter of debate (see Pantano *et al.*, 1995). In fact, the case presented above is atypical in that most reported cases with prolonged flaccid paralysis after stroke show involvement of the lentiform nucleus by the infarct. The issue is raised here only to make the reader aware that not all cerebral infarcts are accompanied by spasticity and typical upper motor neuron signs, and that some strokes may show prolonged flaccid paralysis.

- The primary motor cortex contributes only about 40 percent of the fibers in the pyramidal tract. The remaining fibers come predominantly from the sensory areas of the parietal lobe and from the premotor cortex. However, the primary motor cortex, in the fifth cortical cellular layer, contains the characteristic large pyramidal motor neurons known as the Betz cells. The Betz cells account for about 4 percent of the fibers in the pyramidal tract, and are thickly myelinated, rapidly conducting axons.

- The somatotopic organization of the motor cortex, as depicted by the homunculus (see Fig. 7.5), explains the so-called Jacksonian march seen in some seizures caused by a nidus in the motor cortex. Such seizures manifest an orderly progression of motor seizure activity through the regions of the homunculus, such as contralateral facial grimacing, followed by seizure activity progressing to the thumb, hand, arm, and leg, in an orderly fashion.
- Finally, the layout of the homunculus explains why middle cerebral artery infarcts tend to involve the contralateral face and arm, with sparing of the leg. The lower extremity projects over the medial-most aspect of the precentral gyrus, along the interhemispheric fissure. This is the territory of the anterior cerebral artery. Conversely, isolated weakness of the lower extremity raises the possibility of a contralateral anterior cerebral artery infarct (see Fig. 7.7). This division of

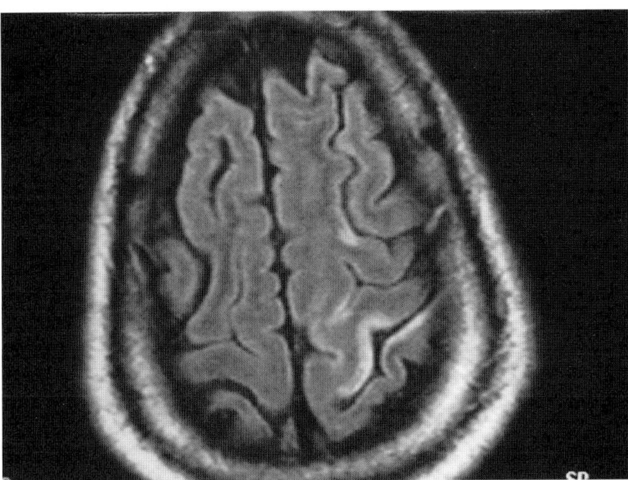

Fig. 7.6. **FLAIR axial image shows a subacute infarct involving only the cortical ribbons of the motor and sensory strips surrounding the central sulcus. The patient manifested with flaccid paralysis and numbness of the right arm and hand.**

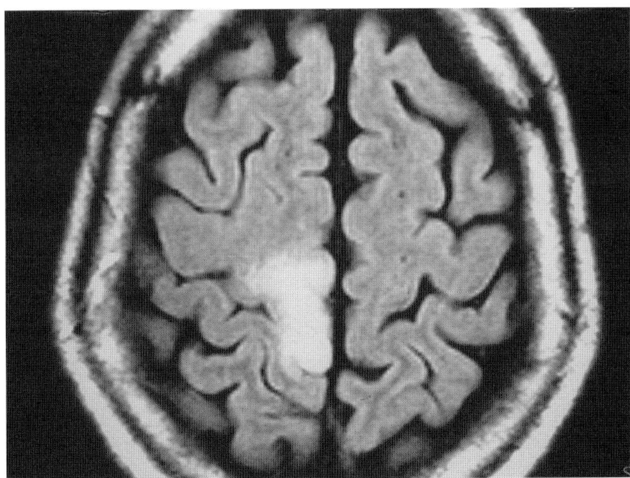

Fig. 7.7. **FLAIR axial image shows a subacute infarct in the right anterior cerebral artery territory along the medial margin of the right posterior frontal lobe in the depth of the right motor strip in this patient presenting with left leg weakness.**

the homunculus across vascular territories explains why, when a patient presents with hemiparesis that involves both the arm and the leg, neurologists almost instinctively localize the lesion to subcortical structures such as the corticospinal tract, either in the posterior limb of the internal capsule or in the brainstem, rather than localizing the lesion to the motor cortex.

Discuss some other motor cortical areas in the brain, focusing on function and clinical relevance.

Along with the primary motor cortex, which is sometimes referred to as MI (M "one"), there are two other major motor areas in the brain, which can be thought of as motor association cortex. These are the supplementary motor area (MII) and the premotor cortex. Both of these are part of Brodmann's area 6 (see Fig. 7.2). They differ from primary motor cortex in their threshold of electrical excitability, as well as in inputs, outputs, and in the general types of motor responses which they subtend.

The premotor cortex lies immediately anterior to the motor cortex, making up most of Brodmann's area 6. The main function of the premotor cortex seems to be in coordinating the vast array of voluntary motor activities which occur in response to sensory inputs, such as visual, auditory, and somatosensory stimuli. Examples of such motor activities would include grasping an object that we see, playing catch, obeying a spoken command, or turning the head and eyes toward a sound. The importance of this area in humans is vast, as evidenced by a comparison of monkeys and humans. In monkeys, the premotor cortex is about the same size as the primary motor cortex, whereas in humans, the premotor cortex is nearly six times as large as the primary motor cortex. It is noted that the premotor cortex outputs both to the motor cortex as well as directly to the pyramidal tract, with approximately 30 percent of pyramidal tract fibers arising in the premotor region. Lesions of the premotor cortex, thus, tend to produce deficits in complex, sequential, compound movements. If there is no associated motor paralysis, such deficits

are known as apraxias. The term "apraxia," often causes some confusion, so it is worth spending a few minutes on this topic. Apraxia implies the inability to deliberately perform a learned, compound, motor task in the absence of motor weakness or sensory, attention, or comprehension deficits. There are different types of apraxia corresponding to lesion location (this will be covered in some more detail later). The type of apraxia caused by lesions in the premotor area is known as ideomotor apraxia. This is the inability to perform a complex task when instructed to do so, even if the task can be performed spontaneously or automatically. A good example would be the inability to stick out the tongue and move it from side to side when commanded, but performing the same action spontaneously when licking one's lips. Lesions in the premotor cortex presumably produce ideomotor apraxia because commands need to be processed through the premotor region to call up the relevant motor engrams necessary to obey the command, and then send them to the primary motor cortex to produce the necessary movements.

The supplementary motor area (MII), is roughly composed of the medial aspect of Brodmann's area 6. The main role of the supplementary motor area seems to be in sequencing complex motions as well as in calling up motor engrams for previously learned activities. Lesions of the supplementary motor area, in the acute phase, produce akinesia (lack of spontaneous movement) in the contralateral body. This, however, is a transient deficit. The major lasting deficits seem to be hypertonia, clonus, and a positive Babinski sign, as well as a disturbance in motor sequences that require alternation of both hands (playing patty-cake, perhaps?).

Reference

Pantano, P., Formisano, R., Ricci, M. *et al.* Prolonged muscular flaccidity after stroke. Morphological and functional brain alterations. *Brain* 1995; **118** (5): 1329–1338.

Case 7.2

67-year-old right-handed male with a 15-year history of progressive weakness and spasticity. The patient's symptoms initially began with right leg weakness and stiffness, leading to a noticeable limp. Within 2 years, the patient developed weakness first in the right upper extremity, then the left lower extremity, and finally in the left upper extremity. Within 4 years of the onset of symptoms, the patient was confined to a wheelchair. Recently, the patient has also begun to have dysarthria. The patient reports no cognitive or memory deficits. On examination, there was motor weakness in all four extremities, marked in the lower extremities and in the distal upper extremities. The deep tendon reflexes were quite brisk throughout, and there were bilateral positive Babinski signs and clonus. Significantly, there was no gross motor wasting, and no evidence of fasciculations.

MRI examination is presented below (Fig. 7.8). What are the findings? What is your diagnosis?

The MRI images show marked atrophy of the motor cortex bilaterally, with expansion of the central sulci. There is abnormal T2-weighted hyperintensity in the subcortical white matter of the motor strips. This abnormal T2-weighted hyperintensity continues into the posterior corona radiata, and into the corticospinal tracts along the posterior portions of the posterior limbs of the internal capsules.

The imaging findings are consistent with selective involvement of the motor cortex and the corticospinal tracts. Such selective involvement of the motor pathways would be suggestive of a diagnosis of amyotrophic lateral sclerosis (ALS, Lou Gehrig's disease), the most common degenerative motor neuron disease. In fact, the findings displayed above are precisely the expected findings in ALS (see Terao *et al.*, 1995). However, our patient presents a somewhat different clinical picture than that typically seen in ALS. Most striking is the duration of disease, as well as the lack of lower motor neuron findings such as muscle wasting and fasciculations. The MRI, in conjunction with the clinical findings, suggest a pure upper motor neuron syndrome. Do you know such a syndrome?

Diagnosis

Primary lateral sclerosis (PLS).

Discuss primary lateral sclerosis.

Primary lateral sclerosis is a rare, idiopathic, neurodegenerative disorder which appears to selectively involve the upper motor neurons in the primary motor cortex, with degeneration along the corticospinal tracts. There is sparing of the lower motor neuron anterior horn cells, distinguishing this disease from ALS, which typically shows both upper and lower motor

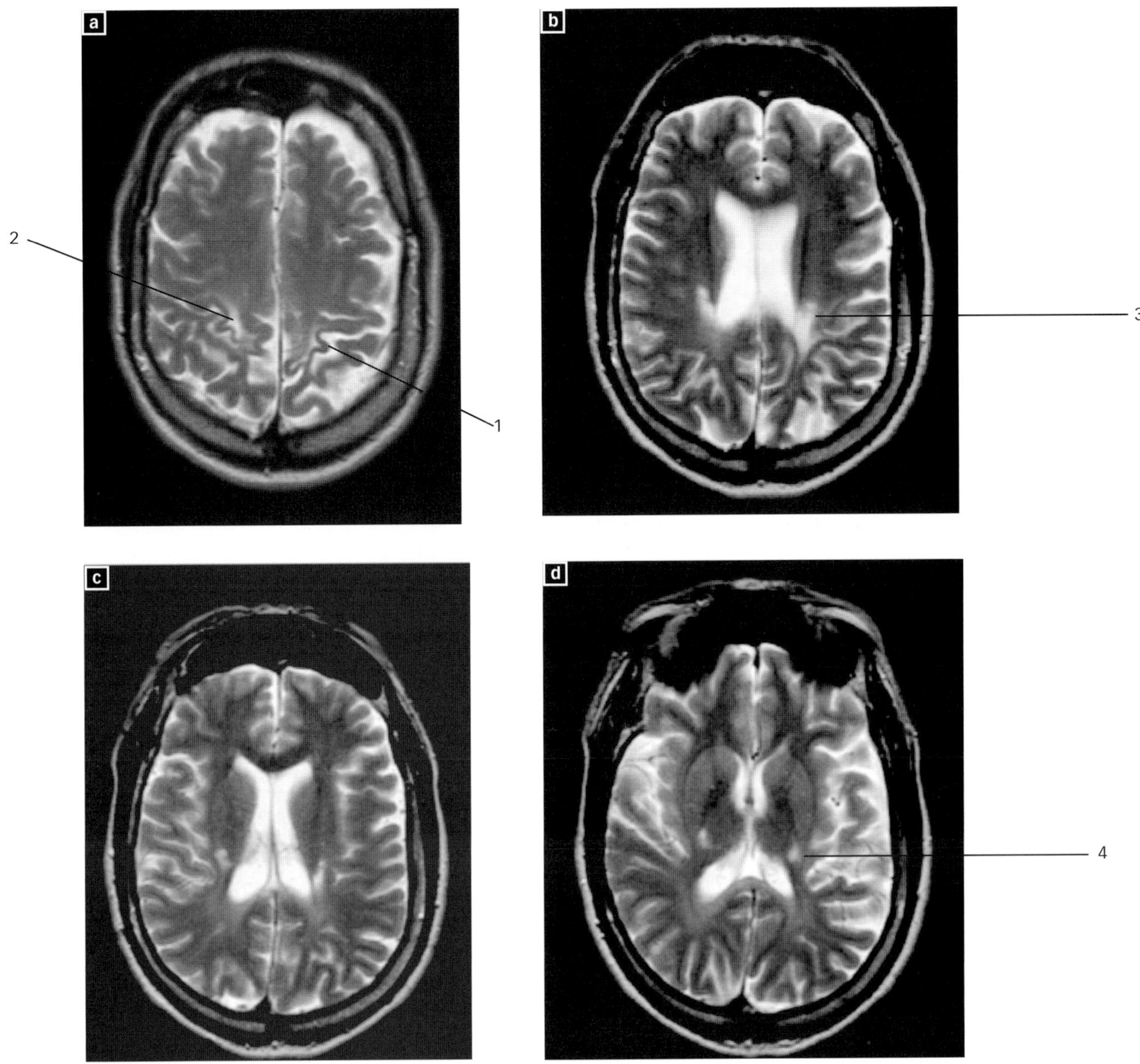

Fig. 7.8. **(a)–(d) T2-weighted axial images of the brain are presented. (1) Widened central sulcus; (2) atrophic motor strip with subcortical hyperintensity; (3) abnormal signal in posterior corona radiata along motor pathways; (4) abnormal signal in corticospinal tracts in posterior portion of the posterior limbs of the internal capsules.**

neuron degeneration. The upper motor neuron histopathological changes, however, are very similar to those of ALS, with a severe depletion of the Betz cells in layer 5 of the motor cortex, and a significant depletion as well in the smaller pyramidal neurons of the motor strip. PLS typically progresses as in our patient, usually beginning insidiously in the sixth decade with stiffness of the legs, which progresses to weakness, and then involvement of the upper extremities. Eventually, there is development of severe spastic paraparesis or quadraparesis, often also with a pseudo bulbar palsy. It is noted that the imaging findings in our case are somewhat atypical in that there is marked abnormal T2-weighted hyperintensity along the corticospinal tracts. The few reported cases in the literature have tended to show only atrophy of the perirolandic regions, without such significant signal abnormalities (Peretti-Viton *et al.*, 1999).

Discuss the differential diagnosis of progressive upper motor neuron disease.

Most patients with such a presentation do not have primary lateral sclerosis, which is rather a rare disease. Such a presentation is often secondary to multiple sclerosis, particularly with cord involvement, or to spinal cord myelopathy, often secondary to degenerative spondylosis or compression by a slow-growing tumor of the spinal canal such as a meningioma. Other cases may be secondary to HTLV infection and tropical spastic paraparesis, or vacuolar myelopathy of AIDS, or may be seen in patients with a progressive familial spastic paraparesis. One such disorder is known as Strumpell–Lorrain disease. There are also a variety of rare familial spastic paraplegias which occur with ocular symptoms, but these do not pertain to our patient. In a small percentage of cases with progressive bilateral upper motor neuron disease, patients will be given a diagnosis of primary lateral sclerosis, as in the case above.

The diagnostic criteria for PLS, and its relationship to ALS, are topics of interest and debate. One of the most definitive papers on primary lateral sclerosis seems to be the one by Pringle *et al.*, 1992. The authors make a strong case that PLS is a distinct entity from ALS, particularly given the sparing of lower motor neurons. Interestingly, however, there have also been reports of long-standing cases of PLS which have developed late-onset lower motor neuron signs, and progressed to assume a clinical picture similar to that of ALS. This, of course, has led to debate as to whether PLS and ALS do indeed belong to the same spectrum of disease (see Bruyn *et al.*, 1995).

What does this case reflect regarding the location of the corticospinal tracts in the posterior limb of the internal capsule?

This is another topic of considerable interest. Many of you may recall being taught that the corticospinal tract runs in the anterior half of the posterior limb of the internal capsule, beginning at the genu, with a somatotopic organization of the head, arm, and leg fibers. However, further neuroanatomic studies and MRI imaging, along with autopsy correlation in such diseases as ALS, has corrected that misconception. We now know that the corticospinal tracts, in fact, run in the posterior portion of the posterior limb of the internal capsule. This matches precisely the location seen in the MRI images above (Fig. 7.8(d)), as well as the descriptions which have appeared in the literature regarding the location of the corticospinal tracts within the internal capsules as shown by MRI imaging (Yagishita *et al.*, 1994).

Finally, a note for the real aficionados of motor neuron disease: there is a very rare form of motor neuron disease which is, essentially, a unilateral form of PLS. For all the big prizes, can you name it? Good job: it is called Mills' syndrome (see, for example, Gastaut *et al.*, 1994).

References

Bruyn, R. P. M., Koelman, J. H., Troost, D. *et al.* Motor neuron disease (amyotrophic lateral sclerosis) arising from long-standing primary lateral sclerosis. *Journal of Neurology, Neurosurgery, and Psychiatry* 1995; **58**: 742–744.

Gastaut, J. L., Bartolomei, F. Mills' syndrome: ascending (or descending) progressive hemiplegia: a hemiplegic form of primary lateral sclerosis? *Journal of Neurology, Neurosurgery, and Psychiatry* 1994; **57**(10): 1280–1281.

Peretti-Viton, P., Azulay, J. P., Brunel, H. *et al.* MRI of the intracranial corticospinal tracts in amyotrophic and primary lateral scelrosis. *Neuroradiology* 1999; **41**: 744–749.

Pringle, C. E., Hudson, A. J., Munoz, D. G. *et al.* Primary lateral sclerosis: clinical features, neuropathology and diagnostic criteria. *Brain* 1992; **115**: 495–520.

Terao, S., Yasuda, T., Kachi, T. *et al.* Magnetic resonance imaging of the corticospinal tracts in amyotrophic lateral sclerosis. *Journal of the Neurological Sciences* 1995; **133**: 66–72.

Yagishita, A., Nakano, I., Oda, M. *et al.* Location of the corticospinal tract in the internal capsule at MR imaging. *Radiology* 1994; **191**: 455–460.

Case 7.3

72-year-old male who presents with rightward eye deviation and mild left-sided incoordination for fine motor movements.

MRI images are presented (Fig. 7.9). Where is the lesion located? What is your diagnosis?

There is a subacute infarct in the right premotor area, predominantly along the right middle frontal gyrus.

Discuss why the patient has rightward gaze deviation. In other words, what specific area is involved?

To finish up our discussion of motor areas in the cortex, we need to discuss the cortical eye fields. This patient's infarct involves the right frontal eye field, which is located at the anterior edge of the premotor cortex in the middle frontal gyrus (see Fig. 7.10). The frontal eye fields correspond to Brodmann's area 8.

The control of eye movements is an extremely important cortical function, which we often take for granted. It involves a variety of tasks, including generating both saccades and smooth pursuit movements, and requires the integrated action of several different cortical regions, such as the frontal eye fields, the supplementary eye fields, the parieto-occipital eye fields, as well as regions in the prefrontal cortex, inferior parietal lobule, and the hippocampus.

One of the most important eye movements is known as saccadic eye movement, or saccades for short. These are rapid eye movements, which quickly take the vision from one point in space and fix it on another, without interest in visualizing the points in between. Voluntary saccades can take the eyes from one visible target to another, or from one location to an expected location of where the target might move (such as when shifting the eyes quickly to see where a tennis ball is expected to land after a smash), or to a remembered location of where the target was. The frontal eye fields are critical in the control of such voluntary saccades, which form a very important part of the way we visually explore our environment, and for such activities as reading.

Another type of eye movement is smooth pursuit eye movement, where a target is followed throughout its course, such as watching a bird as it flies through the air. This involves a slow eye movement and visually tracking an object. The cortical areas mediating smooth pursuit eye movements are not as well delineated as those involved in generating saccades, but are thought to primarily involve temporo-occipito-parietal cortex, with some interaction with the frontal eye fields.

In generating voluntary saccades, the frontal eye fields communicate with the nuclei of the extraocular muscles through neuronal relays, which involve the paramedian pontine reticular formation (PPRF) for horizontal saccades as well as the midbrain tectum and the rostral interstitial nucleus of the MLF for vertical saccades. The frontal eye fields trigger voluntary saccades to the contralateral side, and each frontal eye field can be thought of as maintaining an active "tone" to the contralateral side. In simpler terms, the right frontal eye field functions in triggering saccades to the left, and can be thought of as "pushing" the eyes to the left. Thus, a lesion in the right frontal eye field takes away the leftward "tone," and leaves the left frontal eye field unopposed. The left frontal eye field, then, pushes the eyes to the right without opposition, with a resultant rightward gaze deviation, as in our patient. Thus, in cortical infarcts, the eyes are said to look towards the lesion (see Fig. 7.11).

Conversely, with epileptic foci involving the region of the frontal eye fields, there is excess "tone" to the contralateral

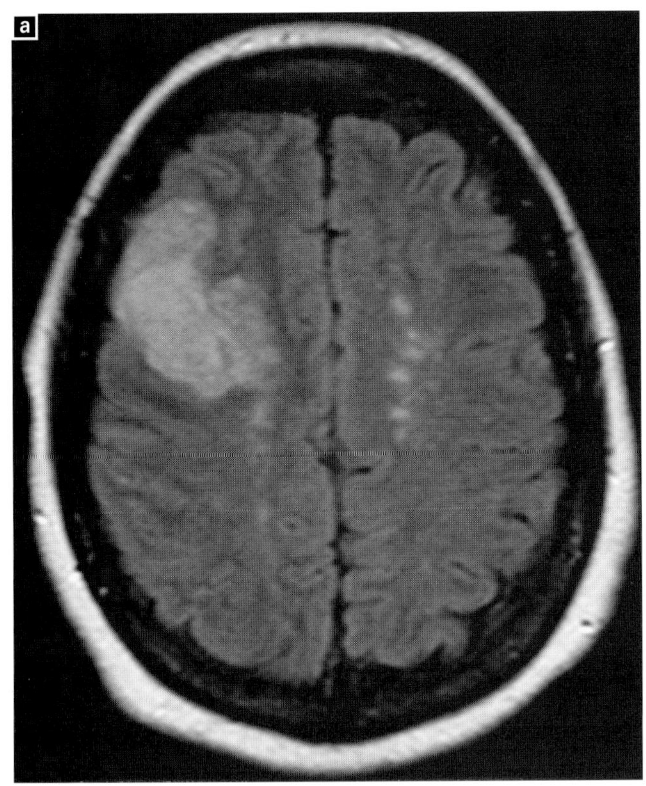
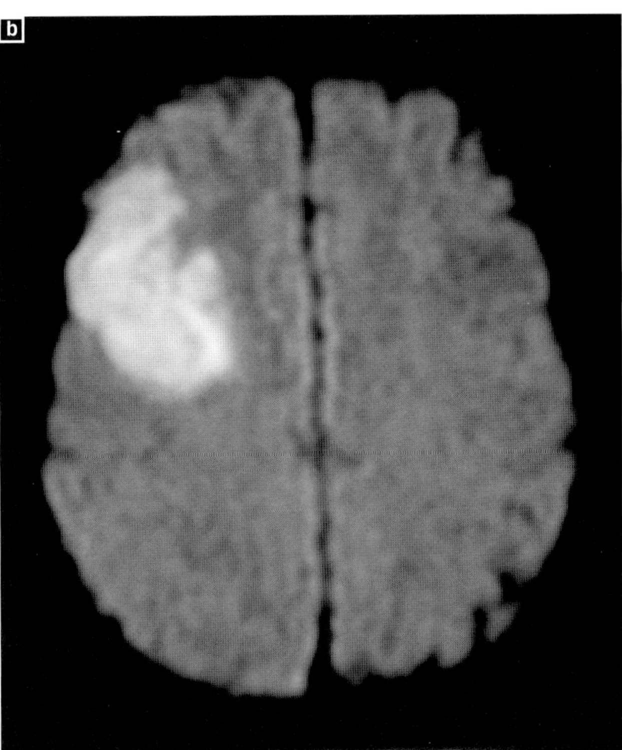

Fig. 7.9. **(a) Axial FLAIR and (b) DWI images.**

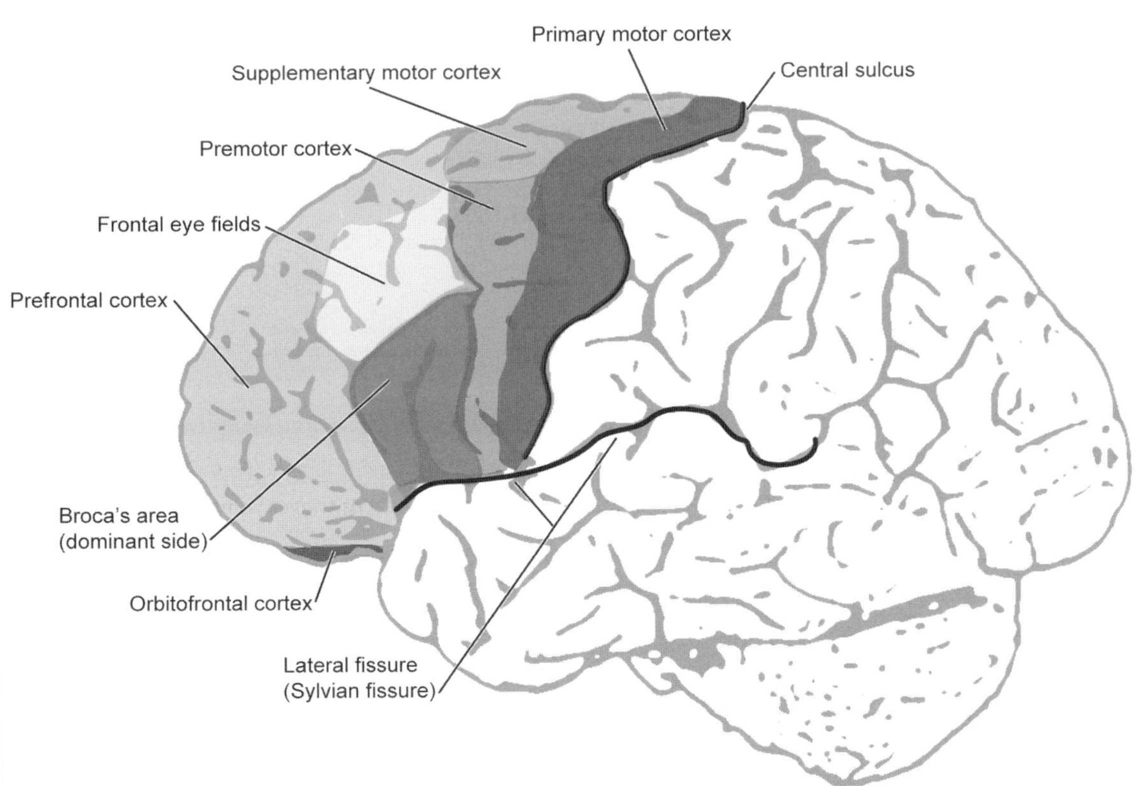

Fig. 7.10. **Location of the frontal eye field in the right middle frontal gyrus.**

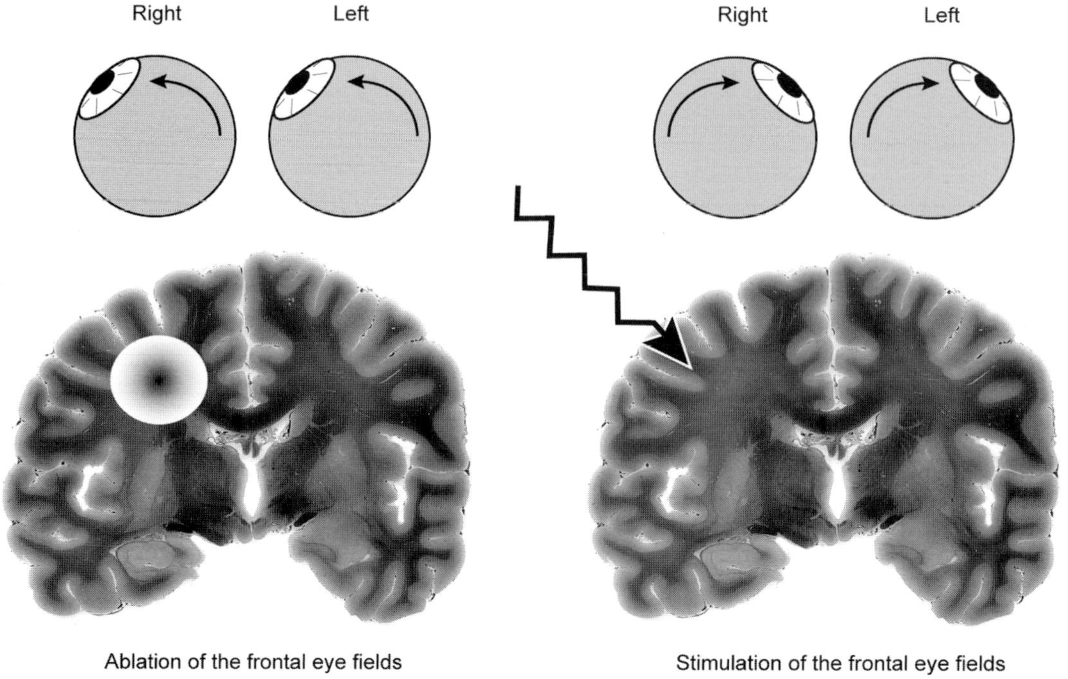

Fig. 7.11. **Gaze deviation toward the side of the lesion (to the right) with ablation of the right frontal eye field, as may occur with stroke, and gaze deviation away from the side of the lesion (to the left) with excess stimulation of the right frontal eye field, as may occur with a seizure focus.**

side, and there is contralateral eye deviation with seizures. For an interesting discussion, the reader is referred to Tijssen's paper (Tijssen, 1994).

Finally, we need to point out that there is currently some controversy in the world of neuro-ophthalmology regarding the precise location of the frontal eye fields in humans. Above, we glibly stated that the location is in Brodmann's area 8. This assertion is based primarily on animal studies. More recent functional imaging studies now suggest that, in humans, the frontal eye fields may lie a bit more posteriorly, along the anterior edge of the premotor cortex in Brodmann's area 6, at the junction of the superior frontal sulcus with the precentral

sulcus (see, for example Petit *et al.*, 1997). We will leave the particularly interested readers to follow this controversy on their own.

References

Petit, L., Clark, V. P., Ingeholm, J. *et al.* Dissociation of saccade-related and pursuit-related activation in human frontal eye fields as revealed by fMRI. *Journal of Neurophysiology* 1997; **77**(6): 3386–3390.

Tijssen, C.C. Contralateral conjugate eye deviation in acute supratentorial lesions. *Stroke* 1994; **25**(7): 1516–1519.

Case 7.4

59-year-old man presents with sudden onset of left arm numbness and tingling, as well as mild facial numbness. Sensory testing showed significant deficits in all sensory modalities involving the right hand and arm.

MRI images are presented below. What are the findings? Where is the lesion located?

In Fig. 7.12, the central sulcus is labelled. Posterior to it is the postcentral gyrus, where the primary sensory strip is located. The FLAIR and diffusion weighted images reveal a small infarct involving the right sensory strip, consistent with the patient's left-sided sensory symptoms.

Discuss the cortical sensory areas.

Somatosensory information from the body is carried via the medial lemniscus (the continuation of the posterior columns which carry sensory information for vibration, proprioception, and two-point discrimination) and the spinothalamic tract (mediating touch, pain, and temperature) to the ventral posterolateral nucleus of the contralateral thalamus (VPL). Similar information

from the head is carried via the trigeminothalamic tract to the ventral posteromedial nucleus of the thalamus (VPM). This sensory information is relayed from the VPL and the VPM to the primary somatosensory cortex (SI), which is located in the postcentral gyrus of the parietal lobe, directly behind the central sulcus. The primary somatosensory area corresponds to Brodmann's areas 1, 2, and 3 (see Fig. 7.1 and 7.2). Areas 1, 2 and 3 form long thin parallel strips, each of which contains neurons with slightly different functions. For example, the neurons in Brodmann's area 1 reflect activity in rapidly adapting cutaneous receptors, while those in area 2 are concerned with deep receptors such as those in the joints. This level of detail, though, is beyond what is typically clinically relevant. It is important to know, however, that the body is mapped along the somatosensory cortex in a manner very similar to that along the motor cortex, with a sensory homunculus which projects different areas of the body along different regions of the cortical ribbon (Fig. 7.13).

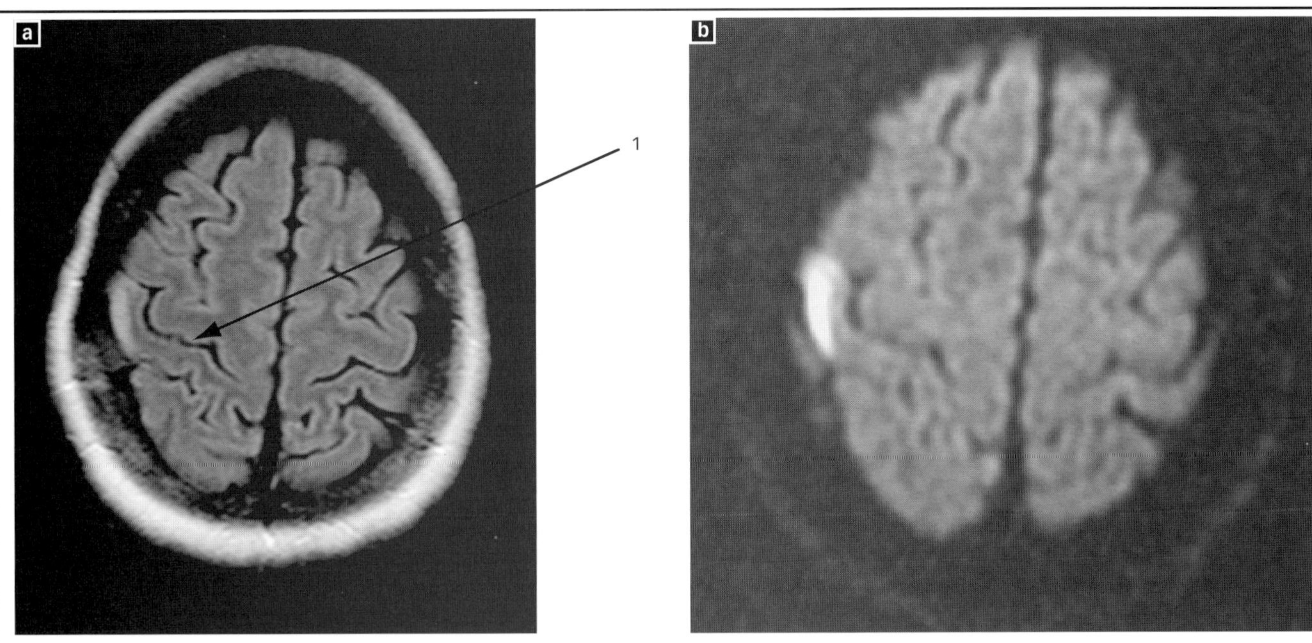

Fig. 7.12. **(a) FLAIR and (b) diffusion-weighted MR images are presented. Label #1 indicates the central sulcus.**

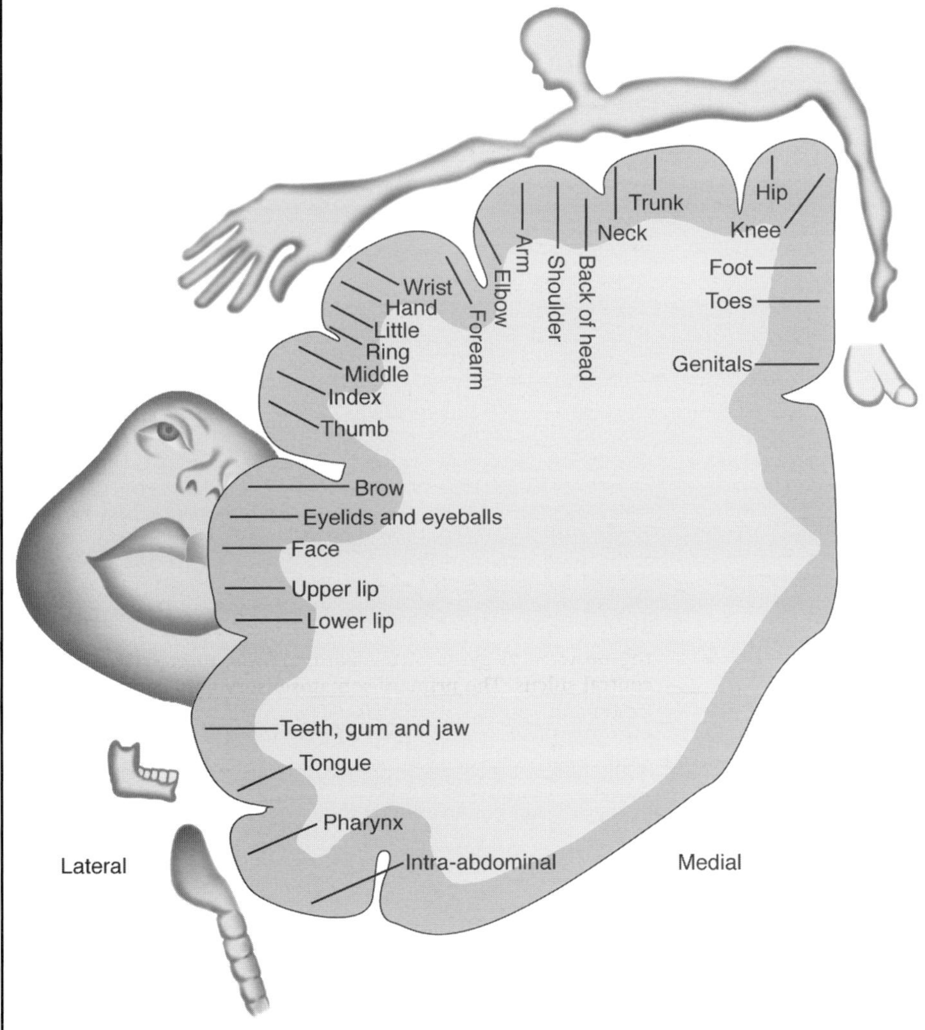

Fig. 7.13. **Representation of sensory homunculus along the right postcentral gyrus.**

The pharynx and tongue are represented along the inferior-most portion of the lateral parietal convexity along the sensory strip, followed by the face, hand, arm, and trunk. The leg and foot area are represented along the medial surface of the somatosensory cortex, in the posterior portion of the paracentral lobule. The anal and genital regions are just inferior to the foot area, along the medial surface of the sensory strip. As is the case with the motor homunculus, there is an exaggerated representation of the face, lips, hand, and finger areas, particularly the index finger.

Electrical stimulation of the primary sensory cortex in patients causes sensations of tingling, or sensations of movement without actual movement being elicited. These sensations occur in the contralateral body. It is noted, however, that the face and tongue have a bilateral representation.

What happens with lesions of the somatosensory cortex?

According to some authors, lesions of the sensory cortex, such as infarcts, typically present with loss of all sensory modalities in the contralateral body corresponding to the area of the lesion. Over time, though, there is some recovery of pain, touch, and temperature sensation, although these sensations are more vague than normal. The patient, however, will have loss of discrimination. In other words, he or she will have difficulty localizing the source and the severity of pain sensations, although they will have awareness of pain. The patient will also have difficulty with two-point discrimination, body position and proprioception, as well as difficulty recognizing objects by feel (astereognosis). This constellation of findings is sometimes referred to as the Verger–Dejerine cortical sensory syndrome. The dissociation between relatively intact sensations of pain, temperature, and touch, but loss of discrimination and position sense may be because pain, temperature, and touch are processed at the thalamic level, and also have some representation in the secondary sensory area SII (to be discussed below). Thus, after a stroke, for example, there may be some recovery of pain, temperature, and touch sensations. Interestingly, however, there is little recovery of proprioception or two-point discrimination, since two-point discrimination and proprioception seem to depend on an intact cortex, and joint receptors do not seem to project to the secondary sensory area (see Fig. 7.14).

The above discussion, though, gives only one possible scenario of deficits following a lesion of the sensory cortex. There are actually a number of so-called cortical sensory syndromes, and parietal lobe lesions may present with a complex array of clinical findings. For example, in the Dejerine–Mouzon "syndrome," there is loss of pain, touch, temperature, vibration, and proprioception in the contralateral body. While usually due to thalamic lesions, it has also been described with large parietal lesions which involve cortex and white matter. Other described deficits include a pseudothalamic pain syndrome, as well as a pseudocerebellar syndrome with incoordination of the contralateral limbs. Finally, since the sensory strip supplies a significant number of fibers to the corticospinal tract, lesions there may have motor manifestations such as hemiparesis, poverty of movement without gross weakness, or sometimes hypotonia.

Discuss the secondary sensory area.

A secondary somatosensory area (SII) has also been described in humans. It is located deep in the parietal operculum, along the superior lip of the Sylvian fissure, along the posterior-inferior margin of the sensory strip. The body is represented in this area in a homunculus-like fashion as well, but in the opposite order to the representation in the primary somatosensory area. Thus, the two face areas end up being adjacent to each other. Interestingly, the body is represented bilaterally in SII, and the neurons have large receptive fields, which overlap with each other. The secondary somatosensory area receives input both from the primary

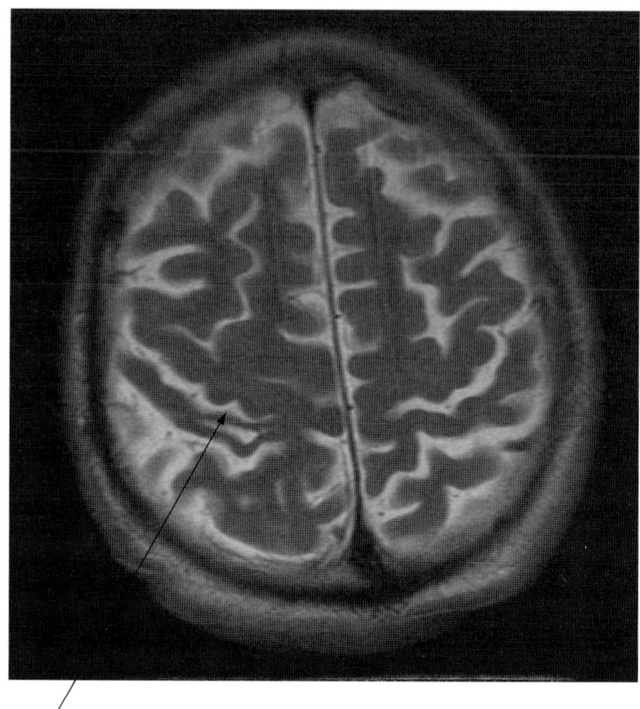

Fig. 7.14. **Patient with an old infarct involving the right sensory strip (arrow). The patient recovered vague sensations of touch, pain, and temperature in the left arm, but had significant impairment with two-point discrimination and proprioception in the left arm and hand, illustrating that these modalities depend on an intact cortex, and do not recover well after infarct.**

somatosensory cortex, as well as from the VPL and VPM nuclei of the thalamus. This area seems to be extremely important in the perception of pain, and its precise role is now a subject of intense study. For an excellent and in depth review of the role of SII in pain perception, the reader is referred to Treede *et al.*, 2000. A very interesting neurological condition, called asymbolia for pain, has also been related to lesions in this area. This condition entails the absence of appropriate emotional responses to pain (such as psychological discomfort, fear, or withdrawal), although the patient is aware of the presence of pain. Some authors have speculated that this condition, typically seen with lesions of the insula and surrounding operculum, apparently more frequently on the left, is actually a disconnection syndrome, possibly separating SII from the limbic system (see Berthier *et al.*, 1988).

In general, we note that, although the primary and secondary sensory areas are key to processing somatic sensations, there is still a great deal to be understood about the integration of sensory stimuli into a conscious sensory experience, and this is probably a distributed function involving multiple cortical areas. A recent paper, for example, begins as follows: "There is a severe lack of knowledge regarding the brain regions involved in human sexual performance in general, and female orgasm in particular." This paper presents a study of cerebral blood flow changes during female orgasm, and attempts to provide an integrated theory of how different cortical regions participate in the experience of orgasm (see Georgiadis *et al.*, 2006). I mention this for two reasons: to show that there is much left to learn about how sensations are integrated into a full "sensory experience" at the cortical level, and to show that some people get all the really cool research projects – while others of us are stuck writing and reading clinical neuroanatomy!

References

Berthier, M., Starkstein, S., and Leiguarda, R. Asymbolia for pain: a sensory-limbic disconnection syndrome. *Annals of Neurology* 1988; **24**(1): 41–49.

Georgiadis, J. R., Kortekass, R., Kuipers, R. *et al.* Regional cerebral blood flow changes associated with clitorally induced orgasm in healthy women. *European Journal of Neuroscience* 2006; **24**(11): 3305–3316.

Treede, R.-D., Apkarian, A. V., Bromm, B. *et al.* Cortical representation of pain: functional characterization of nociceptive areas near the lateral sulcus. *Pain* 2000; **87**: 113–119.

Case 7.5

70-year-old male patient brought in by family because "he is just not himself." When pressed for details, the family stated that the patient was apathetic, and had become bland in his interactions. On examination, the patient was lying in bed with his eyes closed, and initially refused to open them. The patient exhibited left-sided hemineglect on both visual and tactile stimulation, ignoring stimuli from the left visual field and showing left-sided extinction with bilateral simultaneous tactile stimulation.

From the provided history and physical findings, where would you place the lesion? An MRI is provided (Fig. 7.15). What do you see?

The patient has an early subacute right parietal infarct involving both the somatosensory association cortex (Brodmann's area 5) as well as the large region of temporo-parieto-occipital multimodal association cortex which makes up the bulk of the parietal lobe.

Discuss the manifestations of right (more correctly, non-dominant) parietal infarcts.

Correlative neuroanatomy has certainly come a long way from a century ago, when the parietal lobes, particularly the non-dominant one, were considered "silent areas" of the brain. We now realize that the non-dominant hemisphere in general, and the non-dominant parietal lobe in particular, are very important in attention functions, as well as in integrative visuospatial functions, such as ascertaining the orientation of the body in space, or drawing figures. For the remainder of the discussion, we will assume that the non-dominant parietal lobe is the right one. It can be fairly stated that, while the left hemisphere attends to the right side of the body and the right external space, the right hemisphere attends to both sides of the internal and external space, but attends more strongly to the left side. This notion is corroborated by functional experiments, which show that the left hemisphere activates with right-sided stimulation, but the right hemisphere activates with both right- or left-sided stimuli, but responds more strongly to left-sided stimulation. This is the flip side of the left hemispheric dominance in motor planning, where it has been shown that the left pre-motor cortex is active in planning motion with either hand, but that the right pre-motor cortex activates only for left-sided motion (see Blumenfeld, 2002). Not only does the right parietal lobe attend to the right as well as to the left sides, it is also hypothesized that the right parietal lobe attends to the left side more strongly than the left parietal lobe attends to the right side, again underscoring the predominance of the right hemisphere in attention functions.

This long-winded exegesis explains two important clinical points: (1) parietal lobe lesions can present with contralateral hemineglect; (2) hemineglect occurs much more commonly with right parietal lobe lesions than with left. That is because, when the left parietal lobe is infarcted, for example, the right parietal lobe still partially attends to the right side, and because attention functions in general are more localized to the right hemisphere as mentioned above (see Weintraub and Mesulam, 1987).

Discuss the different manifestations of hemineglect.

Hemineglect is a complex and fascinating topic (see, for example, Kerkhoff, 2001). There are several forms of hemineglect, but we can classify them broadly into sensory hemineglect, motor hemineglect, and conceptual hemineglect. Patients with sensory hemineglect tend to ignore stimuli, usually visual and tactile, on the side contralateral to the lesion. Tactile hemineglect can be tested by checking for extinction with double-simultaneous stimulation. For example, when the patient is touched on both arms, they neglect the touch on the left side. Another manifestation of sensory hemineglect is called allesthesia, where the patient, when touched on the left, reports the stimulus on the right. Motor hemineglect manifests with ignoring the contralateral body in making motor movements, so patients, for instance, barely move their left arm, although it is not paralyzed. Alternatively, patients may not make movements within the contralateral hemispace. This can be tested, for instance, by asking patients to collect coins from a table while blindfolded, and observing that they do not collect coins toward the left. A nice test for combined sensory and motor hemineglect is the line-cancellation test, where the patient is asked to cross out lines on a piece of paper (to make them into

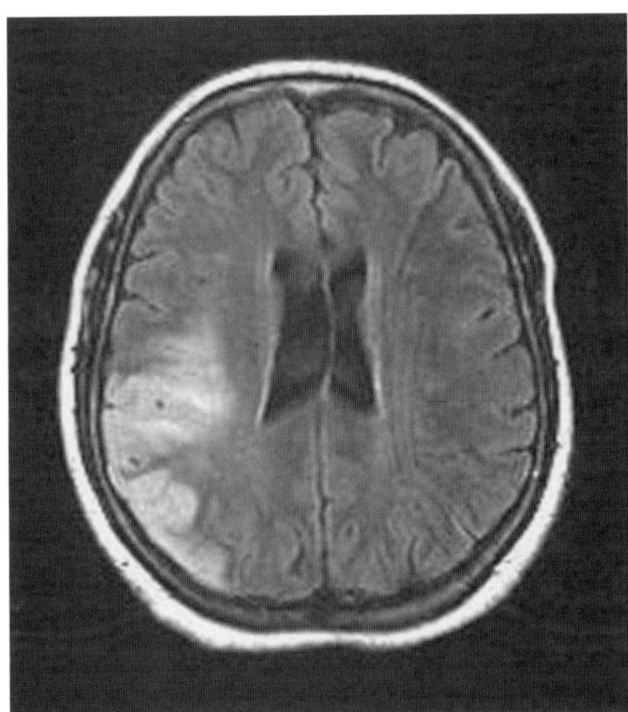

Fig. 7.15. **FLAIR axial MRI.**

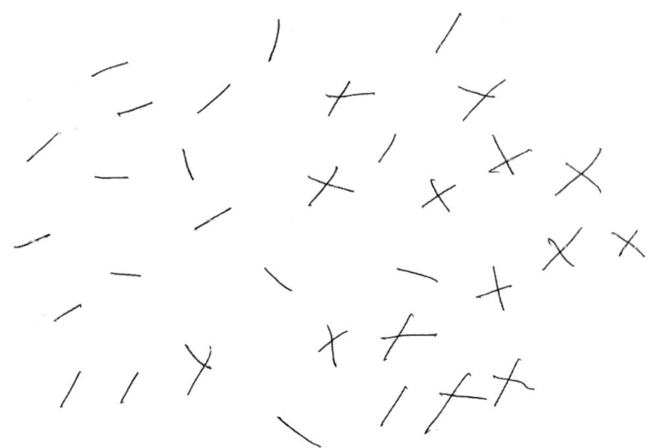

Fig. 7.16. **Typical line-cancellation pattern in a patient with combined sensory and motor left hemineglect after a right parietal infarct. The lines on the left are ignored.**

Xs). Patients will ignore the lines on the left side of the paper (Fig. 7.16).

The most interesting form of hemineglect is conceptual hemineglect, where a patient's internal representation schema of either their own body or of the external world becomes disrupted. There have been reports of patients who comb only one side of their head, or shave only one side of their face! A fairly common presentation of conceptual hemineglect is anosognosia, where the patient is unaware of his or her deficit on the contralateral side. For instance, a patient with profound left hemiparesis may deny entirely that anything is wrong with them. They wonder why they are in the hospital, and when asked to lift the left arm, they lift the right instead (this is called allokinesia), or make excuses such as, "I'm tired now." For a bit of gamesmanship on rounds, do you know the eponym associated with anosognosia? It is sometimes referred to as the Anton–Babinski syndrome. For an interesting discussion of the confabulation that occurs with anosognosia, see Feinberg *et al.*, 1994.

A truly unusual and fascinating presentation of conceptual hemineglect is hemiasomatognosia, where the patients entirely lose awareness that the left side of their body belongs to them. In one case, a woman would repeatedly wake up screaming, "someone left a leg in my bed," because she did not recognize that her left leg was part of her body.

References

Blumenfeld, H. *Neuroanatomy Through Clinical Cases*. Sinauer Publishers, Sunderland, MA, 2002; 839.

Feinberg, T. E., Roane, D. M., Kwan, P. C., *et al*. Anosognosia and visuoverbal confabulation. *Archives of Neurology*. 1994; **51**(5): 468–473.

Kerkhoff, G. Spatial hemineglect in humans. *Progress in Neurobiology* 2001; **63**(1): 1–27.

Weintraub, S., and Mesulam, M.M. Right cerebral dominance in spatial attention: Further evidence based on ipsilateral neglect. *Archives of Neurology* 1987; **44**: 621–625.

Case 7.6

64-year-old male patient presented with a progressive onset of inability to express his thoughts in writing. On clinical examination, the patient also displayed right–left disorientation upon motor testing.

An MRI examination is presented (Fig. 7.17). What are the findings?

The MRI shows a subacute infarct in the left parietal lobe. The location of the lesion suggests that the inferior parietal lobule, in the area of the left angular gyrus and surrounding subangular white matter, is involved (see Fig. 7.1(a)).

What other findings should you test for?

The presence of agraphia and right–left disorientation brings to mind an unusual tetrad of findings which sometimes occur together: (1) agraphia; (2) right–left disorientation; (3) acalculia (the inability to do mathematical calculations); and (4) finger agnosia (the inability to name or identify the fingers of either hand).

A bright resident was aware of this unusual tetrad, and upon testing our patient, found all components present. The patient had no other motor, sensory, or visual deficits.

What is your diagnosis?

The tetrad of clinical findings described above is known as Gerstmann's syndrome. It is quite rare, but fairly distinct. It is typically secondary to a lesion in the left inferior parietal lobule, particularly in the left angular gyrus. While there has been some controversy as to whether such a syndrome truly exists, and whether it can be due to localized inferior parietal lobule lesions, the preponderant opinion seems to be that Gerstmann's syndrome is indeed a distinct, albeit unusual, entity. For an excellent review of this syndrome, please see Mayer *et al.* (1999). The underlying neuropsychiatric basis for this syndrome, and how the angular gyrus contributes to each of the four disrupted functions, is still under investigation. However, a recent cortical electrostimulation study provides strong evidence that the tetrad of Gerstmann's syndrome indeed maps to the region of the left angular gyrus (Roux *et al.*, 2003). Another interesting line of support that there is a genuine association between the four entities which constitute Gerstmann's syndrome can be found in the pediatric neurology literature, where a developmental form of Gerstmann's syndrome has been described (Suresh and Sebastian, 2000). Children afflicted with this disorder have difficulty with spelling and writing, learning basic mathematics, as well as with right–left orientation and finger recognition. They also often have an associated constructional apraxia, with difficulty reproducing figures. This cluster of findings is sometimes seen in children who are otherwise highly intellectually functioning. However, as with adult Gerstmann's syndrome, the developmental variant is also a controversial entity, with some authors stating that the occurrence of the symptoms is a chance association (Miller and Hynd, 2004).

It is noted that other than strokes and tumors, Gerstmann's syndrome has been described in association with herpes simplex encephalitis, progressive multifocal leukoencephalopathy, subdural hematoma, and tumors (Fig. 7.18).

Now that we have surveyed some of the findings associated with right and left parietal lobe lesions in the last two cases, *please give a synopsis of the manifestations of lesions in the parietal lobes.*

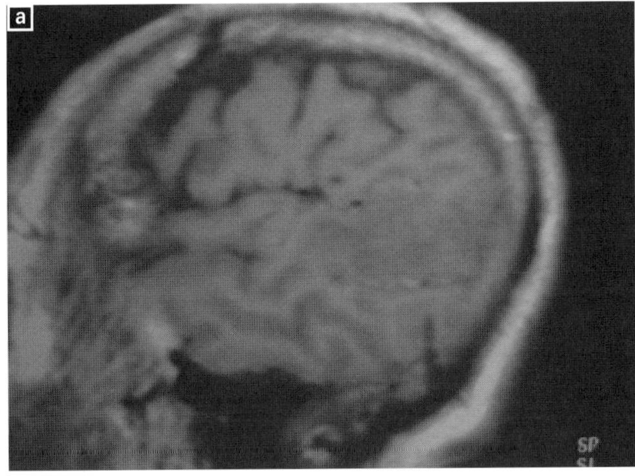

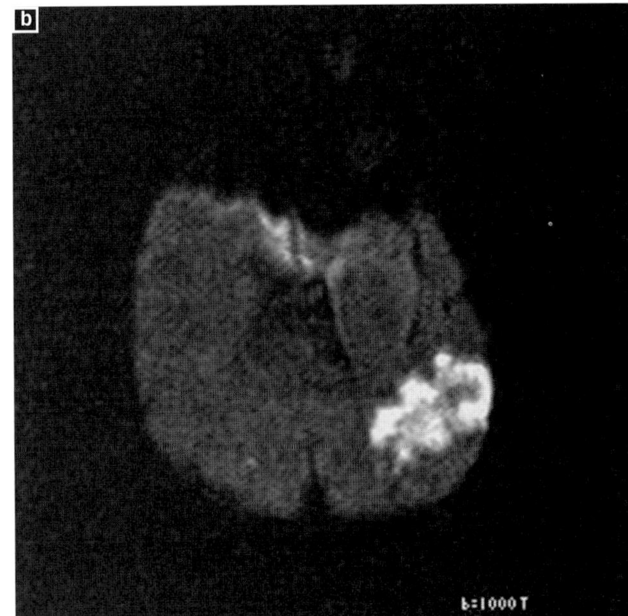

Fig. 7.17. **(a) T1-weighted sagittal and (b) DWI axial MRI images.**

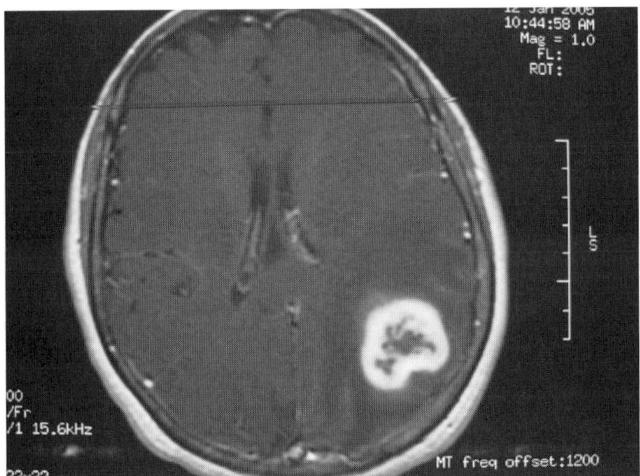

Fig. 7.18. **T1-weighted axial post-contrast image reveals an enhancing tumor in the left inferior parietal lobe in this patient, who presented with the classic tetrad of Gerstmann's syndrome.**

This question is even more difficult than it looks. It evokes a few lines from Adams and Victor's well-known textbook, *Principles of Neurology*: "Within the brain, no other territory surpasses the parietal lobes in the rich variety of clinical phenomena that are exposed under conditions of disease." (Victor and Ropper, 2001). We present here the more common entities, partially based on their summary of the variety of neurologic disorders caused by lesions of the parietal lobes.

(1) Lesions of either the right or left parietal lobe
   (a) Cortical sensory syndromes, such as hemianesthesia and loss of discriminative functions, contralateral to the lesion.
   (b) Motor findings on the contralateral side, such as mild hemiparesis, hypotonia, poverty of movement, or hemiataxia

(2) Lesions of the left (dominant) parietal lobe – additional manifestations
   (a) Gerstmann's syndrome
   (b) Astereognosis (inability to recognize objects by touch using either hand).
   (c) Bilateral ideational apraxia (loss of ability to conceptualize the use of common instruments, such as a pen or screwdriver).
   (d) Alexia (inability to read).
(3) Lesions of the right (non-dominant) parietal lobe – additional manifestations
   (a) Hemineglect, including sensory, motor, and conceptual, with such manifestations as anosognosia and hemiasomatognosia.
   (b) Visuospatial disorders, including constructional apraxia
   (c) Loss of geographic and topiographic orientation
   (d) Apathy
   (e) Tendency to keep the eyes closed and to resist opening them, without motor weakness

References

Mayer, E., Martory, M. D., Pegna, A. J., *et al.* A pure case of Gerstmann syndrome with a subangular lesion. *Brain* 1999; **122** (6): 1107–1120.

Miller, C. J., and Hynd, G. W. What ever happened to developmental Gerstmann's syndrome? Links to other pediatric, genetic, and neurodevelopmental syndromes. *Journal of Child Neurology* 2004; **19**(4): 282–289.

Roux, F. E., Boetto, S., Sacko, O. *et al.* Writing, calculating, and finger recognition in the region of the angular gyrus: a cortical stimulation study of Gerstmann syndrome. *Journal of Neurosurgery* 2003; **99**(4): 716–727.

Suresh, P. A., and Sebastian, S. Developmental Gerstmann's syndrome: a distinct clinical entity of learning disabilities. *Pediatric Neurology* 2000; **22**(4): 267–278.

Victor, M. and Ropper, A. *Adams and Victor's Principles of Neurology*, 7th edn. McGraw-Hill Publishers, 2001; 483.

Case 7.7

58-year-old patient presents with an acute onset inability to speak. Testing revealed that the patient had very little spontaneous speech, using only single or very few words, such as "yes" and "no." The patient grunted and was frustrated by his inability to speak. He could not repeat words. However, his comprehension was relatively intact, and he was able to obey commands. There was moderate right-hand and right lower facial weakness.

From the history and physical findings, what is your diagnosis? Where do you expect the lesion to be?

The patient appears to have a primary disturbance of language, with markedly impaired expression, and relatively intact comprehension. This suggests a so-called "expressive" or Broca's aphasia. This typically occurs with lesions involving Broca's area, along the posterior aspect of the left frontal operculum (Fig. 7.19).

An MRI examination is provided (Fig. 7.20). What are the findings?

There is an early subacute infarct involving the left frontal operculum (Broca's area), left insula and left peri-insular region. The left postero-superior temporal region, corresponding to Wernicke's area, is spared.

Describe the main language areas in the brain.

Language is a very complex function. It resides predominantly in the dominant (usually left) hemisphere. In fact, in 90–95 percent of right-handed individuals and in 60–70 percent of left-handed individuals, almost all language functions are in the left hemisphere.

In broad terms, we can consider that the brain has two main centers, or better yet, systems, involved in language processing. There is an expressive, or executive system, responsible for language production, and a receptive system, involved in language comprehension. Integral to the expressive system is Broca's area (Brodmann's areas 44 and 45), which correspond to the triangular and opercular portions of the left frontal operculum (Fig. 7.19). Integral to the receptive system is Wernicke's area (the posterior aspect of Brodman's area 22, along the posterior aspect of the left superior temporal gyrus – Fig. 7.19). Broca's and Wernicke's areas are part of a larger region which surrounds the insular cortex, considered to be the main language region of the brain.

In the 1860s and 1870s, when Broca and Wernicke described the types of aphasia named for them, it was felt that language functions in the brain resided in specific anatomic areas, much like movement is associated with the motor cortex. In the early to mid 20th century, this view fell out of favor, and gave way to a more systems-oriented holistic approach, which treated language as a distributed brain function predominantly in the left hemisphere. The last few decades have seen a compromise view arise, where it is felt that Broca's and Wernicke's areas indeed do have specificity for expressive and receptive language functions respectively, but that they work in close conjunction with adjacent association cortex in the frontal and temporal-parietal-occipital regions as part of an entire language system. This language system also communicates with homologous areas in the right brain, which has some role in the emotional aspects connected to language (Fig. 7.21).

This system, displayed in Fig. 7.21, is perhaps the best available simple model to understand the various types of aphasia, and to attempt to correlate them to the different locations of lesions which produce them. It is stressed, however, that this correlation is much looser than the pathologic correlation seen with modality-specific areas of the brain such as the motor

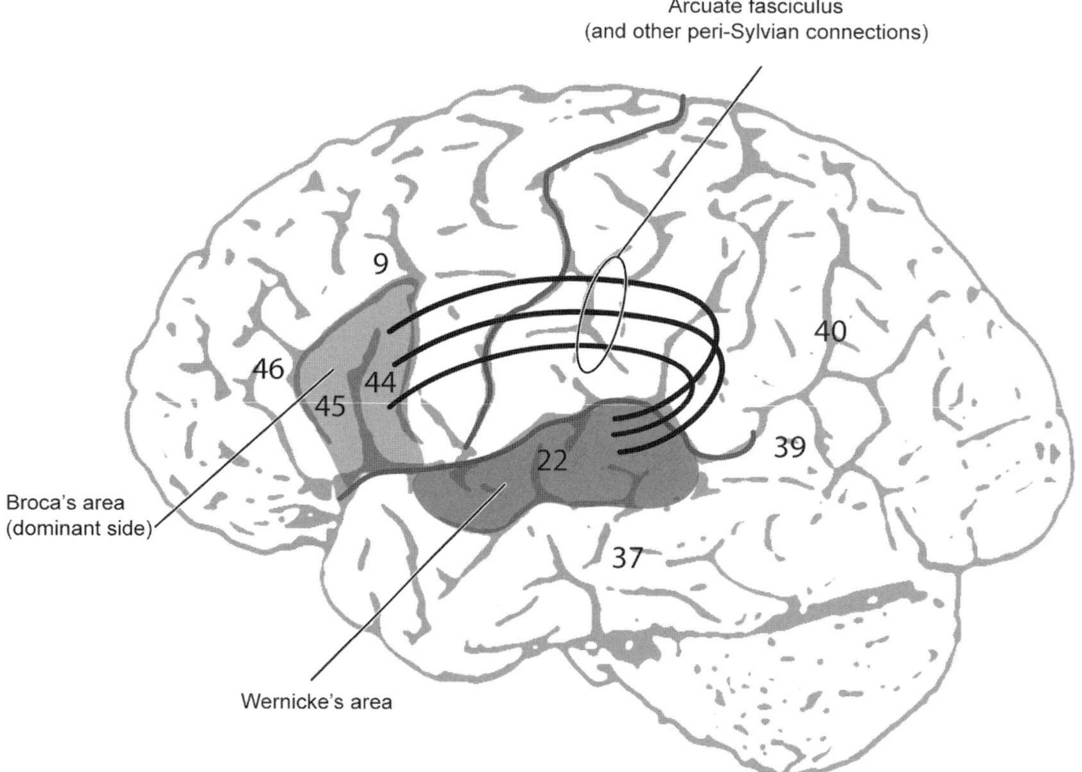

Fig. 7.19. **A schematic diagram showing the location of Broca's and Wernicke's regions, with corresponding Brodmann's area numbers. These two regions are connected by the arcuate fasciculus.**

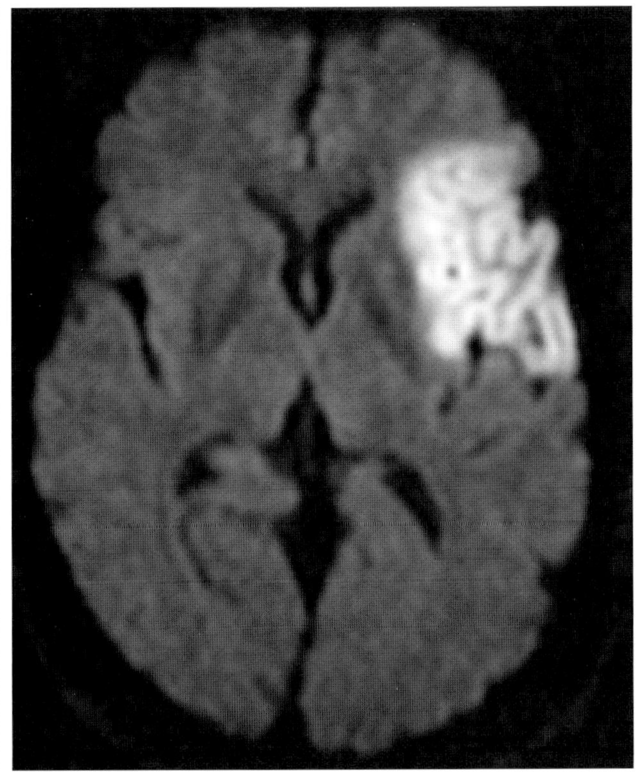

Fig. 7.20. **DWI MR image.**

cortex or the visual cortex. Hence, it is not always possible to predict either the location of the lesion from the observed deficit, or the type of deficit from an observed lesion. General correlations, though, are possible, and that is what we will attempt to do in this and the next few cases related to language.

Describe, in very general terms, the anatomy of language processing involved in repeating a phrase.

Referring to Fig. 7.19, we will break down the basic steps involved in repeating a phrase, and look at the language functions and brain regions that subserve this task. First, the phrase must be heard, which is a function of the auditory apparatus, ending in Heschel's area in the mid-aspect of the left superior temporal gyrus. The sounds which are heard are then decoded as words in the auditory association cortex (Wernicke's area), along the posterior aspect of the left superior temporal gyrus, posterior to Heschel's gyrus. Broca's area, in the left frontal operculum, is where the motor engrams for producing words reside. Impulses travel from Wernicke's area to Broca's area through the arcuate fasciculus, which curves along the posterior margin of the insula (Fig. 7.19). Broca's area then communicates with the facial region of the motor cortex, activating the necessary phonation apparatus of the mouth, tongue, and larynx, using the proper engrams to produce the words just heard, rather than inarticulate sounds.

More advanced linguistic functions, such as those needed to answer a question, require the larger language system in the left hemisphere (Fig. 7.21). Wernicke's area decodes sounds as words, and works closely with the adjacent left temporal–parietal association cortex, including such regions as the angular gyrus and the supramarginal gyrus, for full comprehension of meaning. This includes drawing up mental images of the nouns involved

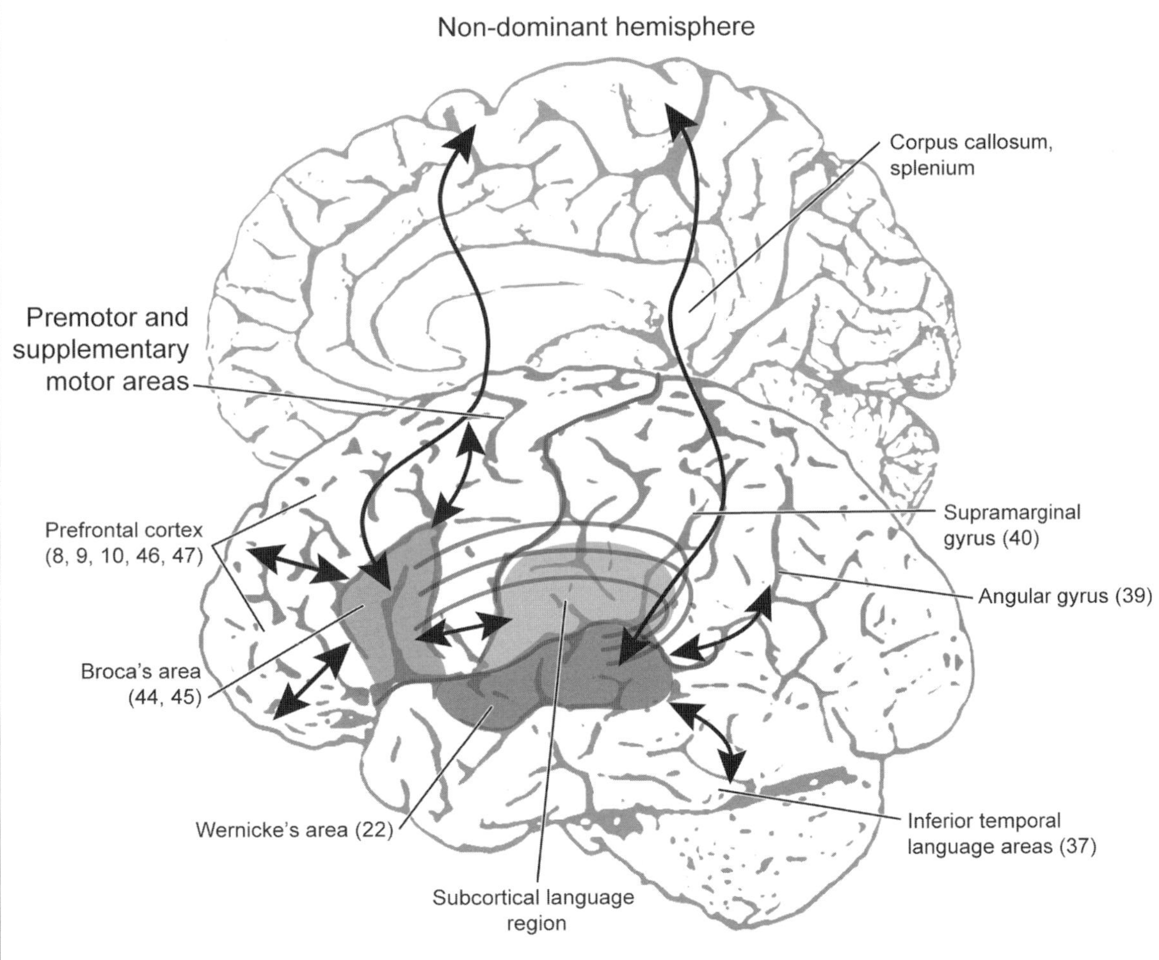

Fig. 7.21. **Schematic diagram showing Broca's and Wernicke's areas working in conjunction with multiple regions of adjacent association cortex and with homologous areas in the right hemisphere, as part of a larger language system based primarily in the peri-Sylvian left hemisphere.**

in the sentence, as well as understanding the actions connoted by the verbs in the sentence. Once the question is comprehended, the answer is formulated, presumably relying on the frontal association cortex, and the answer is then translated into word engrams in Broca's area, which then communicates with the appropriate motor regions to produce the words. Therefore, as shown in Fig. 7.21, Wernicke's and Broca's areas work closely with adjacent association cortex to subserve the complex linguistic functions which we take for granted. Figure 7.21 also shows connections between the primary language regions in the left hemisphere and homologous areas in the right hemisphere. Although we say that language is predominantly a left hemisphere function, there is interaction with the right hemisphere which appears to contribute to the emotional aspects of language.

The sort of model displayed in Figs. 7.19 and 7.21, albeit vastly oversimplified, will allow us to develop a basic schema to discuss the various types of aphasias, and relate them to commonly observed lesion locations.

Discuss Broca's aphasia.

First, aphasias must be distinguished from other speech problems. We must be clear that aphasia is a defect in language (either speech production or speech comprehension), and that this is very different from a defect in speech articulation, known as dysarthria.

After this distinction is made, we will divide the aphasias into two main types, Broca's (also sometimes called expressive, motor, anterior, or non-fluent aphasia), and Wernicke's (also called receptive, sensory, posterior, or fluent aphasia). We will describe the other types of aphasias, in later cases, in relation to Broca's and Wernicke's aphasias, which we consider as the two main prototypes.

As we have already discussed, Broca's area is integral in the expressive part of linguistic function. Therefore, the salient abnormality in Broca's aphasia is loss of the ability to produce language, most obviously marked by a decrease in the fluency of spontaneous speech. In severe cases, the patient may appear to have lost all power of speech, or may preserve only a very few words, such as our patient above. Typically, there is a significant paucity of language, with a word frequency of 10–15 per minute, compared to normal speech, which contains between 100 and 120 words per minute. Patients with Broca's aphasia tend to have what is called "telegraphic" speech, relying on basic nouns and verbs to try to express what they mean, and dropping such things as prepositions, articles, and adjectives. The speech of such a patient seems to be very labored and very sparse. Also, patients with Broca's aphasia will show marked naming difficulties, and because Broca's area is involved, repetition is also markedly impaired. If the patient is asked to write, written language will show the same defects as spoken language, with very few words, and an agrammatical structure.

In examining a patient with Broca's aphasia, however, it becomes clear that even with the paucity of words, patients are often able to bring across at least some of what they mean, and the examiner has a definite sense that the patient is both purposeful in his linguistic attempts, and has a relatively intact comprehension of language. Therefore, patients with Broca's aphasia are typically able to obey spoken or written commands, and comprehend speech directed at them. Patients are also typically aware of their expressive deficits, and become quite frustrated by them.

These sorts of deficits can be understood using the simple model of Fig. 7.21. Wernicke's area is intact, so language comprehension is expected to be unaffected. Broca's area is involved, so language production is expected to be impaired, including repetition, since the impulses traveling from Wernicke's area cannot be received. As we will see, repetition is one of the key parameters used in classifying aphasias. Once again, though, it is stressed that this model – classifying Broca's aphasia as expressive and Wernicke's as receptive – is an oversimplification. The frontal association areas adjacent to Broca's area, for example, are critical in decoding complex syntactical structure. Thus, patients with Broca's aphasia often have some impairment in comprehension when the syntax is complex. Thus, in a sentence such as, "The cat was bitten by the dog," a patient with Broca's may think that the dog is the one who was bitten.

Interestingly, although we equate Broca's aphasia with Broca's area in the brain, it must be noted that most neurologists recognize that lesions confined just to Broca's area produce only mild expressive linguistic impairment. The typical Broca's aphasia is caused by a larger lesion which not only involves Broca's area, but the surrounding regions in the left frontal and left insular cortex as well, as in our patient. The distinction is thus sometimes drawn between a "big Broca's aphasia" versus a "little Broca's aphasia." Part of the confusion, of course, stems from the fact that, when Broca described his aphasia, he imputed it to the region of the brain which has since come to be called Broca's area. Those interested in the history of neurology, though, are quick to point out that in one of Broca's original patients, anatomic examination of the brain showed a fairly extensive lesion that involved the frontal and parietal operculum as well as the peri-insular regions. Broca, however, attributed the patient's expressive aphasia to the lesion of the frontal operculum alone, considering the remainder of the stroke as non-contributory. Thus, even in Broca's own patient, Broca's aphasia was caused by a lesion that extended beyond Broca's area.

The most common etiology of Broca's aphasia is a left middle cerebral artery territory infarct. However, a slowly developing Broca's aphasia may be caused by tumor growing in the region of the left frontal operculum (see Fig. 7.22).

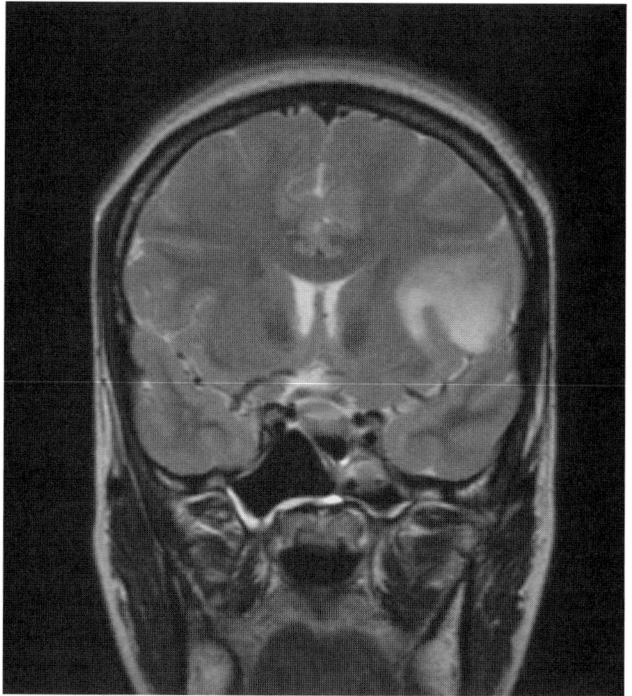

Fig. 7.22. **T2-weighted coronal image of a 26-year-old female patient with slowly progressive Broca's aphasia, which began as a naming difficulty. The patient has a glioma involving the left frontal operculum**.

Case 7.8

54-year-old hypertensive patient who developed sudden onset of "inability to communicate." While at home, the patient began speaking nonsensically, and was brought to the emergency room by his wife. Neurological examination was quite difficult, as the patient was unable to follow commands. He moved all extremities spontaneously. His speech was fluent, but made no sense. He was unable to repeat, name objects, or to read. The patient was pleasant, and seemed unaware of his remarkable deficits!

Based on the above, what is your diagnosis? Where do you think the lesion is?

The patient's main problem seems to be a receptive aphasia. He has no gross motor deficits, and displays fluent, although nonsensical speech, along with gross comprehension deficits. These signs suggest a Wernicke's aphasia, and a lesion in Wernicke's area (Brodmann's area 22 in the left superior temporal gyrus. See Fig. 7.19).

A follow-up MRI obtained during the patient's hospitalization is presented adjacent (Fig. 7.23). What are the findings?

MRI examination shows a hemorrhage in the left superior temporal gyrus, consistent with the above analysis, and with the diagnosis of Wernicke's aphasia.

Discuss Wernicke's aphasia.

Wernicke's aphasia, sometimes also called receptive or sensory aphasia, is most commonly caused by infarcts involving the inferior division of the left middle cerebral artery, but may be caused by tumor, bleed, or infection. It is characterized by the following:

(1) A severe impairment in the comprehension of spoken and written language.

(2) Fluent but nonsensical speech. The patient's speech usually has normal melody and rhythm, with a normal word frequency (about 120 words per minute), but is typically meaningless. Speech is filled with literal paraphasias (substituting sound-alike words, such as "nar" for "car") and neologisms (made-up word sounds which have no meaning).

(3) Marked impairment in naming of objects.

(4) Markedly impaired repetition (because Wernicke's area is disconnected from Broca's).

(5) The patient often seems unconcerned or unaware of his or her deficits (anosognosia). This is in sharp contrast to the typical presentation of Broca's aphasia, where the patient is aware of, and frustrated by, their inability to speak.

Another interesting facet of Wernicke's aphasia is that the patient can often easily understand commands given in sign language; thus, the comprehension deficits seem to be confined to spoken and written language, and do not extend to all communication. Patients with Wernicke's aphasia do not typically have significant motor weakness or dysarthria, but they may have a right homonymous hemianopsia secondary to involvement of the left optic radiations as they pass through the temporal lobe (most commonly a right superior quadrantanopsia from interruption of the geniculo-temporal radiations).

Although typically oblivious to their deficits but otherwise pleasant, patients with severe Wernicke's aphasia may present with jargon aphasia or "word salad" (completely incomprehensible speech), increased word output (known as logorrhea), and paranoia. This constellation can lead to a mistaken diagnosis of schizophrenia.

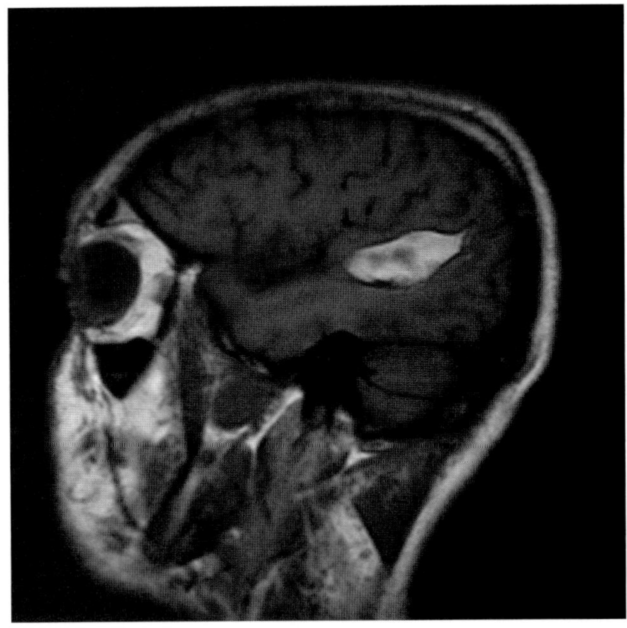

Fig. 7.23. **Left parasagittal T1-weighted MRI image.**

While classic Wernicke's aphasia typically entails severe comprehension deficits in both spoken and written language, one or the other facet may predominate. If the patient has much greater difficulty understanding written language, this is referred to as Wernicke's aphasia with predominant word blindness. It is more often seen with lesions that extend to the inferior parietal lobule and the angular gyrus. If the patient's comprehension of spoken language is significantly more affected, this is called Wernicke's aphasia with predominant word deafness. The lesions here tend to be in the depth of the superior temporal gyrus. This latter condition though, needs to be distinguished from a much rarer language disorder, known as "pure word deafness." In that syndrome, patients cannot understand spoken language and cannot repeat, but have no impairment in understanding written language, and no impairment in perceiving and identifying nonverbal sounds, such as a telephone ring. Pure word deafness usually results from bilateral superior temporal gyrus lesions involving Heschel's gyrus, but can result from left temporal lesions alone that involve Heschel's gyrus and/or the radiations from the left medial geniculate nucleus to Heschel's gyrus. Wernicke's area is typically spared. This syndrome, thus, is not a true aphasia or language disorder, but rather a defect in transmitting verbal auditory signals to the language areas for interpretation. Therefore, it is a form of auditory verbal agnosia, closer to deafness than to aphasia. The interested reader may refer to Coslett *et al.*, 1984.

Reference

Coslett, H. B., Brashear, H. R., and Heilman, K. M. Pure word deafness after bilateral primary auditory cortex infarcts. *Neurology* 1984; **34**: 347.

Case 7.9

57-year-old patient presents with "speech disturbance." Motor and sensory examination is unremarkable. The patient has intact comprehension, and follows commands. On language testing, speech is fluent, although with slightly decreased verbal output. Repetition, however, is markedly impaired.

MRI is presented (Fig. 7.24). What are the findings? What is your diagnosis?

There is a subacute infarct along the left posterior insular margin. The patient displays intact comprehension and intact verbal output, but has a marked defect in repetition.

Diagnosis

Conduction aphasia.

Conduction aphasia occurs when Broca's area is disconnected from Wernicke's area, but both areas remain intact. This occurs with lesions of the arcuate fasciculus (Fig. 7.19). Such lesions are typically along the posterior margin of the upper bank of the left Sylvian fissure, because the arcuate fasciculus bends around the posterior end of the left Sylvian fissure as it goes from Wernicke's

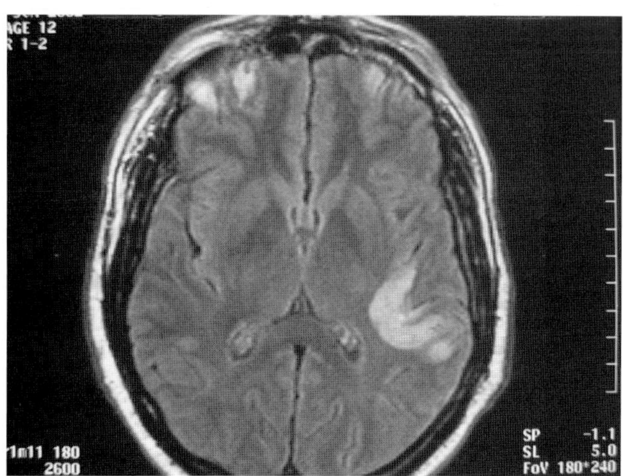

Fig. 7.24. **FLAIR axial MRI.**

area in the left superior temporal gyrus to Broca's area in the left frontal operculum (Fig. 7.19). Because Wernicke's area is intact, comprehension is preserved. Because Broca's area is intact, speech is fluent. However, repetition is impaired, as expected from a disconnection between the two areas. Also, speech contains frequent paraphasic errors. Not surprisingly, reading aloud is also impaired, with many paraphasic substitutions. Patients, however, can read silently with good comprehension. As opposed to Wernicke's aphasia, patients are typically aware of their deficits. This syndrome – conduction aphasia – originally described by Wernicke, lends support to the notion that language function is somewhat compartmentalized into receptive and expressive regions.

We have now discussed Broca's, Wernicke's and conduction aphasia. Do you know any other types? Please describe them, as well as a functional scheme for classifying aphasias.

The main types of aphasia are as follows:

(1) Broca's aphasia
(2) Wernicke's aphasia
(3) Conduction aphasia
(4) Global aphasia
(5) Transcortical aphasia
    (a) Transcortical motor aphasia
    (b) Transcortical sensory aphasia
    (c) Mixed transcortical aphasia
(6) Anomic aphasia

Global aphasia is a severe language disturbance, involving all of its aspects. Specifically, the patient shows severe deficits in speech output, speech comprehension, and in repetition. Global aphasia usually occurs secondary to large infarcts involving the bulk of the left MCA territory, including both Broca's area and Wernicke's area. Such an aphasia is typically associated with a right hemiparesis (Fig. 7.25a). Rarely, even in

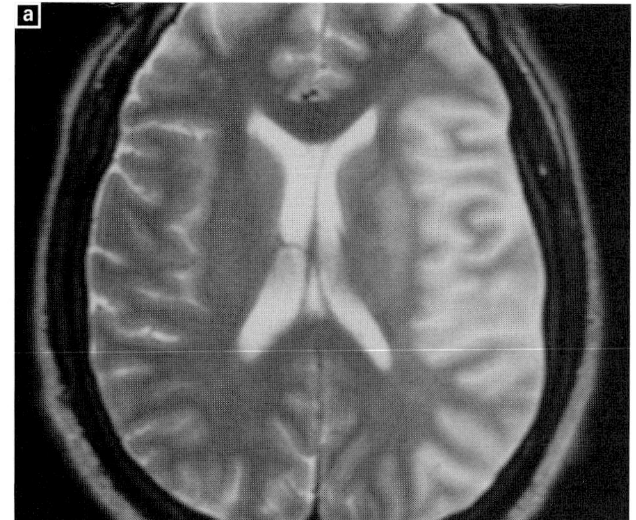
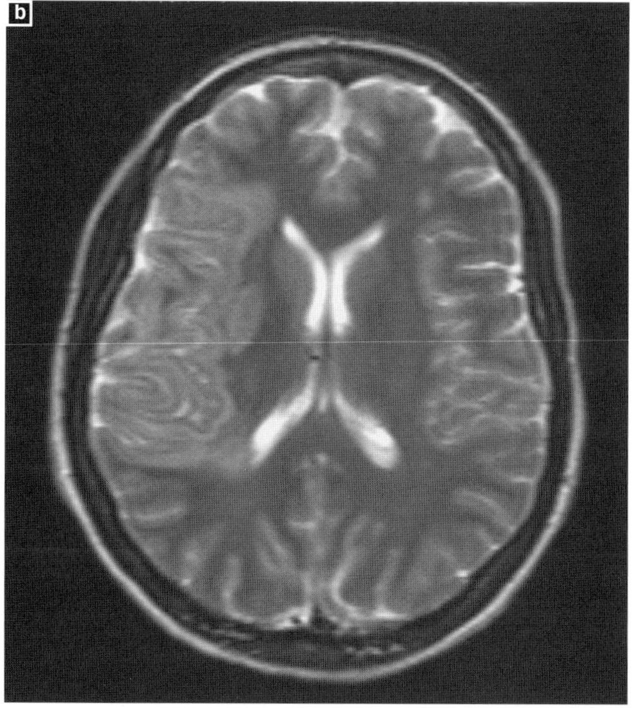

Fig. 7.25. **(a) T2-weighted axial MRI shows a large early subacute left MCA infarct extending from the left frontal operculum through the left temporo-parietal region, spanning Broca's and Wernicke's areas. (b) T2 axial MRI shows a large right MCA infarct involving the right Broca's and Wernicke's homologs. This 42-year-old female was right handed, and presented with a dense global aphasia.**

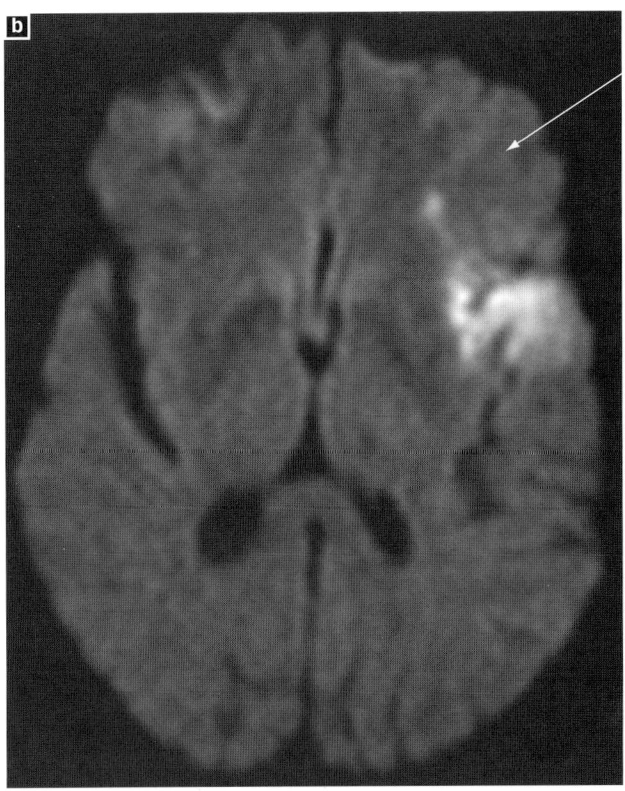

Fig. 7.26. **(a), (b) 50-year-old female patient presenting with sudden-onset echolalia. DWI images shows an infarct slightly posterior and superior to Broca's area, extending into the deep left frontal white matter and presumably disconnecting Broca's area from adjacent language areas in the frontal cortex. The expected location of Broca's area in the left frontal operculum is shown by the arrow. Compare with Fig. 7.20.**

right-handed individuals, there is right hemisphere language dominance, and a global aphasia results from a right MCA infarct (Fig. 7.25b).

Transcortical aphasia is of three main types, and represents the disconnection of Broca's or Wernicke's areas from the other regions of the cerebral cortex central for language processing. While the existence of conduction aphasia supports some compartmentalization of language, as discussed above, transcortical aphasias support the notion that language is also a distributed function in the brain, involving more than just Wernicke's and Broca's areas. Transcortical motor aphasia is similar to Broca's aphasia, except that repetition is spared. The typical cause is an infarct which disconnects Broca's area from the other regions of the frontal cortex which are needed for Broca's area to function in language production. Therefore, such a patient may present with a condition known as echolalia, where essentially the only speech the patient is capable of is repeating what they have just heard (Fig. 7.26).

In the patient presented above, the infarct which caused echolalia was a left frontal infarct adjacent to Broca's area. However, according to textbooks, the most common cause of transcortical motor aphasia is an ACA–MCA watershed infarct (Fig. 7.27).

Transcortical sensory aphasia is quite similar to Wernicke's aphasia, with markedly diminished comprehension, and fluent, meaningless, jargon-filled speech. However, in contradistinction to Wernicke's aphasia, patients with transcortical sensory aphasia show intact repetition. One possible cause of this disorder is watershed infarction in the MCA–PCA territory, which disrupts connections between Wernicke's area and the adjacent temporal-parietal-occipital association cortex needed for Wernicke's area to function in language comprehension. Both

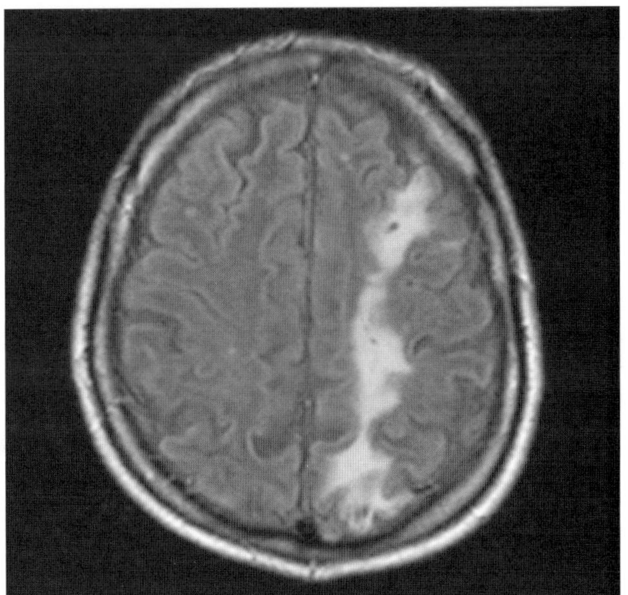

Fig. 7.27. **FLAIR axial image showing a left ACA–MCA watershed infarct.**

Wernicke's area and the arcuate fasciculus are intact, so repetition is preserved.

Mixed transcortical aphasia resembles global aphasia, except that repetition is preserved. Such a patient has impaired

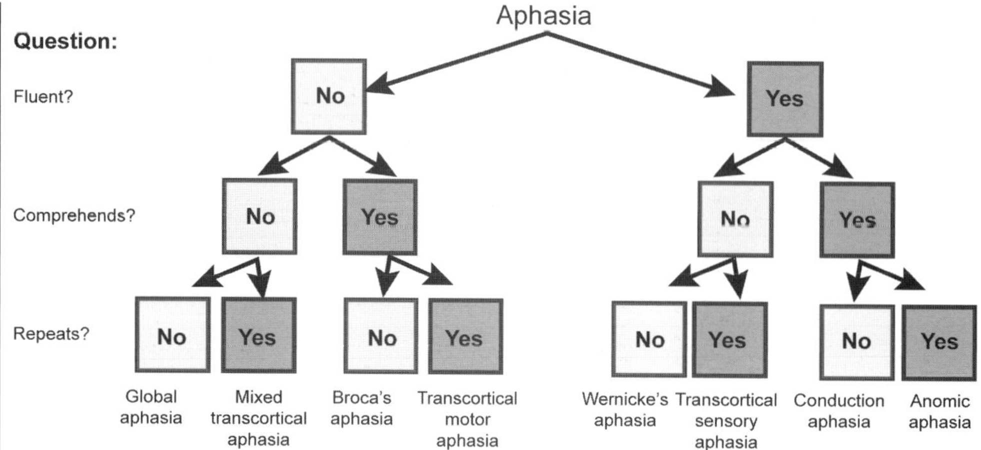

Fig. 7.28. **Tree diagram of the aphasias based on assessing across the three main parameters of speech fluency, language comprehension, and repetition.**

fluency and impaired comprehension, but maintains intact repetition. This condition is also known as isolation of the language areas, and is often due to large left-hemispheric infarcts which involve the ACA–MCA and the MCA–PCA watershed territories.

There is a final type of aphasia which displays fluent speech, intact comprehension, and intact repetition. Such a patient sounds normal, right? Certainly, the main deficiencies in aphasia involve either speech fluency, comprehension, or repetition. However, there is one final parameter important in normal speech, and that is "naming." Patients who have isolated naming difficulties are said to have an anomic aphasia. Certainly, anomia is part of all of the other aphasias, but the term "anomic aphasia" is reserved for patients who have no deficits except in the naming. Such patients cannot name simple objects, like a pen or a key, or have trouble naming parts of an object, like the buckle on a belt. Some authors do not consider anomic aphasia as a separate aphasia, because we cannot easily localize pathology to a specific part of the brain. In other words, it does not fit the anatomical model presented in Fig. 7.21. This is a reasonable objection, since all of the other types of aphasia we have discussed seem to have an anatomic–pathologic correlation. Anomic aphasia, in fact, is typically seen in the recovery phase from one of the other aphasias, or as part of global dementia syndromes.

A simplified model to classify the aphasias we have discussed thus far relies on sequentially assessing three parameters: Is the speech fluent? Is comprehension intact? Is repetition intact?

Based on the binary "yes" or "no" answers to these three questions, a tree diagram of the aphasias is presented to greatly simplify their classification (Fig. 7.28).

Case 7.10

48-year-old male patient with end-stage renal disease and diabetes, who is 6 days status post-CABG. The patient complains that he has lost control of his left hand, which now "has a mind of its own."

What do you think so far? Perhaps it is better to examine the patient before making a snap judgment.

On examination, the patient displays tactile anomia, unable to name objects placed in the left hand. The left hand is observed to make complex movements, not under the patient's control. For example, when handed a piece of paper in his right hand, the left hand grabs it as well, and tries to pull it away. The left hand also spontaneously scratches the patient's head. The patient complains that he has no volitional control over these activities. There is no grasp reflex by the left hand, and no evidence of motor deficits.

After your examination, you immediately send the patient for an MRI, shown below (Fig. 7.29). What are the findings? What is your diagnosis?

Diagnosis

Alien hand syndrome.

Alien hand syndrome (sometimes also called anarchic hand syndrome or Dr. Strangelove syndrome) is a rather bizarre neurological disorder where the patient feels that they have lost control of one of their hands, which now seems to act of its own volition, and often undertakes complex motor tasks. The disorder was first described by Goldstein in 1908, who reported the case of a patient who lost control of her left hand following a stroke. The left hand acted on its own, and sometimes would try to choke the patient, and would have to be pried off. The term "alien hand," was coined by Brion and Jedynak in 1972. In the century since that first report by Goldstein, there has been intense interest and study of this unusual syndrome, and it has become apparent that "alien hand" is not a syndrome, but actually a group of syndromes, each with its own characteristic findings, lesion location, and putative neuroanatomical basis.

Discuss the different types of alien hand syndrome (AHS).

There are three main types of alien hand syndrome: the callosal type, the frontal-callosal type, and a more recently described posterior type.

Callosal type

The callosal form typically affects the non-dominant (usually left) hand, and is the classic form of AHS. It has been described in patients who have had sectioning of the corpus callosum to treat intractable seizures, as well as in patients with tumors of the

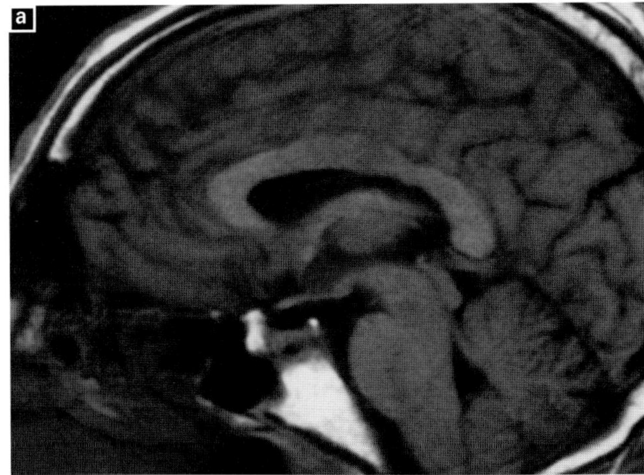

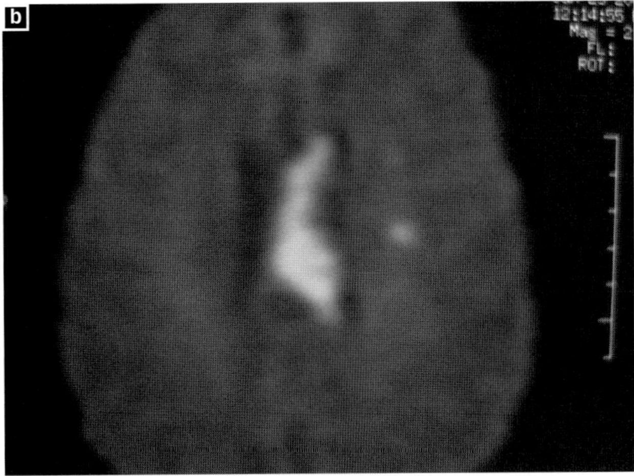

Fig. 7.29. **(a) Sagittal T1-weighted and (b) axial DWI images are provided. The images reveal a large infarct involving the body of the corpus callosum. Given the history, clinical examination, and MRI findings, you reach a diagnosis. Please identify the diagnosis, and discuss this entity.**

corpus callosum who underwent surgical resection. This form represents a classic disconnection syndrome, where the left hand is disconnected from the conscious motor planning and sense of voluntary action subserved by the left motor association cortex in the left hemisphere. Recall that functional imaging studies have shown that the left hemisphere premotor and supplementary motor areas are active in movements not only of the dominant right hand, but also of the left hand. The right premotor and supplementary motor regions, though, activate only with left hand motor tasks (Kim *et al.*, 1993). This left hemsiphere motor dominance over both sides of the body is the flip side of the right hemisphere's sensory dominance over both sides of the body, which correlates with left hemineglect in right parietal lesions. Therefore, with lesions of the corpus callosum, the dominant left motor association cortex is disconnected from the right brain, which controls the left hand. One way to think about the syndrome is that the "subconscious" of the right hemisphere is now controlling the left hand, unchecked by the "conscious" volition which resides in the left hemisphere. Thus, patients claim that their left hand has "a mind of its own." Some people even personify the left hand, giving it a name, or punishing it, because it is "naughty," or "disobedient." It is this variant which leads to the most interesting neurological manifestations, such as intermanual conflict, where the left hand acts at opposing purposes to the right. For example, in one reported patient, every time the right hand put a cigarette in the patient's mouth, the left hand would take it out and throw it away before the patient could light it. The patient would say, referring to the imagined alien power controlling the left hand, "I guess 'he' doesn't want me to smoke."

Frontal-callosal variant

This variant involves the dominant (typically right) hand, and is associated with damage to the left medial frontal lobe and the adjacent genu and anterior body of the corpus callosum. In this variant of AHS, the right hand engages in compulsive exploratory and grasping behavior, as if the grasping reflex normally inhibited by the left frontal lobe has now been released. The right hand will clutch at objects in its vicinity, and the objects often have to be peeled away from the fingers of the right hand by force. All of this occurs outside of the patient's conscious control.

Posterior variant

This is the most recently described and the most unusual variant. It typically, although not exclusively, involves the non-dominant hand, and occurs secondary to parietal/occipital strokes, but has also been reported in such entities as corticobasal degeneration. In this form, the alien hand behaves essentially opposite to the frontal form. Instead of grasping, the hand shows avoidance behavior, levitating upward with the palm up and the fingers extended backward to avoid contact with objects (a so-called "parietal" hand posture). There may also be writhing motions, and the hand motion may be somewhat ataxic (see Fig. 7.30). Some authors have speculated that the posterior alien hand syndrome, as opposed to types where the corpus callosum is involved, represents a loss of a sense of either body topography or proprioception secondary to parietal infarcts.

For an excellent review of alien hand syndrome and the full spectrum of literature reports, please see Scepkowski and Cronin-Golomb, 2003. For more focused reports on the posterior form, since it is new and unusual, see Bundick and Spinella, 2000 and Ay *et al.*, 1998.

Before leaving our main case (Fig. 7.29), it is important to point out that it is quite unusual in its own right, even within the spectrum of a rare entity such as AHS. Most cases of callosal AHS have lesions which involve the anterior aspect of the corpus callosum. In this case, the mid-body and posterior aspect of the corpus callosum are the involved portions, not the anterior. This subvariant of the callosal type, with involvement of the midbody of the corpus callosum, has already been reported in a handful of cases, with an MR appearance essentially identical to our current case. The interested reader is referred to Geschwind *et al.* (1995) and Suwanwela and Leelacheavasit, 2002.

References

Ay, H., Buonanno, F. S., Price, B. H., *et al.* Sensory alien hand syndrome: case report and review of the literature. *Journal of Neurology, Neurosurgery, and Psychiatry* 1998; **65**: 366–369.

Bundick, T., Spinella, M. Subjective experience, involuntary movement, and posterior alien hand syndrome. *Journal of Neurology, Neurosurgery, and Psychiatry*, 2000; **68**(1): 83–85.

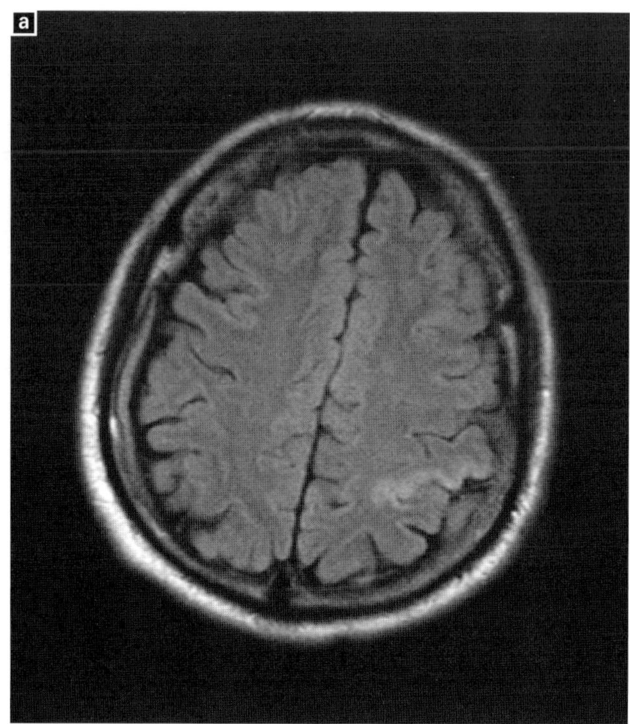
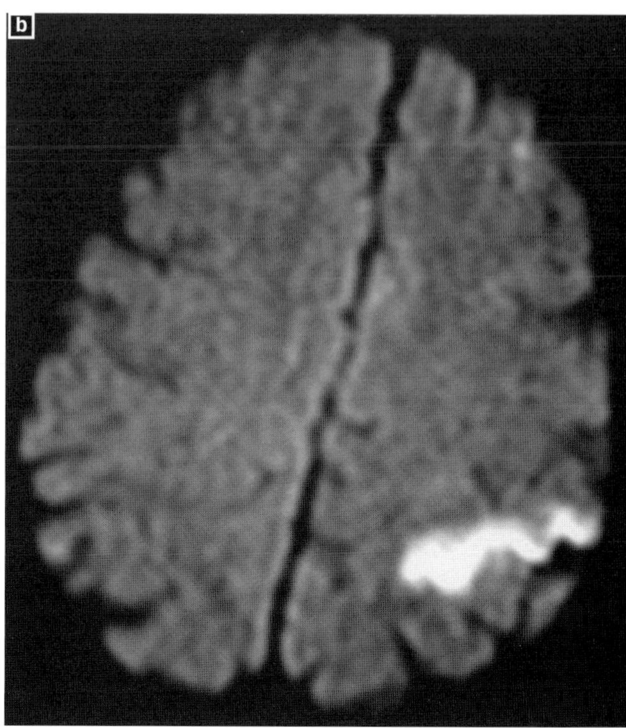

Fig. 7.30. **(a) FLAIR and (b) DWI axial images. This case illustrates a very unusual right-hand posterior alien hand syndrome in a patient with a left parietal infarct.**

Geschwind, D. H., Iacoboni, M., Mega, M. S. *et al*. Alien hand syndrome: interhemispheric motor disconnection due to a lesion in the midbody of the corpus callosum. *Neurology* 1995; **45**: 802–808.

Kim, S. G., Ashe, J., Hendrich, K. *et al*. Functional magnetic resonance imaging of motor cortex: hemispheric asymmetery and handedness. *Science* 1993; **261**: 615–616.

Scepkowski, L. A., and Cronin-Golomb, A. The alien hand: cases, categorizations and anatomical correlates. *Behavioral and Cognitive Neuroscience Reviews* 2003; **2**: 261–277.

Suwanwela, N. C. and Leelacheavasit, N. Isolated corpus callosal infarction secondary to pericallosal artery disease presenting as alien hand syndrome. *Journal of Neurology, Neurosurgery, and Psychiatry* 2002; **72**: 533–536.

Case 7.11

64-year-old male patient, scanned for headache. The patient had normal motor function, and normal cognitive function, and was not perceived to have deficits by the ward team.

MRI examination is presented (Fig. 7.31). What are the findings?

The MRI images reveal a large subacute infarct of the corpus callosum, extending from the mid-body through the splenium. The brain was otherwise unremarkable (do not be confused by the bright T2 signal overlying the frontal regions on the T2 sagittal image – it is partial voluming artifact with CSF in the interhemispheric fissure).

Diagnosis

Infarct of the corpus callosum. Interhemispheric disconnection syndrome.

After the diagnosis of infarct of the corpus callosum was made, more specialized testing was undertaken by the neurology team, who found evidence of interhemispheric disconnection. This case can be considered a follow-up to our previous patient with alien hand syndrome, since alien hand syndrome motivates the study of colossal disconnection syndromes in general. These syndromes, while not typically of strong clinical import, are of significant neuropsychological interest, as they underscore the different functions of the cerebral hemispheres.

Although the two large cerebral hemispheres are directly contiguous to each other, they are anatomically separate, and are connected by only three structures: the corpus callosum, and the anterior and posterior commissures. The large corpus callosum contains the bulk of the interhemispheric connections. The anterior commissure connects the bilateral olfactory regions and portions of limbic system, and the posterior (or hippocampal) commissure interconnects portions of the limbic system as well.

As described previously in the discussion of alien hand syndrome, interhemispheric disconnection syndromes have been mainly studied in the epilepsy population, where patients would sometimes undergo sectioning of the corpus callosum to prevent intractable seizures from spreading from one hemisphere to the other. However, disconnection syndromes may also be seen in tumors or infarcts of the corpus callosum.

Interestingly, if the lesion is isolated to the corpus callosum, patients seem to function quite normally. They seem to retain normal motor skills and normal cognitive function. The manifestations of interhemsipheric disconnection are elicited only by specialized testing. In our patient, such specialized testing revealed some of these manifestations: the patient had left-hand tactile anomia (he could not name an object placed in his hand), left-hand somesthetic alexia (he could not identify words

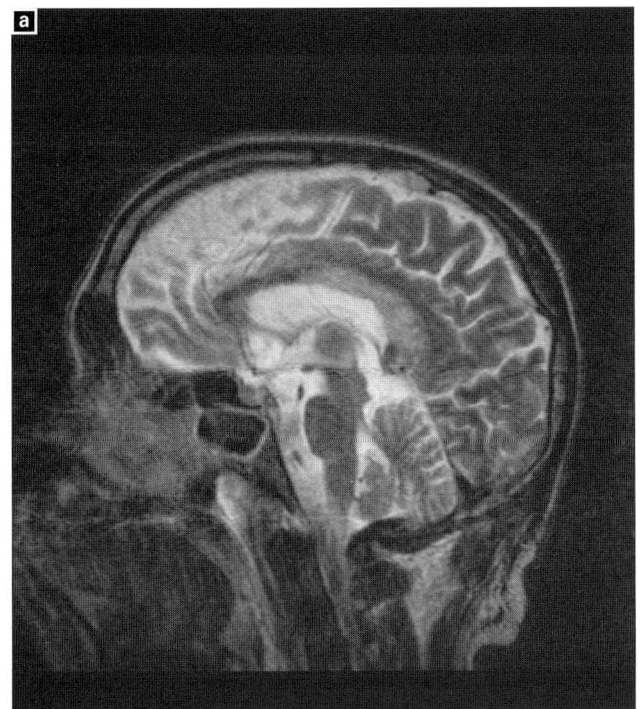
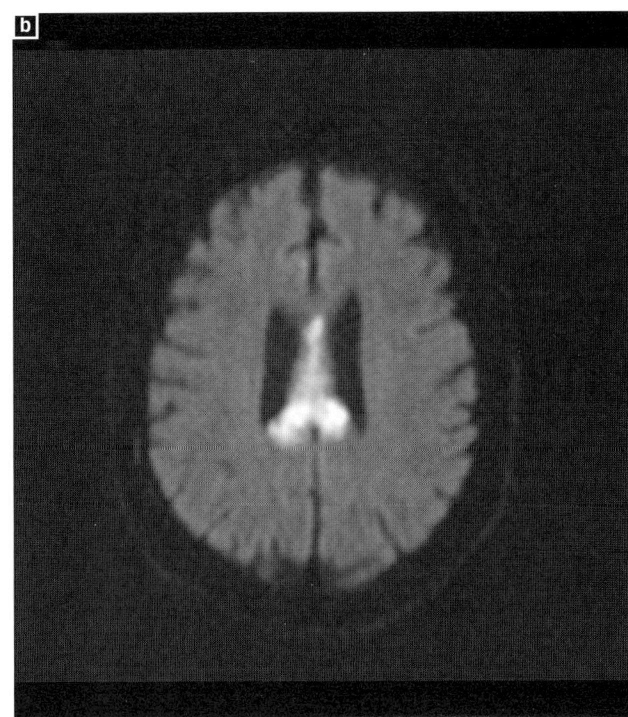

Fig. 7.31. **(a) T2 sagittal and (b) DWI axial MRI images.**

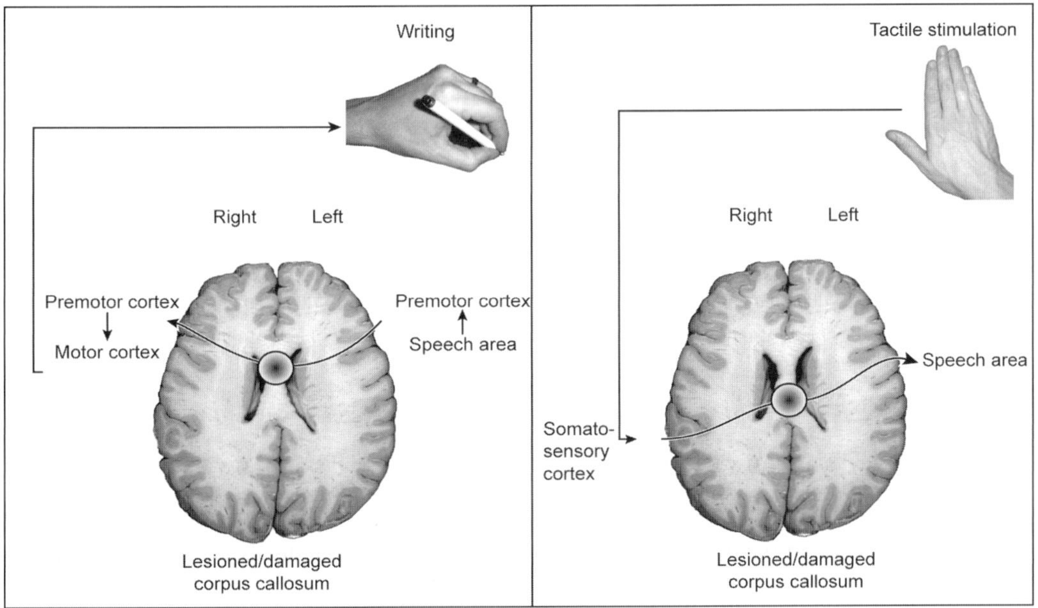

Fig. 7.32. **Schematic diagram illustrating, in a highly simplified fashion, a possible basis of some disconnection syndromes secondary to lesions of the corpus callosum. The figure on the left illustrates the interruption of information flow which leads to left-hand ideomotor apraxia, while the figure on the right illustrates the putative basis for left-hand tactile anomia.**

scratched into his palm), and apraxia confined to the left hand. No such manifestations were evident on the right.

Discuss some of the manifestations of callosal disconnection syndromes.

Callosal disconnection syndromes can be thought of as an interruption of information flow between the hemispheres (see Fig. 7.32).

Therefore, possible manifestations include the following.

Tactile anomia

If an object is placed into the patient's left hand, sensory impulses travel to the right somatosensory cerebral cortex. However, impulses cannot travel to the left hemisphere, which therefore is unable to participate in either identifying or naming the object (see Fig. 7.32).

Somesthetic alexia

Although the pathway to the right sensory cortex is intact, impulses cannot be sent to the left hemisphere language areas. Patients, though, can easily identify words scratched into their right hand.

Unilateral left hand apraxia

In this situation (a form of ideomotor apraxia), the patient is unable to perform tasks with his left hand upon verbal commands. For example, a patient may be unable to mime the use of a key or a screwdriver when asked to do so. The verbal order, comprehended in the left hemisphere, and the action plan, presumably formulated in the left hemisphere, cannot be transferred to the right motor and premotor cortex, which control the left hand (see Fig. 7.32).

Unilateral left hand agraphia

For similar reasons as above, particularly disconnection of the left hemisphere language areas from the right motor and premotor cortex, the patient is unable to write with his left hand (Fig. 7.32).

Right ear preference with dichotic listening

When different words are simultaneously presented to the right and left ear, verbal information is very poorly perceived by the left ear. This is because the pathway from the right ear to the left hemisphere language areas seems to be dominant, and suppresses the pathway from the left ear to the left hemisphere language areas. Since we consider auditory impulses to be bilaterally distributed, it is unclear how a lesion in the corpus callosum would produce this defect. We can hypothesize that there is asymmetry in the auditory pathway, with the left ear projecting more to the right hemisphere auditory cortex, which is then unable to adequately communicate with the left auditory association cortex due to the callosal lesion.

Verbal anosmia for the right nostril

Recall that olfactory information is the single sensory modality which is not crossed in the brain. Therefore, information from the right nostril is conveyed to the right olfactory cortex, and this information may not cross to the left hemisphere, particularly if there is involvement of the anterior commissure.

Right hand constructional apraxia

This is included to highlight the fact that not all of the disconnection deficits involve the left hand. Since the right hemisphere is dominant in visuospatial processing, the patient may display difficulty with copying figures or constructing figures which require depth and perspective. The visuospatial planning in the right hemisphere cannot be transmitted to the left motor and premotor areas, which would control the right hand.

As stated at the outset, most of these manifestations may be subtle, and without significant clinical impact (left ear deficit with dichotic listening – please!). However, hopefully the topic adds some depth to our appreciation of cerebral function.

Case 7.12

55-year-old patient who presents with headaches and visual difficulties. On direct confrontation visual examination, the patient's lateral visual fields appear compromised.

What is the proper term for the patient's visual deficit? Where do you think the lesion is?

The "lateral" visual fields are more properly termed the "temporal" visual fields, whereas the "medial" visual fields are called the "nasal" fields. The patient, then, has a bitemporal hemianopsia (or bitemporal hemianopia – both terms are used). Everyone remembers from medical school that bitemporal hemianopsia is caused by a lesion which impinges upon the optic chiasm. The explanation for this lies in the unusual organization of the visual pathway. As you recall, things are projected onto the retina "upside down and backwards." Objects in the right visual field fall on the left half of each retina. This means that objects in the right visual field fall on the nasal half of the right retina and the temporal half of the left retina. Also, objects in the superior aspect of the visual field fall on the inferior portion of each retina.

The retina is organized in a very interesting and complex fashion, with three layers of neurons. The first layer (deepest layer) is the rods and cones, followed by a second layer of neurons known as bipolar cells, and a third layer of neurons known as ganglion cells. Axons of the ganglion cells are collected together at the optic disk in the posterior pole of the eye, and exit the globe as a bundle known as the optic nerve, which has a meningeal sheath. The somatotopic organization of the visual pathway is maintained in the optic nerve. The two optic nerves come together at the optic chiasm, where fibers from the nasal portion of each retina decussate to the contralateral side (see Fig. 7.33). Fibers from the temporal halves of each retina remain uncrossed. Therefore, optic nerve fibers derived from the nasal half of the right retina will cross over to the left in the optic chiasm to join the uncrossed fibers from the temporal half of the left retina and form the left optic tract. The left optic tract, containing fibers from the nasal half of the right retina and the temporal half of the left retina will then represent the patient's right visual field. Thus, it is fairly straightforward to localize, in a rough fashion, lesions of the visual pathway based on the patient's visual deficit. This will be described further below.

Currently, however, we want to focus on lesions of the optic chiasm. A lesion impinging the chiasm will affect the decussating fibers from the nasal half of each retina. These fibers are responsible for the temporal visual fields, and therefore the patient will present with a bitemporal hemianopsia (see Fig. 7.33). The most common lesion to present in this fashion is a pituitary macroadenoma. Other lesions in the area of the sella turcica, such as a craniopharyngioma, or meningioma of the tuberculum sellae, may have a similar effect. The resultant bitemporal hemianopsia is sometimes referred to as the "blinker phenomena," referring to the blinkers put on race horses so that they cannot see in their lateral field of vision and are not distracted by the other horses, but can see only centrally along the track that they must run.

An MRI image is presented below (Fig. 7.34). What are the findings?
Two quick clinical pearls:
(1) As the pituitary macroadenoma begins to grow, fibers in the lower portion of the optic chiasm are affected first. These come from the inferior half of each retina, which as you recall represent the superior visual fields. Thus, the initial visual

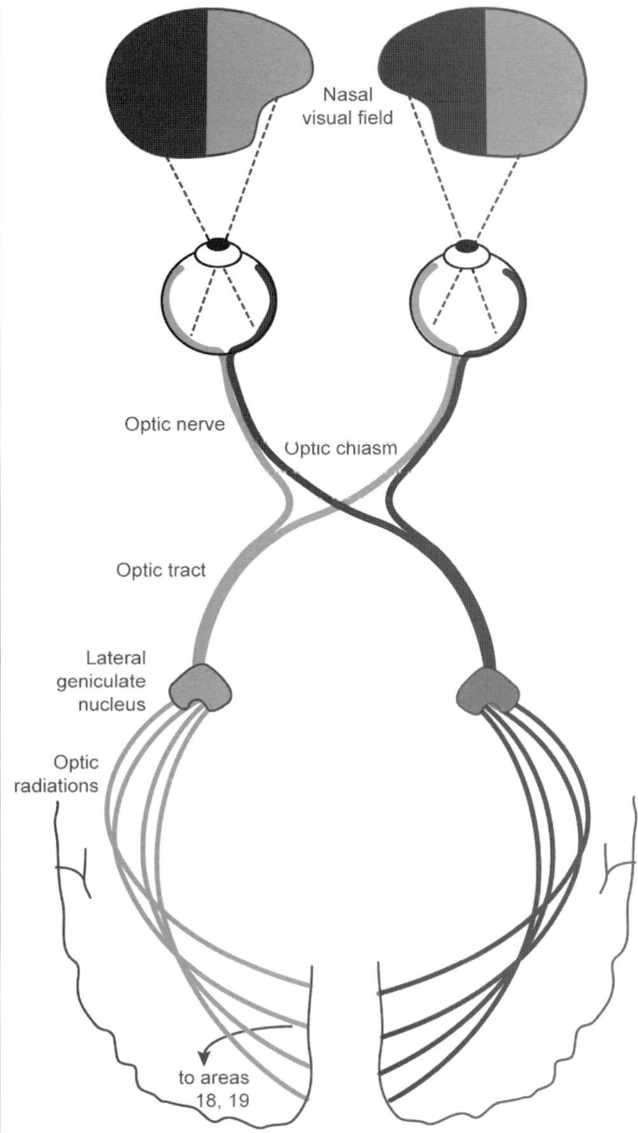

Fig. 7.33. **The somatotopic organization of the visual pathway is shown, with decussation of the fibers from the nasal half of each retina at the optic chiasm.**

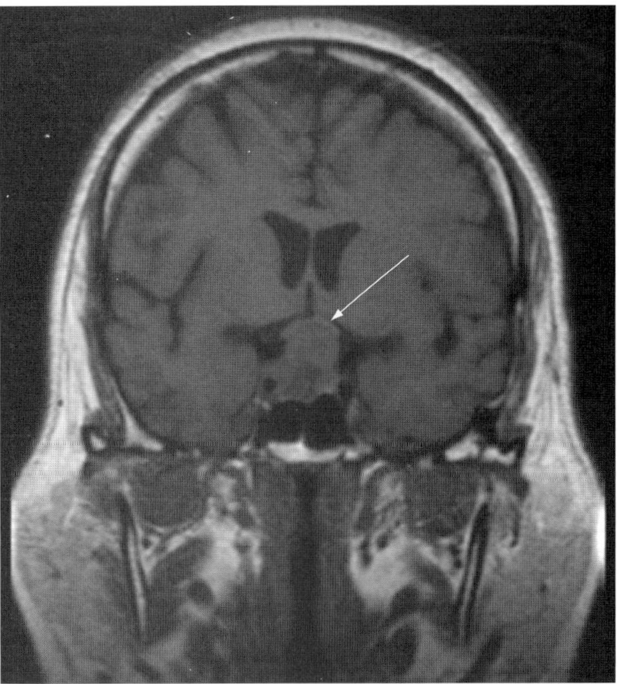

Fig. 7.34. **T1-weighted coronal MRI shows a large mass in the expanding sella turcica and growing into the suprasellar cistern to impinge the optic chiasm (arrow). The images are consistent with a large pituitary macroadenoma and confirm our clinical suspicion.**

deficit may be a bitemporal superior quadrantanopsia rather than a full-blown bitemporal hemianopsia. Also, because color vision is so intensive in its neural representation, only color vision may be initially impaired.

(2) Much less commonly, a patient may present with a binasal hemianopsia. According to some textbooks, this rare clinical finding is often caused by a tumor which has grown around the optic chiasm, and which compresses it from both sides. Thus, the laterally located uncrossed fibers from the temporal halves of the retinas may tend to be affected first, and therefore produce visual deficits in the nasal field of each eye. Careful review of the literature, however, discloses that binasal hemianopsia is usually secondary to an ocular problem (such as ischemic optic neuropathy or glaucoma) rather than to an intracranial problem (see Salinas-Garcia and Smith, 1978.).

Please review briefly the visual deficits produced by lesions along specific portions of the visual pathway.

To begin this review, let us look at Fig. 7.35, which provides an overall summary.

(1) Lesions of the optic nerve will result in monocular blindness or an afferent papillary defect (otherwise known as the Marcus Gunn pupil). This means that the optic nerve fibers are not conducting impulses to the brain. To better understand the implications of this, a very brief recap of the visual pathway is in order. The optic nerve goes through the chiasm, with a partial decussation as described above. From the chiasm, fibers from the left half of the retina of each eye end up in the left optic tract, while fibers from the right half of each retina form the right optic tract. As you recall, the optic tract projects mainly to the lateral geniculate nucleus of the thalamus, and from there to the primary visual (calcarine) cortex via the geniculostriate pathway composed of the optic radiations. However, a small number of fibers in the optic tract travel in the so-called extrageniculate pathway, bypassing the lateral geniculate of the thalamus, and relaying in the pretectal area and the superior colliculus. Each pretectal nucleus then projects to both Edinger–Westphal nuclei in the midbrain, which provide parasympathetic innervation to the ciliary ganglia, which then innervate the papillary constrictor muscle. Therefore, a light shone in one eye produces pupillary constriction in that eye (direct light reflex) and in the other eye (consensual light reflex). This is demonstrated by the swinging flashlight test, where a light is shone in each eye back and forth, and both pupils constrict when the light is shone in either eye. With an afferent pupillary defect, when light is shone in the affected eye, neither pupil constricts, and when light is shone in the normal eye, both pupils constrict. Thus, with the swinging flashlight test, when the light is shone in the bad eye, the pupil dilates (because it had been constricted when the light was shining in the normal eye). Of

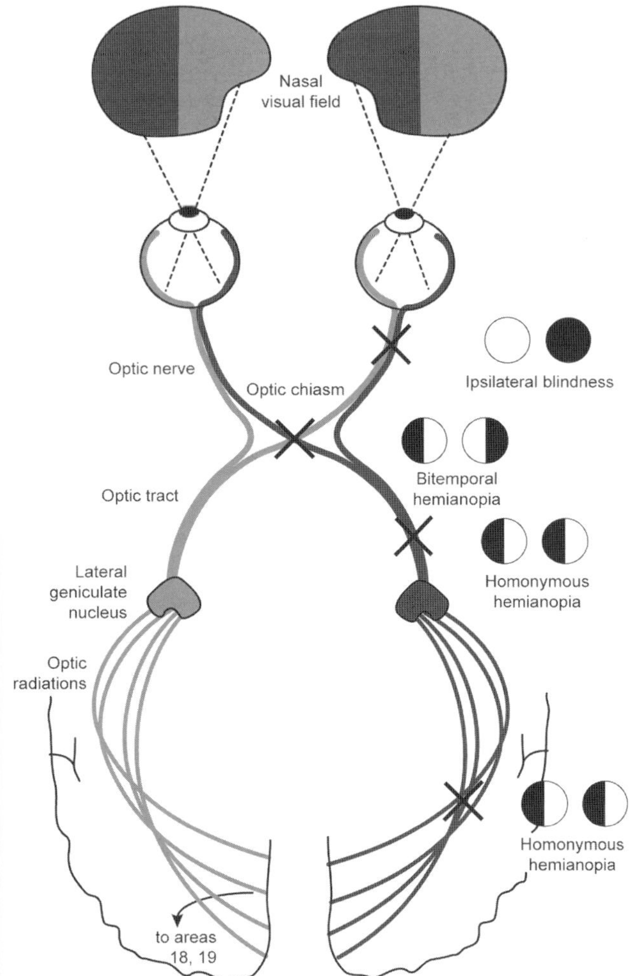

Fig. 7.35. **Lesions of the visual pathway and the deficits which they produce.**

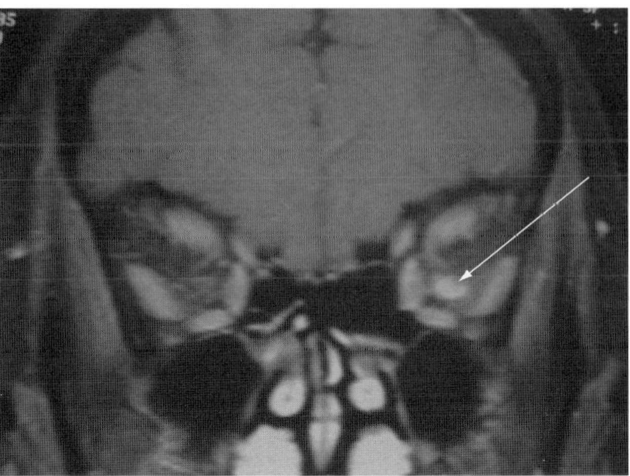

Fig. 7.36. **T1 post-contrast fat saturation coronal image shows abnormal enhancement of the left optic nerve (arrow), compared to the non-enhancing right optic nerve. This is consistent with optic neuritis. Recall that, within 5 years of initial presentation, a large portion of patients with isolated optic neuritis will carry the diagnosis of multiple sclerosis.**

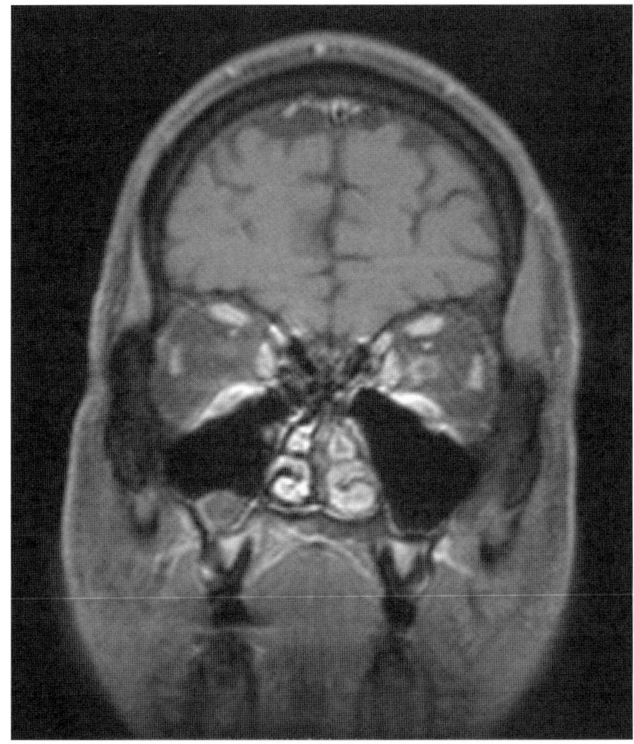

Fig. 7.37. **There is abnormal enhancement of the left optic nerve sheath, surrounding the centrally located non-enhancing left optic nerve (compare to Fig. 7.36, where the core of the optic nerve enhances). This "tram track" sign is highly suggestive of optic nerve sheath meningioma.**

course, monocular blindness and afferent papillary defects do not need to result from optic nerve lesions. They often result from ocular lesions, such as retinal bleeds. We will leave those causes to the ophthalmologists. Our territory begins with the optic nerve. Common optic nerve lesions include ischemic optic neuropathy, optic neuritis (Fig. 7.36), or optic nerve sheath tumors (Fig. 7.37).

(2) Retrochiasmatic lesions, involving the optic tract, lateral geniculate body, or the visual cortex, all result in a contralateral homonymous hemianopsia (see Fig. 7.35), due to involvement of crossed nasal fibers from the contralateral retina and uncrossed temporal fibers from the ipsilateral retina. There are a few clinical pearls here as well:

(a) Lesions of the occipital cortex sometimes show a phenomenon known as "macular sparing." This refers to preserved vision in the center of the visual field, where macular retinal fibers project onto the occipital pole. The occipital pole is sometimes spared because it receives collateral blood supply from the middle cerebral artery. Therefore, infarcts of the posterior cerebral artery may sometimes spare the occipital pole, leading to "macular sparing."

(b) Nerve fibers from the lateral geniculate body project to the calcarine cortex along two pathways (see Fig. 7.38). There is a so-called direct pathway to the upper lip of the calcarine cortex, along the superior bank of the calcarine fissure. There is also the indirect pathway, commonly known as Meyer's loop, which travels inferiorly in the temporal lobe

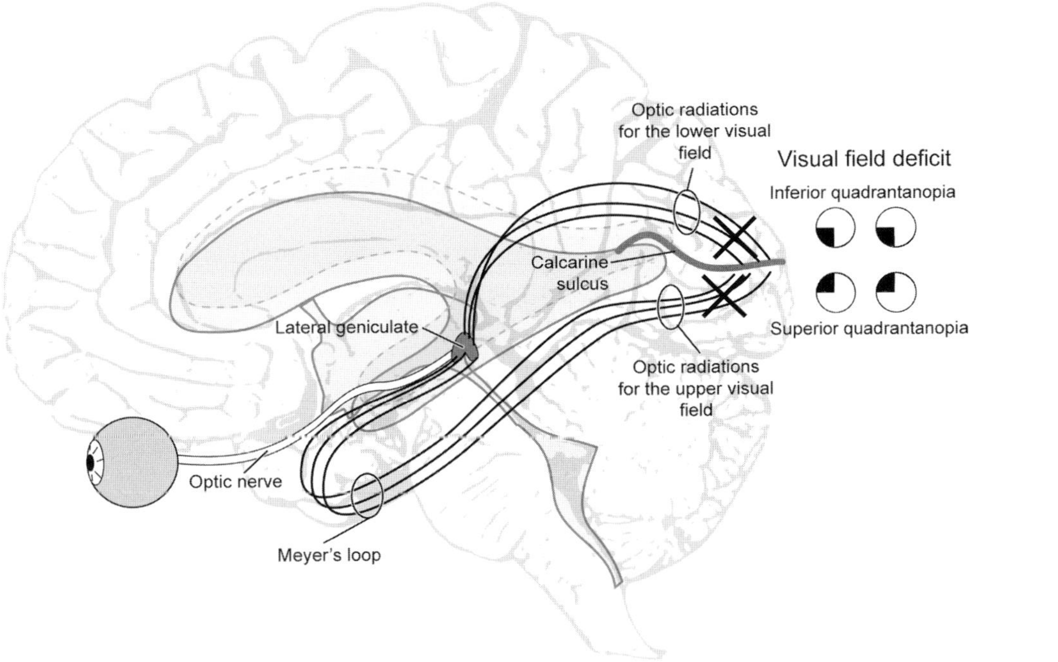

Fig. 7.38. **The two divisions of the geniculostriate pathway, and their associated visual field deficits.**

to the lower lip of the calcarine cortex. This loop initially travels forward, looping along the temporal horn of the lateral ventricle, and then turns and travels posteriorly in the temporal lobe to reach the inferior lip of the calcarine fissure. Thus, temporal lobe lesions may affect Meyer's loop, which carries inferior retinal fibers. Recall that the superior visual field is projected onto the inferior portion of the retina. Therefore, lesions involving Meyer's loop will produce a contralateral homonymous superior quadrantanopsia. (The same deficit will also occur with lesions along the inferior bank of the calcarine fissure, involving the lingual gyrus of the occipital lobe.) These lesions are more common than those affecting the superior or direct

pathway. However, if that pathway is involved in parietal lobe lesions, a contralateral homonymous inferior quadrantanopsia will result. Finally, a fun fact to torment your fellow residents with: ask them about the other eponyms for Meyer's loop. It is sometimes also referred to as Flechsig's loop or Archambault's loop.

Reference

Salinas-Garcia, R. F. and Smith, J. L. Binasal hemianopia. *Surgical Neurology* 1978; **10**(3): 187–194.

Case 7.13

70-year-old right-handed woman with a long history of peripheral vascular disease presented to the emergency room with decreased mentation. She was oriented to time, place, and person. She was unable to read, although she could identify individual letters, spell, speak, and write normally. Visual field tests are shown adjacent (Fig. 7.39).

Where do you think the lesion is?

The above visual field test reveals a right homonymous hemianopsia. This type of visual field defect appears with lesions in the retrochiasmatic pathways including the optic tract, lateral geniculate body, optic radiations, or occipital lobe. Hence, a left retrochiasmatic lesion is suggested.

The patient underwent MRI examination, shown (Fig. 7.40). What are the findings?

There is abnormal T2-weighted hyperintensity in the left mesial occipital lobe, involving the gray and the white matter, sharply defined and in the distribution of the left posterior cerebral artery. The findings are consistent with a subacute left PCA infarct.

What additional findings are there on the MRI? What is the diagnosis?

In addition to the left mesial occipital lobe, abnormal signal is seen involving the left aspect of the splenium of the corpus callosum (arrow in Fig. 7.40(b)) indicating infarction there as well. This may occur secondary to occlusion of an inconstant

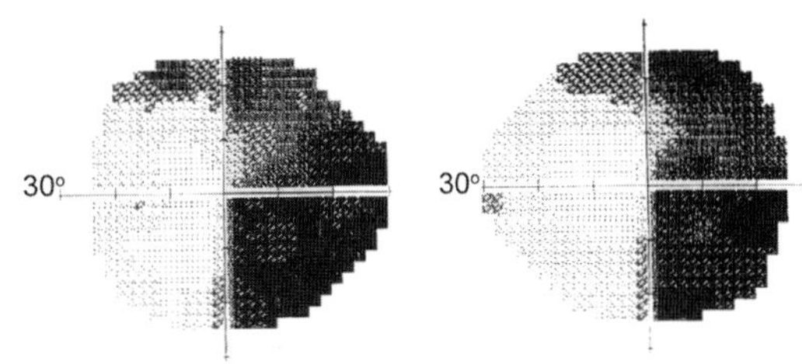

Fig. 7.39. **Visual field tests for the patient above. The dark areas represent defects in the visual field.**

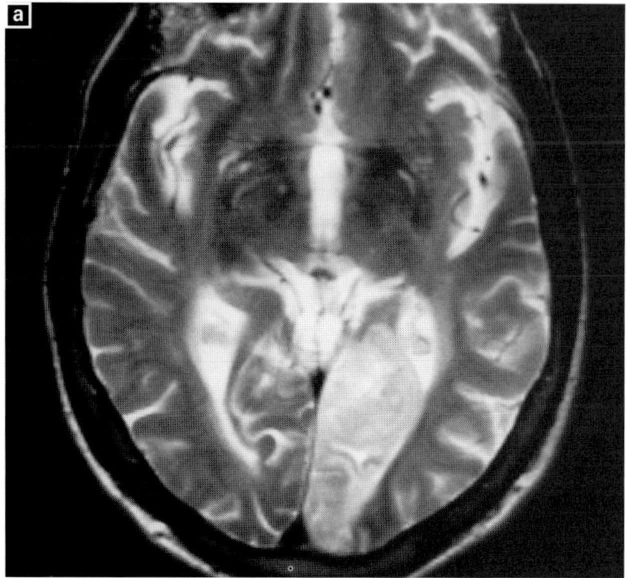
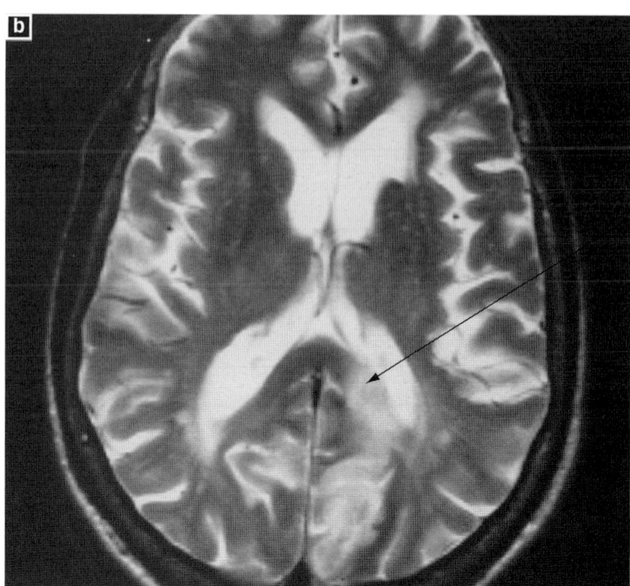

Fig. 7.40. **(a), (b) T2-weighted axial images. Note the arrow in (b).**

branch of the posterior cerebral artery, known as the dorsal splenial, retrosplenial or recurrent splenial branch.

Infarction involving the left mesial occipital lobe as well as the splenium of the corpus callosum may sometimes produce the syndrome of *alexia without agraphia*.

Discuss this diagnosis.

The patient had a right homonymous hemianopsia. The patient was unable to read; however, the patient could write, spell and speak, and even recognize individual letters. If the patient was asked to write a sentence, and it was shown to her later, she could not even read what she herself had written. This syndrome is called alexia without agraphia, but is also called pure alexia, or pure word blindness. It is a classic disconnection syndrome, and results from the disconnection of the dominant angular gyrus from all visual input. It was initially described by Dejerine in 1892.

The left (dominant) angular gyrus is part of the inferior parietal lobule, capping the end of the superior temporal sulcus. It is necessary for the comprehension of written language. In normal comprehension of written language, visual information reaches the left (dominant) angular gyrus from both visual areas.

In this case, we have a lesion in the dominant visual cortex, as well as the splenium of the corpus callosum (see Fig. 7.41). The lesion in the left visual cortex prevents the processing of visual information there. The lesion in the splenium of the corpus callosum prevents visual information entering the intact right visual cortex from reaching the left angular gyrus as well, since fibers from the right visual cortex, and visual association cortex, travel to the left angular gyrus via the inferior portion of the splenium. Therefore, the intact angular gyrus is disconnected from all visual input, resulting in alexia. Since the angular gyrus itself is intact, as well as its connections to Wernicke's and Broca's areas, normal language production, such as writing, remains possible.

As in this case, alexia without agraphia is usually caused by an infarct in the left occipital lobe with an accompanying infarct in the left aspect of the splenium. Therefore, most cases have an associated right homonymous hemianopsia. Any lesion along

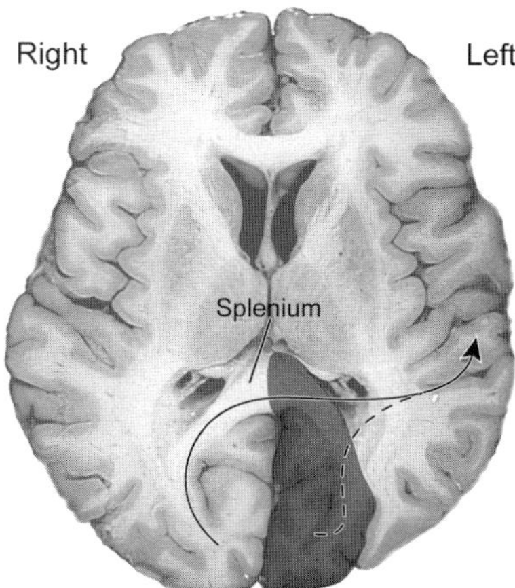

Fig. 7.41. **Diagrammatic representation of alexia without agraphia.**

the pathways conveying visual input from both hemispheres to the dominant angular gyrus, however, will cause this syndrome. Thus, it may also occur with infarction of the left lateral geniculate body and the splenium of the corpus callosum, or with lesions of the deep white matter of the left parieto-occipital region, again disconnecting the left angular gyrus from the visual areas. These latter lesions produce alexia without agraphia or hemianopsia, since the primary visual cortex on the left is spared. Interestingly, an alternative theory has been presented: that pure alexia can be caused by a lesion which damages the extrastriate visual area in the left occipital lobe responsible for word recognition, rather than by disconnection of the dominant angular gyrus. On the basis of PET studies, such an area has been demonstrated in the left medial extrastriate visual cortex (see Petersen *et al.*, 1990). Thus, there are rare reports of patients who have alexia without agraphia or hemianopsia but with lesions which are too ventral in the temporo-occipital area to

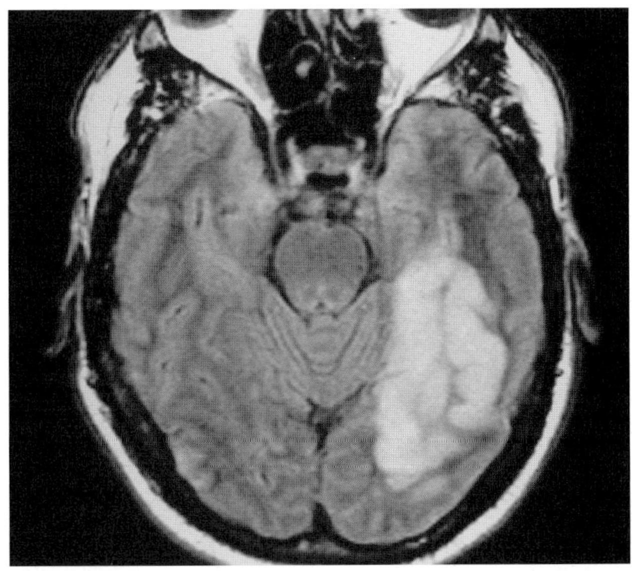

Fig. 7.42. **47-year-old male patient with pure alexia without agraphia and without complete homonymous hemianopsia. FLAIR MRI shows a left temporo-occipital subacute infarct with sparing of the calcarine cortex. The lesion is well below the splenium of the corpus callosum and the left angular gyrus.**

involve the pathways from the visual cortex to the dominant angular gyrus (Benito-Leon *et al.*, 1997). Exclusively for your pleasure, such a rare case is presented here (see Fig. 7.42).

A related syndrome of *alexia with agraphia* can now also be understood. In that syndrome, there are defects in both reading and writing, with the writing defect usually severe. It is produced by a lesion in the dominant angular gyrus itself.

If this patient could not recognize colors, why do you think that is?

Sometimes, a color anomia or color agnosia is seen as part of the alexia without agraphia syndrome, where patients cannot verbally identify the color of an object which they are, shown. They are, however, able to tell what color something should be when asked (i.e., grass is green). Color agnosia should be distinguished from achromatopsia, which will be discussed in the next case.

References

Benito-Leon, J., Sanchez-Suarez, C., Diaz-Guzman, J. *et al*. Pure alexia could not be a disconnection syndrome. *Neurology* 1997; **49**: 305–306.

Petersen, S. E., Fox, P. T., Snyder, A. Z. *et al*. Activation of extrastriate and frontal cortical areas by visual words and word-like stimuli. *Science* 1990; **249**: 1041–1044.

Case 7.14

85-year-old female patient presents with "confusion," as per her family. The family members state that she seems confused as to who they are. Neurological examination reveals a right homonymous superior quadrantanopsia as well as difficulty in recognizing her family by sight. When a family member spoke, she was more successful at recognizing them by voice.

MR images are shown (Fig. 7.43). What are the findings?

The patient has an early subacute infarct in the left inferior occipital lobe, involving both the inferior lip of the primary visual cortex, and the visual association areas along the inferior occipital temporal region, including portions of the fusiform gyrus and the inferior occipital gyrus, as well as a right temporo-occipital infarct.

The inability to recognize familiar faces is a named neurological syndrome. What is this syndrome called? What are the typical lesions that underlie this syndrome?

The inability to recognize familiar faces is an interesting neurological syndrome called *prosopagnosia* (from the Greek *prosopon*,

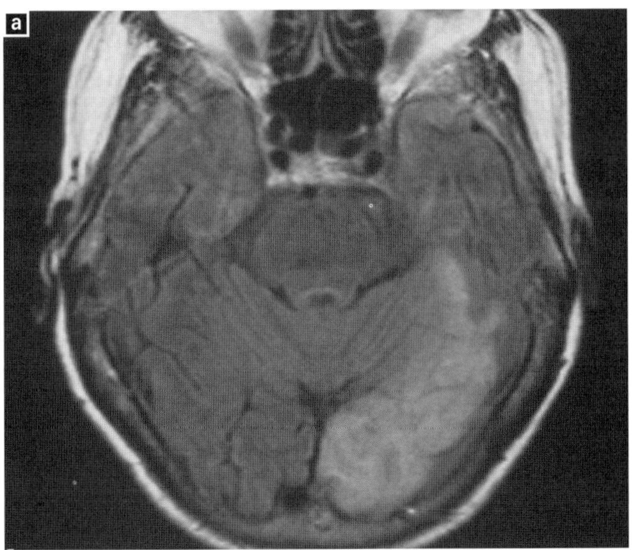

Fig. 7.43. **(a), (b) FLAIR MRI images.**

"face," and *gnosis*, "knowledge"), which is what our patient has. A significant amount has been written in the neurology and neurobehavior literature about this condition, since facial recognition is an important feature of human interaction, and is a complex neurological function. Recent research has revealed that, in most cases, acquired prosopagnosia is due to damage in the bilateral infero-medial occipito-temporal regions, with a right-sided predominance. Some authors have implicated Brodmann's area 37, while others have implicated area 39. Functional MRI research has shown that there seem to be two important areas in face recognition: one of these is in the fusiform gyrus, known as the fusiform face area (FFA); posterior to this, there is a second area in the inferior occipital gyrus, known as the occipital face area (OFA). Damage to these regions can produce a specific visual agnosia involving face recognition, where, in severe cases, patients cannot even recognize their own pictures.

Typically, such patients can recognize a face in general, meaning that they can recognize that they are being shown a face, but cannot put together the features of the face to recognize it as an individual familiar to them. This is despite the fact that they are able to name the different parts of the face, such as ears, nose, and mouth. The interested reader is referred to the articles in the references section to follow the debates and developments in this very interesting neurological condition.

In many cases, the visual agnosia extends beyond faces, to any form-specific recognition. For example, a former automobile enthusiast may be able to tell that he is being shown a picture of a car, but can no longer identify the particular make and model of the car.

It is noted that our case is unusual in that the patient did not exhibit bilateral inferior occipito-temporal lesions, but rather only a left-sided inferior occipito-temporal lesion and a right-sided temporo-occipital lesion. This falls outside the spectrum of the typical cases of prosopagnosia and underscores the fact that there is still much that we do not understand about the widely distributed mechanism of face recognition. For example, there are reported cases of post-traumatic prosopagnosia with isolated left hemisphere lesions (Mattson *et al.*, 2000).

Also, there are described cases of congenital prosopagnosia, where patients exhibit a developmental deficit in face recognition. There are now many such described cases, and the condition appears to run in families. It is often severe enough that a wife, for example, cannot recognize her own husband. An excellent article detailing the human side of growing up with prosopagnosia can be found in one of my favorite medical journals, *People Magazine* (see Hewitt, 2007). In terms of the more conventional scientific literature, the article by Behrmann *et al.* (2007) examines putative alterations in the brains of patients with congenital prosopagnosia.

Please discuss the syndrome of prosopagnosia in the context of the broad scheme of classifying the visual association cortex functions into a dorsal stream and a ventral stream. What are the main functions of the dorsal stream? What syndromes do lesions in the dorsal stream tend to produce? What syndromes do lesions in the ventral stream tend to produce?

As we have seen in the previous three cases, there are specific visual deficits (e.g., unilateral blindness, afferent papillary defects, bitemporal hemianopsia, homonymous hemianopsia) as well as neurobehavioral correlates (e.g., alexia without agraphia) associated with lesions of the primary visual pathways, from the retina through the calcarine cortex. There is also a host of interesting syndromes associated with lesions of the visual association cortex, which we will now explore. After information arrives in the primary visual cortex, it undergoes higher-order processing in the visual association cortex, which can in a very gross way be divided into two main streams: a dorsal stream,

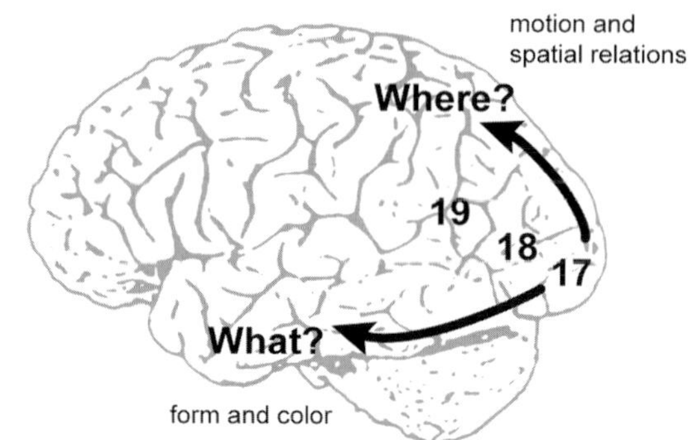

Fig. 7.44. **Conceptual diagram showing the general functions of the ventral and dorsal visual streams.**

which is the parieto-occipital association cortex, and a ventral stream, which is the inferior occipito-temporal association cortex (Fig. 7.44).

The dorsal stream seems to function mainly in visuospatial processing – the spatial relationships between different objects, the spatial relationship between external objects and the body, and how these relationships are altered by motion. This stream has been referred to by some authors (e.g., Blumenfeld), as processing the "Where," part of visual information. This is the sort of information, for example, critical to catching a ball thrown to us. The ventral stream, conversely, processes the "What," aspect of visual information, such as the recognition of form, color, faces, and letter strings.

Lesions in the dorsal association cortex can produce a number of different disturbances, which may be seen alone or in concert. Because these lesions involve the dorsal parieto-occipital regions, they can be associated with hemineglect, apraxia, and inferior quadrantanopsias. Some of the clinical deficits are as follows:

Simultagnosia

This is the classic "can't see the forest for the trees," syndrome, and consists of an inability to put together the individual parts of a visual scene as a meaningful whole. Therefore, patients will perceive and describe small isolated parts of a complex scene, without being able to put the whole picture together. Part of the problem is that patients are not able to accurately scan the different parts of a complex scene in a systematic fashion. Another contributing factor is a difficulty in perceiving moving objects (known as cerebral akinetopsia).

Optic ataxia

This is the inability to reach out and touch an object under visual guidance. This may be secondary to a defect in spatial perception of the relationship between external objects and the self. The false localization of objects in space is known as optic allesthesia. Optic ataxia can be distinguished from cerebellar ataxia in that once the object has been touched (the patient ascertains the needed spatial relationships using the sense of touch), the patient can then move the hand smoothly back and forth to it, which would be impossible with cerebellar ataxia.

Ocular apraxia

This is the inability to smoothly direct one's gaze to objects in the visual field through saccades.

The constellation of the above findings (simultagnosia, optic ataxia, and ocular apraxia) is known as Balint's syndrome. A classic example of Balint's syndrome would be the case of a patient asked to pour juice from a pitcher into an adjacent cup. Although the patient has no motor or primary visual deficit, the patient has trouble reaching out and grasping the pitcher, and ends up pouring the juice outside the cup. This makes us realize how complex the processing involved in such a simple task, which can routinely be done "unconsciously," while carrying on a conversation with a guest, actually is.

Lesions in the ventral stream typically cause visual agnosias, as in our case of prosopagnosia. Since color perception seems to be part of the ventral stream, patients may also develop achromatopsia, which is cortical color blindness. In these cases, patients cannot perceive colors, and hence cannot identify the color of an object, name the color, or match it to a similar color. Anatomical and functional imaging studies indicate that color is processed by a large network of structures. Nevertheless, the lesions causing achromatopsia are rather restricted and usually affect the ventro-medial sector of the occipital lobe in the lingual and fusiform gyri. This abnormality is usually associated with infracalcarine lesions that damage the middle third of the lingual gyrus and also with infracalcarine lesions that damage the white matter lying immediately behind the posterior tip of the lateral ventricle. A subtle distinction should be made between achromatopsia and color agnosia, which occurs in conjunction with alexia without agraphia. In color agnosia, patients cannot verbally identify the color of an object, but can match objects of the same color, indicating that color perception is intact.

There are a variety of other bizarre disorders associated with the ventral stream that we mention simply because they are fascinating. They include *erythropsia*, where things appear colored with a reddish (or sometimes purplish) hue, *cerebral diplopia* or *polyopia*, where two or more copies of the same object are seen (to be distinguished from diplopia caused by conjugate gaze palsies, which typically resolves when one eye is covered), *palinopsia*, where the image of an object seen previously reappears in the visual field when the object is not there, *micropsia* and *macropsia*, where objects appear uniformly smaller or bigger than they should, and *metamorphopsia*, where objects are distorted in appearance.

Another fascinating and rare disorder which occurs secondary to lesions of the bilateral primary visual cortex as well as the visual association cortex is Anton's syndrome, otherwise known as visual anosognosia for cortical blindness. In such cases, bilateral occipital lesions cause cortical blindness, and lesions of the visual association cortex somehow disconnect the visual cortex from the remaining cortical areas, such that patients are unaware of their blindness (Fig. 7.45).

They may confabulate about what they are "seeing," – i.e., the number of fingers which an examiner is holding up, and make excuses for why they got the answer wrong. Part of the anosognosia may be secondary to memory deficits and a confusional state that sometimes accompanies Anton's syndrome, while part of it may be due to the phenomenon of "blindsight," where cortically blind patients seem to have some preserved visual functions, such as recognizing the color of an object or the number of fingers held up with a higher than chance frequency. This phenomenon may be subtended by so-called extrageniculate visual pathways, where some visual information is processed through accessory pathways which bypass the lateral geniculate bodies and the primary visual cortex. An example of this is the accessory pathway to the superior

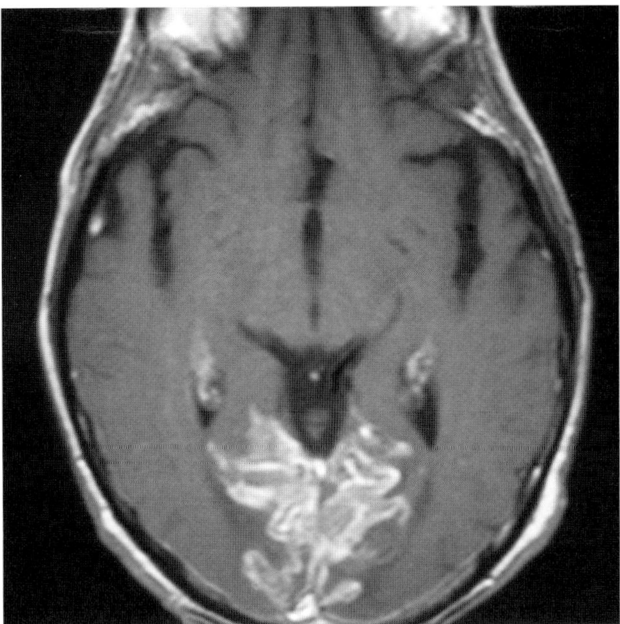

Fig. 7.45. **T1-weighted post-contrast axial MR image shows gyriform enhancement in bilateral subacute occipital infarcts. This 53-year-old patient had cortical blindness with significant denial of his visual deficits.**

colliculi. Thus, cortically blind patients still have a pupillary light response. Another explanation for blindsight is that even with severe bilateral occipital lesions, there may be small spared islands of visual cortex with some live neurons that can subtend some visual function, but their volume is too small to allow conscious visual perception. However, there is enough rudimentary visual function left such that patients deny that they are blind. For an interesting case report on this phenomenon, see Goldenberg *et al.* (1995).

References

Behrmann, M., Avidan, G., Gao, F. *et al.* Structural imaging reveals anatomic alterations in inferotemporal cortex in cogential prosopagnosia. *Cerebral Cortex*, advance access published online January 11, 2007. *Cerebral Cortex*, doi:10.1093/cercor/bhl144.

Damasio, A. R., Damasio, H., and Van Hoesen, G. W. Prosopagnosia: anatomic basis and behavioral mechanisms. *Neurology* 1982; **32**(4): 331–341.

Goldenberg, G., Mullbacher, W., and Nowak, A. Imagery without perception – a case study of anosognosia for cortical blindness. *Neuropsychologia* 1995; **33**(11): 1373–1382.

Hewitt, B. When every face is unfamiliar. *People Magazine* December 24, 2007; 106–110.

Mattson, A. J., Levin, H. S., and Grafman, J., A case of prosopagnosia following moderate closed head injury with left hemisphere focal lesion. *Cortex* 2000; **36**(1): 125–137.

Rossion, R., Caldara, R., Seghier, M. *et al.* A network of occipito-temporal face-sensitive areas besides the right middle fusiform gyrus is necessary for normal face processing. *Brain* 2003; **126**(11): 2381–2395.

Sorger, B., Goebel, R., Schiltz, C. *et al.* Understanding the functional neuroanatomy of acquired prosopagnosia. *Neuroimage* 2007; **35**(2): 836–852.

Case 7.15

32-year-old male transferred from a private hospital after a respiratory arrest from opiate overdose. At the time of transfer, the patient had been extubated, and his sensorium was clear. Neurologic testing showed that the patient was awake and alert, with intact language functions. However, the patient was oriented only to self. His attention was normal, with a forward digit span of 6 and a backward digit span of 4. Memory testing revealed immediate recall of 3 objects. However, within 5 minutes, the patient could not recall any of the objects presented, or even being asked to remember them. The patient's memory for past events was likewise disturbed, with the patient having no recollection of events for approximately 2 weeks before his admission.

What is your assessment? Where in the brain might the patient's lesions be located?

The patient presents with a profound anterograde amnesia, unable to retain new information. The patient also has some retrograde amnesia for recent events. Given the absence of other focal or global symptoms, we would consider lesions in the mesial temporal lobes at the top of our differential. However, we are also aware that amnesia often has no imaging correlate, such as in cases of concussion with no visible traumatic brain injury, or global anoxia without imaging manifestations.

An MRI of our patient is provided, with a normal control for comparison (Fig. 7.46). What are the findings? What is your most likely diagnosis?

In comparison to a normal control (Fig. 7.46(c)), the MRI of our patient clearly shows abnormal FLAIR hyperintensity in the bilateral mesial temporal lobes, which appears to selectively involve the hippocampal formations (Fig. 7.46(a),(b) – arrows).

Diagnosis

Given the patient's history, as well as the vulnerability of the hippocampal formations to ischemia, anoxic damage to the hippocampal formations is the leading differential diagnosis.

The hippocampal formations are part of the limbic system. Discuss the main elements of limbic system.

As mentioned previously, the Latin word "limbus" means ring or border. The "limbic lobe" is a C-shaped set of structures along the medial edge of the cortical mantle. The "limbic system" is a broader concept, and denotes a complex network of connections between structures in the "limbic lobe," the basal forebrain, the diencephalon, the basal ganglia, and the brainstem (Fig. 7.47).

Among the major functions of the limbic system are memory, and emotions and drives. Some authors also consider olfaction as a limbic function, but it is not typically considered so. The main components of the limbic system are:

(1) The limbic cortex, which is a combination of both archicortex and allococortex, including the hippocampal formation, the parahippocampal gyrus, the cingulate gyrus, and the amygdala.

(2) The basal forebrain and the septal nuclei. These structures lie just ventral to the inferior edge of the septum pellucidum and anterior to the hypothalamus on the ventral surface of the brain. They include the substantia innominata which contains the nucleus basalis of Meynert, the nucleus of the diagonal band of Broca, and the medial and lateral septal nuclei.

(3) White matter connecting pathways, particularly the columns of the fornix, which form one of the main output pathways of the hippocampal formations, and which serve as their main connection to the diencephalon.

Briefly discuss short-term memory, long-term memory, and the concept of memory consolidation.

Clearly, one of the most important and mysterious functions of the brain is memory. Otherwise, there would be no point in reading this book, for example, since you would remember none of it (some will claim that there is no point anyway, but as they say in television, that's another Oprah altogether). There are many complex models of memory, but we will consider the simplest classification – that memory is divided into two broad types: (1) declarative, or explicit memory, which has to do with learning facts or recalling events, and (2) non-declarative or implicit memory, which has to do with such things as learning new skills, conditioning, or priming.

Correlation studies of both pathologic and surgical lesions have shown that there are two main areas of the brain critical to memory consolidation: the hippocampal formations and the anterior and medial thalamic nuclei. These two memory areas have rich connections to each other and to extensive areas of association cortex.

The hippocampal formations, particularly, are integral to declarative memory, principally to the function known as consolidation of memory. When new facts are learned, three sequential processes take place: (1) the facts are "registered," – i.e., we become consciously aware of them. In the example of a three object recall, we comprehend the three objects, and hold them for a few seconds in what is called "working memory," or "short-term memory." Hence, the objects can be immediately recalled. Working memory is sometimes also called "attention," and can be tested with forward and backward digit spans. Hippocampal lesions do not affect attention, and a person with hippocampal lesions will often have a normal forward and backward digit span and intact immediate recall of three objects. The dorsolateral frontal lobes seem to play an important part in this phase, and their integrity is important for normal "working memory." (2) The facts are "consolidated," which means that they are shifted to a longer-term memory. If the facts are to be stored for only a few minutes or hours (like a typical three object recall in the neurology examination), they are stored in recent memory. If the facts are to be learned permanently, they are further consolidated into "permanent memory." The hippocampal formations are integral for this process of consolidation, and hippocampal lesions prevent the storage of new facts in long-term memory (either recent or permanent). (3) Facts which are to be with us for the long haul are stored in long-term permanent memory, which appears to be a broadly distributed function of the brain's association cortex. Thus, hippocampal lesions cannot erase someone's store of memories. This statement, however, needs some qualification. Stored memories, to be useful to us, need to be recalled. Sometimes, this process seems to happen automatically, while at other times, there is a conscious search of our memory to recall some fact. The hippocampal formations also seem to have a significant role in this recall process, especially for facts learned more recently. It is less important for core facts, which we have known for years.

Therefore, hippocampal lesions will typically present with anterograde amnesia (the inability to consolidate new facts or events), and a variable component of retrograde amnesia, where some facts and events for a period of time before the lesion may also be forgotten.

Discuss the anatomy and connections of the hippocampal formation.

The hippocampal formation derives its name from the Greek word for "sea horse," indicating its curved inverted S-shaped structure on coronal sections. This shape also inspired the term cornu Ammonis, which is Latin for the horn of the ancient Egyptian ram-headed god, Ammon. Personally, I prefer to think of the shape as resembling a jelly roll. The hippocampal formation consists of three components: the hippocampus, the dentate gyrus, and the subiculum. Looking at a coronal section, the

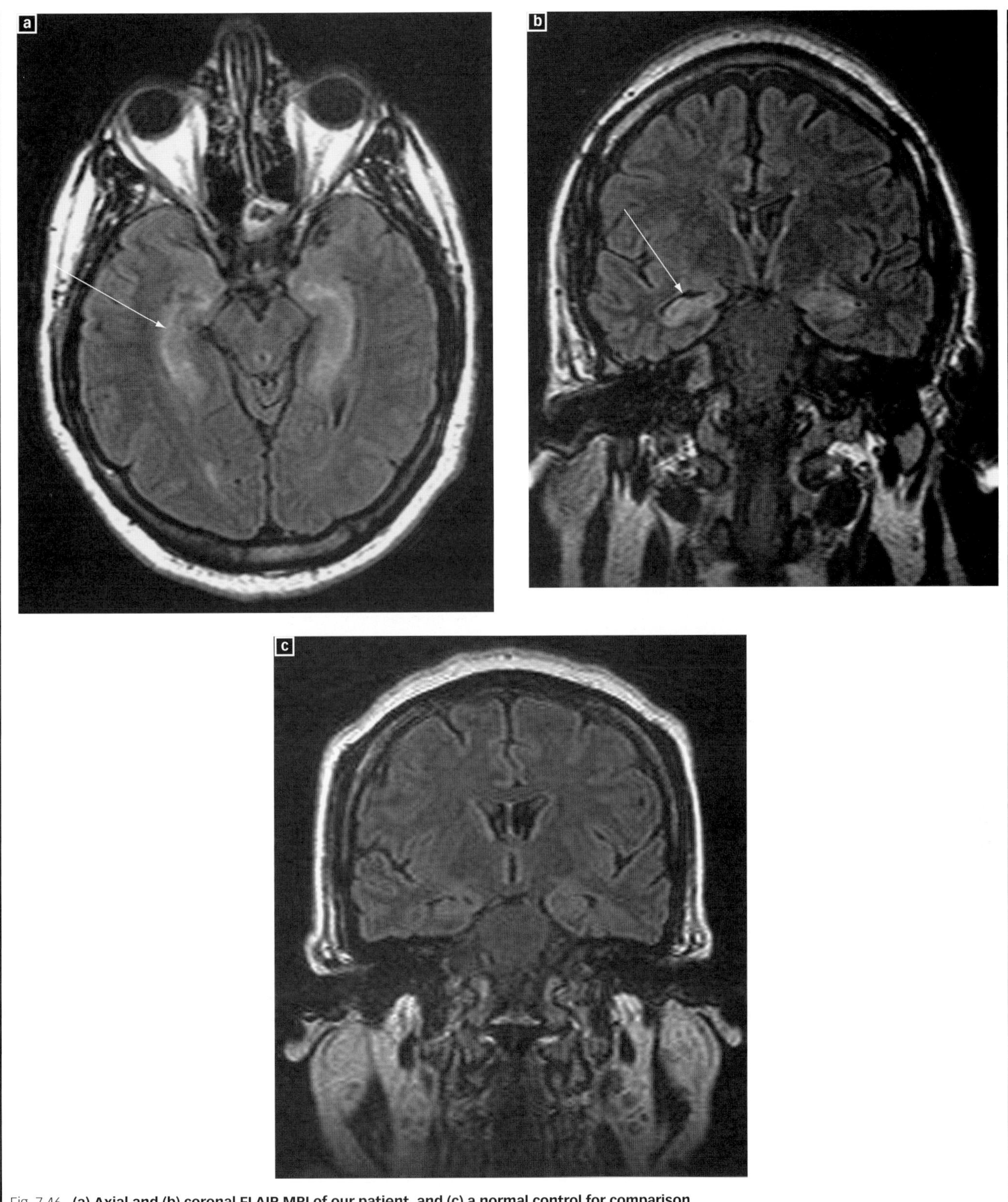

Fig. 7.46. **(a) Axial and (b) coronal FLAIR MRI of our patient, and (c) a normal control for comparison.**

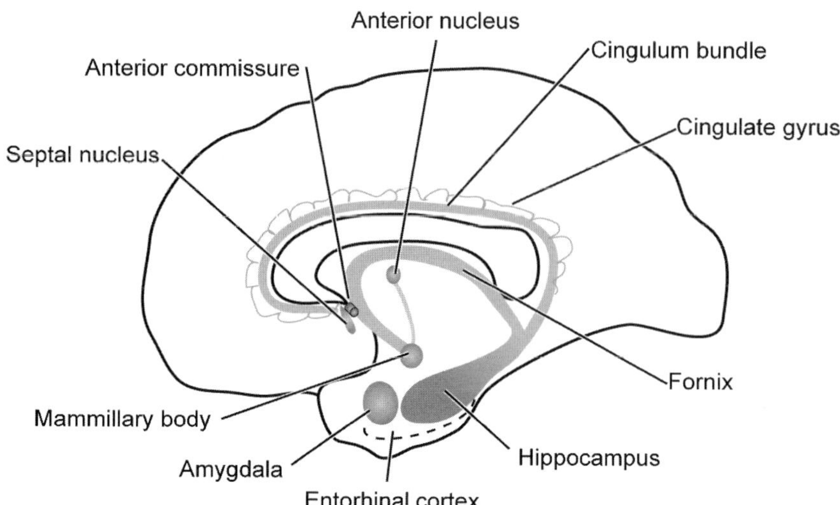

Fig. 7.47. **Schematic diagram outlining some of the main elements of the limbic system.**

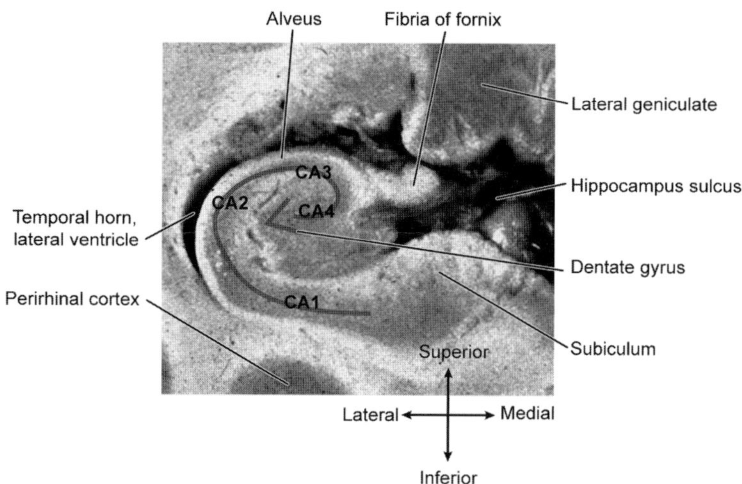

Fig. 7.48. **Coronal section of the right temporal lobe showing the anatomy of the hippocampal formation and adjacent structures. Notice how the hippocampal head lies inferomedial to the temporal horn of the right lateral ventricle.**

hippocampal formation lies ventromedial to the temporal horn of the lateral ventricle, invaginating the temporal horn (Fig. 7.48).

Both the hippocampus and the dentate gyrus are made up of three cell layers. Each contains a polymorphic cell layer, and a molecular cell layer. The hippocampus also contains a pyramidal cell layer, while the dentate gyrus contains a granule cell layer. There are different types of pyramidal cells, and depending on the cell type, the hippocampus has been divided into four sectors, CA1, CA2, CA3, and CA4, where the "CA" stands for cornu Ammonis. Deep within the heart of the jelly roll of the hippocampal formation is the dentate gyrus (Fig. 7.48). Abutting the hilus of the dentate gyrus is CA4, and spiraling outward are sequentially CA3, CA2, and CA1, which lies most inferiorly and superficially. The CA1 sector is the most vulnerable to ischemic damage, as well as to neurodegenerative diseases such as Alzheimer's disease. It directly abuts the third component of the hippocampal formation, known as the subiculum. The subiculum, in turn, transitions into the parahippocampal gyrus through areas known as the presubiculum and the parasubiculum. The parahippocampal gyrus is separated from the neocortex of the remainder of the temporal lobe by the collateral sulcus.

Most of the input to the hippocampal formation comes from an adjacent area of the parahippocampal gyrus known as the entorhinal cortex (Brodmann's area 28). The entorhinal cortex functions as the filter and gatekeeper between the rest of the cerebral cortex and the hippocampal formation. It receives numerous inputs both from modality-specific cortex, and unimodal and heteromodal association cortex. It filters these inputs and conveys them to the hippocampal formation through two pathways: the perforant pathway from the parahippocampal gyrus to the hippocampus and the dentate gyrus (which perforates directly through the subiculum), and an alvear pathway through the alveus. The hippocampus has two main output pathways: a pathway of efferents back to the entorhinal cortex (coming predominantly from the subiculum), and a white matter tract which begins on the ventricular surface of the hippocampus as a flat sheet known as the alveus, and which becomes the fornix. The fornix receives fibers from both the hippocampus and the subiculum (which in turn receives fibers from the hippocampus). The paired fornices curve in a C-shape like the parahippocampal gyrus and the hippocampal formation, except that they travel beneath the corpus callosum. As the columns of the fornix

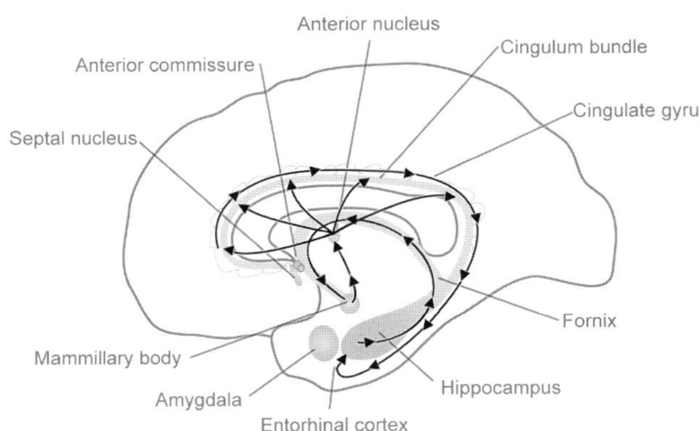

Fig. 7.49. **Simplified diagram of the Papez circuit: hippocampal formation —> fornix —> mammillary body —> anterior nucleus of the thalamus —> cingulate gyrus —> parahippocampal gyrus —> entorhinal cortex —> hippocampal formation.**

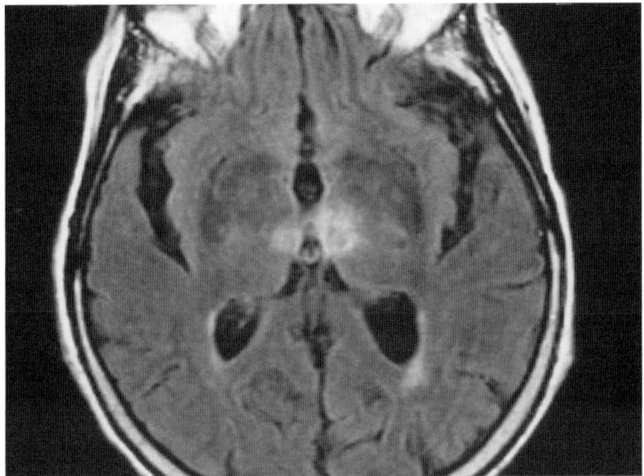

Fig. 7.50. **64-year-old man who suddenly developed apathy and memory deficits, being oriented only to person. MRI shows bilateral anterior paramedian thalamic infarcts.**

descend, most of the fibers travel behind the anterior commissure (forming the post-commissural fornix) and terminate in the mammillary bodies, while a small proportion of the fibers travel in front of the anterior commissure (pre-commissural fornix) to terminate in the septal nuclei, medial frontal cortex, anterior hypothalamus and ventral striatum. This pathway is part of a limbic circuit known as the Papez circuit, after the American neuroanatomist James Papez (Fig. 7.49). To summarize the Papez circuit, fibers begin in the hippocampus and flow through the postcommissural fornix to the mammillary bodies. From there, fibers travel via the mammillothalamic tract to the anterior thalamic nuclei. Fibers then project via the thalamocortical fiber tracts to the cingulate gyrus, which is the anterior continuation of the parahippocampal gyrus (the forward portion of its C loop). From the cingulate gyrus, impulses travel back to the parahippocampal gyrus, and then back to the hippocampal formation through the entorhinal area of the parahippocampal gyrus.

This is a very simplified picture of the circuitry, but it gives a rough idea of how the hippocampal formation communicates with the rest of the brain. In some fashion yet to be understood,

it is able to consolidate memories through these connections, as well as to participate in emotional behavior, core functions known as homeostatic responses which are important to species preservation (like feeding), and to contribute to motivation.

Thus, hippocampal lesions can cause profound memory deficits, as in our patient with anterograde amnesia in the aftermath of anoxic injury to the hippocampus. Moreover, from the above description of hippocampal connections, we can appreciate that lesions involving the so-called diencephalic memory pathways (fornix–mammillary bodies–anterior thalamic nuclei) can also cause similar memory deficits. An example is the mammillary body atrophy associated with Korsakoff's syndrome, and the attendant memory deficits. Also, lesions of the paramedian thalami, as you recall, can cause a combination of apathy and anterograde amnesia, reflecting the role of the limbic system in motivation and memory (Fig. 7.50).

To end our review of the hippocampal formation, let us quickly preview a few additional interesting cases:

(1) A 60-year-old man survived herpes encephalitis and was left with profound anterograde amnesia. His MRI, shown below (Fig. 7.51), reveals liquefactive change of both mesial temporal lobes with destruction of the hippocampal formations.

This MRI looks remarkably similar to that of perhaps the most famous patient in neurology, known as H.M. This patient, at 27 years of age, underwent bilateral medial temporal lobectomies in an attempt to control refractory epilepsy (see Corkin *et al.*, 1997). The surgery left H.M. with a profound anterograde amnesia. He had a normal IQ, and intact immediate recall, but within five minutes of being given three words to remember, he not only forgot the words, but forgot even being asked to remember them. H.M. could converse normally with his doctor, but when his doctor left the room and returned a few minutes later, H.M. would forget ever having seen him, and was frustrated at constantly having to talk to new doctors. It was H.M.'s experience, to some degree, which called attention to the fact that bilateral temporal lobectomies should not be performed to treat epilepsy.

(2) An important condition to be familiar with in the setting of epilepsy is hippocampal sclerosis, also known as Ammon's horn sclerosis. This condition, which entails loss of the pyramidal cells in the hippocampus, is found in 65 percent of cases of temporal lobe epilepsy (typically characterized by complex partial seizures). The hallmark of hippocampal sclerosis on MRI is shrinkage and abnormal FLAIR and T2-weighted hyperintensity of the involved hippocampus (Fig. 7.52).

This condition is important to identify on MRI, since if there is a concordance between MRI, EEG and PET findings, surgical therapy has a greater than 90 percent success rate in curing temporal lobe epilepsy.

(3) The case below (Fig. 7.53) is that of a 76-year-old male with Alzheimer's disease and consequent profound memory impairment. The coronal MRI (Fig. 7.53) reveals marked atrophy of the hippocampal formations bilaterally, and this sort of hippocampal atrophy is the best diagnostic MRI finding for Alzheimer's. Indeed, neuropathologists have found that the hippocampal formations are heavily impacted in Alzheimer's disease, with an especially high concentration of neurofibrillary tangles and senile plaques. The resultant hippocampal atrophy, of course, correlates with the marked memory deficits characteristic of Alzheimer's dementia. The pattern of hippocampal damage, now that we have reviewed some hippocampal anatomy and circuitry, becomes particularly interesting. For example, we know that the efferent projections of the hippocampus – both directly back to broad areas of the cortex via projections from the hippocampus to the

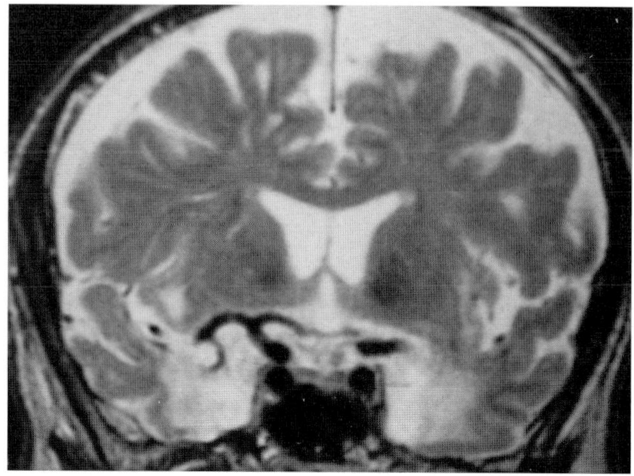

Fig. 7.51. **Coronal T2-weighted image shows bilateral mesial temporal lobe encephalomalacia status post herpes encephalitis.**

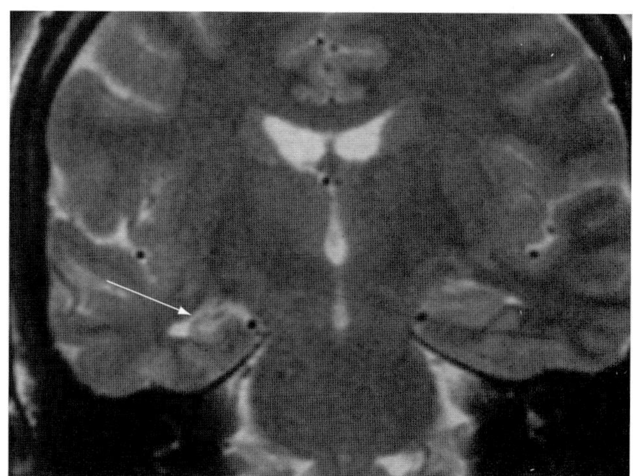

Fig. 7.52. **Coronal T2-weighted MRI in a patient with right hippocampal sclerosis. The right hippocampal formation is shrunken and abnormally hyperintense compared to the normal left side (arrow).**

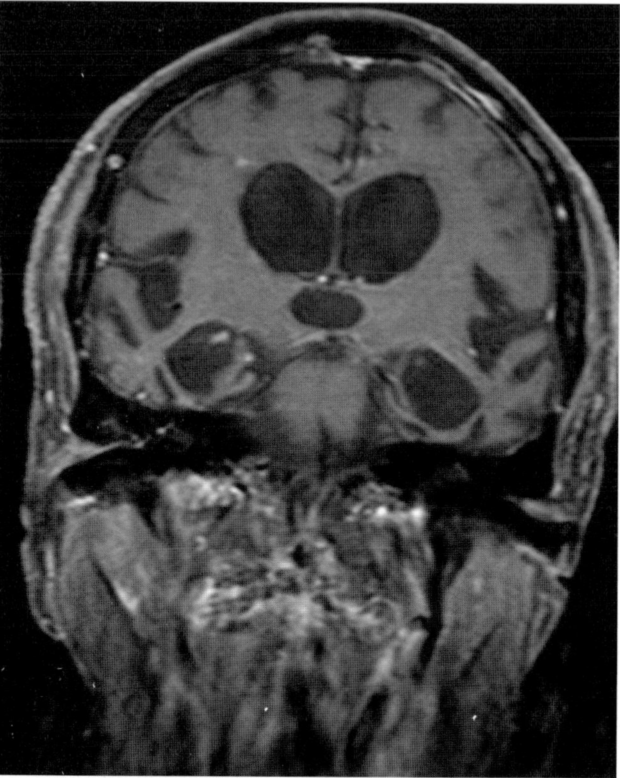

Fig. 7.53. **T1-weighted post-contrast coronal MRI reveals marked hippocampal atrophy with compensatory dilatation of the temporal horns of the lateral ventricles.**

Alzheimer's not only damages the hippocampus, but also isolates it from the rest of the brain by cutting off its efferent and afferent pathways, and this likely contributes to the marked memory degeneration (see Van Hoesen and Hyman, 1990 and Hyman *et al.*, 1984).

References

Corkin, S., Amaral, D. G., Gonzalez, R. G. *et al.* H.M.'s medial temporal lesion: findings from magnetic resonance imaging. *Journal of Neuroscience* 1997; **17**(10): 3964–3979.

Hyman, B. T., Van Hoesen, G. W., Damasio, A. R. *et al.* Alzheimer's disease: cell-specific pathology isolates the hippocampal formation. *Science* 1984; **225** (4667): 1168–1170.

Van Hoesen, G. W. and Hyman, B. T. Hippocampal formation: anatomy and the patterns of pathology in Alzheimer's disease. *Progress in Brain Research* 1990; **83**: 445–457.

entorhinal cortex, and to the diencephalon and basal forebrain through the fornix – emanate mainly from the subiculum and the CA1 hippocampal sector. These two regions, it turns out, are the most severely affected in Alzheimer's. Also, layer II of the entorhinal cortex suffers severe neurofibrillary degeneration. It is in this layer that the perforant pathway into the hippocampus predominantly originates. Thus,

---

Case 7.16

66-year-old male patient referred for new onset complex partial seizures which begin with an olfactory aura (the patient senses an extremely unpleasant odor), accompanied by extreme fear and anxiety.

Given the above history, where do you think the patient's lesion is located?

The presence of an olfactory aura strongly suggests a lesion in the anteromedial temporal lobe, in the region of the olfactory cortex. To review briefly, olfactory nerves pass through the cribriform plate, synapse in the olfactory bulb on each side, and nerve fibers travel from the olfactory bulbs through the olfactory tracts to reach the primary olfactory cortex. This organization is unique, since olfaction is the only sensory modality which does not pass through the thalamus before it projects to cortex, and most of the nerve fibers pass to ipsilateral rather than contralateral cortex. The primary olfactory cortex is made up of the piriform cortex and the periamygdaloid cortex, located just rostral to the amygdala in the anteromedial temporal lobe.

The amygadala, in turn, is part of the limbic system, as described in the previous case. It lies just anterior and dorsal to the hippocampal formation in the anteromedial temporal lobe, adjacent to the primary olfactory cortex. As stated before, the limbic system works as a whole, along with numerous other brain areas, to accomplish its main functions of memory, emotions, drives, and adjusting appetitive states and maintaining homeostatic functions. However, just as we say that the hippocampal formations are central to the limbic system's memory function, we state that the amygdala is central to emotions and drives. In particular, the amygdala seems key in mediating the fear response, and it is well known that seizures arising in the amygdala can be accompanied by feelings of panic and extreme fear.

On the basis of these considerations, we would place the lesion in the anteromedial temporal lobe, particularly in the amygdala and adjacent olfactory cortex.

The patient's MRI is presented (Fig. 7.54) What are the findings?

The MRI reveals a ring-enhancing lesion in the left anteromedial temporal lobe, anterior and rostral to the hippocampal formation. This lesion is located in the amygdala and adjacent cortex.

Briefly describe the anatomy and connections of the amygdala.

Through a set of complex interactions with multiple cortical and subcortical structures, the amygdala has a central role in mediating emotions and drives. It is composed of three main nuclei, and the neural connections of each of these nuclei seems geared towards helping with a certain facet of the amygdala's functions. These three nuclei are the central nucleus, the corticomedial nucleus, and the basolateral nucleus. The basolateral nucleus is the largest, and communicates with diverse cortical areas including multiple regions of heteromodal association cortex, other regions of limbic cortex including the hippocampus, the basal forebrain, and the medial thalami. This latter set of connections to the medial thalami may explain, in part, why lesions of the bilateral amygdala lead to placidity and lesions of the bilateral medial thalami lead to apathy. The connections to the hippocampus seem important in attaching emotional significance to memories, particularly to fearful memories.

The corticomedial nucleus interacts with the olfactory cortex. Also, some fibers of the olfactory tract project directly to the corticomedial nucleus. The corticomedial nucleus also interacts with the hypothalamus. This set of connections probably plays a role both in attaching emotional significance to odors and in appetitive responses of the hypothalamus in response to olfactory stimuli (like feeling hungry when we smell a great dish being prepared, although we did not feel hungry before!).

The central nucleus is the smallest of the amygdaloid nuclei, and interacts with the hypothalamus and brainstem. It seems important in mediating the autonomic and neuroendocrine responses associated with emotion, such as the sympathetic response which accompanies fear.

The neuronal connections of the amygdala will be touched upon only very briefly, looking at cortical and subcortical

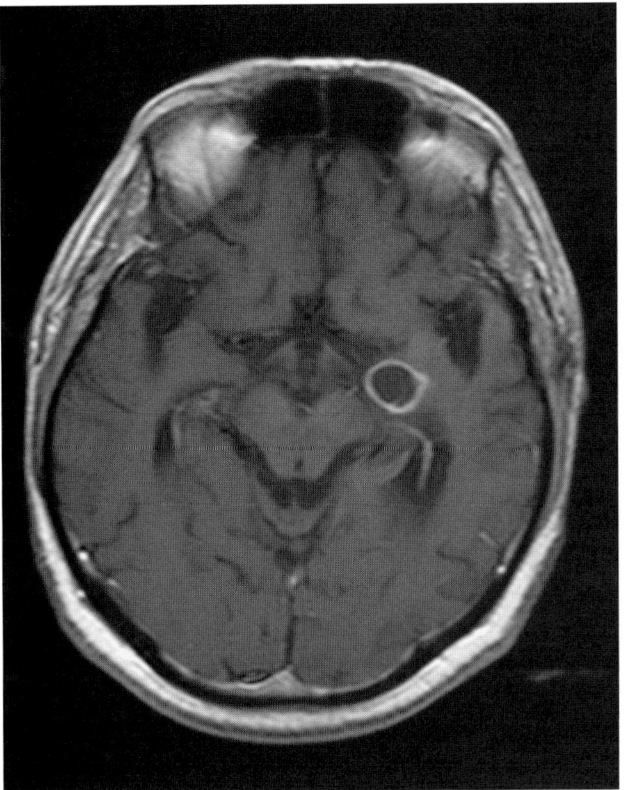

Fig. 7.54. **Axial T1-weighted post-contrast image.**

connections in turn. The amygdala sends fibers posteriorly and laterally through the temporal lobes to interact with multiple cortical areas, including reciprocal connections with the hippocampus. It also sends fibers anteriorly through a white matter tract known as the uncinate fasciculus to the cingulate cortex and the inferomedial frontal lobes. The subcortical connections of the amygdala to the thalamus, hypothalamus and brainstem are important for the motivational, neuroendocrine and autonomic facets of emotional response as mentioned above. These connections occur via two main pathways: the stria terminalis and the ventral amygdalofugal pathway. The stria terminalis is another C-shaped structure (following the theme of the limbic system), which runs along the inferolateral wall of the lateral ventricle, from the amygdala to the hypothalamus and spetal regions. It is a main output pathway of the amygdala, analogous to the fornix in relation to the hippocampus. The ventral amygdalofugal pathway connects the amygdala with the basal forebrain, ventral striatum, brainstem, and the medial thalami.

Through this web of connections, once again in a fashion not yet understood, the amygdala is central in producing in us the powerful array of emotions and drives which both characterize us as humans and link us with the remainder of the animal kingdom.

Case 7.17

41-year-old male patient presents with progressive dementia over several months. Neurological examination reveals profound memory deficits, with significant anterograde amnesia manifested as 0/3 object recall at 5 minutes. The patient also had visual agnosia, with a markedly diminished ability to recognize familiar objects. The patient also showed pronounced behavioral changes over the span of the last several months. The most pronounced of these was extreme hypersexuality. The patient also developed hyperorality (putting objects into the mouth) and marked hyperphagia (extreme food consumption), with rapid weight gain.

There were no focal motor deficits. The patient's sensorium was clear.

What does the constellation of findings suggest?

As described previously, profound anterograde amnesia suggests involvement of the hippocampal formations, or possibly the medial thalami. The patient also seems to have profound disturbances that can be characterized as an increase in the basic drives for sex and food. We have previously discussed the role of the amygdala in motivations and drives. Therefore, temporal lobe damage would seem the most reasonable possibility.

MRI images are presented (Fig. 7.55). What are the findings?

The MRI image shows profound hippocampal atrophy bilaterally. There is also extensive gliosis in the right temporal lobe, with similar but less pronounced changes on the left. The findings raise the possibility of an infectious encephalitis. Cerebrospinal fluid analysis and PCR viral typing did not yield any definite infectious agent, although there was some oligoclonal banding in the CSF, suggesting an inflammatory response. A right temporal lobe brain biopsy was performed, which revealed non-specific encephalitis.

Diagnosis

Kluver–Bucy syndrome, secondary to non-specific bilateral temporal lobe encephalitis.

Discuss the Kluver–Bucy syndrome.

This is a very rare neurological syndrome, which manifests with:

(1) Severe memory deficits, with anterograde amnesia
(2) Hypersexuality
(3) Hyperorality and hyperphagia

Other manifestations may include dementia, visual agnosia, placidity with loss of fear and anger responses, easy visual distractibility, and seizures.

This syndrome is thought to be secondary to anteromedial temporal lobe lesions, particularly involving the amygdala and the hippocampal formations. It ties in the two previous cases nicely, as it shows the clinical manifestations of damage to both regions. The most common etiology of the Kluver–Bucy syndrome is post herpes encephalitis. It has also been described secondary to trauma, and in the settings of such dementing illnesses as Pick's disease with frontotemporal atrophy.

This syndrome was actually initially described based on animal experiments (in monkeys) with surgical lesions involving the mesial temporal lobes. There has been some debate over whether the syndrome actually exists in humans. Certainly, there are several human case reports, although most of these tend to be isolated cases, or very small series. The number of reports, though, has increased in recent years with improved survival of herpes encephalitis patients.

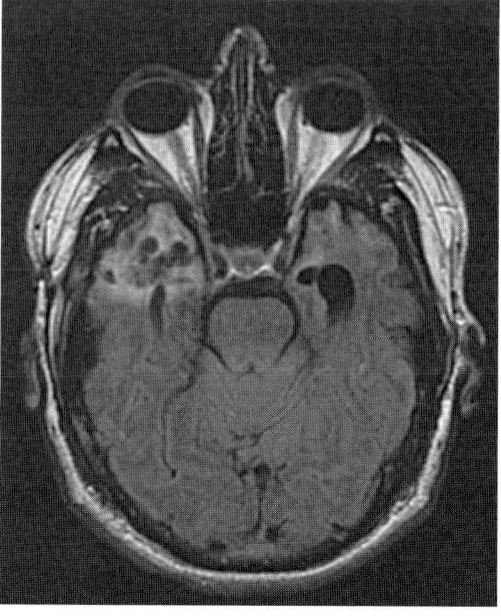

Fig. 7.55. **Axial FLAIR MRI image. Case courtesy of Dr. Mario Mendez, UCLA Department of Neurology, Division of Neurobehavior.**

This case is presented here because it is a rare and interesting syndrome which correlates with our study of the limbic system (the above case is the only one I have ever seen!). However, the precise neuroanatomic basis of the syndrome remains elusive.

There have been attempts to treat this syndrome with selective serotonin reuptake inhibitors and carbamazepine.

The interested reader is asked to refer to the references below.

References

Goscinski, I., Kwiatkowski, S., Polak, J., *et al.* The Kluver–Bucy syndrome. *Journal of Neurosurgical Science* 1997; **41**(3): 269–272.

Pradhan, S., Singh, M. N., and Pandey, N. Kluver–Bucy syndrome in young children. *Clinical Neurology and Neurosurgery* 1998; **100**(4): 254–258.

Slaughter, J., Bobo, W., and Childers, M. K. Selective serotonin reuptake inhibitor treatment of post-traumatic Kluver-Bucy syndrome. *Brain Injury* 1999; **13**(1): 59–62.

Case 7.18

53-year-old patient with a subtle gradual personality change, brought in by his wife. Apparently, the patient is displaying some emotional lability, with poor impulse control. The patient, by report, has become socially inappropriate, often making tactless and sexually explicit remarks to strangers. The patient also sometimes flies into fits of rage.

Neurologic testing displayed some evidence of disinhibition, with the patient often interrupting the examiner with inappropriate comments. No focal motor or sensory deficits are elicited. No language deficits are appreciated. The patient's recent and remote memory appeared intact.

Based on the history and exam findings, where in the brain do you think the lesion might be located?

The patient seems to be displaying lack of judgment and socially inappropriate behavior. Such a history makes us consider frontal lobe lesions involving the large cortical areas anterior to the premotor regions, which are collectively known as the prefrontal cortex. These areas are significantly larger in humans than in other mammals, and are thought to underlie many of the cerebral functions which distinguish our species. More specifically, we note that the prefrontal cortex is not involved in concrete functions, such as perception of a specific sensory modality or performance of motor tasks, the way other regions of the cortex are. Instead, the prefrontal cortex, in broad terms, may be stated to have three significant abstract functions:

(1) Judgment and insight (including a sense of self-inhibition which prevents socially inappropriate behavior).
(2) Reasoning and planning.
(3) Motivation and initiative. This particular aspect of frontal lobe functioning is also linked to the limbic system, as described previously.

The patient's MRI examination is presented (Fig. 7.56). What are the findings? What is your diagnosis?

There is a large extra-axial midline lesion along the region of the olfactory groove, causing significant displacement and mass effect on the gyri recti and the orbitofrontal gyri bilaterally. Post-contrast images show uniform enhancement of this lesion. The imaging characteristics are consistent with a large meningioma along the floor of the anterior cranial fossa.

How can the patient's symptoms be linked to this lesion? Specifically, discuss the notion of three main frontal lobe circuits and their putative functions.

Now that we have characterized the three main domains of function of the prefrontal cortex, the question naturally arises as to whether specific lesion locations selectively affect each of the three domains. It turns out that the answer is "yes and no." Neuroanatomists and behavioral neurologists have mapped the main functions of the prefrontal cortex into three distinct neural loops or circuits, each circuit preferentially associated with a particular domain. However, lesions do not typically tend to respect the anatomic boundaries of a circuit, and the neural pathways in the separate circuits often run quite close together, so that a particular lesion may simultaneously affect several domains. Even this explanation is quite simplistic, since identical looking lesions in different patients often have opposite clinical effects, causing disinhibition in one patient while leading to apathy in another. More confusing still, the same patient can episodically manifest opposing behavior patterns.

All that being said, however, we note that some useful generalizations are possible, and that it is quite interesting and instructive to review the three functional circuits of the prefrontal cortex, keeping in mind that they do not work in isolation, and that the correlation between lesion location and behavioral disturbance is a loose one.

The circuits have a characteristic overall general organization which should be familiar to us from our prior study of the basal ganglia. Each circuit begins and ends in a specific region of the prefrontal cortex, and goes through the caudate nucleus, globus pallidus, and thalamus, prior to returning to its cortical field of origin. The three circuits are named according to the location of the prefrontal cortex in which they originate, and are traditionally described as follows:

The dorsolateral circuit

This neural loop begins and ends in the dorsolateral prefrontal cortex in Brodmann's areas 9 and 10. Neurons from these regions project to the dorsolateral caudate nucleus. From the caudate, there are direct and indirect pathways to the globus pallidus interna, with balancing excitatory and inhibitory functions. The indirect pathway gets to the globus pallidus interna by way of the subthalamic nucleus. This follows the scheme which we encountered when we discussed the interaction of the motor cortex and the basal ganglia. From the globus pallidus interna, the circuit continues to the ventral anterior and dorsomedial nuclei of the thalamus, and then returns to the dorsolateral prefrontal cortex. During its course, the circuit has reciprocal connections with multiple other cortical regions. The dorsolateral circuit is thought to function primarily in reasoning and planning. Lesions in this circuit cause loss of the so-called "executive

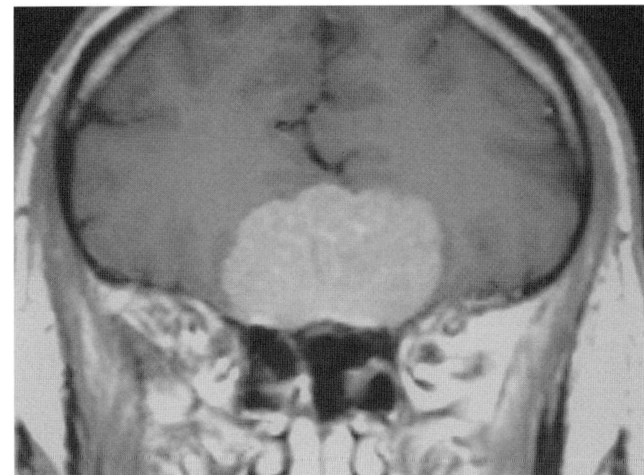

Fig. 7.56. **Post-contrast coronal T1-weighted image.**

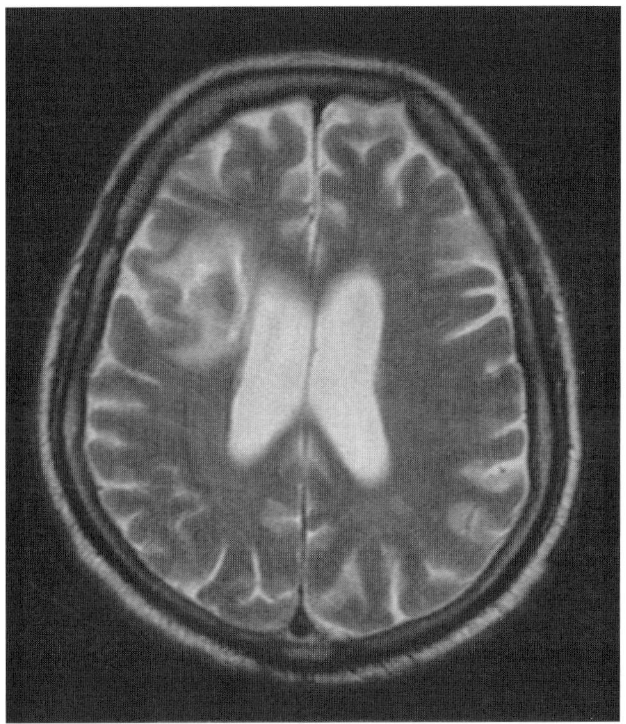

Fig. 7.57. **Unusual deep right frontal lobe hemorrhagic infarct which clinically seemed to involve the dorsolateral frontal circuit.**

functions." Patients are very concrete in their thinking, and are unable to plan the sequential steps in a multi-step task. Also, patients may be unable to focus on a task, and are unable to shift from one task to another, so they may show perseveration. The dorsolateral frontal lobes are also important for the function of "attention," or "working memory," as described in Case 7.15. That is why lesions in this area may cause inability to focus and easy distractability; the patient cannot keep in mind that they are involved in a specific task.

A nice example is the patient displayed above (Fig. 7.57). He was a 71-year-old male who suffered an unusual deep right frontal lobe hemorrhagic infarct involving the dorsolateral prefrontal

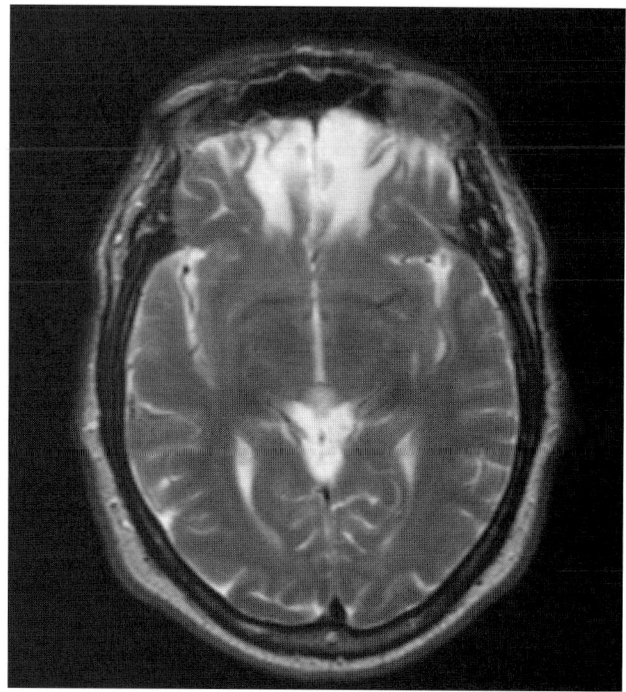

Fig. 7.58. **Patient with post-traumatic encephalomalacia involving the inferomedial frontal lobes. The patient was disinhibited and socially inappropriate.**

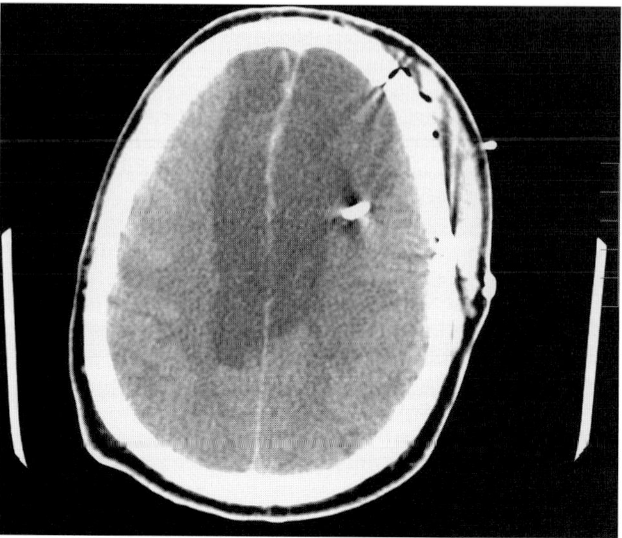

Fig. 7.59. **Devastating case of a 42-year-old male who suffered bilateral high anteromedial frontal lobe infarcts following a subarachnoid bleed. The patient was reduced to a state of lethargy, akinetic mutism, and incontinence secondary to involvement of the bilateral anterior cingulate circuits.**

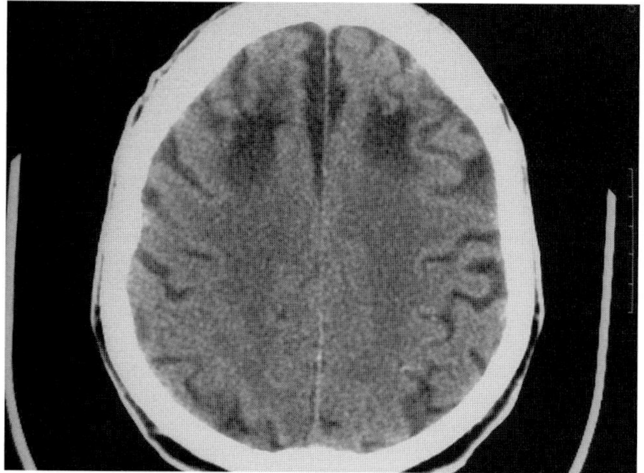

Fig. 7.60. **One of the few surviving lobotomy patients at our hospital. Note the focal leukomalacia of the white matter in the bilateral frontal lobes.**

cortex. The patient developed profound difficulties with executive function. For example, he would feel cold, and would turn on the air conditioner, then the heater, then the air conditioner, then the heater, and so on, unable to stick to the simple plan of putting on a sweater, and turning on the heater and waiting for the room to warm up.

The orbitofrontal circuit

This neural loop begins and ends in the inferomedial prefrontal cortex, involving the inferomedial aspect of Brodmann's area 10, and Brodmann's area 11, along the medial base of the frontal lobes, including the regions of the gyrus rectus and the orbitofrontal gyri. Axons from these cortical regions project to the ventromedial caudate nucleus, and from there to the globus pallidus interna through direct and indirect pathways similar to the dorsolateral circuit. From there, axons project to the ventral anterior and dorsomedial thalamic nuclei, and back to the orbitofrontal cortex. This neural circuit also receives significant input from the amygdala, and anterior temporal lobes. The orbitofrontal circuit is thought to function in judgment and self-restraint. It helps us conduct ourselves in a socially appropriate fashion. Therefore, lesions of this circuit produce disinhibition, loss of impulse control, emotional lability and explosiveness, as well as crude and tactless behavior.

Our patient presented above has a lesion impinging the inferomedial frontal lobes, involving primarily the orbitofrontal circuit. This particular patient displayed the expected disinhibition and loss of orientation to "socially appropriate" cues. The most common cause of such findings, though, seems to be post-traumatic frontal lobe injury, which tends to involve the inferomedial frontal lobes and anterior frontal poles (Fig. 7.58).

The anterior cingulate circuit

This circuit begins and ends in Brodmann's area 24, known as the "ventral anterior cingulate" area, which comprises much of the anterior cingulate gyrus and portions of the adjacent frontal lobe. This circuit is closely linked to the limbic system, and fibers from the anterior cingulate gyrus course to the "limbic striatum," i.e., the ventral caudate and putamen and the region of the nucleus accumbens. From there, the circuit continues to both the ventral and rostromedial globus pallidus interna, then onto the dorsomedial thalamus, and finally back to the anterior cingulate cortex. Like the others, this circuit also likely has an indirect pathway which utilizes the subthalamic nucleus. This circuit receives significant limbic input in the form of connections between the amygdala, hippocampus, and entorhinal cortex and the limbic striatum. The main function of this circuit is felt to be motivation and initiative. Thus, lesions here (particularly bilateral lesions) produce marked apathy and abulia (lack of will or initiative), which in the severest forms may manifest as akinetic mutism. Patients may not have enough initiative to eat and drink on their own, and may become incontinent (Fig. 7.59).

A final interesting and pertinent aside is a brief digression to the topic of frontal lobotomy. This procedure, performed on as many as 40 000 people in the U.S. in the mid 1900s, was meant to disconnect the prefrontal cortex from the rest of the brain (see Fig. 7.60).

Even in its most refined form, it was a very crude procedure, where long sharp instruments were placed into the anterior frontal lobes through the orbital roofs or the frontal bones, and moved around to sever the white matter tracts (hence the procedure's original name of "leukotomy"). It is not, as many people conceive, an open craniotomy with surgical removal of the frontal lobes, but rather a functional disconnection of the frontal lobes from the rest of the brain by severing their afferent and efferent white matter pathways. This procedure became popular long before detailed knowledge of the separate prefrontal circuits described above was attained, and was far too crude to lesion a particular circuit. Now we know that its presumed target was mainly the anterior cingulate circuit, to produce apathy in those with mental illness and violent tendencies. Seemingly, however, this drastic procedure was abused beyond its role as an extreme, last resort sort of measure. It took until the late 1970s or early 1980s for this procedure to become discredited, but for many decades, it was considered legitimate medicine. In fact, it may interest the reader to know that the Portuguese physician and neurologist, António Egas Moniz, was awarded the 1949 Nobel Prize in Medicine for his discovery and refinement of the frontal lobotomy as a useful therapy in the treatment of certain kinds of mental illness!

For further study of the anatomy and functional correlations of the prefrontal circuits, please see the provided references.

References

Burruss, J. W., Hurley, R. A., Taber, K. H., *et al.* Functional neuroanatomy of the frontal lobe circuits. *Radiology* 2000; **214**(1): 227–230.

Cummings, J. L. Frontal-subcortical circuits and human behavior. *Archives of Neurology* 1993; **50**(8): 873–880.

Mega, M. S. and Cummings, J. L. Frontal-subcortical circuits and neuropsychiatric disorders. *Journal of Neuropsychiatry and Clinical Neuroscience* 1994; **6**: 358–370.

Introduction

Stroke is overall the leading cause of adult disability and the third leading cause of adult mortality in the United States. The term "stroke," denoting a sudden neurologic ictus, is of two main types: ischemic and hemorrhagic. Ischemic strokes are much more common, making up about 85–90 percent of the stroke population. Of course, ischemic strokes may later undergo hemorrhagic conversion, but this is a different entity than hemorrhagic stroke, which is really a primary intracerebral bleed causing neurologic deficit.

Ischemic strokes, most of which occur secondary to vessel occlusion, can be caused by emboli traveling to the cerebral vessels from distant sites, such as from atherosclerotic plaques in the cervical internal carotid arteries or the aortic arch, thrombus in the cardiac chambers, or vegetations on cardiac valve leaflets. Strokes may also be caused by local vascular thrombosis potentiated by hyalinoid degeneration of perforating vessels secondary to hypertension, by vascular abnormalities secondary to vasculitis, or by decreased perfusion pressure secondary to high grade stenosis, dissection, vasospasm or systemic hypotension.

To get a sense of the relative importance of each of these causes, we note that data from the Massachusetts General Hospital (Romero *et al.*, 2005) indicates that the etiologies of ischemic stroke break down roughly as follows:

30 percent secondary to carotid atherosclerotic disease

30 percent secondary to cardioembolic causes

20 percent secondary to small vessel disease (i.e., lacunar infarcts)

20 percent due to other causes; of this group, about 40 percent of strokes are secondary to aortic arch atherosclerotic disease, and about 20 percent have no identifiable cause.

If we wish to approach the issue of stroke coherently, there are several questions we must explicitly address, even if we are unable to answer some of them; at least this will structure our thinking. In the early 1990s, neuroradiologists typically looked at CT exams of the head for stroke patients in a fairly abbreviated fashion. If there was no gross blood in the brain, we often dictated something to the effect of, "re-image in 24 hours. The stroke will likely be evident then." Now, we carefully scrutinize the films, wringing them for very subtle signs of acute infarct. Why the drastic change in emphasis over little more than a decade? The answer, most fundamentally, is that there is now a potential for stroke treatment. Most of this treatment centers around thrombolysis to recanalize occluded vessels and restore cerebral perfusion.

Certainly, most readers of this book (I mean by this presumably neurology residents and radiology residents and neuroradiology fellows) are already familiar with how to diagnose acute stroke on imaging as well as with the concept of thrombolytic therapy. There is, however, less familiarity with the actual data which support the algorithms we learn for diagnosis and treatment. Therefore, in this chapter, we hope to review in slightly deeper fashion the data on stroke imaging, stroke therapy, and most importantly, the interaction between the two. In other words, how does imaging guide therapy? More briefly, we wish to cover some "clinically relevant stuff."

Basics of stroke imaging

As stated, we are less interested in describing how to diagnose stroke on imaging than in understanding the interplay between imaging and potential therapy. Therefore, the discussion of imaging findings will be brief and restricted to clinically relevant aspects.

The two main imaging modalities used in the evaluation of acute stroke patients are non-contrast CT and MRI, including diffusion-weighted images (DWI) and perfusion-weighted images (PWI). Of course, many other adjunctive imaging techniques are available, and there are multiple studies on the use of other CT techniques, such as CT angiography and CT perfusion, SPECT scanning, PET scanning, Xenon CT, and transcranial Doppler in the evaluation of acute stroke patients. Particularly promising among these are CT perfusion studies.

For now, however, we'll stick to looking at non-contrast CT and MRI.

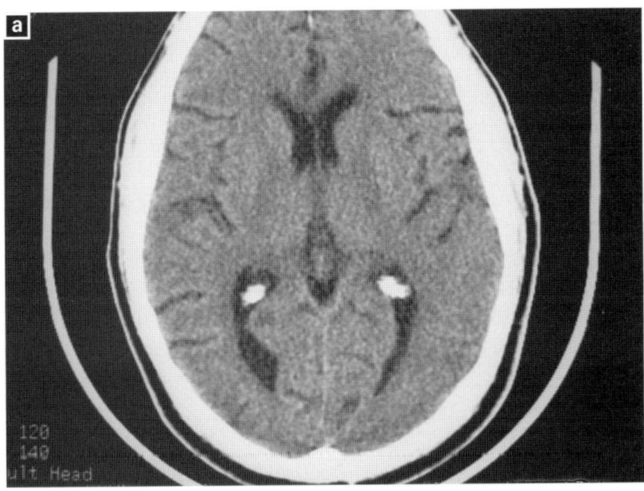

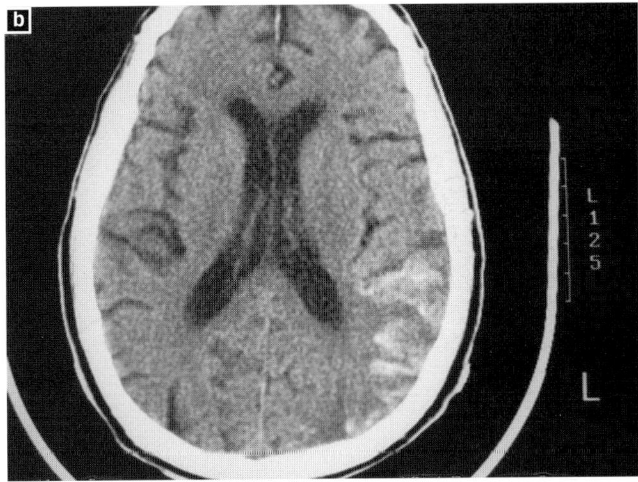

Fig. 8.1. (a) Initial CT scan shows subtle loss of sulci and subtle hypodensity in the left temporo-parietal region, consistent with an early infarct. (b) Images obtained 2 weeks later show gyriform petechial hemorrhage in the infarct zone, confirming the presence of a large infarct.

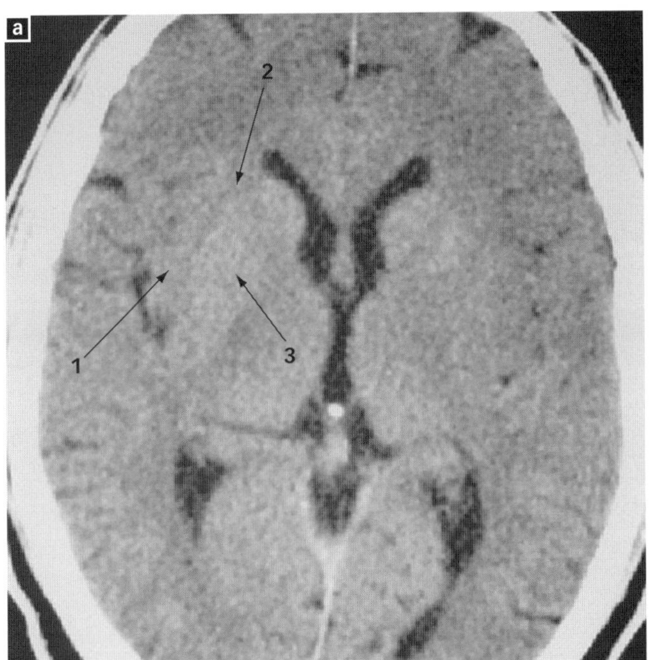

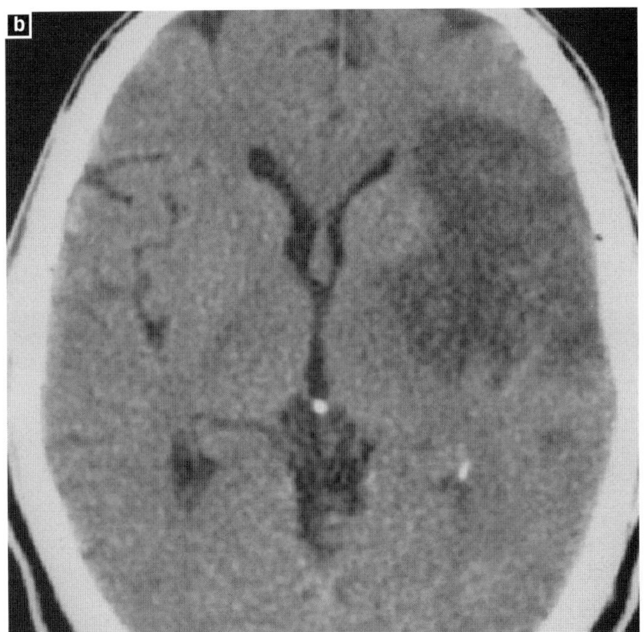

Fig. 8.2. (a) On the initial CT, there is relative hypodensity of the left insular ribbon. The right side shows the normal anatomic landmarks of a bright insular ribbon (arrow 1), a thin dark external capsule (arrow 2) and a bright putamen (arrow 3). This "bright–dark–bright" striation is lost on the left. Repeat scan 3 days later confirms a large left MCA infarct.

Non-contrast CT in acute stroke

In brief, there are three main findings on CT that aid in the diagnosis of early stroke:

Sulcal effacement

This occurs when cytotoxic edema causes enough mass effect to efface sulci in the infarct zone (Fig. 8.1). This is the latest of the early signs to appear, but may still sometimes be seen within three hours of ictus.

Hypodensity of the gray matter and loss of the gray–white matter differentiation

This occurs when cytotoxic edema begins to accumulate in the neurons, causing hypoattenuation of the gray matter so that it matches the white matter in density. A good place to look for this is along the insular ribbon; loss of the distinction between the insular cortex and the adjacent white matter of the external capsule is known as a "positive insular ribbon sign" (see Fig. 8.2).

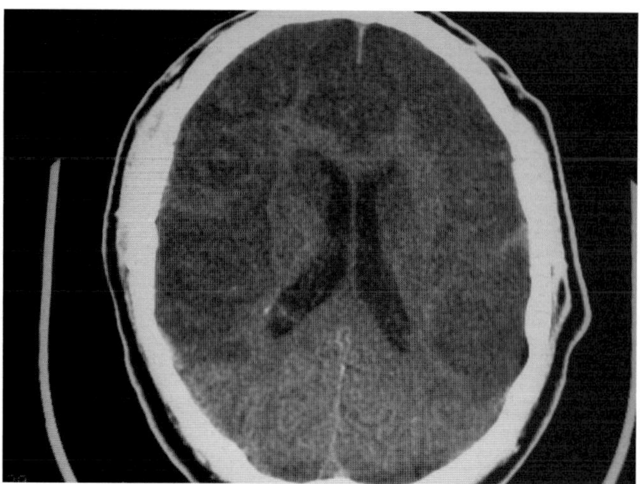

Fig. 8.3. **In this patient with bilateral anterior circulation infarcts, there is marked gray matter edema, such that the gray matter is now hypodense to the white matter.**

CT scanning works by measuring the attenuation of X-ray photons by tissue. This attenuation can be measured in terms of CT Hounsfield units (HU), which are defined relative to the linear X-ray attenuation coefficient of water, such that $HU = 1000 \times [(u_v - u_{H_2O})/u_{H_2O}]$, where u_v is the linear X-ray attenuation coefficient of the voxel of tissue being measured, and u_{H_2O} is the linear X-ray attenuation coefficient of water. Thus, according to this scale, water, by definition, has a density of 0 HU. The scale goes from about -1000 HU for air to about 3000 HU for cortical bone. Gray matter typically has an attenuation of about 40 HU, while white matter typically measures about 30 HU (thus, they are quite close, but the gray matter is a bit brighter than white matter). With early edema, the gray matter loses density, becoming iso-dense to white matter – i.e., loss of gray–white matter differentiation. As the edema becomes more pronounced, the gray matter may actually become hypodense to white matter (Fig. 8.3).

There have been passing claims that CT typically cannot diagnose these changes of early infarct in the acute (less than 3 hour) time frame, since edema will not accumulate quickly enough to produce the necessary decrease in density. Thus, some have suggested that a CT with evidence of gray matter edema should prompt a re-evaluation of the time of ictus, despite what is claimed by the patient. Experimental data, however, show that CT is well capable of diagnosing acute infarct. With severe perfusion deficits, edema begins to accu-mulate quickly in the ischemic brain. For every 1 percent increase in local water content, there is a corresponding decrease in tissue density of approximately 2.6 HU. For those with keen eyes, a visually detectable decrease in density requires a drop of at least 4 HU. In cases of severe hypoperfu-sion caused by MCA occlusion, cytotoxic edema can produce a 3 percent increase in water content in one hour (i.e., a drop of about 8 HU), and a 6 percent increase at 2–4 hours. Therefore, at least in cases of severe perfusion deficit, CT is certainly capable of detecting evolving cytotoxic edema (see Gaskill-Shipley, 1999; Unger et al., 1988; Garcia, 1984).

Dense vessels indicating intravascular clot

This sign is typically seen in the middle cerebral artery, where it is known as a "hyperdense MCA sign." It can also occur in the carotid artery terminus, where it is sometimes referred to as a "carotid T" occlusion. Uncommonly, it is seen in the basilar artery (see Figs. 8.4–8.6).

The dense vessel sign is the earliest possible CT sign of acute stroke, and may be seen prior to the development of cyototoxic edema leading to loss of the gray–white matter distinction, and prior to frank hypodensity or sulcal effacement. Unclotted blood typically measures in the 30–60 HU range, depending on such factors as hematocrit and hydration. As the blood clots, its density increases to the 60–90 HU range, making the dense vessel stand out. However, because of the broad ranges of HU, the dense vessel sign is often a difficult radiographic call. In fact, the sensitivity of this sign varies anywhere from 5 to 50 percent in the literature. One large series (Leys et al., 1992) examining 272 consecutive unselected first-time stroke patients found that the prevalence of a dense MCA sign was about 27 percent.

Overall, using these early ischemic signs (EIS), the sensitivity of non-contrast CT in diagnosing early infarct is, as a reason-able estimate, about 31 percent in the first 3 hours, and about 40–60 percent in the first 6 hours (see Schellinger, 2005).

MRI in stroke

The sensitivity of FLAIR and T2-weighted MRI, surprisingly, has been shown to be no better than conventional CT in the acute stroke setting. Increasing edema produces hyperintensity on these sequences, but usually in a time frame of about 6 hours. In one study from Massachusetts General Hospital, CT, in fact, did significantly better than conventional MRI in diagnosing acute stroke (within 6 hours). In that study, CT had a sensitivity of 45 percent, while conventional MRI had a sensitivity of only 18 percent (Gonzalez et al., 1999). Fear not, though; DWI had a sensitivity of 100 percent in that study. DWI, of course, is not 100 percent sensitive, but multiple studies have shown an excellent sensitivity in the first 6 hours, and reasonable values are prob-ably in the 94–97 percent range (Fig. 8.7) (see Mullins et al., 2002). Therefore, we will focus here on DWI and PWI techniques.

Diffusion-weighted (DWI) MRI

For those of us who work with stroke patients on a daily basis, it is probably worthwhile to know how DWI works at a slightly deeper level than, "the bright stuff means stroke." To achieve this level of understanding actually requires reviewing only a few basic principles of MRI physics and stroke physiology:

(1) MR is an imaging method which visualizes hydrogen pro-tons. Most of these hydrogen protons are part of water molecules. Thus, to some extent, MR images water mol-ecules in their different environments.

(2) Hydrogen protons behave, in some sense, like small com-pass needles – that is, they have a magnetic moment. When placed within a strong magnetic field, the protons spin, or precess, around the axis of the magnetic field at terrifically high speeds (Fig. 8.7).

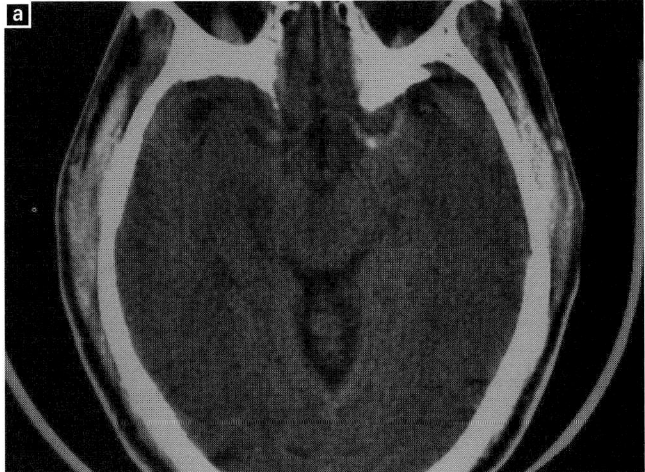

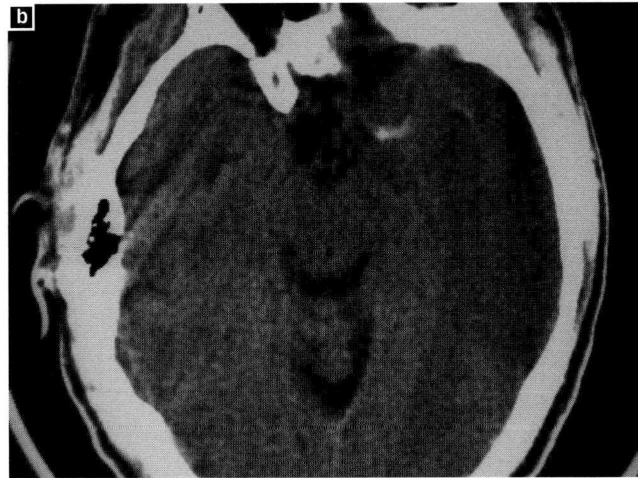

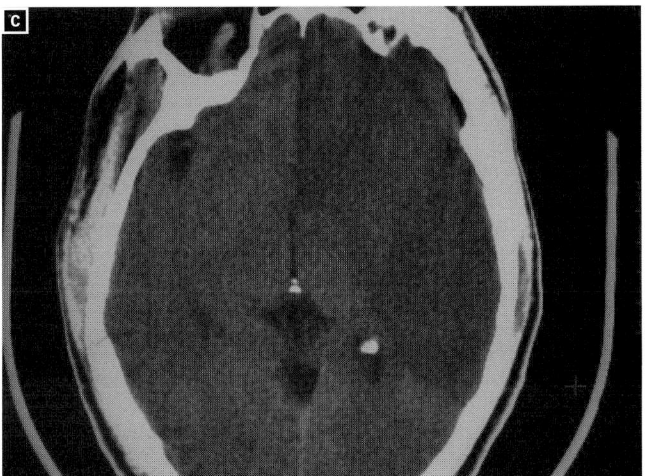

Fig. 8.4. **(a) Initial CT scan is obtained 30 minutes post-ictus. There is hyperdensity in the left carotid terminus, left A1 segment and left M1 segment consistent with a carotid T occlusion. There is no significant gray matter edema at this time. Images (b) and (c), obtained 6 hours later, show the hyperdense vessel sign and an extensive infarct of the left ACA and MCA territories.**

(3) The electrical signal which is spatially encoded to generate MR images results when the protons spin together, or in MR parlance, when they are "in phase." To picture the concept of phase, imagine each proton as a second hand on a large wall clock. If we start them all at 12:00 o'clock and let them spin around the clock face at the same speed, then they are all spinning in phase. Let's say one of the second hands starts ahead of the others, say at 3:00 o'clock, while the others are at 12:00. This particular second hand is then said to be 90 degrees out of phase with the others. Now, let us talk about protons instead of second hands. MR signal is maximal when all of the protons are in phase. If we imagine that suddenly, while the protons are at 12:00, we instantaneously switch half of them to 6:00, then one half of the protons are 180 degrees out of phase with the other half. In this case, the horizontal component of the magnetic vector of each proton at 12:00 would be cancelled by the oppositely directed magnetic vector from a proton pointed at 6:00. In such a situation, there would be no MR signal, because the protons are out of phase with each other. If instead of being split into two halves, the population of protons is now randomly and uniformly distributed around the clock face, there would again be no MR signal, because the protons would again be completely out of phase. In terms of magnetic vectors, those at 12:00 would be cancelled by those at 6:00, those at 3:00 would be cancelled by those at 9:00, etc. (see Fig. 8.8).

(4) MRI signal is generated when radiofrequency pulses, such as the so-called 90 degree pulse, force the protons into phase. When these pulses are stopped, the protons begin to slowly dephase from each other, and so the MR signal starts to decay (Fig. 8.9).

This MR signal decay occurs with an exponential time constant known as $T2^*$. Thus, dephasing leads to a decrease in MR signal. That is the key point to take away.

(5) Now, let us look at water molecules. We know that such molecules undergo Brownian motion. Each molecule, if it starts in a specific location, undergoes a random walk, wiggling and jiggling in small straight-line path segments, and over time ends up in a different location from which it started. How far the water molecule gets is governed by something called its diffusion coefficient, D. To get a sense of what this diffusion coefficient entails, imagine observing the random walk of a single water molecule for 1 second, and then covering this walk with the smallest possible disk which contains the entire path (Fig. 8.10). Molecules with a high diffusion coefficient (large value of D) require a larger disk, while those with a smaller diffusion coefficient (small value of D) require a smaller disk.

The area of the disk containing the random walk would be measured in mm². This, recall, is for a random walk which lasted 1 second. Therefore, we can see that the

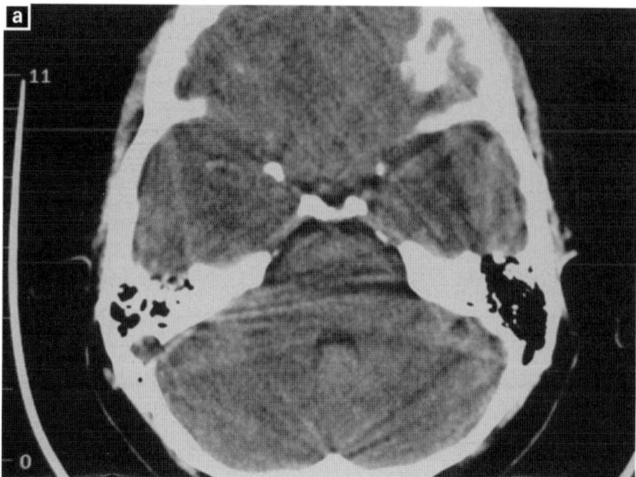

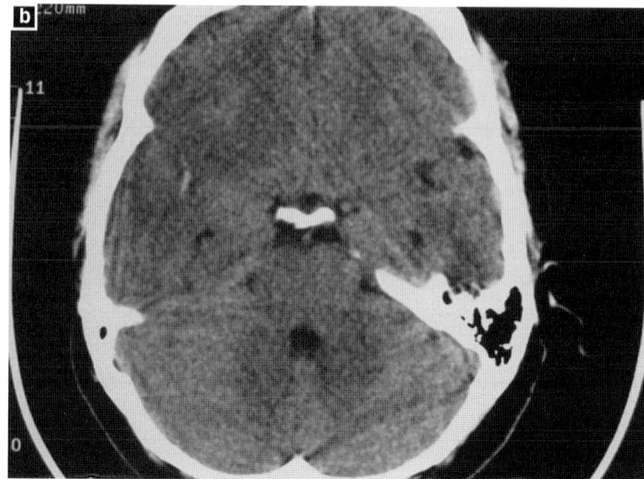

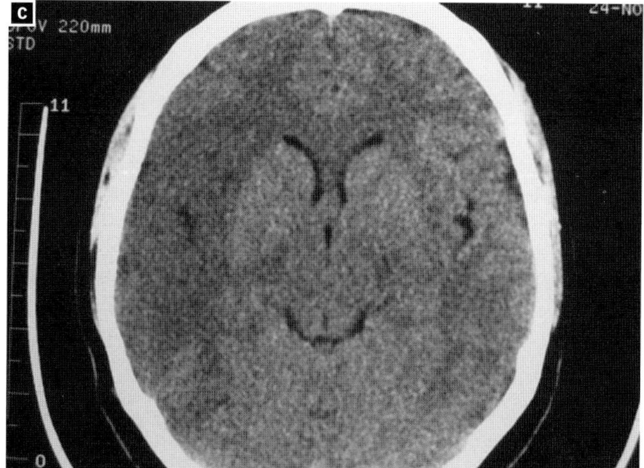

Fig. 8.5. **(a)–(c). This 33-year-old female was imaged 3 hours after ictus. There is a right-sided hyperdense MCA sign, with a large right MCA early subacute infarct. There is gray matter edema and a positive insular ribbon sign. Subsequent investigation revealed a patent foramen ovale.**

units of D are mm^2/s. For the sake of accuracy, the scenario we have just conjured is not precisely the definition of D. The precise definition was actually derived by none other than Albert Einstein (the great ones always keep popping up), but our scenario certainly captures the spirit of D sufficiently for our purposes. The bottom line is that D is measured in units of mm^2/s, and reflects how far a water molecule drifts per unit time. Water molecules with high values of D travel far and their random walks are contained in a disk of large area, while those with small values of D do not travel very far and their random walks can be contained in a disk of smaller area.

(6) Diffusion-weighted (DWI) sequences are designed to measure and reflect the diffusion coefficient D of water molecules. The DWI sequence starts with a spin echo–echo planar MRI sequence, and adds "diffusion gradients" onto that sequence. The DWI sequence is designed in such a way that water molecules with high D undergo significant dephasing from each other, while those with low D undergo less dephasing. Let us now look at two regions, HD where the water molecules have a high D, and LD, where the water molecules have a low D. Based on what we have said so far about how dephasing of protons lowers MR signal, we can understand that when the diffusion gradients are turned on, the hydrogen protons in water molecules in region HD dephase significantly from each other, and this produces a large drop in MR signal. Conversely, the protons in region LD dephase less, so their MR signal drops less. These effects become more pronounced with increasing strength of the applied diffusion gradients. This gradient strength is traditionally referred to as "b." With $b = 0$, there are no diffusion gradients applied. The DWI sequence we usually look at in clinical practice has a b value of 1000, considered to be a strong diffusion gradient. A medium b value is $b = 500$. You may have seen DWI scans acquired in this way, where there are three different sequences ($b = 0$, $b = 500$, and $b = 1000$), and the radiologist looks only at the last one. The units of b, which we will understand better later, are s/mm^2, the reciprocal of the units for D.

We can see how this DWI process works by looking at Fig. 8.11.

At $b = 0$ (Fig. 8.11 (a)), there are no diffusion gradients applied. The baseline sequence, then, is seen to be a T2-weighted sequence (the CSF is bright). A baseline T2-weighted sequence is used because it is more sensitive to the dephasing effects that diffusion gradients have. As b increases, the images become progressively darker, with all tissues losing MR signal. This fact is often not appreciated because the images are re-windowed for display. It is important, though, to understand this fact, and to get some sort of numerical sense for it. To achieve this, we will look at MR signal using the images in Fig. 8.11 in two representative regions: an area of brain

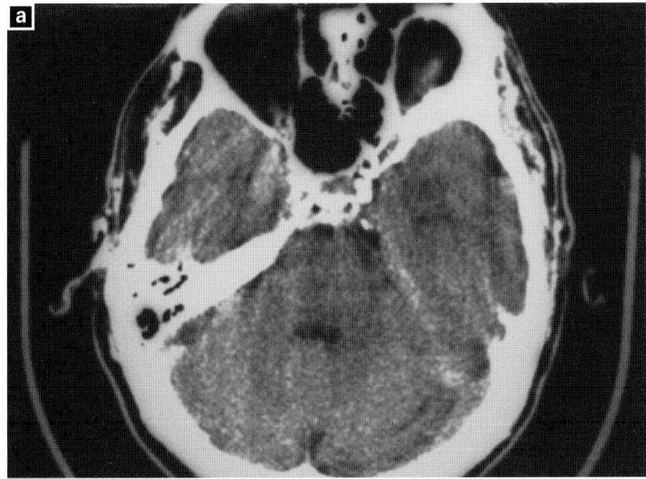

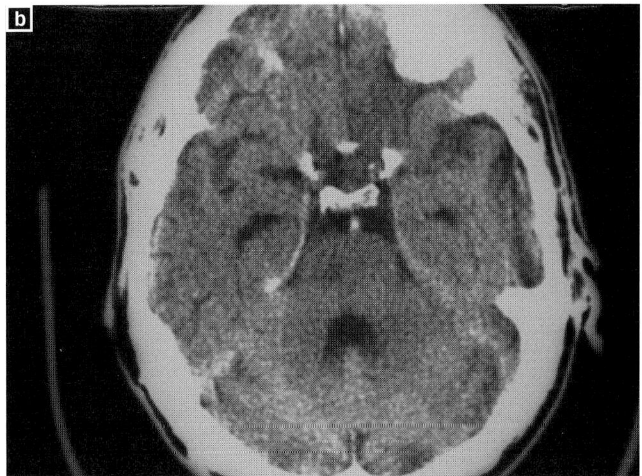

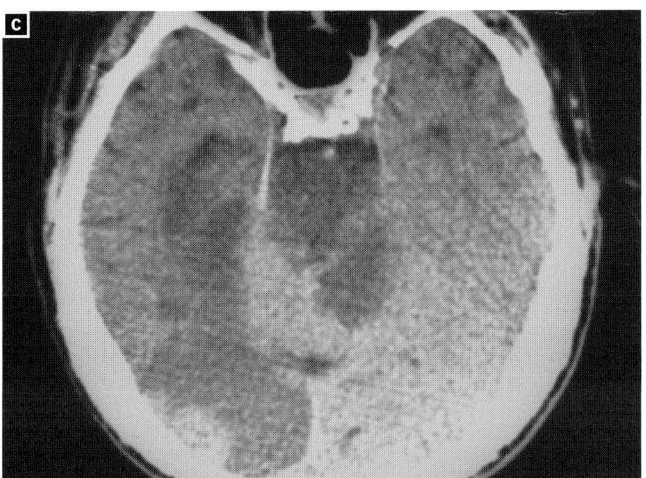

Fig. 8.6. **(a) CT obtained 1 day prior to ictus. The basilar artery is normal in density. (b) CT obtained 1 hour after the patient became unresponsive. Notice that the basilar artery has now become hyperdense. (c) Image obtained 12 hours later reveals extensive infarcts throughout the pons, right PCA territory and left superior cerebellum. The basilar artery remains dense.**

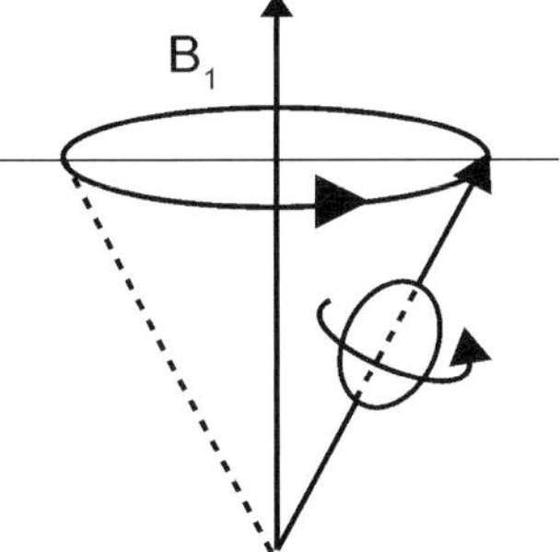

Fig. 8.7. **A hydrogen proton spins on its axis, giving it a magnetic moment, which behaves like a compass needle. This precesses around the main magnetic field B1 at a frequency of about 63.9 Megahertz (million cycles per second) in a 1.5 tesla magnet.**

parenchyma in the right frontal lobe, and a region of CSF in the third ventricle. The measured MR signal for the different b values is graphed as well as tabulated below in arbitrary MR signal units (see Fig. 8.12 and Table 8.1).

As we can see, at $b = 0$, the CSF has a significantly higher MR signal than the brain parenchyma. As b increases, both compartments lose MR signal. However, the CSF signal drops more sharply than the brain parenchyma because free water in the ventricles has a significantly higher D value than water in the brain parenchyma, much of which is intracellular and bound to intracellular organelles, cell membranes, etc. The end result is that at $b = 500$ and $b = 1000$, the parenchyma ends up higher in signal than the CSF – because it dropped signal less.

With this, we have finished our review of MR physics, and are finally in a position to understand how DWI works in stroke. With ischemia, the normal cellular ion pumps, such as the Na–K pump, fail. When this happens, ions and accompanying water molecules shift from the extracellular space to the intracellular space, producing cytotoxic edema. It is estimated that, in normal brain, approximately 80 percent of water is intracelleular while 20 percent is extracellular. In regions of cytotoxic edema, the proportion of intracelleular water increases to about 95 percent. Intracellular water, for a variety of reasons, has a much lower D than extracellular water. Thus, water molecules in the infarct zone have, on average, a significantly lower D value than those in normal brain parenchyma. Hence, with the application of diffusion gradients, water molecules in the infarct zone dephase less and so drop signal less than their counterparts in normal brain. Therefore, the infarct zone (see Fig. 8.13) stands out as relatively bright!

If you think about it, this is rather ingenious. Normally, we want to make something happen to the abnormal area to make it stand out – like have it enhance with contrast while the rest of the brain does not. With DWI sequences, it is the reverse. We make all normal brain drop signal. The infarct zone drops signal less, and so stands out as bright in comparison. This is analogous to a situation where a group of radiology residents are asked, "Who wants to volunteer to do this rectal fistulogram?" Everyone takes a step back, recoiling at the thought, except you. Therefore, it now appears that you have stepped up to volunteer. The value of this strategy cannot be overestimated. Most people think that DWI simply lets us see infarcts earlier than we otherwise would (e.g., Fig. 8.13). What they fail to realize, however, is that DWI does this by looking at a completely unique parameter – the D value of tissue. Thus, while two lesions may appear identical on FLAIR or T2

sequences (because they have the same T2 time), they may look completely different on DWI, because of different D values. This gives us the capacity to distinguish infarcts from identical-appearing chronic microvascular ischemic changes on conventional sequences (Fig. 8.14).

Now that we have a conceptual understanding of DWI, let us cover some of the more hardcore specifics for those who are interested. The diffusion sequence commonly used is known as the Stejskal–Tanner diffusion spin-echo sequence (Fig. 8.15).

The sequence works like a spin-echo pulse sequence, with a 90 degree and 180 degree pulse resulting in a spin echo which is used to form the MR image. On either side of the 180 degree pulse, identical diffusion gradients G are turned on for a period of time δ, and then turned off. The first gradient makes the hydrogen protons spin faster for a brief period based on their

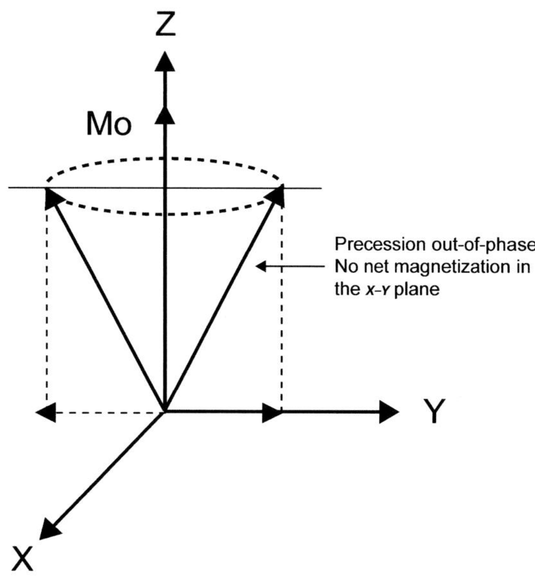

Fig. 8.8. **Two protons 180 degrees out of phase. The horizontal components of their magnetization vectors cancel each other out completely, and there is no MR signal.**

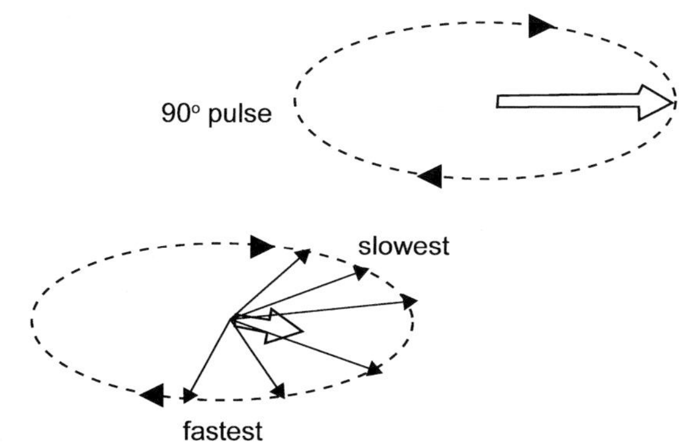

Fig. 8.9. **After the 90 degree pulse, the protons are in phase, and MR signal (thick arrow, top diagram) is maximal. Over time, because of intrinsic variations in precession speed, the protons begin to dephase from each other, and MR signal diminishes (bottom diagram).**

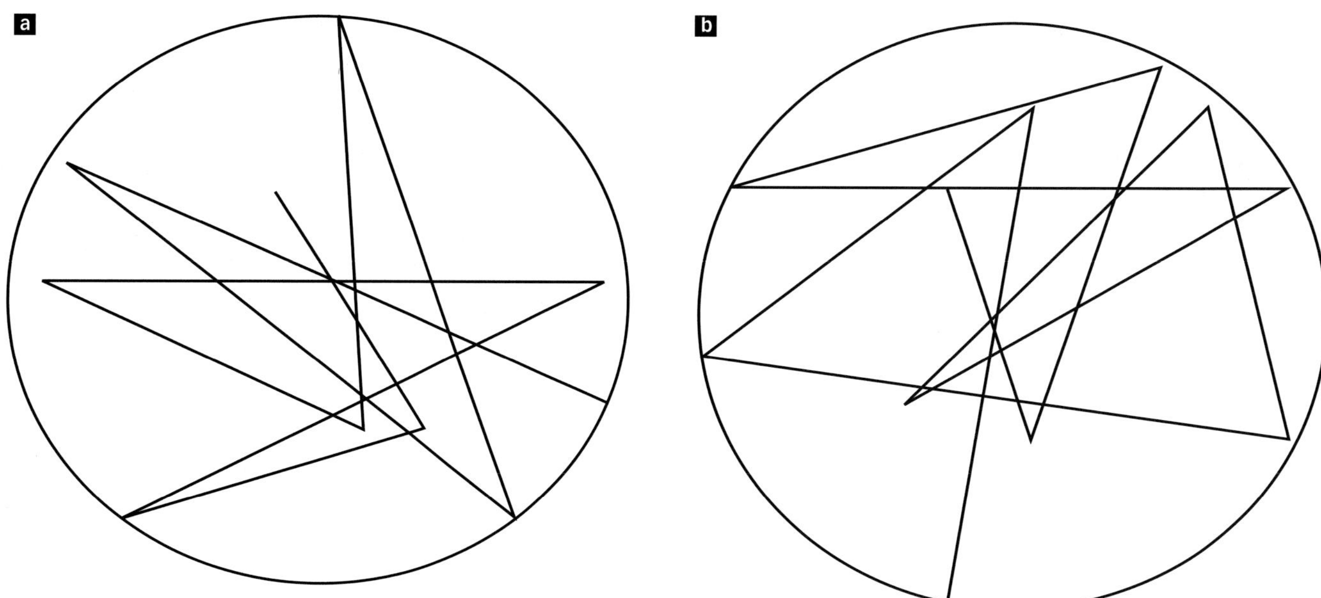

Fig. 8.10. **The sequential straight line segments of a water molecule's random walk are diagrammed. (a) A random walk for a water molecule with a high diffusion coefficient (D) requires a disk of larger area to contain its path, while (b) a random walk for a molecule with a small D requires a disk of smaller area.**

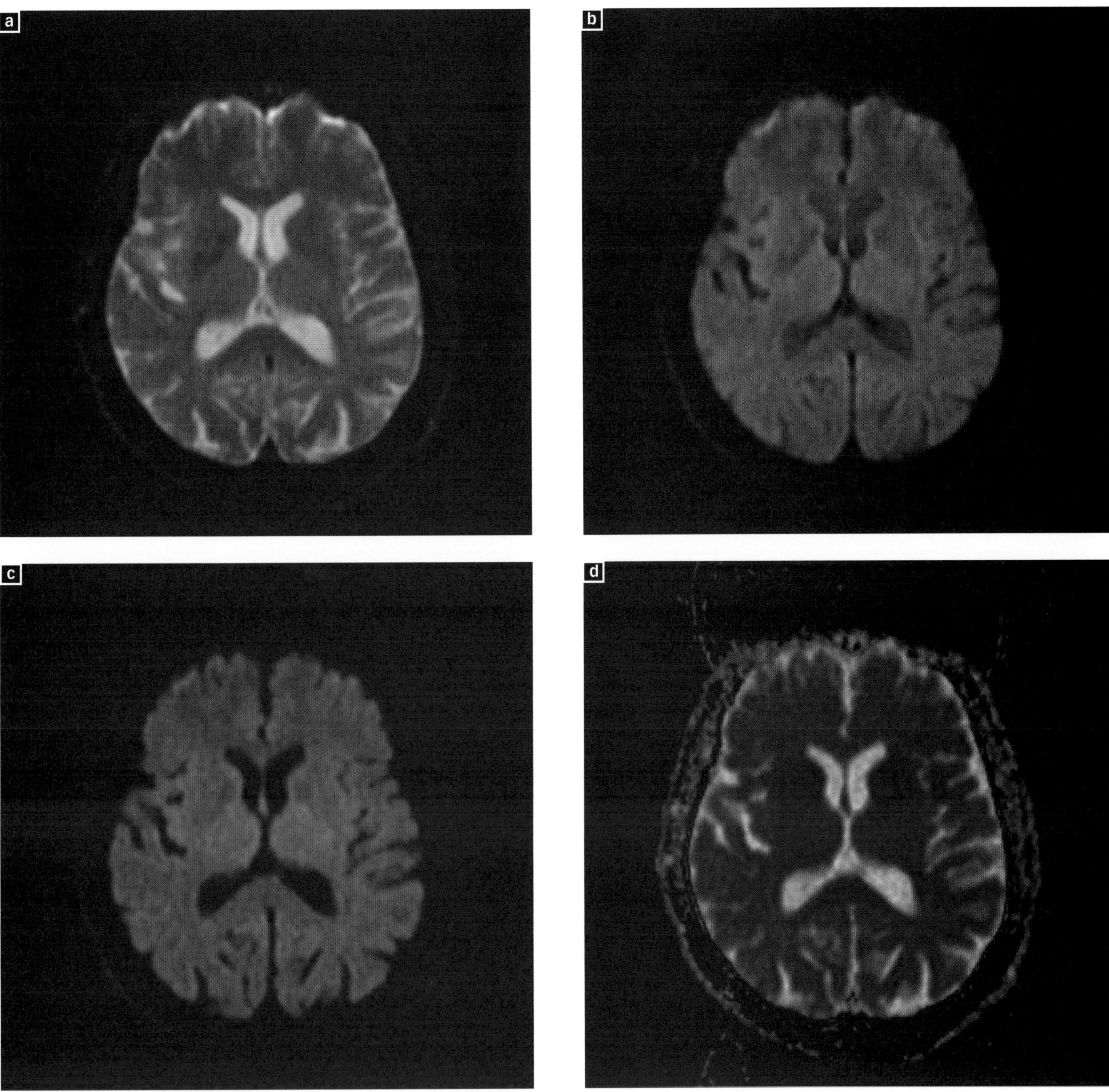

Fig. 8.11. **The various parts of a DWI sequence. Images are obtained with (a) $b = 0$, (b), $b = 500$, and (c) $b = 1000$. (d) An ADC map (D) is then calculated from these various b-value images.**

location along the gradient axis. The gain in precession frequency ω is proportional to γB where γ stands for the gyromagnetic ratio of hydrogen protons (42.6 MHz/tesla) and B is the strength of the magnetic field seen by the protons. When a gradient G is turned on in the x direction, $B = Bo + G(x)$, where Bo is the baseline magnetic field, say 1.5 tesla, and $G(x)$ is the incremental magnetic field added by the diffusion gradient, varying in strength based on the location x along the gradient axis. Because of this incremental magnetic field, the protons spin faster for a brief period. When the gradient is turned off,

the protons return to precessing at the same rate, but now some of them are ahead of others in phase – how much ahead depending on their position x at the time the gradient was turned on. After the first gradient $G1$ is turned off, a 180 degree pulse is applied, which reverses the direction in which the protons spin. After a time period Δ from the first gradient $G1$, a second identical gradient $G2$ is again turned on. Now, however, the protons are spinning in the reverse direction because of the 180 degree pulse. Therefore, if they have not moved in position during this acquisition period, they now

Table 8.1. MR signal vs. *b* value

b value	Brain MR signal	Ventricle MR signal
0	254	592
500	159	108
1000	106	25

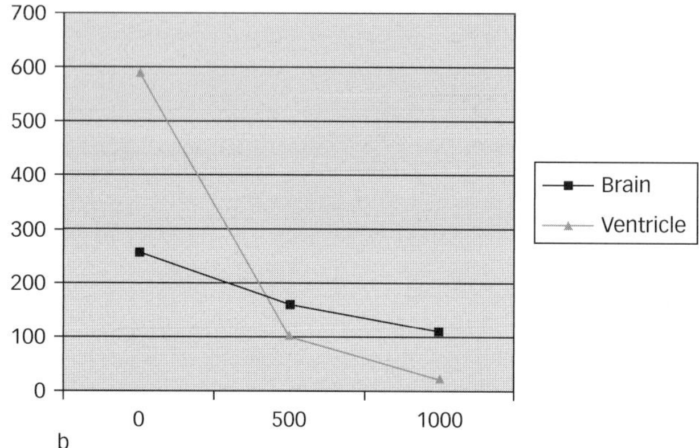

Fig. 8.12. **Signal changes (in arbitrary MR signal units) versus *b* values for brain parenchyma and lateral ventricle.**

acquire a negative phase shift identical in magnitude but opposite in sign to that given by G_1. For example, a proton acquires a phase shift of 30 degrees after G_1. After G_2, if this proton has remained stationary, it gets a phase shift of negative 30 degrees. These two cancel each other out, and it is as if G_1 and G_2 had never happened, i.e., there is not net phase shift. This precise cancellation depends on the proton being stationary during the time period Δ between G_1 and G_2. If the proton moves, then it is in a different location along the gradient axis, so the phase shift given by G_1 is not precisely cancelled by the negative phase shift given by G_2. Thus, the protons dephase from each other, causing MR signal to drop. All protons move to some extent, and that is why some dephasing always happens, and signal always drops with a DWI sequence, as we have seen above. The more protons diffuse (the bigger D), the less cancellation occurs, and the more net phase shift of protons from each other. This is synonymous with more dephasing and more MR signal drop with higher D. That is how diffusion gradients cause MR signal to drop, with the degree of signal drop being proportional to D.

This proportionality can be expressed quantitatively in terms of the following equation:

$$S_{DWI} = S_0 e^{-bD} \tag{8.1}$$

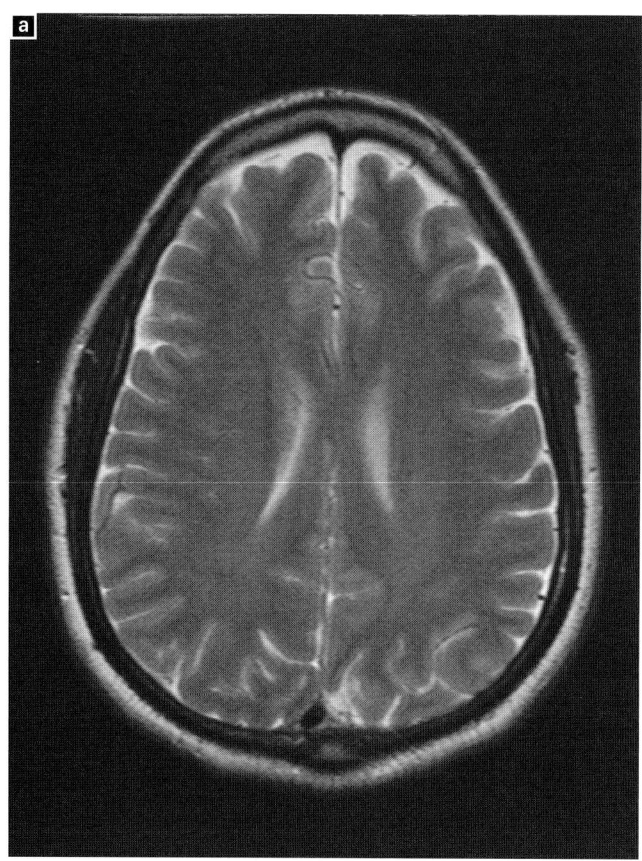

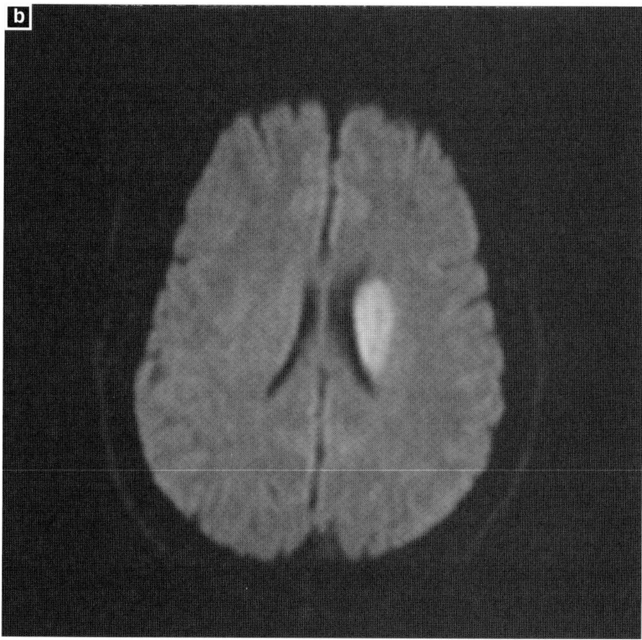

Fig. 8.13. **Images from a patient with acute left corona radiate infarct. (a) The infarct is invisible on T2, but (b) bright on DWI. In the infarct zone, the diffusion coefficient *D* is lower, so there is less MR signal loss, and the infarct stands out as the rest of the brain drops signal around it.**

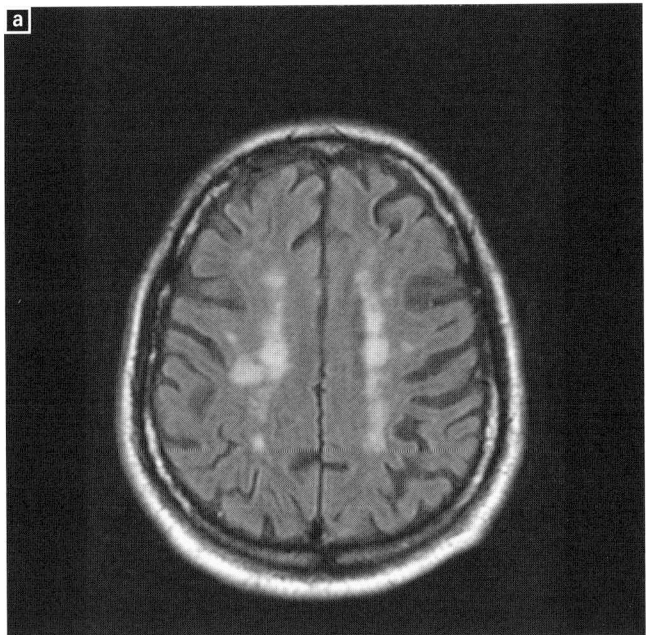
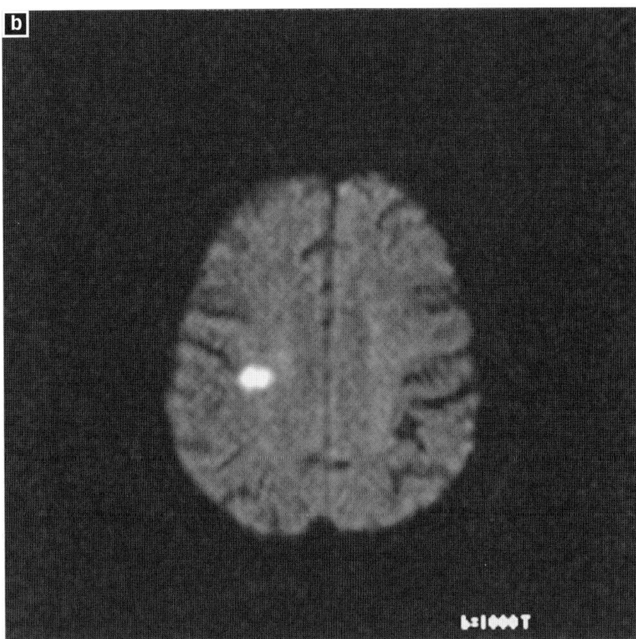

Fig. 8.14. **Patient presents with left-sided weakness. (a) FLAIR image shows multiple identical-appearing foci of microvascular deep white matter ischemic disease. (b) DWI reveals that one of these foci is actually a subacute infarct in the right centrum semiovale subjacent to the motor strip.**

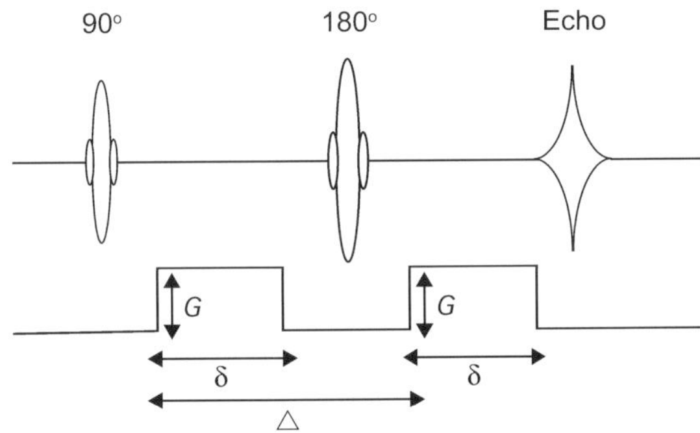

Fig. 8.15. **Diagram of the Stejskal–Tanner diffusion spin-echo sequence.**

Here, S_{DWI} is the signal intensity of a voxel on the DWI pulse sequence. S_o is the baseline MR signal which would be obtained without diffusion gradients. In this equation, e is the natural logarithm base which equals about 2.718. Recall that $e^{-bD} = 1/e^{bD}$. Thus, for a given b value, say $b = 1000$ s/mm^2, we see that the larger the value of D, the smaller the value of e^{-bD}, and hence the smaller the MR signal S_{DWI}. Conversely, S_{DWI} will be relatively large (bright signal on DWI) if D is small, such as in an infarct zone. However, if we look carefully at Eq. 8.1, we see that S_{DWI} may conceivably be large not because D is small, but because S_o, the baseline MR signal, is itself large. In other words, something may end up being bright on DWI because it is bright on the baseline $b = 0$ T2-weighted image. This is known as T2 shine-through artifact.

Now, we understand why we obtain images at multiple b values, including a $b = 0$ image. If we obtain and look at only the $b = 1000$ DWI image, we do not know whether a region is bright because it is a zone of truly restricted diffusion, such as

an infarct with a low D value, or because it is intrinsically bright on T2 (high S_o), without a particularly low D value. Obtaining images with at least two b values allows us to resolve this dilemma. You have undoubtedly heard of this solution – it is the ADC map. The ADC map (see Fig. 8.11) is a calculated image which reflects the D value of each voxel of tissue; things with low D values are dark on the ADC map. Thus, if something is bright on DWI but dark on the ADC map, we know that it represents a zone of true diffusion restriction (Fig. 8.16).

If something is bright on DWI but not correspondingly dark on ADC, then we surmise that it represents shine-through artifact (Fig. 8.17).

Thankfully, shine-through artifact is an uncommon phenomenon. Most of the time, zones of T2-weighted hyperintensity without true diffusion restriction, although bright on the baseline $b = 0$ image, are not bright on the DWI image. This is because the high value of S_o is more than compensated for by the low value of e^{-bD} caused by the high D often found in these zones. A great example of this is the behavior of vasogenic edema on DWI images (Fig. 8.18).

Although bright on T2, the edema zone becomes slightly dark on DWI because of the high D values caused by a significant increase in interstitial (extracellular) water as compared to intracellular water. The ADC map is bright in this region, reflecting the high D values. At the risk of being repetitive, we stress that this is essentially the opposite phenomenon of cytotoxic edema in infarcts. In that case, once again, an increase in intracellular water over extracellular water leads to a low D, with hyperintensity on DWI and hypointensity on ADC (Fig. 8.19).

Understanding the physics and pathophysiology underlying DWI and ADC maps also allows us to better understand the

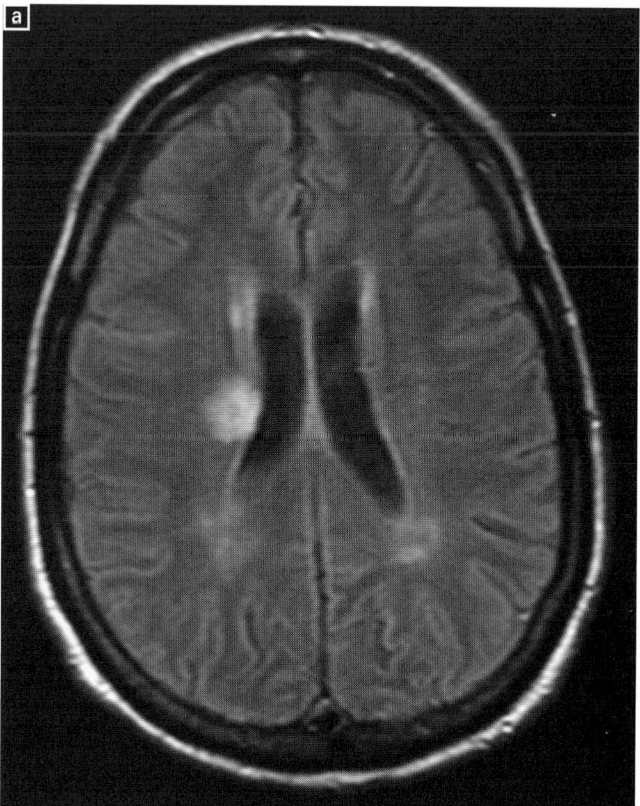

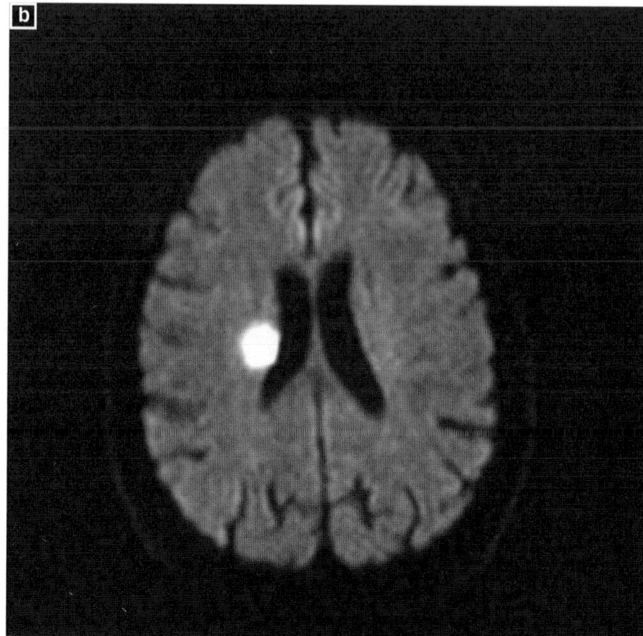

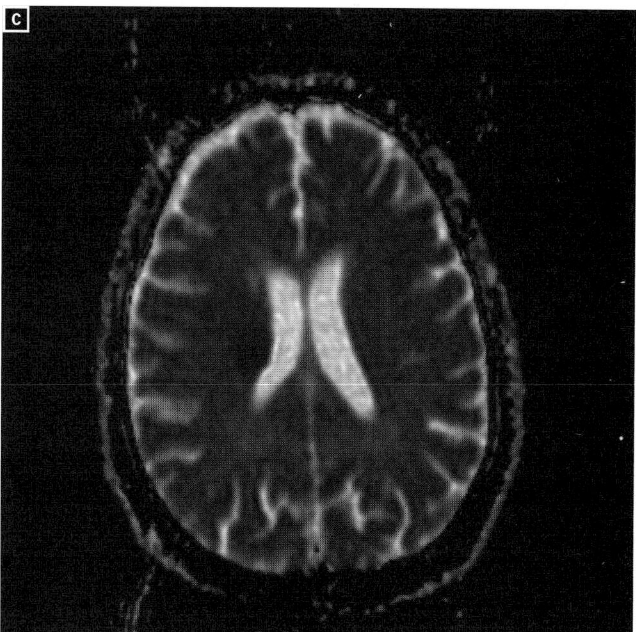

Fig. 8.16. **(a) FLAIR, (b) DWI, and (c) ADC map images of a subacute right caudate body/corona radiata infarct. The infarct is bright on DWI and dark on ADC, indicating a zone of true diffusion restriction.**

time course of signal changes with stroke. After 1 to 2 weeks, cells begin to rupture in the infarct zone, increasing the extracellular water. Thus, the local D value begins to increase, and the ADC changes begin to resolve, going from dark to isointense to bright in that time span. The time course and final fate of the infarct on the DWI images are less certain, because the increasing extracellular water caused by cell rupture is bright on T2, and therefore may cause shine-through brightness that may last for several weeks (see, for example, Desmond *et al.*, 2001).

"How is this ADC map calculated?" you may ask. The calculation of the ADC map is actually quite easy. All we need is two images obtained with different b values – let's say $b=0$ and $b=1000$. Our DWI signal equation, $S_{DWI} = S_0 e^{-bD}$, tells us that, for $b=0$, $S_{DWI} = S_0$ because $e^{-bD} = e^0 = 1$. Thus, from the $b=0$ image, we get, on a voxel by voxel basis, the value of S_0. Now, we obtain the DWI image with a gradient of $b = 1000$. We measure the signal S_{DWI} in each voxel, and we know that $S_{DWI} = S_0 e^{-1000D}$. Thus, we now have values for S_{DWI} and S_0, as well as an equation that links the two through the parameter D. Now, all that remains is to solve for D, which is done on a voxel-by-voxel basis as follows:

$$\left(\frac{S_{DWI}}{S_0}\right) = e^{-1000D} \qquad (8.2)$$

Now, we take the natural log of both sides, and we get

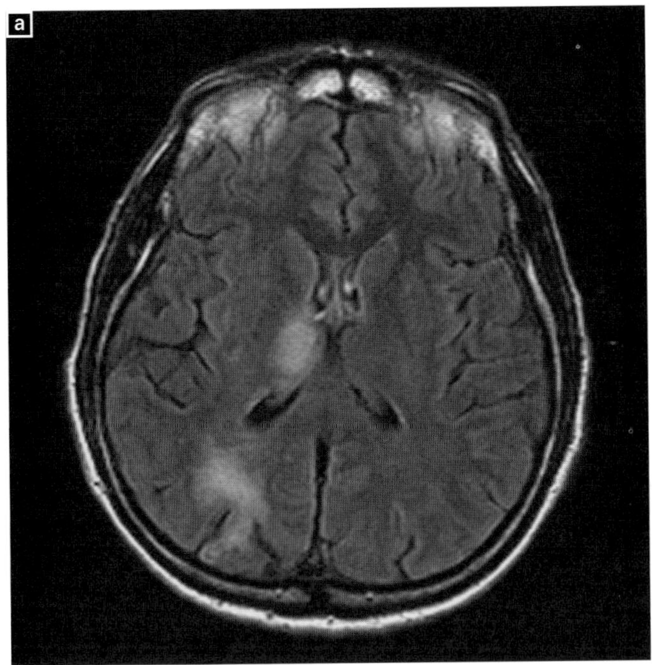

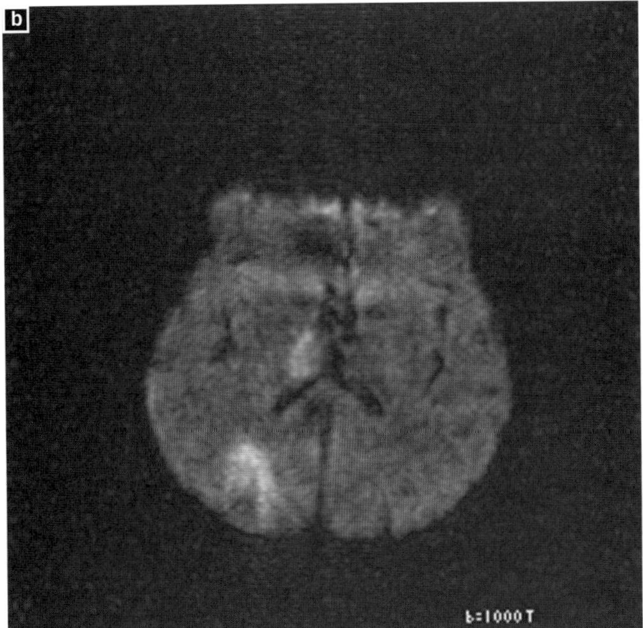

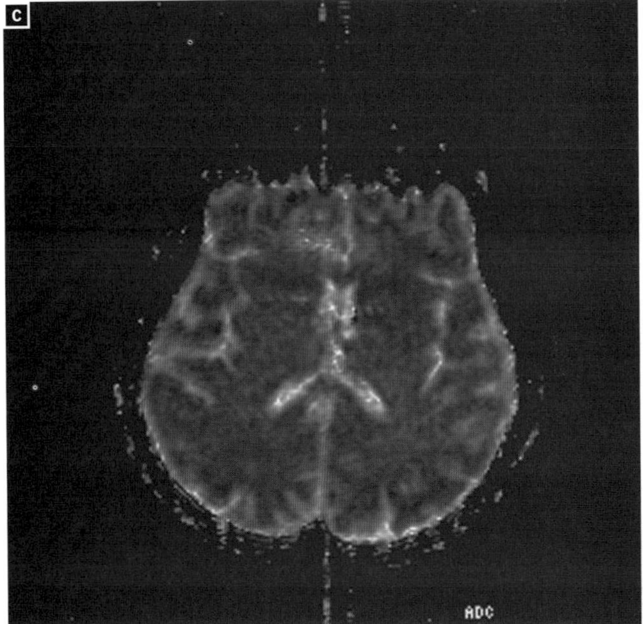

Fig. 8.17. **(a)–(c) Zones of demyelination in this patient with PML are evident in the right thalamus and right parieto-occipital region. They are bright on FLAIR (a) and DWI (b), but not dark on ADC (c). The right thalamic lesion, in fact, is slightly bright on the ADC map. The DWI brightness is a shine-through artifact.**

$$D = -\ln\left(\frac{S_{DWI}}{S_0}\right)/1000 \qquad (8.3)$$

or

$$D = \ln\left(\frac{S_0}{S_{DWI}}\right)/1000 \qquad (8.4)$$

From these values of D, calculated for each voxel, we form an image where each pixel's brightness is directly proportional to the calculated value of D in the corresponding tissue voxel. Low values of D are dark, and high D values are bright. For example, using the data in Fig. 8.12, we can see that for the brain displayed in Fig. 8.11, the calculated values of D are $870 \times 10^{-6}\,\mathrm{mm^2/s}$ for the brain parenchyma, and $320 - 10^{-5}\,\mathrm{mm^2/s}$ for the CSF – a significantly higher value. Thus, in the ADC map (Fig. 8.11(d)), the CSF is significantly brighter than the brain parenchyma. For the image data shown in Fig. 8.19, similar calculations show a D value of $760 \times 10^{-6}\,\mathrm{mm^2/s}$ for the normal brain parenchyma and a D value of $470 \times 10^{-6}\,\mathrm{mm^2/s}$ in the right temporal lobe infarct. Thus, the infarct is dark on the ADC map (Fig. 8.19(c)).

Finally, since we have decided to take a rigorous approach, let us look a little more closely at the parameter b. We see from our DWI signal equation that e^{-bD} must be a dimensionless quantity, since it represents the ratio of S_0 to S_{DWI}. Thus, since the units of D are $\mathrm{mm^2/s}$, the units of b must be the reciprocal of this ($\mathrm{s/mm^2}$) so that the units cancel. We can confirm this understanding by looking again at Fig. 8.15 and reviewing the actual mathematical expression for b derived by MR physicists:

$$b = \gamma^2 G^2 \delta^2 (\Delta - \delta/3)$$

Here, γ stands for the gyromagnetic ratio of hydrogen protons, whose units are Hz/tesla. The unit Hz (hertz), of course, is equivalent to "per second," or 1/s. Therefore, the units of γ are

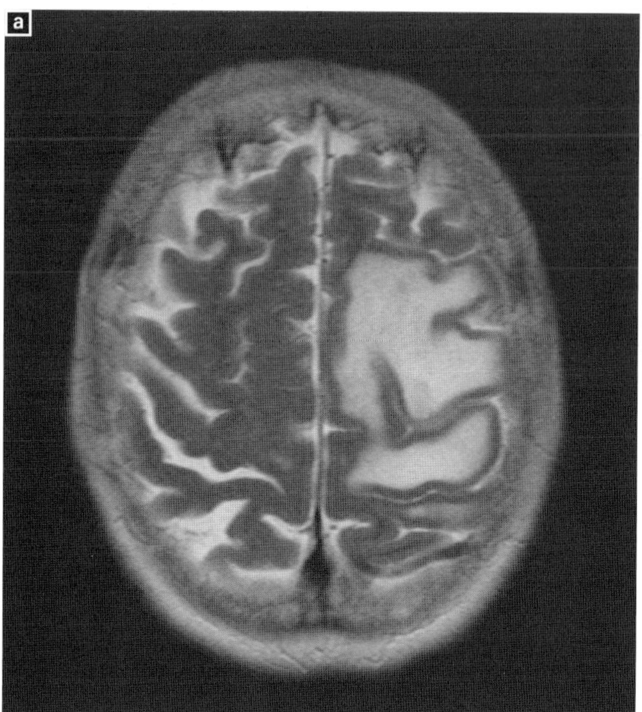

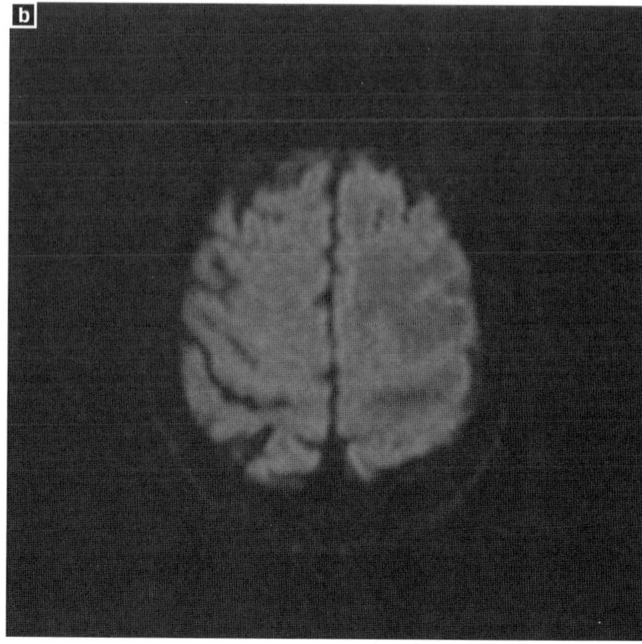

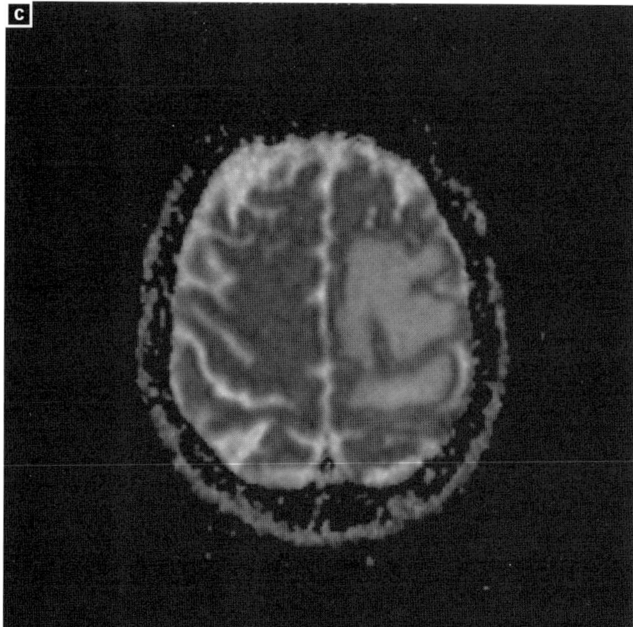

Fig. 8.18. **(a) T2, (b) DWI and (c) ADC map images show a large zone of vasogenic edema in the left frontal lobe secondary to underlying metastatic disease.**

1/(tesla s). G is the strength of the imposed diffusion gradient, i.e., how much the magnetic field changes per unit distance along the axis of our gradient. Its units can be expressed as tesla/mm. The terms δ and Δ are just measures of time, whose units are seconds. δ represents how long the gradient G is turned on, while Δ represents the time interval separating the two lobes of the diffusion gradient, which we have referred to as G_1 and G_2, but which are both referred to as G in Fig. 8.15. If we do dimension analysis on the units for the equation of b, we see that $b = \gamma^2 G^2 \delta^2 (\Delta - \delta/3)$ leads to units of

$$b = \frac{1}{s^2 \, \text{Tesla}^2} \cdot \frac{\text{Tesla}^2}{\text{mm}^2} \cdot s^2 \cdot s$$

Doing the needed cancellations, we get

$$b = \frac{1}{\cancel{s^2} \, \cancel{\text{Tesla}^2}} \cdot \frac{\cancel{\text{Tesla}^2}}{\text{mm}^2} \cdot \cancel{s^2} \cdot s$$

This leaves us with the units of b as s/mm², just as advertised!

Before we leave the discussion of DWI imaging, we must discuss a few small pitfalls. We have pointed out how the ADC map can help us detect T2 shine-through artifact, because such lesions will not be dark on ADC, although they are bright on DWI. Thus, the ADC map allows us to confirm true diffusion restriction. However, we must note that there are lesions other than infarct which show true diffusion restriction, although this is uncommon. Among these lesions are hematoma (Fig. 8.20), bacterial abscess (Fig. 8.21), status epilepticus (Fig. 8.22), and some cases of encephalitis (Fig. 8.23), including Creutzfeldt–Jakob prion disease. Thus, on DWI imaging, all of these may be stroke mimics.

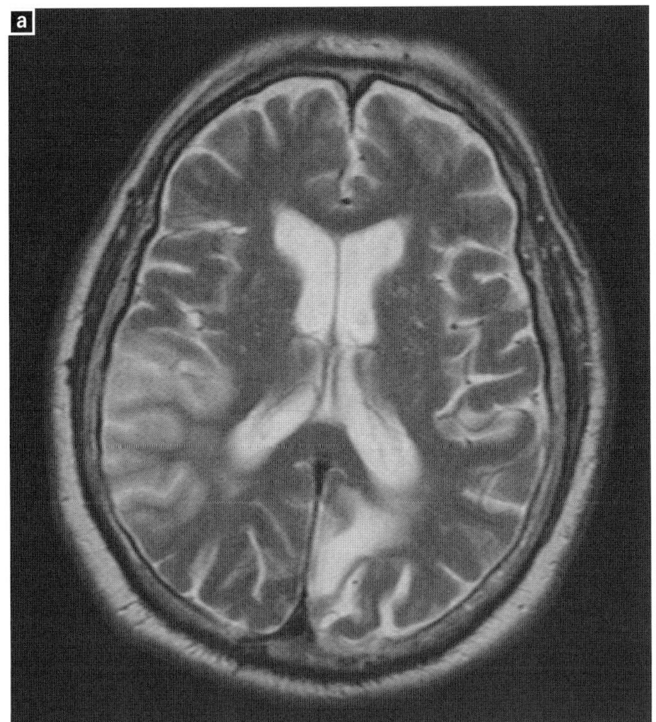

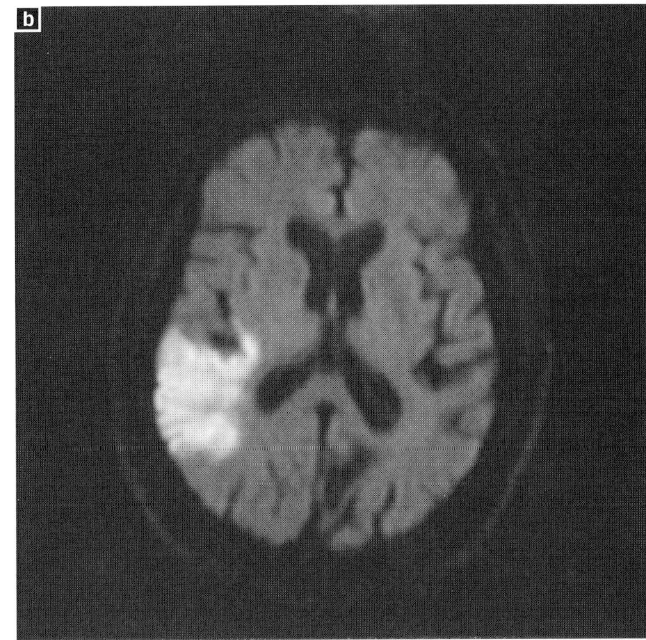

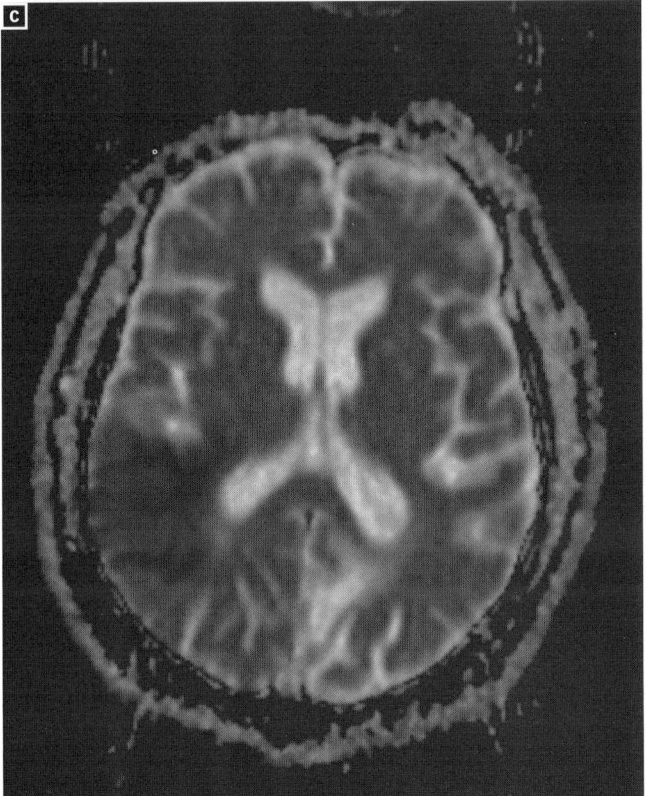

Fig. 8.19. **(a) T2, (b) DWI and (c) ADC map images. The patient has an early subacute right temporo-parietal infarct and an old left mesial occipital infarct. Both are bright on T2. The subacute infarct is bright on DWI and dark on ADC due to low _D_. The old infarct with encephalomalacia, conversely, is dark on DWI and bright on ADC due to a high _D_ sufficient to overwhelm the baseline T2 brightness.**

Perfusion-weighted (PWI) MRI

Perfusion-weighted (PWI) MRI is a much more complex topic than DWI. It is a technique which estimates a variety of flow parameters. It is usually performed by repeatedly imaging the brain as a bolus of contrast (typically Gadolinium–DTPA) is injected intravenously and circulates into and then out of the brain.

We are familiar with gadolinium as a contrast agent used with T1-weighted images to make lesions enhance (Fig. 8.24). It does this by shortening the T1 time of local hydrogen protons.

An underappreciated fact is that gadolinium also shortens the T2* time of hydrogen protons. Thus, on T2*-weighted images, such as T2 gradient echo sequences, gadolinium causes a signal drop. PWI imaging characterizes the dynamics of this signal drop as an intravenously injected gadolinium bolus "hits" the brain and then washes out. As the gadolinium arrives in the brain, signal drops sharply (Fig. 8.25).

As the bolus leaves the brain, the signal rises again but not quite to baseline, because the gadolinium bolus now mixes with the entire blood pool, mildly decreasing MR signal. The signal in each voxel of brain is measured over time. The images in Fig. 8.25 are obtained at 1 second intervals. Therefore, on a pixel-by-pixel basis, a signal–time curve is obtained, characterizing the passage of the gadolinium bolus into and out of the brain. These signal–time curves can then be mathematically manipulated to yield a variety of perfusion maps (Fig. 8.26).

We can imagine that the more vigorous the inflow of gadolinium, the faster and larger the MR signal drop. Areas which are well perfused will show a rapid and profound signal drop. Areas which are less well perfused will have a broader and shallower signal–time curve (Fig. 8.26).

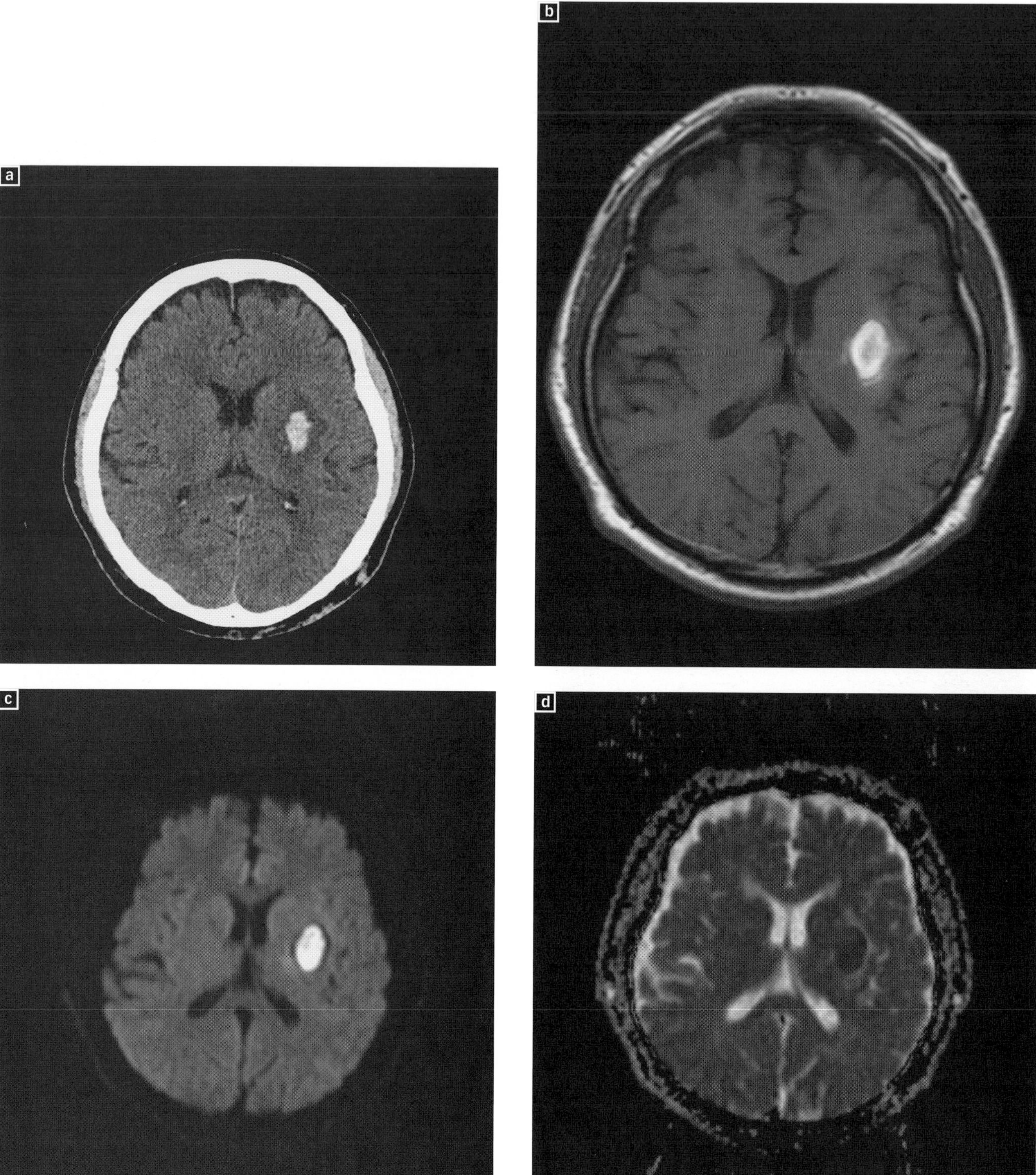

Fig. 8.20. **Patient with a hypertensive left basal ganglia hemorrhage. (a) CT and (b) T1-weighted MRI show a bleed, seen to be subacute on MRI. It is a zone of true diffusion restriction, (c) bright on DWI and (d) dark on ADC.**

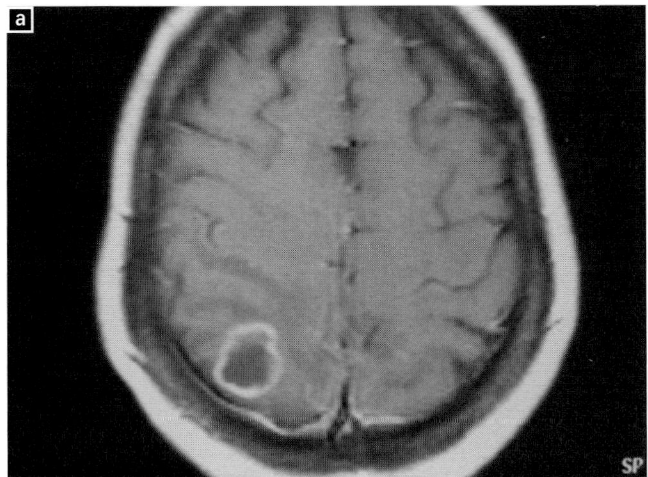

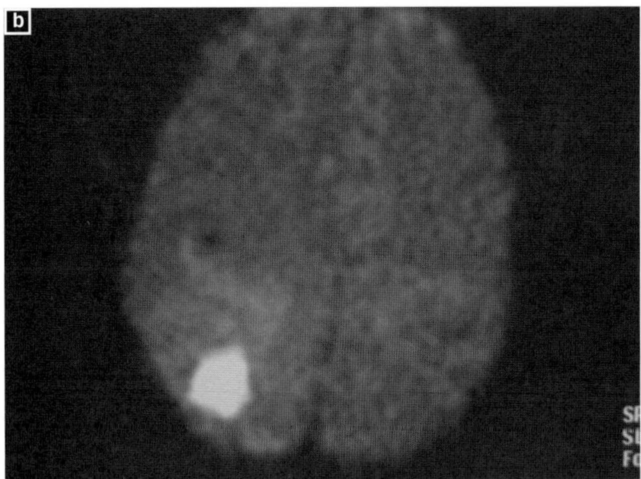

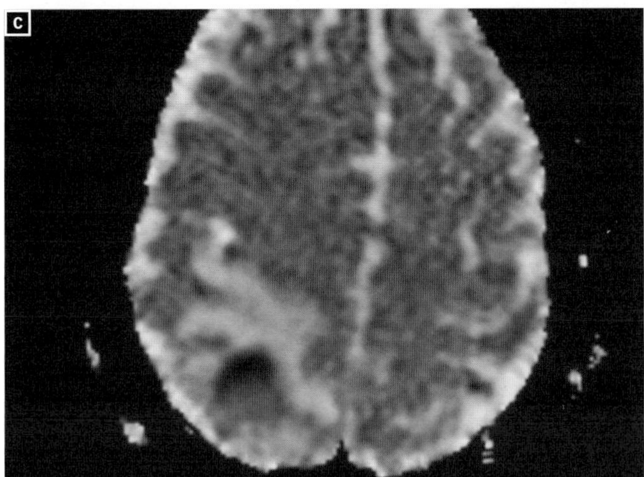

Fig. 8.21. **Patient with right parietal pyogenic abscess. The abscess is (a) ring enhancing on T1 post-contrast, (b) bright on DWI and (c) dark on ADC, indicating true diffusion restriction. The edema surrounding the abscess is minimally bright on DWI (very subtle T2 shine-through), and quite bright on ADC, indicating a high *D* value in the zone of vasogenic edema.**

The easiest flow parameter to understand is the time-to-peak or TTP (Fig. 8.26). For each pixel, the signal–time curve is digitally analyzed, and the time at which the MR signal reaches its nadir is determined. This is the TTP for that pixel. The better the perfusion, the shorter the TTP. TTP images thus reflect this parameter, with higher TTP values (presumably reflecting decreased CBF) appearing relatively bright (Fig. 8.26).

The remaining flow parameters are harder to understand without some fairly serious mathematics and some knowledge of the theory of tracer kinetics. Therefore, they will be introduced only briefly. As stated, gadolinium shortens the T2* of adjacent protons. The parameter 1/T2* is known as relaxivity, or R2*. As gadolinium enters the cerebral vasculature, there is a shortening of T2* of adjacent hydrogen protons, which can be characterized by a change in relaxivity, i.e., ΔR2*. By making

certain assumptions about the relaxivity, the signal–time curve can be converted to a gadolinium concentration–time curve in the brain using the pair of equations:

$$\Delta R2^*.(t) = -\ln\,(S(t)/S(o))/TE \tag{8.5}$$

and

$$\Delta R2^* = k_2[\text{gadolinium concentration}] \tag{8.6}$$

The first equation relates signal changes compared to baseline signal to a change in relaxivity, while the second equation relates this calculated change in relaxivity to the tissue concentration of gadolinium through a constant that depends on such things as field strength, tissue type, and pulse sequence used.

The area under the signal–time curve or the concentration–time curve provides a measure of relative cerebral blood volume (Fig. 8.27).

Another parameter commonly used to characterize perfusion is the mean transit time or MTT. In general terms, this is the time needed to completely wash out the blood from a certain region of brain and bring in fresh blood. In the presence of a contrast bolus, it measures the time needed to wash out the contrast. It depends on the cerebral blood volume (CBV) and the cerebral blood flow (CBF) as follows: MTT = CBV/CBF. MTT is simply the ratio of cerebral blood volume to cerebral blood flow; this makes intuitive sense that for a given CBF, the MTT is the time needed to bring in a volume of blood CBV. However, the difficulty of the calculation is belied by this simple-appearing equation. The tissue concentration of gadolinium as a function of time is "blurred" by the arterial concentration of gadolinium, washing into the tissue as we are assessing tissue concentration. Removing this blurring effect is known in mathematical terms as "deconvolution," and requires a knowledge of (or certain assumptions about) the arterial concentration–time curve, known as the "input function." Once this deconvolution is performed, the MTT and hence the CBF can be calculated. Conversely, by using the arterial input function and the tissue concentration–time curve, the CBF can be calculated, and then from it and the CBV, the MTT can be obtained. In broad terms, we can say

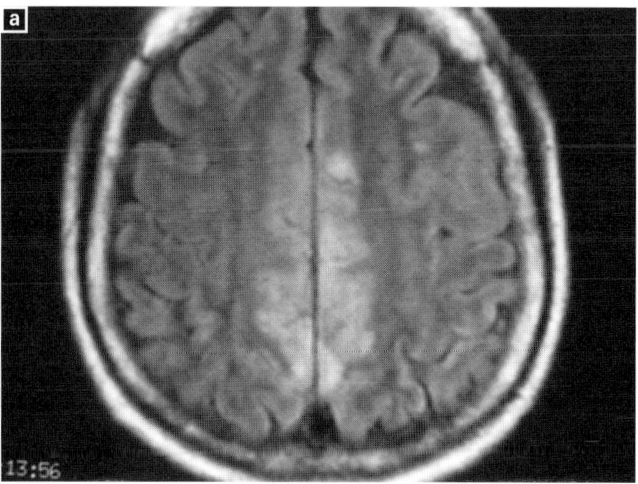 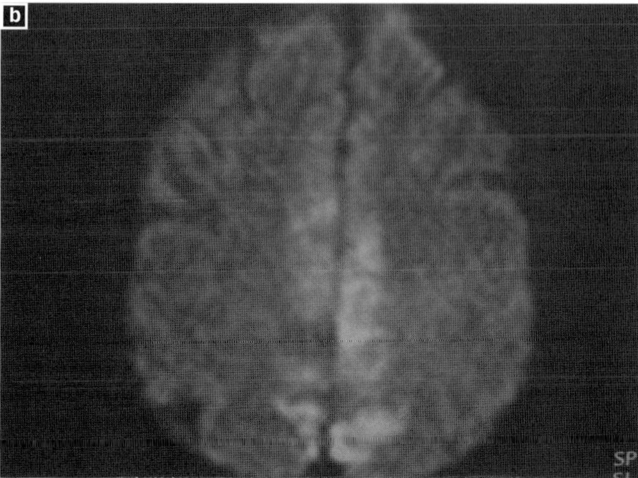

Fig. 8.22. **There is gyriform (a) FLAIR and (b) DWI hyperintensity along the cingulate gyrus bilaterally in this patient with status epilepticus. This is thought to be due to transient cytotoxic edema which may accompany seizures. See Kim *et al.*, 2001.**

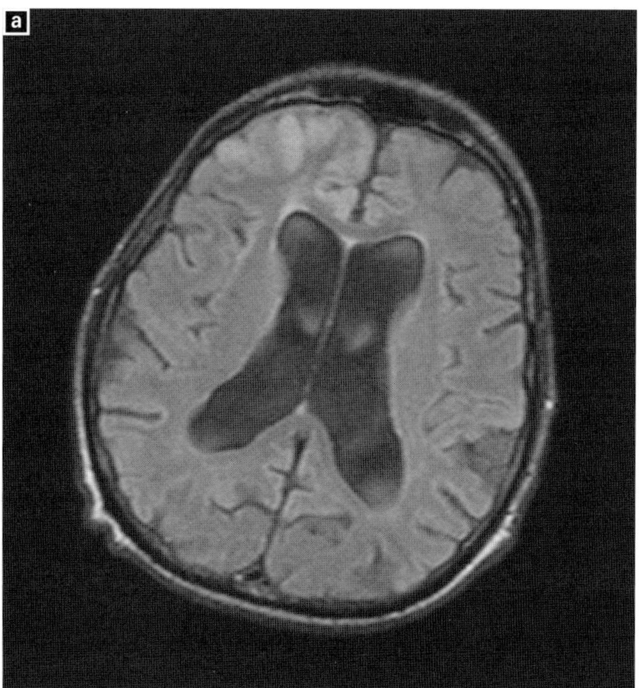 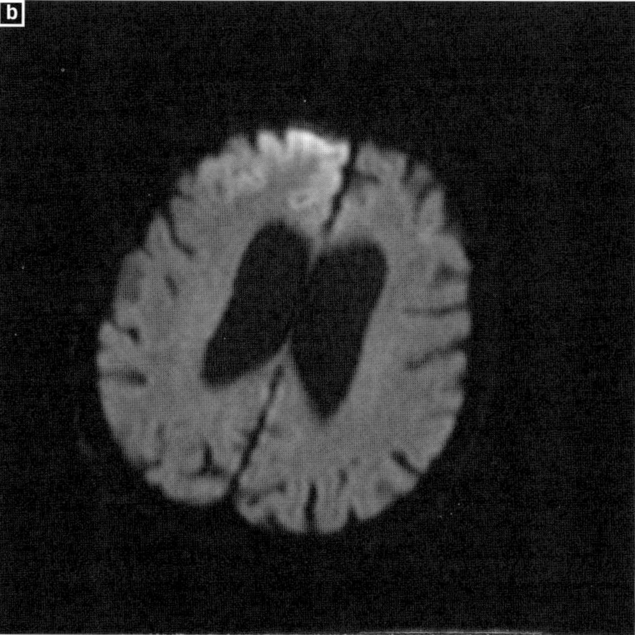

Fig. 8.23. **(a) FLAIR and (b) DWI images show subtle gyriform hyperintensity in the right anterior frontal lobe in this patient with non-specific viral encephalitis.**

that the greater the CBF, the less time it takes to wash in and out a given volume of blood, and hence the shorter the MTT. Conversely, areas of hypoperfusion will be characterized by a prolonged MTT.

Some of these various flow parameters are shown in Fig. 8.27 superimposed on the signal–time curve without the intervening conversion to a concentration–time curve, just to get some conceptual feel for the parameters. For more of the actual mathematics behind PWI MRI, the reader is referred to an excellent article by Wu *et al.* and the references cited therein

(see Wu *et al.*, 2005). What must be remembered is that, at this time, PWI MRI can give only relative flow estimates, not precise quantitative flow information. This is due to a number of causes, the most important of which are non-linearity of the MR signal with gadolinium tissue concentration, and a tremendous difficulty in establishing precise arterial-input functions, due in part to the confounding effects of flow on MR signal.

In summary, typical PWI imaging works by obtaining serial images of the brain using T2*-weighted GRE images obtained before and during the passage of an intravenously injected gadolinium bolus through the cerebral vessels. Four main types of perfusion parameters may be obtained:

(1) TTP images
(2) CBV images
(3) CBF images
(4) MTT images.

Other more advanced parameters are also sometimes derived, only one of which is mentioned here – the T_{max} parameter. This is the time-to-peak of the so-called residue function, obtained by deconvolution of the tissue concentration–time curve and the arterial input function.

TTP images are relatively straightforward to understand, and probably the most commonly used in clinical practice to visually assess perfusion deficits. They are obtained directly from the signal–time curve, and do not require an arterial input function. However, it must be stressed that TTP maps are among the the least accurate of the flow parameters, since

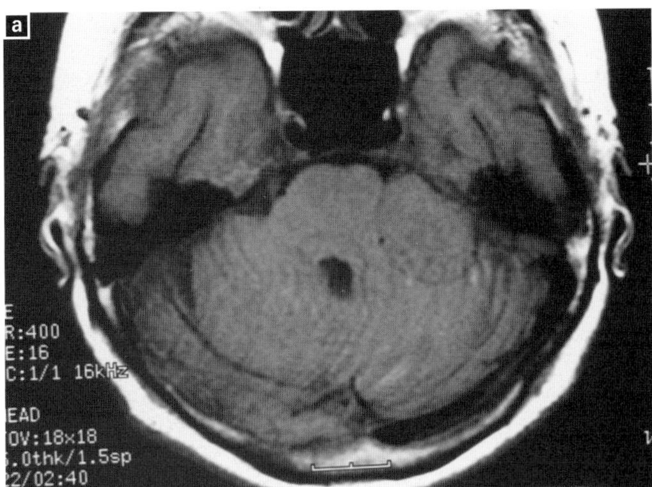
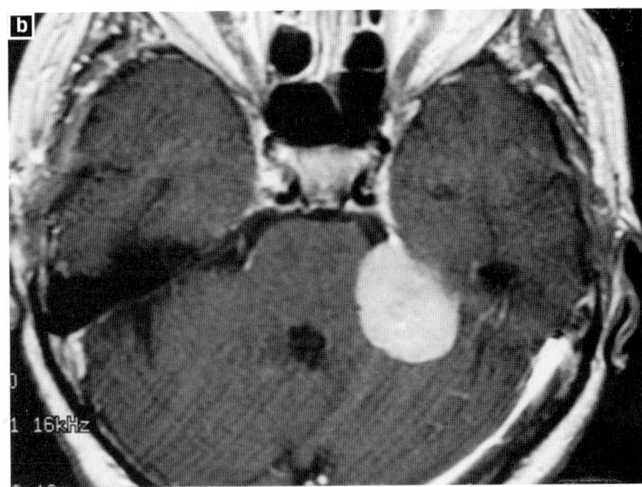

Fig. 8.24. **(a) Pre- and (b) post-contrast T1-weighted axial images reveal a meningioma in the left cerebellopontine angle cistern. The meningioma is isointense to brain on pre-contrast T1, but enhances avidly on post-contrast T1.**

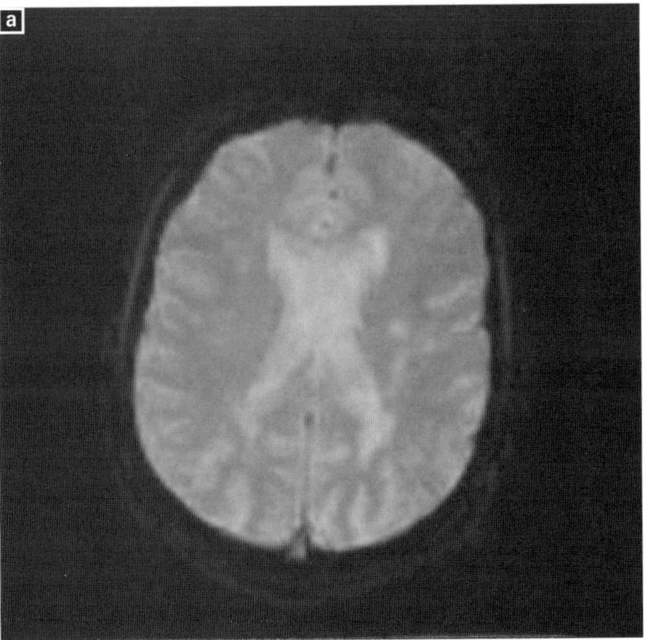
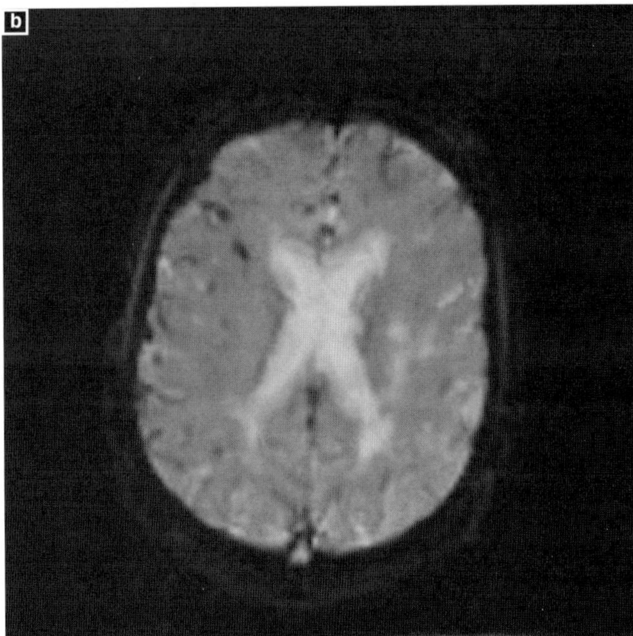

Fig. 8.25. **Raw data from a PWI scan in a patient with left MCA infarct. The images for this sequence are obtained at 1 second intervals, and selected images are shown. Image (a) is the baseline T2 GRE sequence before gadolinium hits the brain. Images (b), (c) show the progressive signal drop that occurs as the gadolinium bolus washes in. The discerning eye will notice less signal change in the left MCA territory, and that the signal drop is delayed compared to the right side (see image (b)). The discerning eye will also notice small foci of hyperintensity in the left deep white matter (a). These represent small deep infarcts.**

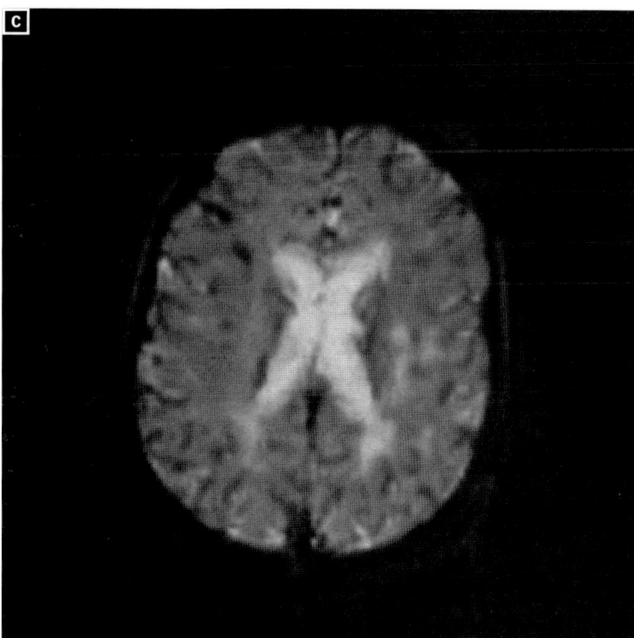

Fig. 8.25. **(cont.)**

collateral flow can cause a delay in TTP, even if in real terms, the brain is adequately perfused by this collateral flow. There is significant evidence mounting that the more complex parameters, although requiring some estimate of an arterial input function (usually from the MCA contralateral to a lesion), more closely predict the fate of ischemic tissue, and are hence more clinically useful. This difficult area is the new frontier in PWI. For a glimpse of that frontier, see Thijs *et al.*, 2004 and Mlynash *et al.*, 2005.

Now that we have finished reviewing some of the clinically relevant basics of CT, DWI and PWI imaging, it is time to discuss stroke therapy and the role of these imaging techniques therein.

Stroke therapy

Why do we need stroke therapy? The answers, in terms of mortality and morbidity, seem obvious. A more fundamental answer, though, is that the body's endogenous thrombolytic mechanisms, while effective, often do not work fast enough in cases of thrombotic occlusion to prevent stroke. On the flip side, they very often do, and those are the patients we refer to as having had transient ischemic attacks (TIAs). In cases of major vessel occlusions, though, data shows that timely spontaneous recanalization of major vessel occlusions such as the ICA or proximal MCA occurs in only 0–14 percent of cases (Meschia *et al.*, 2002). When the body's spontaneous thrombolysis mechanisms do not work, then we intervene! Thus, it is no surprise that current stroke therapy, to a great extent, means thrombolysis.

Before moving on to discuss this topic, it is good to note that there is also a very broad range of evolving stroke therapy

agents based on the complex physiology of cell death and attempts to interrupt or delay the biochemical cascade which results in neuronal demise. Such therapies include hyperoxia and hypertension, as well as a host of biochemical neuroprotectants. Among these are such agents as the antioxidant Ebselen, the AMPA antagonist YM872, and the so-called "free radical spin trap" agent, NXY-059. In fact, preliminary results of the stroke-acute ischemic-NXY treatment (SAINT – don't you just love how creative these names are?) trial were presented in May 2005. In this study, conducted at more than 200 centers worldwide, stroke patients within 6 hours were randomized to receive NXY-059 versus placebo, in addition to possible other treatments. While the agent seems safe, no additional benefit of NXY-059 over intravenous tissue plasminogen activator could be demonstrated. Thus, at this time, we'll focus on thrombolysis.

Intravenous thrombolysis: the basics

As stated earlier, there is no doubt that most readers of this book are already familiar with the fact that ischemic stroke can sometimes be treated with intravenous tissue plasminogen activator (i.v. TPA). However, it is important to be familiar with some of the key data upon which this therapy is based, as well as some of the interesting controversies in the literature regarding some portions of the i.v. TPA treatment algorithm.

We begin by noting that the current treatment algorithms, although in a state of rapid flux, did not come about without some false starts. One such mis-step was the attempt to use i.v. streptokinase as a thrombolytic agent to treat acute ischemic stroke. In the mid 1990s, in fact, there were three randomized trials assessing the use of intravenous streptokinase for thrombolysis of acute stroke: the Multicentre Acute Stroke Trial – Italy (MAST–I), the Multicentre Acute Stroke Trial – Europe (MAST–E) and the Australian Streptokinase Trial (ASK). All three trials were halted due to an increase in mortality and morbidity, including a significant increase in intracranial hemorrhage, in the treatment group compared with the placebo group.

The situation is somewhat better when the data for tissue plasminogen activator (TPA) is considered, but it is also more complex. TPA is a protease, endogenously released from blood vessel endothelium. Unlike more globally acting agents such as urokinase and streptokinase, TPA is more selective, activating only plasminogen which is already bound to fibrin. Streptokinase, by comparison, activates both freely circulating plasminogen, and plasminogen bound to fibrin. Plasminogen is activated to form plasmin, which digests the fibrin strands that hold the clot together, thereby leading to thrombolysis. The greater specificity of TPA may be one key to its more positive results.

With regard to intravenous TPA, there have been two major sets of studies, known popularly as the "European" and the "American." The main American studies are the two NINDS (National Institute of Neurological Disease and Stroke) TPA trials, commonly referred to as NINDS1 and NINDS2. Often, the data from both are lumped together, and the results simply

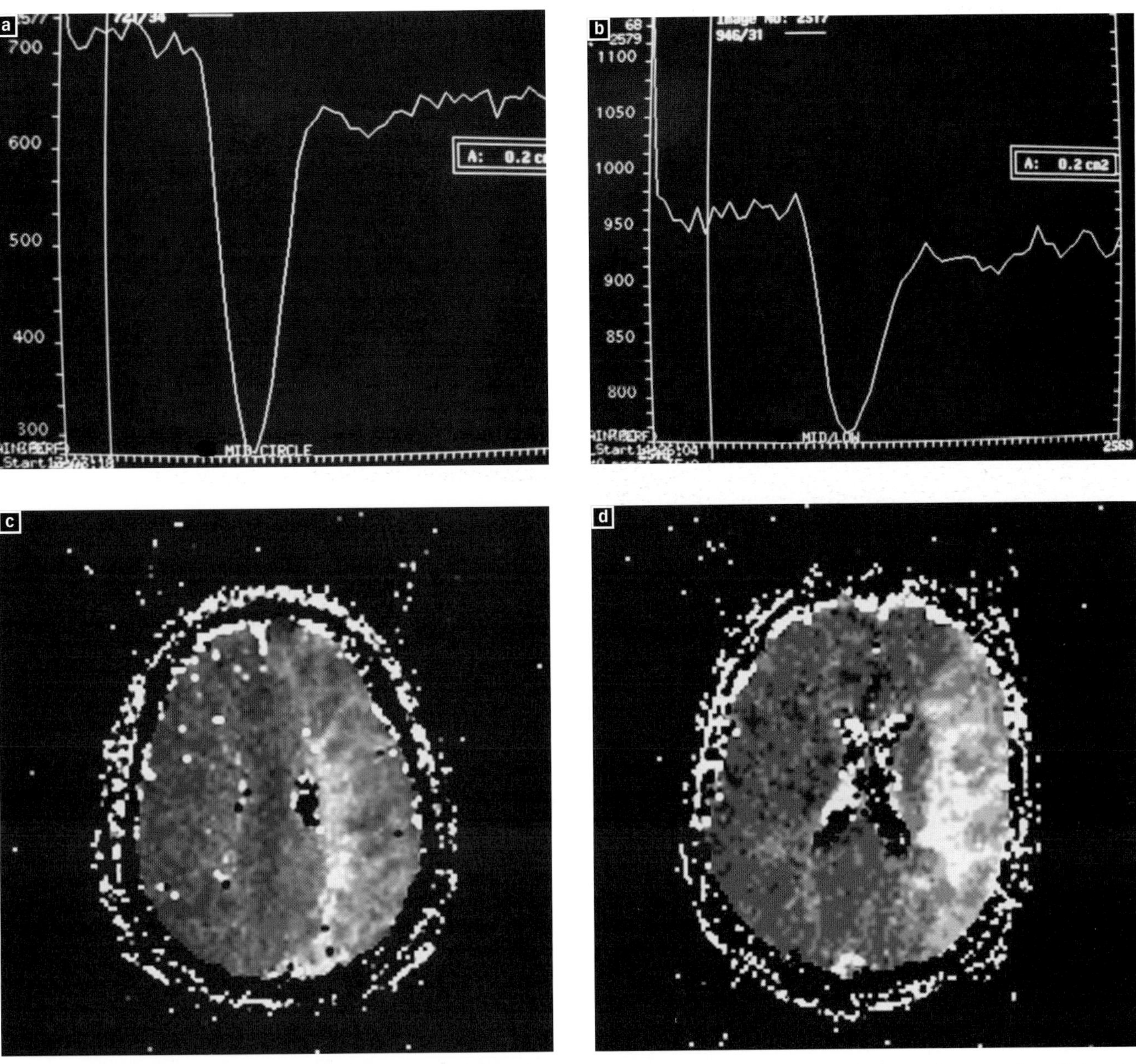

Fig. 8.26. **Signal–time curves and perfusion maps corresponding to the raw image data in Fig. 8.25. (a) Signal–time curve from a region of interest (ROI) in the right hemisphere. There is a brisk wash-in and wash-out of contrast, evidenced by a large signal drop and a narrow signal–time curve. (b) Signal–time curve from a corresponding ROI in an infarct zone in the left hemisphere. Notice the signal begins higher than in A (approximately 950 versus 700 signal units) because the infarct is bright on the baseline T2 image. However, the signal drop is much less, and the signal–time curve is significantly broader than in (a). This indicates significant hypoperfusion. (c), (d) Time-to-peak perfusion maps generated from the signal–time curves on a pixel-by-pixel basis. There is significant hypoperfusion (bright signal) throughout the left MCA territory.**

referred to as the NINDS study (National Institute of Neurological Disorders and Stroke rt-PA Stroke Study Group, 1995). Together, these trials enrolled 624 patients, who were randomized, if eligible, to treatment with i.v. TPA versus placebo. A key eligibility criterion was that the time between ictus and treatment could not exceed 3 hours. If time of ictus could not be determined, such as in strokes that occurred while patients were asleep, the patients were not eligible for the study. The i.v. TPA was administered at a dose of 0.9 mg/kg, with 10 percent of the dose given as a bolus and the remaining 90 percent infused intravenously over 60 minutes. The trials assessed outcome for treatment with intravenous TPA in both the immediate/early post-treatment phase (within 24 hours), and a late subacute phase (90 days post-stroke).

Whenever we are assessing outcomes in scientific trials, it is important to have at least a vague notion of the outcome scale – in other words, what precisely is being measured. There are different outcome measures and different endpoints

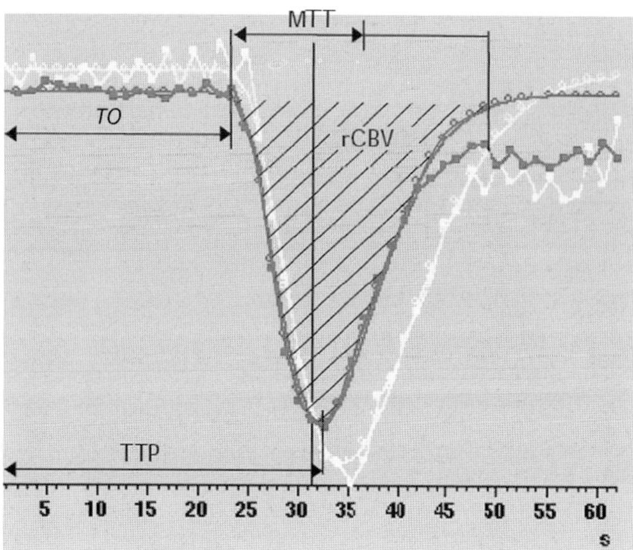

Fig. 8.27. **Some of the main parameters in PWI. Solid curves are original and recirculation-corrected signal–time curves resulting from a gadolinium bolus. These can be used to calculate $T0$, the time of arrival of the bolus, and time to peak (TTP). The negative integral of the signal–time curve (area under the curve) yields an estimate of cerebral blood volume (CBV). The dashed curve is the tissue signal–time curve de-blurred from the arterial inflow by deconvolution with the arterial input function. This yields the mean transit time (MTT). The ratio of CBV and MTT can be used to calculate CBF. (Courtesy of Philips MR Inc.)**

that have been employed in the multiple scientific thrombolysis trials. Yet, we rarely stop to ask ourselves what does it mean, in a rigorous fashion, that a patient improved or did not improve after thrombolytic therapy? In the NINDS1 trial, the primary outcome measure was the percent of patients who showed significant early improvement, defined as either complete resolution of neurologic symptoms or an improvement of at least 4 points on the NIH stroke scale (NIHSS) at 24 hours. The NIHSS is an important scale to know; it measures the severity of neurologic deficit using a standardized physical examination. Using this measure, 46 percent of patients in the TPA group improved, versus 39 percent of the placebo group. This finding did not reach statistical significance, so according to its own endpoints, the study did not demonstrate a significant difference in favor of i.v. TPA at 24 hours. However, some other measures, such as the average NIH stroke scale decline at 24 hours between the treatment group and control group, did show statistically significant differences. Both the control and treatment arms had an average NIH stroke scale score of 14 at randomization. At 24 hours, the treatment group had an average NIHSS rating of 8, while the control group was at 12. Also, when assessed at 3 months, the i.v. TPA group did better on a variety of outcome scales. These positive findings were considered sufficient to be "hypothesis generating" for the premise that i.v. TPA leads to an improved outcome in ischemic stroke. Therefore, the Data and Safety Monitoring Committee for NINDS1 recommended a second part to the trial. The study design was identical to NINDS1,

but the primary endpoint was assessing the percentage of patients who had little or no neurologic deficit at 3 months post-treatment. Before we discuss the results of NINDS2, we need to briefly familiarize ourselves with some of the major stroke assessment scales:

The NIHSS, described above
Minimal or no neurologic deficit equates to an NIHSS score of 0 or 1. Very severe strokes, for example, may have an NIHSS of greater than 20.

The modified Rankin Score (mRS)
This scale measures patient disability. A score of 0–1 indicates little or no deficit, while an mRS of 3–5 means that the patient does not have the capacity for independent living.

The Barthel Index
This index also measures the degree of independence in performing the activities of daily living. A good score is considered a Barthel Index of 95–100.

The Glasgow Outcome Scale
This scale measures the patient's functional status. A score of 1 means recovery with minimal or no deficit.

While the details of these outcome criteria are beyond the scope of this book, it is important to be familiar with their names and to have a vague notion of what constitutes a good outcome.

The NINDS2 trial used each of the above scales as a separate primary endpoint, as well as a composite global statistic combining all of them. Using these outcome measures and assessing the patients at 90 days, there was now a significant benefit in favor of the TPA treatment group compared to the placebo control group. Using the NIHSS, 31 percent of the TPA group showed minimal or no disability compared to 20 percent of the control group. On the Barthel Index, minimal or no disability was present in 50 percent of the TPA group versus 38 percent of the control group. As an aside, the difference in numbers – e.g., 50 percent vs. 31 percent in the treatment arm – using the same group of patients and the same general endpoint but a different evaluation scale underscores the importance of such issues as the choice of evaluation scale and of a close and critical reading of the literature to see how conclusions were reached. In reporting the results of the trial, the NINDS study group concluded that, "As compared with patients given placebo, patients treated with t-PA were at least 30 percent more likely to have minimal or no disability at three months on the assessment scales." To get a slightly different sense of the efficacy of TPA, we can look at a parameter called the NNT, which stands for the "number needed to treat" to make one person better. The 12 percent difference between the TPA and control groups on the Barthel Index translates to an NNT of about 8.3. Thus, we need to thrombolyse about eight patients so that one patient will be left with minimal or no disability at 3 months.

In summary, then, the NINDS studies showed a benefit for the use of TPA. This benefit was marginal in the acute post-stroke period, but was more evident at three months. Even at 3 months, however, the NNT numbers suggest that while there is definite statistical benefit for TPA, it is by no means a miracle therapy for acute stroke.

It was primarily on the basis of these studies that i.v. TPA was granted FDA approval for use in acute stroke. A point often unclear to residents is that, at the time of this writing, intravenous TPA remains the only FDA approved thrombolytic therapy for acute stroke. Yes, this means that intra-arterial TPA is not yet FDA approved, and is used according to internal protocols at various institutions.

To make things interesting, a large European study known as the European Cooperative Acute Stroke Study (ECASS I) was published nearly contemporaneously with the NINDS study. It was also a prospective randomized trial examining the use of intravenous TPA in the setting of acute stroke in 620 patients. It came to an opposite conclusion from the NINDS study that intravenous TPA is not more effective than placebo in improving the outcome of stroke patients, or to quote directly, "intravenous thrombolysis cannot currently be recommended for use in an unselected population of acute ischemic stroke patients" (Hacke *et al.*, The European Cooperative Acute Stroke Study, 1995).

To be more complete, the ECASS study found that i.v. TPA may be useful in a select subset of stroke patients, but that this subset could not be easily identified, leading to the above conclusion.

The fact that two large prospective randomized trials dealing with such an important topic came to different – and nearly opposite – conclusions was a cause for consternation and led to a flurry of *post-hoc* analyses attempting to understand the difference in conclusions and recommendations. The results of these analyses make some critical points about i.v. TPA and highlight as well some of the controversies regarding imaging findings and their role in therapy. Three major issues can be immediately identified:

The dosage of TPA

There are several reasons that a prospective randomized trial may find TPA ineffective when comparing outcomes in the treatment group to the control group. One of the main reasons may be that the hemorrhagic complications of TPA in some patients, in terms of symptomatic intracranial bleeds, may offset the beneficial effects in other patients. This was of particular concern after the intravenous streptokinase trials had to be halted due to unacceptably high rates of death and symptomatic intracranial hemorrhage in the treatment group versus the control group. In the MAST-E trial, for instance, the rate of symptomatic intracranial hemorrhage was 21 percent in the group treated with intravenous streptokinase versus only 3 percent in the control group. The evidence is quite clear, in fact, that i.v. TPA also increases the rate of intracranial bleeds in stroke patients. From the NINDS trials, we know that the rate of symptomatic intracranial hemorrhage in the treatment group was 6.4 percent, versus 0.6 percent in the control group – a ten-fold increase in the likelihood of symptomatic bleeds. The rates of all bleeds (asymptomatic and symptomatic) were even higher. The rates of intracranial hemorrhage are, of course, somewhat related to the dose of thrombolytic agent used. The NINDS trial, as mentioned, used a dose of 0.9 mg/kg i.v. TPA. The ECASS I study, meanwhile, used a higher TPA dose of 1.1 mg/kg. In that study, the rates of symptomatic intracranial hemorrhage were 20 percent in the treatment group versus 7 percent in the placebo group. The high symptomatic intracranial bleed rates in the treatment group were a main reason that, overall, no efficacy for TPA was found in that study. As will be discussed below, these high rates were not just a function of the higher dose of TPA. However, the message was clear to scientists and regulatory bodies, and when it came time for FDA approval, i.v. TPA was approved at a dose of 0.9 mg/kg.

The time to treatment: the 3-hour thrombolysis window

Ischemic strokes occur because of insufficient perfusion to the brain. This, in turn, is a function of two parameters: the severity of the perfusion deficit (i.e., how low the cerebral blood flow falls) and the duration of the perfusion deficit. With severe hypoperfusion (CBF values less than 7 ml/100 g per min), irreversible ischemic damage occurs within 1 hour. If the CBF is a bit higher, say in the range of 12 ml/100 g per min, the brain can tolerate these low rates for a few hours without ischemic damage. If the vascular occlusion is long-lasting, ischemic damage will occur with CBF values as high as 24 ml/100 g per min. Thus, for any given perfusion deficit, there is a critical time window for lysing the clot if the brain is to be saved.

One main difference between the NINDS study and the ECASS I study that likely contributed to the lack of a positive result in ECASS I is the time to thrombolysis. The NINDS study allowed patients to be enrolled only within 0–3 hours of stroke, while ECASS I had a 6 hour time window. The vast majority of patients in ECASS, in fact, were treated between 4–6 hours of stroke onset. It turns out that this time difference is a significant factor in both the efficacy of i.v. TPA and in the avoidance of its complications. To help sort out the effect of dose versus time, a second study, ECASS II was launched. It enrolled 800 patients and used a TPA dose of 0.9 mg/kg (like NINDS), but retained the 6-hour time window. In ECASS II, 80 percent of the patients were treated in the 3–6-hour time window. Like ECASS I, this study also failed to show efficacy of i.v. TPA in improving clinical outcome for stroke patients (Hacke *et al.*, ECASS II, 1998a). A second study examining the issue of extending the i.v. TPA thrombolysis window beyond 3 hours was the Alteplase Thrombolysis for Acute Noninterventional Therapy in Ischemic Stroke (ATLANTIS) study. This study was conducted in two parts, ATLANTIS A and ATLANTIS B, and enrolled 761 patients in a randomized trial using a TPA dose of 0.9 mg/kg. Part A treated patients within 6 hours of stroke, but was halted early due to unacceptably high intracranial bleed rates in the patients treated between 5 and 6 hours after stroke onset. Analysis of preliminary data revealed no positive effect for TPA and a significantly higher mortality in the treatment group (36.1 percent versus 4.2 percent). ATLANTIS B enrolled patients at a time interval between 3 and 5 hours, also using a TPA dose of

0.9 mg/kg. This study was stopped early when data analysis revealed no significant outcome difference between the TPA and control groups, and futility analysis indicated that "treatment was unlikely to prove beneficial" if the study were to continue. Both the ECASS II and ATLANTIS trials confirmed once again that i.v. TPA increased the rates of symptomatic intracranial bleed compared with placebo (ECASS II: 8.8 percent vs. 3.4 percent; ATLANTIS B: 7.0 percent vs. 1.1 percent). However, these bleed rates were significantly better than the 20 percent figure in ECASS I, which had used the higher TPA dose of 1.1 mg/kg.

The aggregate of these studies strongly suggests that the 3-hour deadline is a valid and significant time point, and that there is little gain to be expected in treating patients with i.v. TPA beyond 3 hours. Hence, FDA approval for i.v. TPA is only for a 3-hour time window, and that is why we see neurologists rushing so quickly to treat their patients within this window. While the sight of neurologists frantically checking their watches as perspiration beads on their foreheads is often not understood – sometimes even joked about – by other physicians, the data fully bear the neurologists out: time is brain! In the NINDS study, for instance, about half of the patients were treated ultra-early, at or before 90-minutes. This group did significantly better than the group treated at 91–180 minutes, with the odds ratio for good outcome at 3 months being 2.11 in the former group versus 1.69 in the latter group (Marler *et al.*, 2000). Conversely, when patients are treated with TPA outside the FDA guidelines (this often means later than 3 hours) various studies have documented poor outcomes. For instance, a study by Buchan *et al.* (2000) showed that when patients were treated within FDA guidelines, the rate of symptomatic intracranial hemorrhage was 5 percent while patients treated outside the guidelines had a symptomatic intracranial hemorrhage rate of 38 percent. So, for all the rebels out there, be careful with the FDA guidelines; they actually seem to be there for a reason.

Findings on the pre-treatment head CT and the "1/3 of the MCA" rule

The impact of the findings on the initial non-contrast head CT represents another significant design difference between the ECASS and NINDS studies. Given the limited sensitivity of CT in the first few hours post-stroke, the ECASS investigators reasoned that if a patient already had signs of a large stroke on CT, this indicated a severe perfusion deficit and a high likelihood that the brain had already infarcted. In this circumstance, i.v. TPA would not help, and could hurt by increasing the intracranial bleed rates. Thus, evidence of a large infarct on the initial head CT – defined as an infarct involving more than one-third of a given vessel's territory, usually the MCA – was explicitly stated as an exclusion criterion from the study. Unfortunately, of the 620 patients randomized in ECASS, there were 109 protocol violations – i.e., patients who were included in the study who should not have been. Of these, 52 had early evidence of a large stroke on CT, but the finding was missed by local investigators, and the patients were mistakenly enrolled in the study and randomized. Thus, although

ECASS had intended to exclude such patients, it inadvertently ended up providing data on the efficacy of TPA in patients with a large stroke already visible on CT. The data was not encouraging, and the ECASS investigators arrived at the following conclusion: "Our findings strongly suggest that a parenchymal area of hypoattenuation in excess of one third of the middle cerebral artery territory is indicative of both poor clinical outcome and ineffectiveness of treatment with intravenously administered rt-PA. Moreover, these observations suggest that intravenous rt-PA may be detrimental in patients with a large early edema." (von Kummer *et al.*, 1997). More specifically, in this group of CT protocol violators who showed signs of large infarct and were treated with i.v. TPA, the intracranial bleed rate was 40 percent (Fisher *et al.*, 1995). Retrospective analysis of the NINDS data also showed a significantly higher bleed rate (31 percent) in TPA-treated patients who had evidence of edema or infarct on the initial CT as compared to those who did not (6 percent).

Thus was born the famous "1/3 of the MCA" rule with which most residents are now familiar. On the basis of such data, the Stroke Council of the American Heart Association formally advised that i.v. TPA not be used in patients with evidence of large infarcts on the initial CT scan: "If CT demonstrates early changes of a recent major infarction such as sulcal effacement, mass effect, edema, or possible hemorrhage, thrombolytic therapy should be avoided (Grade A recommendation)." (Adams *et al.*, 1996). This rule has since been widely quoted in both the neurology and the neuroradiology literature. For example, in an article from the Department of Neurology in Heidelberg, Germany, one of the listed exclusion criteria for i.v. TPA is "marked early signs >1/3 MCA hypodensity." (Schellinger 2005). Similarly, in one of my favorite neuroradiology texts of all time, we find the following in the section on stroke treatment: "There is an increased risk of fatal hemorrhage when there is decreased density in greater than one-third of the middle cerebral artery territory (thrombolytics in large MCA infarcts even with an ischemic penumbra are contraindicated)." (Grossman and Yousem, 2003).

Thus, the role of radiologists is obvious. Not only must we detect intracranial hemorrhage, which is an absolute contraindication to thrombolysis, but we can no longer afford to miss those very subtle signs of early stroke on CT, as we did with impunity in the past. The data on the matter seems clear and compelling. Yet, as with many such things in medicine, "clear and compelling" is just code for "questionable and controversial"! The first hint that there is more to the story of the "1/3 rule," is that, despite the data cited above, the actual American Academy of Neurology thrombolysis guidelines do not include evidence of a large infarct on head CT as an exclusion criterion, but only the presence of intracranial blood (see for example the Brain Attack Coalition thrombolysis guidelines, titled TPA Stroke Study Group Guidelines which can be found at http://www.stroke-site.org/guidelines/tpa_guidelines.html).

How can this be? The answer lies in returning to the data. Unlike ECASS, the NINDS study did not employ a "large infarct" exclusion criterion. The only CT exclusion criterion was the presence of intracranial blood. Yet, the NINDS study found TPA useful despite thrombolysing those with evidence of ischemic changes on their head CTs. In fact, after the findings of ECASS regarding the poor outcome of TPA-treated patients with evidence of large stroke on head CT, there have been multiple directed analyses using the NINDS patient group. These have come to a surprising conclusion: patients with evidence of early ischemic changes (EIC) on their head CT, in fact, do worse than those with normal head CTs, but this occurs regardless of whether they are in the TPA group or the control group. It seems that the presence of EIC is simply a marker for the presence of a severe stroke, indicating that these patients will have a poorer outcome regardless of treatment group. However, the ischemic changes, in and of themselves, are not an independent prognostic sign that such patients will do worse with TPA. The NINDS study group found that, in treated patients, there were only two independent variables associated with a risk of increased intracranial hemorrhage: initial severity of stroke symptoms and positive initial head CT with evidence of edema or mass effect. Yet, in both subgroups, the TPA treated patients actually did better than their placebo counterparts, with an odds ratio of 4.3 for the subgroup with severe neurological deficit and an odds ratio of 3.4 for the subgroup with edema or mass effect on their head CT. Thus, the study concluded: "Despite a higher rate of intracerebral hemorrhage, patients with severe strokes or edema or mass effect on the baseline-CT are reasonable candidates for t-PA, if it is administered within 3 hours of onset." (NINDS t-PA Stroke Study Group, 1997). A second analysis of the NINDS data with more careful scrutiny of the head CTs for EIC came to an identical conclusion (Patel et al., 2001). If the effect for initial severity of stroke using the NIH stroke scale is controlled for, there is no independent association between the findings of early ischemia on the initial head CT and the outcome of treatment with i.v. TPA, or to quote the investigators directly: "Our analysis suggests that EICs are prevalent within 3 hours of stroke onset and correlate with stroke severity. However, EICs are not independently associated with increased risk of adverse outcome after rt-PA treatment. Patients treated with rt-PA did better whether or not they had EICs, suggesting that EICs on CT scan are not critical to the decision to treat otherwise eligible patients with rt-PA within 3 hours of stroke onset."

To be rigorous about things, it must be noted that the NINDS investigators who did these analyses on the significance of EIC were not looking at precisely the same issue as the ECASS investigators. The above NINDS *post-hoc* analyses were looking at patients with evidence of early ischemic change on head CT without specific attention to the size of these changes. Once again, even more thorough data analysis is then warranted, which was carried out on two fronts. First, there was an approach to be more rigorous about sizing the early ischemic changes rather than simply the subjective impression of the radiologist or the neurologist that it was greater than one-third of the MCA territory. This was done under the auspices of the Alberta Stroke Program Early CT Score, known as the ASPECTS scoring system. This scoring system divides the MCA territory into ten regions, with one point deducted for each area showing evidence of hypodensity, sulcal effacement or loss of the gray-white matter junction. Thus, a normal head CT would have an ASPECTS score of 10, while moderately severe changes would be an ASPECTS score of less then 7. The ASPECTS scoring system was then applied to the NINDS patient group, seeking to analyze the significance of not only the presence of early ischemic changes but also of their size, with respect to treatment decisions. A second approach was to apply the subjective 1/3 MCA rule to the NINDS data in the same way as ECASS had done. Both approaches once again yielded the conclusion that there was still no treatment modifying interaction between large areas of baseline ischemic change on head CT and the use of TPA, and that patients should not be excluded from TPA based solely on the presence of even large areas of ischemic change (see Lyden 2003, and Demchuk et al., 2005b).

The reader must be clear, however, that there is great prognostic significance to the presence of large areas of EIC on the head CT. Such changes indicate more profound perfusion deficits and more severe infarcts, and are associated with larger areas of DWI positivity and poorer clinical outcomes than in patients with normal head CTs (von Kummer et al., 2001). Such patients also have significantly higher intracranial bleed rates after i.v. TPA. However, this group of patients will do poorly regardless of whether TPA is used or not, and will still tend to do slightly better with TPA than without it, as discussed above. One way to reconcile the findings of the NINDS group regarding the lack of significance of ischemic changes on head CT with the opposite conclusion of the ECASS investigators is to note that the studies had different time windows. It may be that large areas of EIC on head CT are significant at 6 hours for treatment decisions with i.v. TPA but not at 3 hours. Thus, those using i.v. TPA outside of FDA guidelines may choose to avoid thrombolyzing patients with large infarcts evident on CT in the 3–6-hour time window. Before accepting this compromise solution, though, consider the fact that according to some authors, "the importance of the greater than one-third MCA territory rule could not be confirmed in the ECASS-2 trial, however, where no association with increased mortality was seen with rt-PA." (Demchuk et al., Neuroimaging Clinics of North America 2005a). Thus, it may be that even at 6 hours, the venerable "1/3 MCA" rule may have little significance to treatment decisions.

Another significant CT finding in the setting of acute stroke is the dense vessel sign, sometimes referred to in the literature as the hyperdense MCA sign (HMCAS). There is less controversy with this finding than with early ischemic changes, but there is some nonetheless. One immediate controversy is that this is a poor radiographic sign that does not necessarily indicate MCA occlusion, with many false positives such as due to calcification in vessel walls or to elevated hematocrit. Let us deal with this one right off the bat. A study by Tomsick et al. (1990) found that HMCAS is specific enough. This study found that the HMCAS had a sensitivity of 78 percent, specificity of 93 percent and an accuracy of 91 percent in predicting MCA occlusion.

This sign is seen in a significant percent of stroke patients. When seen, it is associated with more severe strokes (higher NIHSS scores) and significantly worse clinical outcomes. In one frequently quoted study by Tomsick *et al.* (1996), one-third of the patients had the HMCAS. The stroke patients were treated with ultra-early TPA, within a 90-minute time window, thus maximizing their likelihood of a good outcome. However, despite ultra-early therapy, HMCAS-positive patients did not fare well. These patients, at presentation, had a median baseline NIHSS score of 19.5, compared to a score of 10 for those without HMCAS. At 3 months, only 6 percent of those with HMCAS had complete neurological improvement compared with 47 percent of the HMCAS negative patients. Even controlling for stroke severity and restricting the analysis to patients with an NIHSS score of greater than 10, the HMCAS positive patients exhibited less neurological recovery. This study concluded that "the presence of the HMCAS on CT scans obtained within 90 minutes of stroke onset is associated with a major neurologic deficit, and in this study it predicted a poor clinical and radiologic outcome after intravenous thrombolytic therapy."

Other studies were not quite as negative, although all agree that HMCAS-positivity heralds a poor outcome. A multicenter European study by Manelfe *et al.* (1999) analyzed the ECASS patient pool with respect to the HMCAS and found that, while HMCAS-positive patients had significantly worse outcomes than those without a hyperdense MCA sign, i.v. TPA actually produced a slight improvement in neurologic outcome at 3 months. This same conclusion was reached in another recently published study addressing the same issue, assessing patients treated with i.v. TPA within 3 hours (Qureshi *et al.*, 2006). The conclusion of this study was the most positive yet, finding a definite improvement in outcome when i.v. TPA was used in the setting of HMCAS. This finding, though, was once again given with the caveat that HMCAS is, in general, associated with a poor outcome. Thus, it is probably fair to say that the general consensus is that if there are no other treatment options, patients with a hyperdense MCA sign may benefit from i.v. TPA. According to several authors, however, because of the likelihood of a poor outcome, such patients should probably be triaged to other therapy if that is available. Among such alternatives is intra-arterial thrombolysis. What a segue!

Intra-arterial thrombolysis

As already mentioned, at this time there is no FDA approval for an agent or regimen of intra-arterial thrombolysis for acute stroke. However, the readers of this book are doubtless aware that such therapy exists and is sometimes used in stroke patients (Fig. 8.28). In whom should it be used, and what data is there in support of its use?

To begin answering these questions, we state that there are two main populations in which intra-arterial thrombolysis is usually considered:

(1) Those outside the 3-hour time window for i.v. TPA

A viable alternative for these patients may be intra-arterial thrombolytic therapy, which in the anterior circulation may traditionally be administered up to 6 hours after stroke onset, significantly expanding the time window available to treat patients. Therapeutic windows for posterior circulation infarcts can be even longer.

(2) Those with a heavy clot burden, such as proximal MCA occlusion or ICA occlusion.

We know that ICA and proximal MCA occlusions are associated with a higher NIHSS score at presentation, indicating a more severe neurologic deficit. Severe stroke at presentation, in and of itself, is a poor prognostic factor, and thus such patients typically do not fare well with i.v. TPA. To be a bit more specific, the NINDS data indicated that with i.v. TPA, 52 percent of the patients with an NIHSS of less than 10 at presentation showed an excellent response, with minimal or no neurologic deficit at 3 months; only 8 percent of those with an NIHSS of 20 or greater showed the same favorable response to i.v. TPA (The NINDS t-PA Stroke Study Group, 1997b). Moreover, in those with major infarcts, angiographic studies in the first 6 hours post-ictus have revealed that a significant portion do have evidence of proximal occlusion and heavy clot burden – again making them less likely to respond well to i.v. TPA, as discussed above. Data from an article by the Executive Committee of the American Society for Interventional and Therapeutic Neuroradiology (ASITN) estimates that in those with major stroke, 30 percent have an M1 occlusion, 25 percent have an M2 occlusion, 10 percent have a carotid "T" occlusion, 15–20 percent have a proximal ICA occlusion or severe stenosis, and 5–10 percent have a vertebrobasilar occlusion. Only 10–20 percent of those with major strokes will not have an obvious thrombo-embolic large vessel occlusion at angiography (Executive Committee of the ASITN 2001a). It turns out, as we will discuss below, that intra-arterial thrombolysis achieves excellent recanalization rates for these occluded vessels. A conglomerate estimate compiled by the ASITN from various series reports that, for MCA occlusions, the average recanalization rate for intra-arterial thrombolysis is about 83 percent (Executive Committee of the ASITN 2001b).

It is difficult to directly compare intra-arterial thrombolysis to i.v. TPA on the issue of vessel recanalization, as the large i.v. TPA studies did not involve angiography to check for vessel recanalization. However, the results of one smaller study suggests a relatively low rate of vessel recanalization with i.v. TPA (Wolpert *et al.*, 1993). The overall partial arterial recanalization rate was only 30 percent, and the complete recanalization rate was only 4.3 percent. Such data indicate that there should be a significant role for intra-arterial thrombolysis in stroke therapy, particularly in patients with a heavy clot burden. The only thing remaining would be some efficacy and safety data, which is what we turn to next.

There have been many small series which have reported the efficacy of intra-arterial thrombolysis. For example, Suarez *et al.* (1999) reported on a group of 54 patients treated with intra-arterial urokinase within 6 hours of stroke onset. Using a Barthel Index of 95–100, 48 percent of their patients had a good

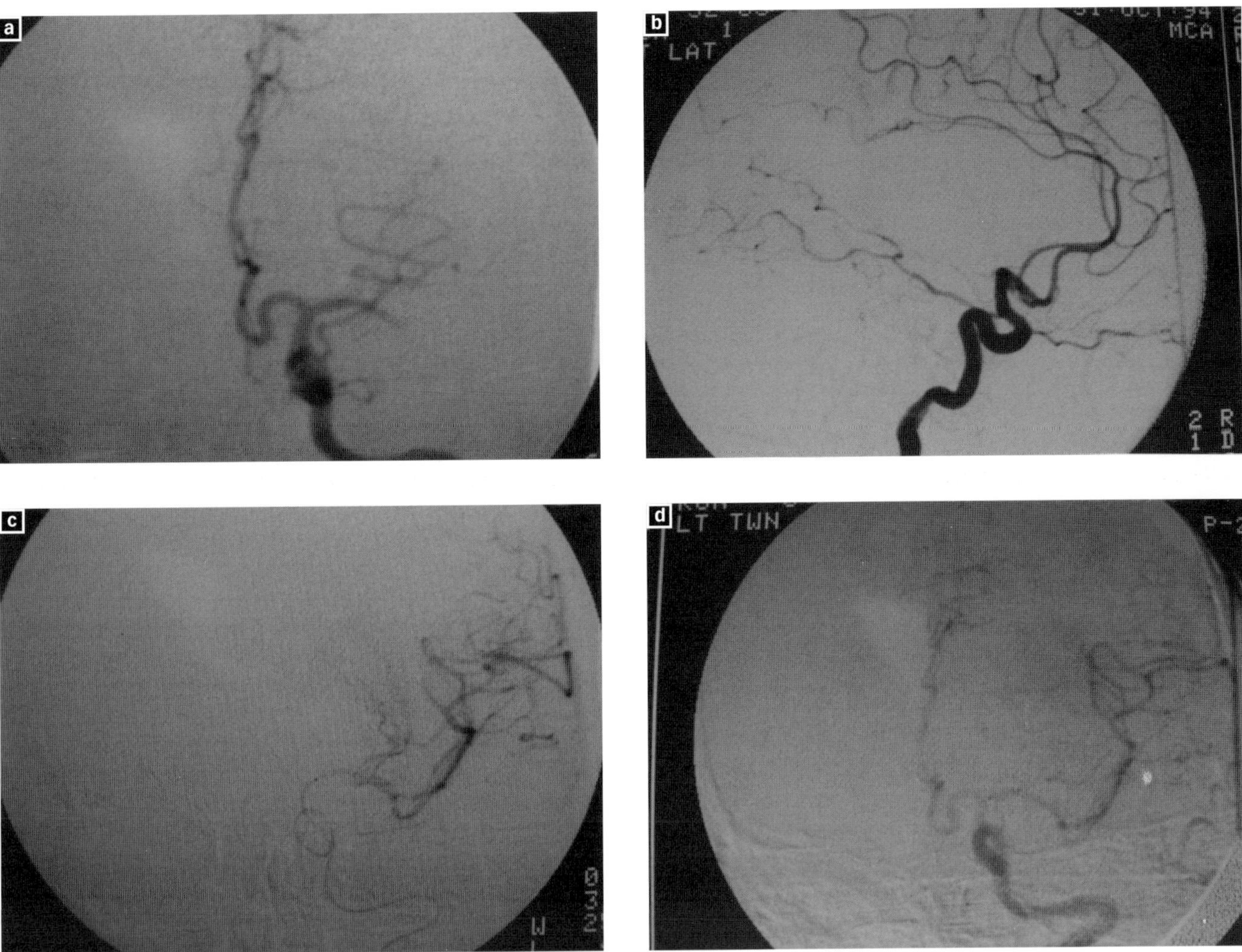

Fig. 8.28. **Patient presents with acute onset dense right hemiparesis and aphasia. (a) AP and (b) lateral angiogram shows occlusion of the distal M1 portion of the left MCA, with absence of the Sylvian branches. (c) A tracker catheter is used for intra-arterial thrombolysis, with (d) recanalization of the left MCA. The patient recovered with no detectable clinical deficit.**

outcome, with a 17 percent intracranial bleed rate. Similarly, Xavier *et al.* (2005) treated 40 patients who were not candidates for i.v. TPA with intra-arterial TPA. Overall, they achieved a 92 percent vessel recanalization rate, and of the patients with an MCA occlusion, 60 percent achieved a good outcome. However, there are very few prospective randomized trials which have assessed the efficacy of intra-arterial thrombolysis. The main study to be aware of in this realm is the Prolyse in Acute Cerebral Thromboembolism Trial (PROACT II). This study represented the first randomized, controlled study of the efficacy and safety of intra-arterial thrombolysis. The patients were a fairly homogeneous group in that they all had M1 or M2 occlusions, were within 6 hours of ictus (mean time to treatment 5.3 hours) and had severe strokes, with a median NIHSS score of 18. In total, 180 patients were randomized in a 2:1 ratio to receive intra-arterial pro-urokinase and heparin (121 patients) or placebo and heparin (59 patients). The pro-urokinase group showed significantly higher vascular

recanalization rates (66 percent versus 18 percent in the control group). These higher revascularization rates translated into better neurologic outcomes. Using an efficacy criterion of a modified Rankin Scale score of 2 or less at 90 days, the treatment group achieved a 40 percent rate of good neurologic outcome versus 25 percent in the control group. This represents an absolute improvement likelihood of 15 percent, and a relative improvement likelihood of 60 percent. These results were achieved despite significantly higher rates of symptomatic intracranial bleeds in the treatment group versus the controls – 10 percent versus 2 percent (see Furlan *et al.*, 1999). The significance of the PROACT II results are difficult to overstate. It was the first randomized controlled trial of thrombolytic therapy to show a statistically significant treatment benefit beyond 3 hours after stroke onset. While the results of this study did not convince the FDA to approve an intra-arterial thrombolytic, they provided what is called a "proof of principle" that intra-arterial thrombolysis may be beneficial.

This is especially in view of the alternative for the patient population enrolled in PROACT II. An ancillary set of results which came out of the study was a reconfirmation of the abysmal natural history of MCA occlusions without aggressive thrombolysis. In the control group of PROACT II , treated only with i.v. heparin, 25 percent were dead and 48 percent disabled at 3 months, with only 25 percent having good outcomes (mRS 0–2).

Thus, despite the lack of FDA approval, data such as that quoted above prompted the American Society of Interventional and Therapeutic Neuroradiology to ask the following: "If 40–66 percent good outcomes with MCA occlusion may be offered to patients with timely treatment, how can that opportunity not be offered to a patient faced with only 25 percent likelihood of good outcome if no intervention is instituted?" (Executive Committee of the ASITN 2001a). The ASITN answered the question, stating that "the results of this [PROACT II] trial are convincing evidence that intra-arterial thrombolytic therapy can now be considered an acceptable and appropriate therapy for acute stroke" (Executive Committee of the ASITN; Intraarterial Thrombolysis 2001b).

At the time of this writing, the field of intra-arterial therapy is thus rapidly evolving, and several variations need to be briefly discussed:

Combination of intra-arterial and intravenous (bridging) thrombolytic therapy

Despite good recanalization rates with intra-arterial thrombolysis, it does not do the brain much good (and may do it harm) to recanalize a vessel after the brain territory which it supplies has already infarcted. Intra-arterial therapy, of course, takes time. Getting the patient to the angio suite, getting a catheter into the vessel, etc., are quite time consuming. One strategy to try to maximize outcome for the patient is to begin therapy immediately with i.v. TPA and then go to intra-arterial thrombolysis. This approach was the basis for the Emergency Management of Stroke (EMS) Bridging Trial. This was a small multicenter prospective randomized trial which assigned 35 patients within a 3-hour time frame to one of two limbs: i.v. TPA (0.6 mg/kg) versus placebo, followed by intra-arterial TPA in both the i.v. TPA and placebo groups. Vascular recanalization rates were better in the combined i.v. TPA–intra-arterial TPA group than in the intra-arterial TPA only group (81 percent versus 50 percent). The intracranial bleed rates were not significantly different between the two groups. The higher recanalization rates, though, did not translate into a better neurological outcome for the combined therapy group, which on clinical outcome measures was equivalent to the intra-arterial only therapy group (Lewandowski et al., 1999). However, the study highlighted that combination therapy was feasible, equivalent in safety and clinical efficacy to intra-arterial thrombolysis, and probably superior in terms of vascular recanalization rates.

Alternative thrombolytic agents

We have already discussed the use of intra-arterial prourokinase/urokinase and intra-arterial TPA. There is now some discussion about using glycoprotein IIb-IIIa inhibitors, such as abciximab, in conjunction with these agents to improve thrombolysis. Abciximab is not a thrombolytic agent. It blocks platelet aggregation, and thus may help in preventing re-thrombosis after thrombolytic therapy ends. This is actually an important issue to which insufficient attention has been paid. Thrombolytics, it seems, cause platelet activation, which may lead to re-thrombosis. A study by Qureshi et al. (2004) found that the rate of re-thrombosis after arterial thrombolysis is 17 percent. Patients with reocclusion did significantly worse clinically than those who did not reocclude. However, abciximab therapy, although theoretically sound, must still be considered experimental at this stage. There has been one randomized trial evaluating abciximab versus placebo (Abciximab in Ischemic Stroke Investigators, 2000). This study showed a reasonable safety profile for abciximab even when used out to 24 hours, and showed a slight trend for improved clinical outcome in patients treated with abciximab compared to placebo.

A new thrombolytic related to TPA is retaplase, which is a recombinant plasminogen activator derived from TPA. It has been studied in the setting of mycardial infarction, and is now being investigated for use in stroke. A small study by Qureshi et al. (2002) showed an over 80 percent recanalization rate using intra-arterial retaplase plus mechanical clot disruption. A significantly larger study evaluating intra-arterial retaplase in comparison to intra-arterial urokinase has very recently been published, and it found higher rates of recanalization using retaplase (82 percent) as compared with urokinase (64 percent). This seemed to come at a cost of higher symptomatic intracranial bleed rates (12 percent with retaplase versus 4.5 percent with urokinase). However, mortality rates and clinical outcomes were comparable between the two agents (Sugg et al., 2006). Therefore, it is likely that retaplase will be added to the list of intra-arterial thrombolytic agents currently in use.

Mechanical clot retrieval

Finally, we must touch on another catheter-based recanalization technique, but one which does not involve thrombolysis. Thromboembolic material obstructs vessels, causing stroke. Therefore, it is an intuitively appealing idea to restore blood flow simply by removing the clot mechanically rather than lysing it; this avoids the dangers inherent in thrombolysis. The FDA has recently approved a clot retrieval device known as the Merci device (Mechanical Embolus Removal in Cerebral Ischemia) that can be used to remove large vessel thrombi up to 9 hours after stroke. The approval was based on the Merci I and Merci II trials, which used the PROACT II placebo group for comparison. The trials found a 54 percent recanalization rate for vessels versus 18 percent in the control group. The overall device and procedure complication rate was 7 percent. The mortality rate overall for the Merci device treatment group with MCA stroke was 32 percent compared to 27 percent in the placebo group of PROACT II. Univariate analysis showed a slightly better neurologic outcome at 90 days for the treatment group, but multivariate analysis did not. The effectiveness of this device is now being evaluated in a prospective randomized trial using MRI for patient imaging called the MR Rescue (MR and Recanalization of Stroke Clots Using Embolectomy) trial. While the data for this trial accumulates, some neurologists have taken a dim view of the results of Merci I and Merci II, expressing the opinion that FDA approval may have been premature (Becker *et al.*, 2005).

Extending the thrombolysis time window: diffusion–perfusion MRI and the ischemic penumbra model

Although i.v. TPA has been approved for a decade, and the data relating to its use has been presented above, one fact which has not been mentioned looms larger than all the rest. Regardless of the potential efficacy of the therapy, it is hardly ever used. Only a very small minority of stroke patients end up receiving i.v.-TPA. There are various estimates on just how small this percentage is. Among the most optimistic estimates is that 4 percent of stroke patients will receive TPA (Kleindorfer *et al.*, 2004). A recent large study (Qureshi *et al.*, 2005) actually put the number at much less. It found that of 1 796 513 admissions for ischemic stroke in the United States between 1999 and 2001 only 0.6 percent underwent intravenous thrombolysis. Various studies have shown that the most common reason patients are excluded from i.v. TPA therapy is that they are evaluated after the 3-hour time window has expired. One alternative for extending the thrombolysis time window to cover some of the 96–99 percent of stroke patients not treated with i.v. TPA is the option of intra-arterial thrombolysis. The PROACT II trial discussed above, which showed a favorable outcome with intra-arterial thrombolysis, had a mean time to treatment of 5.3 hours. Thus, intra-arterial thrombolysis in anterior circulation strokes is typically used out to 6 hours. However, there are various limitations with intra-arterial thrombolysis. It requires dedicated neurointerventional teams often not present at community hospitals. Also, it is usually performed only with proximal vessel occlusions such as ICA or M1 or M2 occlusions; patients with distal small branch occlusions are typically not candidates for intra-arterial thrombolysis. Finally, there are usually CT based exclusion criteria. For example, the PROACT II trial used a criterion similar to ECASS to exclude from intra-arterial thrombolysis patients with infarcts larger than 1/3 of the MCA territory.

Such exclusion criteria, whether the 3-hour time window for FDA-guideline use of i.v. TPA or the 1/3 MCA rule in ECASS and PROACT II, are all basically attempting to achieve one aim: to exclude from therapy patients who would not be benefited and who may be harmed by thrombolysis. For a number of years, though, there has been a strong and growing feeling among stroke specialists that such exclusion criteria as a uniform elapsed time (3 or 6 hours) or the findings on plain CT, are not sufficiently refined for optimum patient selection or exclusion, and that we can now do better. The current notion is that the fate of ischemic brain is determined by multiple factors, including the severity of the perfusion deficit, the duration of the perfusion deficit, the amount of irreversible ischemic damage at the time of therapy, and the state of collateral vascular supply, to name a few. Therefore, investigators are seeking to shift from the "wall clock" to an individualized set of criteria – a "brain clock" – which will look at each individual patient and decide whether they are a candidate for thrombolysis based on their own brain physiology. The types of questions this new criteria would need to answer are:

- Should this particular patient receive i.v. TPA beyond 3 hours?
- Of patients being considered for intra-arterial TPA or other catheter-based therapy because of proximal vessel occlusion or presentation beyond the 3-hour time window, which patients should be selected and which are unlikely to benefit and therefore should not be treated?

What criteria might be able to provide the answers to such questions? The information available through diffusion (DWI) and perfusion (PWI) MR imaging seems to hold much promise and has been the basis of the "ischemic penumbra" model of stroke therapy. This model has actually been around since the 1970s, but advanced MRI techniques have now made it readily applicable. The basic idea is similar to that used in cardiac imaging and the treatment of myocardial infarction. With vascular occlusion and stroke, there will be a zone of tissue which has infarcted secondary to hypoperfusion. This is the core infarct zone, and is, in theory, irreversibly damaged. It is evident on MRI as a zone of DWI positivity. Surrounding this, however, is a larger zone of hypoperfusion, which is positive on PWI but not bright on DWI. It represents hypoperfused but viable brain tissue. This is considered "at risk" brain, and is referred to as the penumbra zone (see Fig. 8.29).

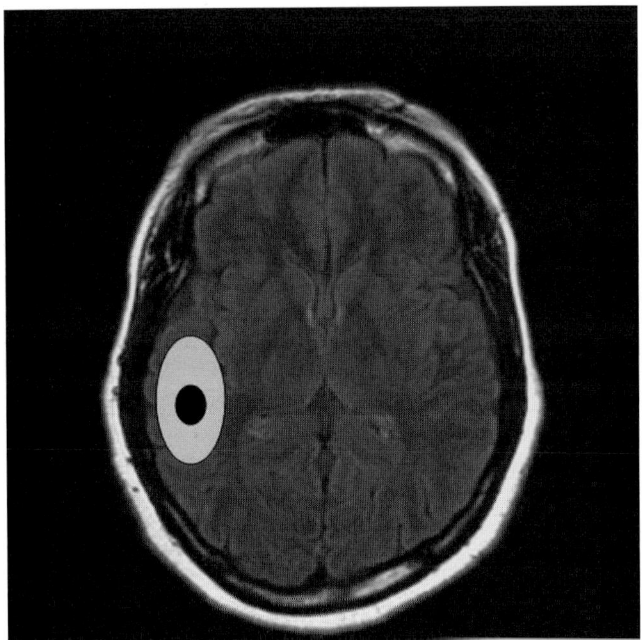

Fig. 8.29. **With MCA branch occlusion, there is a core infarct zone (black oval), which will be DWI positive. This is surrounded by a penumbra zone of hypoperfused but viable brain (gray oval) which is PWI positive but not DWI positive.**

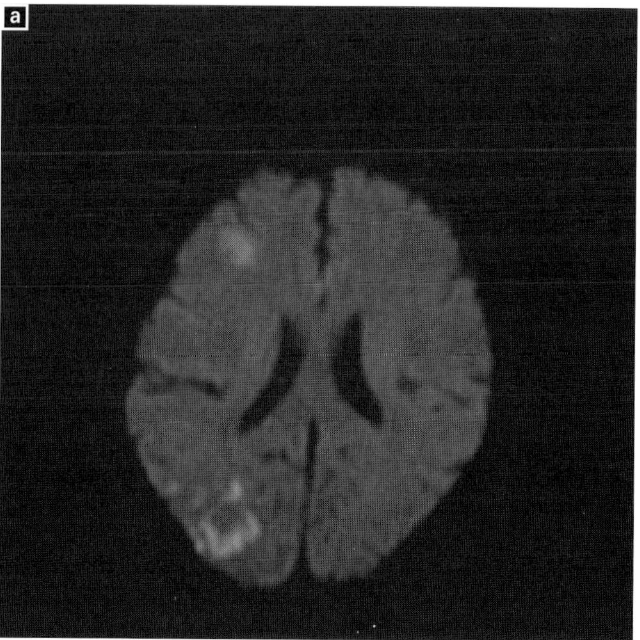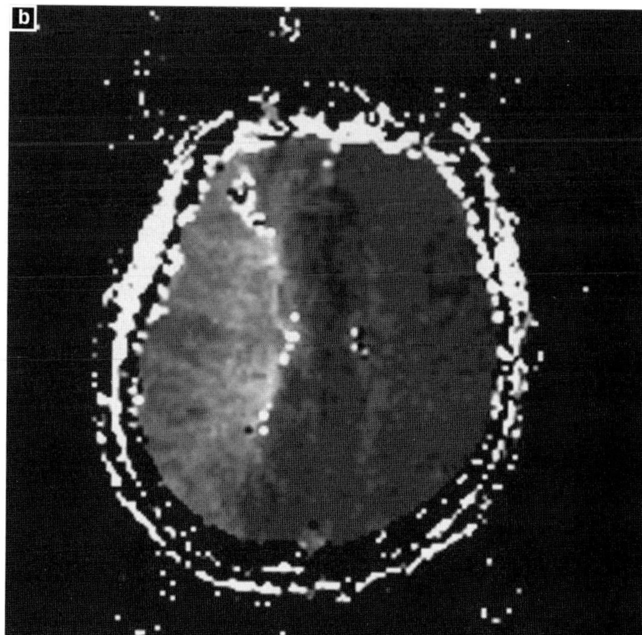

Fig. 8.30. **(a) DWI imaging shows small zones of infarct in the watershed territory of the right cerebral hemisphere in this patient with right MCA occlusion. (b) PWI (TTP) image shows hypoperfusion throughout the right MCA territory. These findings imply a significant PWI–DWI mismatch.**

Patients with a large penumbra zone are said to have a significant PWI–DWI "mismatch," and are considered the ideal patients to thrombolyse, even beyond the 3-hour time window (Fig. 8.30).

The general thinking behind this treatment strategy is that the original TPA data, whether from the NINDS, ECASS or ATLANTIS trials, were based on fairly crude patient selection criteria: the wall clock and the findings on non-contrast CT. If the patients had been selected instead on the basis of PWI–DWI mismatch, the modest benefit of i.v. TPA evident in the NINDS trial would have been significantly enhanced, and the ECASS and ATLANTIS trials would have yielded positive rather than negative results.

When a thrombolysis treatment group is statistically compared to a control group, the relative efficacy of thrombolytic therapy can be offset by two main factors:

(1) Treating patients who would have gotten better on their own, so they do well both with treatment and without.

(2) Treating patients whose condition cannot be improved, because the hypoperfused brain has already infarcted, and there is no significant at risk brain to salvage.

If the patient is in one of these two subgroups, then thrombolysis therapy will provide no benefit, and may do harm, which would offset positive results in other patient subgroups.

The PWI–DWI mismatch criterion seems ideally suited to exclude patients in both of the above subgroups. The mismatch model, of course, rests on the assumption that the penumbra zone of at risk brain is more likely to infarct if the patient is left untreated. In other words, in cases of PWI–DWI mismatch, the DWI lesion will continue to enlarge.

Conversely, if patients have matched PWI–DWI defects, or DWI lesions bigger than PWI, then the DWI lesion will not enlarge over time. These assumptions are open to empiric verification.

A host of small non-randomized MRI studies of the PWI–DWI mismatch hypothesis, in the setting of i.v. TPA therapy within a 6-hour time window, have yielded the following important conclusions regarding extending the intravenous thrombolysis time window.

(1) Approximately 70–80 percent of stroke patients have a PWI–DWI mismatch with PWI > DWI at the time of initial evaluation.

(2) Patients with PWI–DWI mismatch will typically show enlargement of the DWI lesion during the first 3–4 days after stroke onset if the PWI abnormality is not corrected.

(3) If the PWI abnormality is reversed – usually by i.v. TPA within a 6-hour time window, although in a minority of cases through spontaneous recanalization – there is typically little or no growth of the DWI lesion.

(4) In patients with PWI lesions equal to or smaller than DWI lesions, there is typically no further growth of the DWI lesion. These are either patients with small infarcts and early spontaneous recanalization or patients with large infarcts and matched defects (Barber *et al.*, 1998).

(5) Using PWI, DWI, and MRA studies, it has been found that i.v. TPA within a 6-hour time window significantly improves vessel recanalization rates, and that this translates to improved clinical outcome as compared to patients who did not receive i.v. TPA. In an Australian study, the Royal Melbourne Hospital Echoplanar Imaging Stroke

Study Group showed that in patients with PWI–DWI mismatch treated with i.v. TPA, there was a significantly higher vascular recanalization rate compared to similar controls (81 percent versus 47 percent). When severely hypoperfused tissue in the penumbra zone was analyzed, i.v. TPA-treated patients had a significantly larger portion of this at risk tissue not progress to infarct as compared to controls (82 percent versus 25 percent). Overall, despite similar baseline PWI–DWI scans in patients and controls, there was, on average, significantly less infarct extension in the i.v. TPA group when compared with controls (14 cm^3 versus 56 cm^3). These imaging findings translated into improved clinical outcomes for the i.v. TPA group compared to controls and prompted the authors to conclude that, "The natural evolution of acute perfusion-weighted imaging-diffusion-weighted imaging mismatch tissue may be altered by thrombolysis, with improved stroke outcome" (Parsons *et al.*, 2002).

Nice reviews of some of the various MR studies focusing on the PWI–DWI mismatch hypothesis and illustrating the above points are found in Albers (1999), and Hjort *et al.* (2005). The basic conclusions of these various MRI studies provided a strong rationale to launch major randomized prospective trials to test the hypothesis that in properly selected patients (those with PWI–DWI mismatch on MRI), i.v. thrombolysis would be safe and beneficial when used in the 3–6-hour time window, or even beyond.

The attempt to expand the i.v. thrombolysis time window is actually quite rational. In the mid 1990s, when the ECASS I, ECASS II and ATLANTIS studies failed to demonstrate the efficacy of i.v. TPA in the 3–6-hour time window, it was thought that treatment beyond 3 hours was not only futile but probably contra-indicated, as discussed previously.

Once again, however, a closer look at the data, particularly the ECASS data, shows that there might be some flexibility to expand the i.v. TPA time window, even among patients selected using only non-contrast CT. This is an important exercise if, for nothing else, to ingrain the notion that a critical reading of scientific data – rather than a cursory acceptance of conclusions – is a must for those in academics. Two issues regarding ECASS I deserve closer scrutiny. First, as you may recall, among the 620 patients randomized in ECASS I, there were 109 "protocol violations," i.e., patients who were wrongly included in the study. A large portion of these patients had subtle CT findings of large infarcts greater than 1/3 of the MCA territory, but these findings were missed on the initial review, and these patients, who should have been excluded by the study's criteria, were instead mistakenly randomized. As discussed previously, this group of patients had exceptionally poor outcomes, with high intracranial bleed rates and a mortality rate close to 50 percent. If the statistical analysis of the ECASS data is repeated excluding this patient group, it turns out that there is a statisitical significant benefit of i.v. TPA out to 6 hours in one of the two primary endpoints of the study, although not in the other (Meschia *et al.*, 2002). This brings up the second subtle issue with the ECASS I study – the issue of outcome measures. This is a topic which most people do not bother with when quoting study conclusions. ECASS I used two primary outcome measures: a difference in the Barthel Index of 15 points and a difference in the modified Rankin Score of 1 in the treated patients versus the control patients at 90 days. Using these outcome measures, the study could not demonstrate a statistically significant difference in favor of i.v. TPA, and that is why it is considered a negative study. These outcome measures are different than the global end-point analysis used in the NINDS study to demonstrate the efficacy of i.v. TPA. When the ECASS I data is subjected instead to the statistical methodology used in NINDS, it turns out that there is a statistically significant benefit to i.v. TPA in the 0–6-hour time window. The authors of that particular study thus concluded that: "Using the global end-point analysis, ECASS is positive in the intention-to-treat analysis. This may indicate that the time window for thrombolysis may be as long as 6 hours" (Hacke *et al.*, 1998b).

Even without this statistical massaging, a recent meta-analysis study pooling all the data from the NINDS, ECASS and ATLANTIS trials found that the benefit of i.v. TPA may extend beyond the 3-hour time window out to 4.5 hours (Hacke *et al.*, 2004).

Therefore, the initially rigid 3-hour cutoff seems to have some flexibility even when plain old non-contrast CT is used for patient selection. Thus, it is quite rational to try to expand the i.v. TPA treatment window beyond 3 hours when aided by the refined patient selection criteria afforded by MRI and the PWI–DWI mismatch hypothesis. Thus, three major randomized prospective trials were launched specifically testing whether i.v. thrombolysis would be clinically beneficial beyond 3 hours in patients with PWI–DWI mismatch. This is especially pertinent in view of the positive results obtained by Parsons *et al.* (2002) (quoted above). In that study, there was overall no demonstrable benefit to i.v. TPA compared to controls within a 6-hour time window. However, in the subgroup of treated patients and controls with PWI–DWI mismatch, there was a significantly larger area of penumbral salvage (severely hypoperfused tissue not progressing to infarction), decreased infarct growth and final infarct size, as well as improved clinical outcome for those treated with i.v. TPA. This suggests that the PWI–DWI mismatch selection criterion may be what is required to demonstrate clinical benefit of i.v. TPA beyond the 3-hour time window.

This hypothesis has been very recently tested with a randomized prospective study known as the DIAS trial, which stands for Desmoteplase in Acute Ischemic Stroke. This important study used desmoteplase, a new thrombolytic, instead of TPA. Desmoteplase is a new fibrinolytic drug originally isolated from vampire bats (it's now made with recombinant techniques). It is a highly fibrin-specific plasminogen activator with a long half-life. In the DIAS trial, patients were selected for randomization based on PWI–DWI mismatch. The treatment time window was 3–9 hours after stroke onset, representing a significant expansion of the time window. In part I of the DIAS trial, fixed doses of desmoteplase were administered, and this part was terminated due to a high rate of symptomatic intracranial bleeds (27 percent). Part II used several weight-adjusted dose regimens. This produced significantly lower intracranial bleed rates (2.2 percent overall). For the high dose regimen of 125 µg/kg, there was a significantly higher reperfusion rate for the treatment group – 71 percent versus 19 percent for placebo. Favorable 90-day outcomes were found in 60 percent of the high dose treatment group versus 22 percent of the placebo group. Good outcome was strongly related to reperfusion, with good outcomes occurring in 52 percent of patients experiencing reperfusion by MR versus 25 percent in patients without reperfusion (Hacke *et al.*, 2005). The DIAS investigators concluded, "Intravenous desmoteplase administered 3 to 9 hours after acute ischemic stroke in patients selected with perfusion/diffusion mismatch is associated with a higher rate of reperfusion and better clinical outcome compared with placebo. The sICH [symptomatic intracranial hemorrhage] rate with desmoteplase was low, using doses up to 125 µg/kg."

A subsequent very similar placebo-controlled double-blind randomized trial, known as the DEDAS trial, once again evaluated i.v. desmoteplase for treatment of acute stroke in the 3–9 hour time window using doses of 90 µg/kg and 125 µg/kg (Furlan *et al.*, 2006). The results of this trial were similar to DIAS. Reperfusion was achieved in 53 percent of the 125µg/kg desmoteplase versus 37.5 percent in the placebo group. Good clinical outcomes at 90 days, concomitantly, were more common in the high dose treatment group (60 percent versus 25 percent for the placebo group).

With these very recently published trials, it seems that we are at the dawn of a new era of a significantly expanded treatment time window for i.v. thrombolytics, using the MRI PWI–DWI mismatch model as well as the new thrombolytic desmoteplase. Expansion of the time window based on PWI–DWI mismatch seems a conceptually valid model in and of itself, though, independent of what may be a better thrombolytic efficacy of desmoteplase. A recent important study has recently established the validity of the PWI–DWI mismatch criterion for i.v. TPA as well, out to 6 hours (Thomalla *et al.*, 2006). This multicenter study from Germany was conducted with an interesting design. A total of 174 patients were treated with i.v. TPA. Those who came in within 3 hours were treated according to the ECASS II protocol. Those who came in within 3 to 6 hours were treated based on the MRI finding of PWI–DWI mismatch. These data were then compared to both the pooled placebo and pooled i.v. TPA treatment data from the ATLANTIS, ECASS, and NINDS trials. A favorable clinical outcome was more frequent in the MRI-selected patients (48 percent) compared with both the placebo group (33 percent) and the pooled i.v. TPA group (40 percent). Also, the patients selected on the basis of PWI–DWI mismatch showed significantly lower symptomatic intracranial bleed rates than the pooled i.v. TPA group (3 percent versus 8 percent). This low bleed rate was, in fact, comparable to that of 2 percent in the pooled placebo group. The authors concluded that, "This study supports the notion that it is safe and effective to expand the time window for i.v.-TPA up to 6 hours in patients with tissue at risk as defined by MRI." Thus, there seems to be serious validity for the PWI–DWI mismatch model, and it will likely be central in the coming decade's setting of thrombolysis protocols with expanded time windows.

Before leaving this section, we need to explore one additional subtlety regarding the PWI–DWI mismatch model which is seldom discussed in the literature. The way the model is usually phrased, therapy is concerned with salvaging the at risk brain in the penumbra zone so that the DWI abnormality does not expand. This should stop infarcts from growing and patients from getting worse. Thus, thrombolysis makes patients better than they otherwise would have been. Treatment versus placebo trials would then show a significant benefit in favor of thrombolysis. However, what we truly want from therapy in the acute stroke setting is to make the patient better than they are (improve the current neurologic deficit) not better than they otherwise would be (i.e., by saving the penumbra zone from infarcting). The penumbra model, as typically discussed, does not easily describe how we achieve clinical improvement, but rather how we stave off clinical deterioration. This paradox is our first indication that as useful as the PWI–DWI mismatch model is, it needs to be revised. One answer to our dilemma is to look more closely at the correlation between the PWI–DWI examination and the stroke patient. The typical patient presents with a set of clinical deficits (measured by the NIHSS, for example) and a PWI–DWI mismatch. It turns out the degree of clinical deficit at initial presentation is correlated much more closely to the size of the PWI lesion (appropriately defined) than the DWI lesion. Significantly hypoperfused brain, whether or not it is DWI positive, is dysfunctional brain which reflects in the patient's clinical deficits. We have already seen that thrombolysis reverses the perfusion deficit in a majority of cases, and this is the way in which it leads to clinical improvement – at least as much improvement as the size of the DWI lesion will allow. This is because, while the PWI lesion correlates closely to the patient's initial condition, the DWI lesion correlates closely with the final infarct volume as seen on T2-weighted images (Fig. 8.31).

Refining the PWI–DWI mismatch model: DWI reversibility and infarct threshold analysis

The PWI–DWI mismatch model, especially coupled with desmoteplase therapy, is strongly pointing to the conclusion that patients with a mismatch may benefit from i.v. thrombolysis as far out as 9 hours from stroke onset. By implication, it seems that those with a matched defect should not be treated. In those cases, the hypoperfused brain is already DWI positive – the brain is dead, the horse has left the barn, it is too late to do anything. Once again, though, we must not automatically trust implications. The underlying assumption here is that the DWI-positive region represents the irreversibly damaged infarct core. This assumption was taken as fact in many of the early papers on the PWI–DWI mismatch hypothesis.

Under careful scrutiny, however, we see that such an assumption is not theoretically valid – or at least not always valid. The brain suffers irreversible ischemic damage quickly when it is subjected to markedly diminished cerebral blood flow in the range of 8–10 ml/100 g per min (as compared to

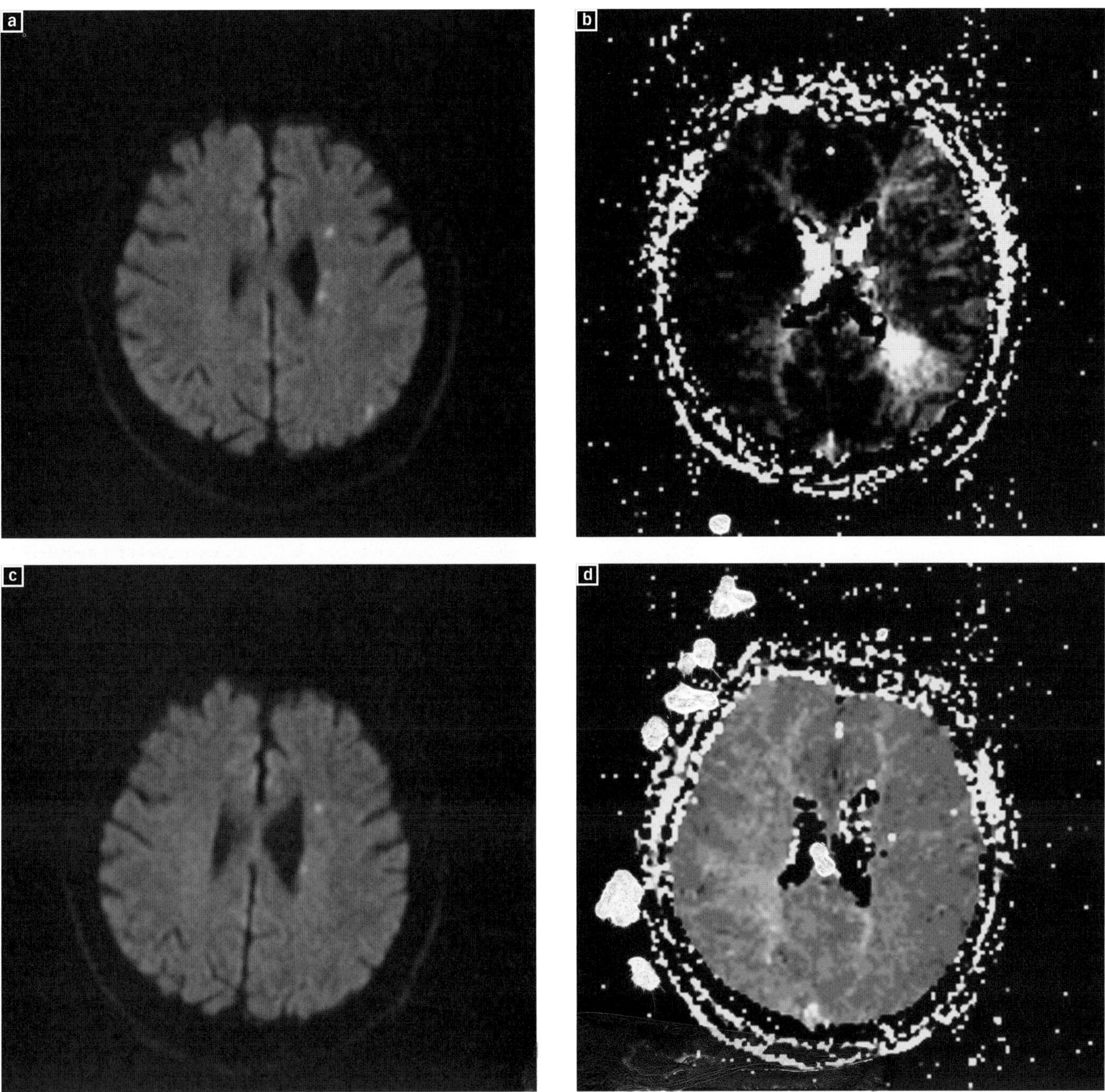

Fig. 8.31. **Patient presents with clinical picture consistent with an acute large left MCA stroke. (a) Initial DWI shows only small foci of hyperintensity in the deep white matter and watershed zones. (b) Poor quality PWI imaging reveals a large area of perfusion deficit in the MCA territory and a significant PWI–DWI mismatch. After i.v. TPA therapy, there was resolution of clinical deficits. (c) Repeat imaging at 24 hours post-presentation reveals only minimal residual DWI abnormality and (d) a resolution of the perfusion deficit on PWI.**

normal cortical CBF, which is in the range of 50–60 ml/100 g per min). Neuronal electrical dysfunction occurs at a CBF rate of about 20 ml/100g per min, and this value of CBF is often quoted as equating to the penumbra zone. Somewhere between these two thresholds, there is failure of the electrolyte pumps, such as the Na–K pump, with resultant development of cytotoxic edema. It is at this point that the scan turns DWI positive. Below this point but above the 8–10 ml/100 g per min

value where the irreversible cell-death cascade initiates, there should be a zone of DWI-positive tissue which can be salvaged if quickly reperfused. Thus, the DWI-positive zone should no longer be considered the infarct core, but should rather be considered to have two compartments:

(1) A central infarct core of irreversibly damaged tissue
(2) A peripheral zone of severely hypoperfused but potentially salvageable cells with electrolyte pump dysfunction.

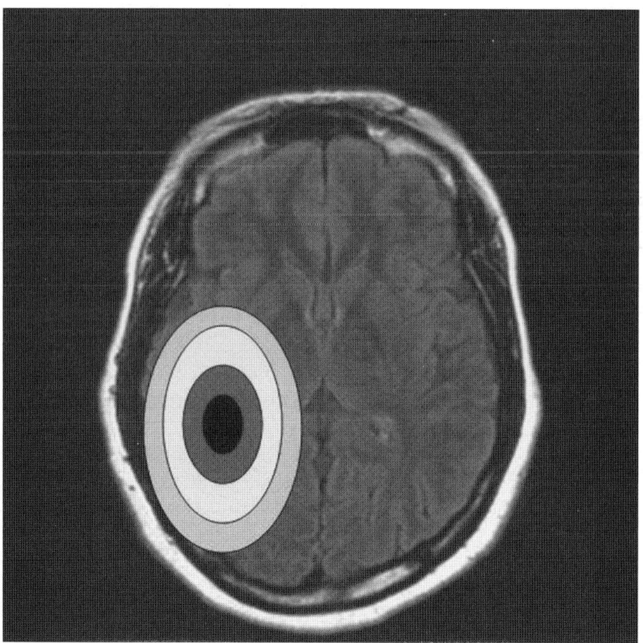

Fig. 8.32. **Refined PWI–DWI four-compartment model. The inner two compartments (regions 1 and 2) together are the DWI lesion. The outer two compartments (regions 3 and 4) together are the PWI lesion outside the DWI-positive area. The innermost region (region 1) is the infarct core, with irreversibly damaged tissue. Region 2 is the DWI-positive but potentially viable tissue. Region 3 is the zone of severely hypoperfused tissue at significant risk for infarction; this is not DWI positive. The outermost region (region 4) is the oligemic tissue not at serious risk for infarction. The penumbra zone now consists of regions 2 and 3.**

Also, the PWI positive zone beyond the DWI lesion should be considered to have two compartments:

(1) A zone of significant hypoperfusion, or true penumbra, corresponding to CBF values of about 20 ml/100 gm per min.
(2) A zone of less severe oligemia where tissue is hypoperfused, but not at serious risk for infarction. It is because of this zone that a number of studies have found that visually demarcated PWI lesions tend to over-estimate final infarct volume (Shih *et al.*, 2003).

If this refined theoretical model (Fig. 8.32) is correct, then with thrombolysis and reperfusion, at least some DWI abnormalities (the DWI-positive tissue outside the core infarct zone) should be reversible. This yields another empirically testable assumption.

Several papers have, in fact, already documented this reversibility of DWI abnormalities with thrombolysis. Probably the first series to report this phenomenon is a pilot study of intra-arterial thrombolysis out of UCLA (Kidwell *et al.*, 2000). In this paper, six out of seven patients showed some reduction in the size of the DWI-positive region with thrombolysis. Initial PWI imaging was obtained in five of the seven cases, and revealed an average PWI–DWI mismatch of 79 percent by size. In four of these cases, there was complete reversal of the perfusion deficits post thrombolysis. A later publication by Kidwell *et al.* (2002a) examining 18 cases of intra-arterial thrombolysis

showed reversal of DWI abnormalities in 8 of the 18 (44 percent). The implications of this DWI reversal are uncertain, as five of the eight patients who showed early reversal of DWI lesions had delayed recurrence of DWI abnormalities, postulated to be secondary to reperfusion injury. Three of the 18 patients, however, had sustained DWI reversal.

Similar DWI reversibility data has been presented for i.v. thrombolysis. Chalela *et al.* (2004) reported partial or complete reversal of DWI abnormalities in 33 percent of patients treated with i.v. TPA.

These results raise the significant question as to whether or not to treat patients with matched PWI–DWI defects. Knowing that the DWI abnormality contains both a core infarct zone as well as a component of the penumbra zone, and that some DWI abnormalities are reversible with treatment, it would make sense that at least some patients with matched defects may reverse with treatment (Fig. 8.33).

At present, there is no randomized trial which gives results as to how such patients – without a PWI–DWI mismatch – would do with thrombolysis versus no treatment. The policy at UCLA, given the current status of the data, is that "cases without mismatch are currently not excluded from endovascular therapy at UCLA" (Liebeskind *et al.*, 2005).

While quite a reasonable stance, this certainly raises the bothersome question as to the value of MRI. Certainly, it gives us significantly more information than non-contrast CT, but if we are going to treat both those with and those without a PWI–DWI mismatch, then what have we achieved with all of the extra information? These are the sorts of questions with which stroke therapy policy will have to grapple in the next decade. In the opinion of the author, those with a PWI–DWI mismatch will be candidates for therapy with an expanded time window, and that further analysis, on a case-by-case basis, will be required for those without a mismatch. One arm of the analysis would determine whether such patients are likely to improve spontaneously, and hence not need thrombolysis. These would be patients without a significant perfusion deficit, such as those with DWI lesions significantly larger than PWI lesions or those with only DWI lesions. This approach is already beginning to take some hold, as the DIAS study, for example, excluded patients with a PWI defect less than 2 cm, since they have probably already spontaneously recanalized.

The second, and more difficult, limb of the analysis are those patients who have matched PWI–DWI lesions with a significant PWI defect. Should all of these patients be treated? Should some of them be excluded, since surely a portion must have completed infarcts without a significant penumbra zone? There is, at present, no consensus on how to triage such patients. One fairly straightforward criterion is that used by the Department of Neurology in Heidelberg, Germany (Hjort *et al.*, 2005). Such patients are treated out to 9 hours if they do not have hyperintensity on FLAIR and T2, as this is taken to indicate completed infarction.

Another approach just beginning to take shape is that of "threshold analysis." Thus far, all of the determinations made by MRI have been qualitative, i.e., done by eyeball. However, it

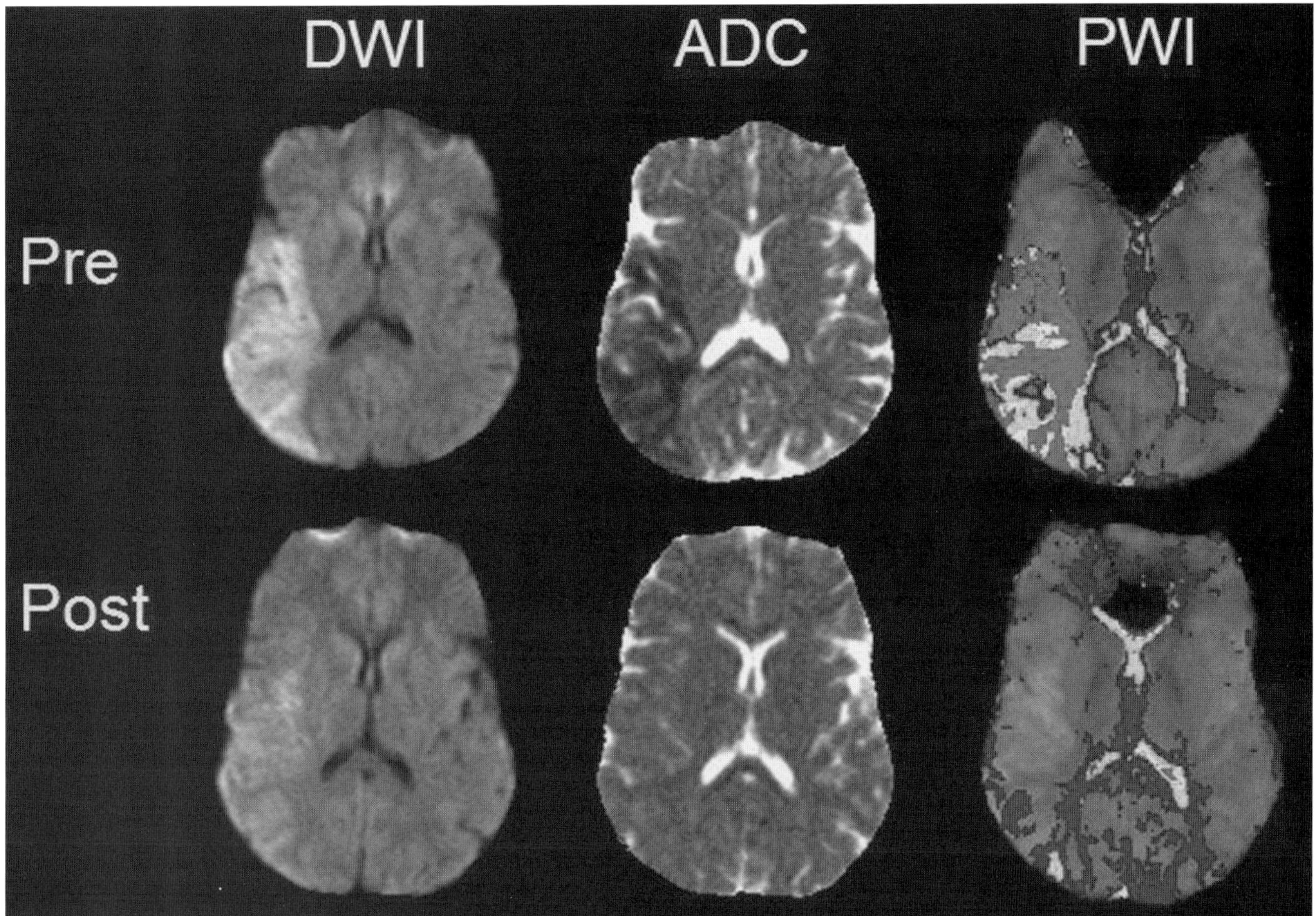

Fig. 8.33. **Pre- and post-thrombolysis images of a patient with right MCA infarct. The pre-treatment images show a matched DWI–PWI defect. Post-treatment, both the PWI and the DWI abnormalities have resolved. (Image courtesy of Dr. Michael Waters, Director of the Stroke Progam, Cedars-Sinai Medical Center, Los Angeles, CA.) See plate section for color image.**

may in the future be possible to use quantitative analysis to determine which tissue is unsalvageable and destined to infarct. Patients with a matched PWI–DWI defect can be analyzed in this fashion. If their tissue is above the infarction threshold (i.e., unsalvageable), they would not be treated; otherwise, they would. The hyperintensity on FLAIR criterion used by the Heidelberg group represents one such infarct threshold.

Various recent papers have looked at quantitative analyisis of both CBF values and ADC values to try to distinguish infarct core, penumbra that progresses to infarct, and penumbra that remains viable. Since MRI has difficulties quantitating CBF, a ratio measure to contralateral brain is used. Various studies have found that, for the infarct core, CBF ratios range from 0.12 to 0.44, for penumbra that progresses to infarction from 0.35 to 0.56 and for penumbra that remains viable, 0.58 to 0.78 (these data and the appropriate citations can be found in Schafer et al., 2005). Application of such threshold values, in general, requires more sophisticated analysis of the PWI studies than just the standard TTP or MTT maps used in most centers, and needs CBF maps. Recall that the higher the MTT, the worse the

perfusion. Some papers have found no statistically significant difference in MTT ratios between infarct core, penumbra that progresses to infarct, and penumbra that remains viable. Other papers, though, have demonstrated differences between all three regions. Reported MTT ratios to contralateral brain range form 1.7 to 2.53 in infarct core, 1.74 to 2.19 in penumbra that progresses to infarct, and are about 1.65 in penumbra that remains viable (this data and the appropriate citations can be found in Schafer et al., 2005).

Some papers have also attempted looking at CBV as a threshold parameter. However, because of an initial compensatory increase in CBV with decreased CBF (as the brain capillary beds maximally dilate), establishing CBV thresholds is much harder. Tissue with significant decreases in CBV is highly likely to infarct, as this indicates that the capillary beds have now collapsed in the face of severe hypoperfusion. However, tissue with normal or elevated CBV ratios is not safe from infarction.

The absolute value of the ADC, as well as ADC ratios, may be more promising parameters. Once again, though, there are mixed results, with some reports showing significantly different values in the three regions of interest, while other studies report no statistically significant difference. One large study that measured absolute ADC values found a value of 661×10^{-6} mm²/s for infarct core and 782×10^{-6} mm²/s and 823×10^{-6} mm²/s for penumbra that progresses to infarct and penumbra that remains viable, respectively (Oppenheim *et al.*,

2001). Others have used an ADC ratio compared to contralateral brain as a threshold parameter, and have found values of about 0.62–0.63 for infarct core, 0.89–0.9 for penumbra that progresses to infarct, and 0.93–0.96 for penumbra that remains viable (see Schaefer *et al.* 2003, and Rohl *et al.* 2001).

In all probability, any serious threshold analysis will probably require a multi-parameter mathematical model

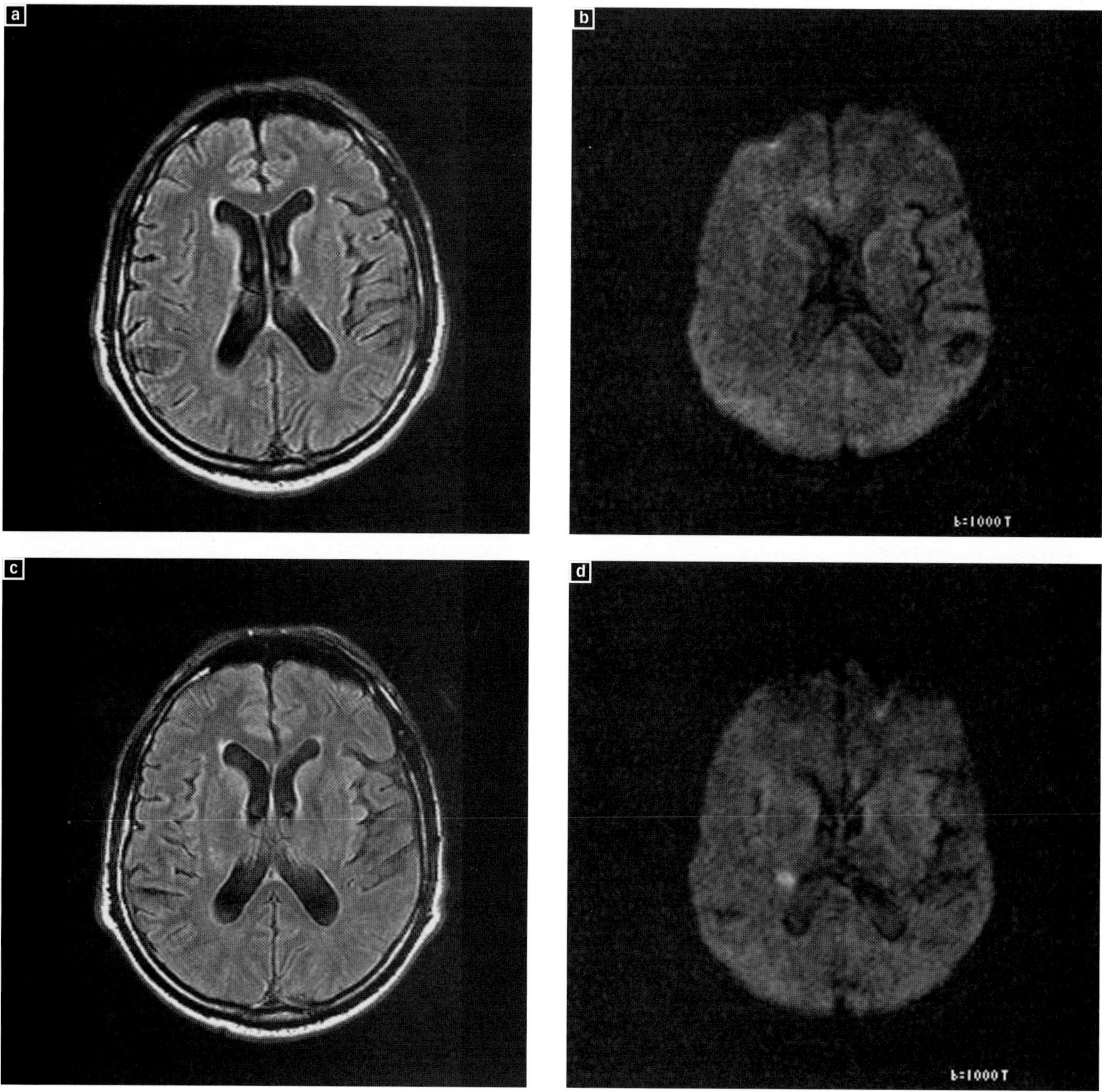

Fig. 8.34 a–f. **Patient presented with left-sided weakness. (a), (b) The initial FLAIR and DWI images obtained at just over 24 hours after ictus are negative. (c), (d) At 48 hours, there is an early infarct evident on DWI with minimal associated FLAIR hyperintensity in the right posterior corona radiata. (e), (f) At 4 days, FLAIR and DWI images now show a more prominent completed right posterior corona radiata infarct involving the descending right corticospinal tract.**

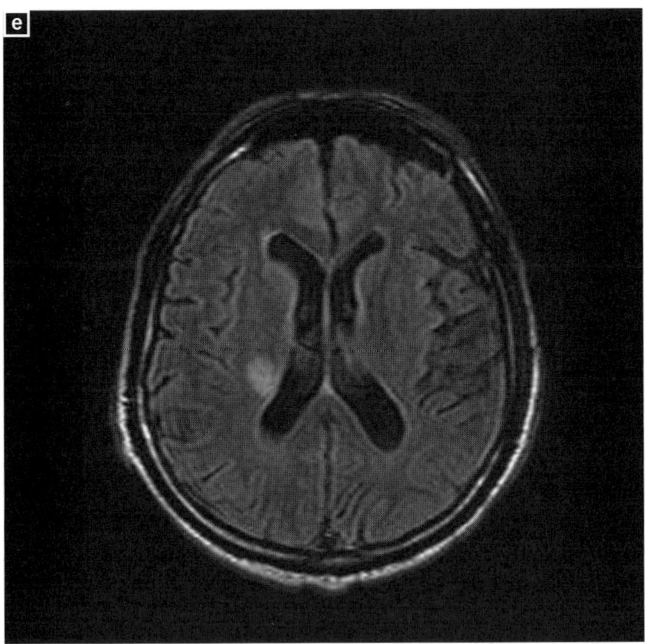

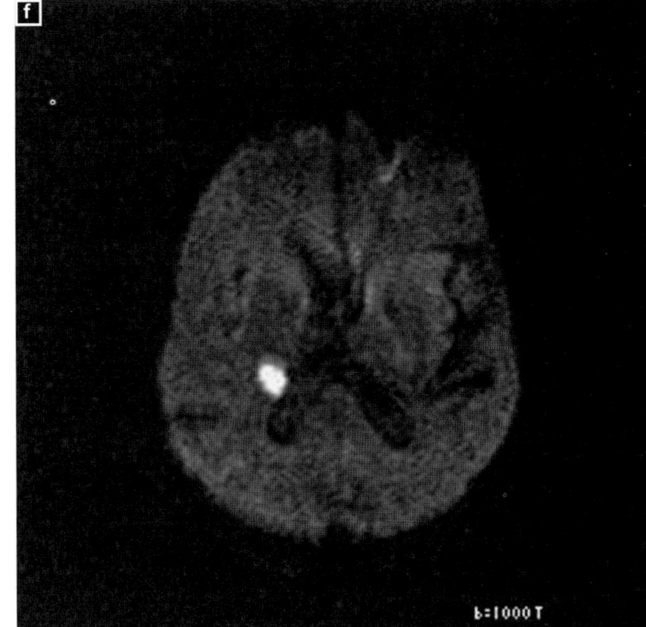

Fig. 8.34. **(cont.)**

incorporating such things as CBF and ADC values to predict the likelihood of infarction. Of course, this sort of research is still in its early stages, and we are some distance yet from a national standard. At this point, each institution needs to establish a stroke treatment policy which takes into account the newest results that allow expansion of the thrombolysis time window, with reasonable inclusion and exclusion criteria, based, as much as possible, on the rapidly evolving results in the literature, such as those we have presented above.

To be concrete, we suggest that a future algorithm might look something like this:

(1) At 0–3 hours, CT and CTA or MRI (including PWI, DWI, and GRE) and MRA are obtained to exclude bleed and assess for proximal vessel occlusion. If there is a bleed, the patient is not a thrombolysis candidate. If there is proximal vessel occlusion, the patient is triaged to intra-arterial therapy, such as thrombolysis or clot retrieval. Otherwise, the patient is triaged to i.v. thrombolysis. However, if there is no significant perfusion deficit, then the patient has probably already recanalized, and the risks of thrombolysis are not warranted. This novel approach of excluding those without a significant perfusion deficit is already in use at the University Hospital, Hamburg-Ependorf, Germany (Hjort *et al.*, 2005).

(2) At 3–6 or 3–9 hours, assess with PWI–DWI MRI for mismatch and MRA for proximal vessel occlusion. If there is significant PWI–DWI mismatch, triage to i.v. or intra-arterial thrombolysis depending on the presence or absence of large vessel proximal occlusion. If there is a matched PWI–DWI defect with a significant PWI component, assess patient using threshold analysis. If there is significant viable penumbra, triage patient to i.v. or intra-arterial

thrombolysis as above. Otherwise, no treatment offered. If there is no significant PWI defect, then no treatment is offered, as the patient has probably spontaneously recanalized, and there is no perfusion deficit to correct.

It must be stressed that this is only a form of what a future algorithm might look like. Before we reach this stage, there are numerous fundamental methodological issues which must be addressed and resolved. Among these are the following:

(1) The sensitivity of DWI MRI in the detection of stroke must be reassessed. If a patient presents with clinical evidence of stroke, but is not DWI positive, should this patient be treated? Some studies have shown a sensitivity of 100 percent for DWI in the acute stroke setting, as indicated above (Gonzalez *et al.*, 1999). The sensitivity, of course, is less than 100 percent, and there are false negative DWI cases even out to 24 hours (Fig. 8.34).

This false-negative phenomenon is particularly true for brainstem strokes. One interesting study is from the Hospitalier Pitié-Salpêtrière in Paris, France (Oppenheim *et al.*, 2000). This paper reviewed initial and delayed MRI images obtained in patients with stroke symptoms lasting more than 24 hours. It concluded that within the first 24 hours, there is a 5.8 percent false-negative rate for DWI overall. In the anterior circulation, the false negative rate was only 2 percent. For posterior circulation stroke, however, the false-negative rate was 19 percent. Shockingly, "31 percent of patients with vertebrobasilar ischemic stroke had a false-negative initial DWI study during the first 24 hours."

(2) If MRI is to be the initial screening modality for stroke therapy, its sensitivity in the detection of acute intracranial hemorrhage must be elucidated. Certainly, GRE sequences are exquisitely sensitive in detecting subacute

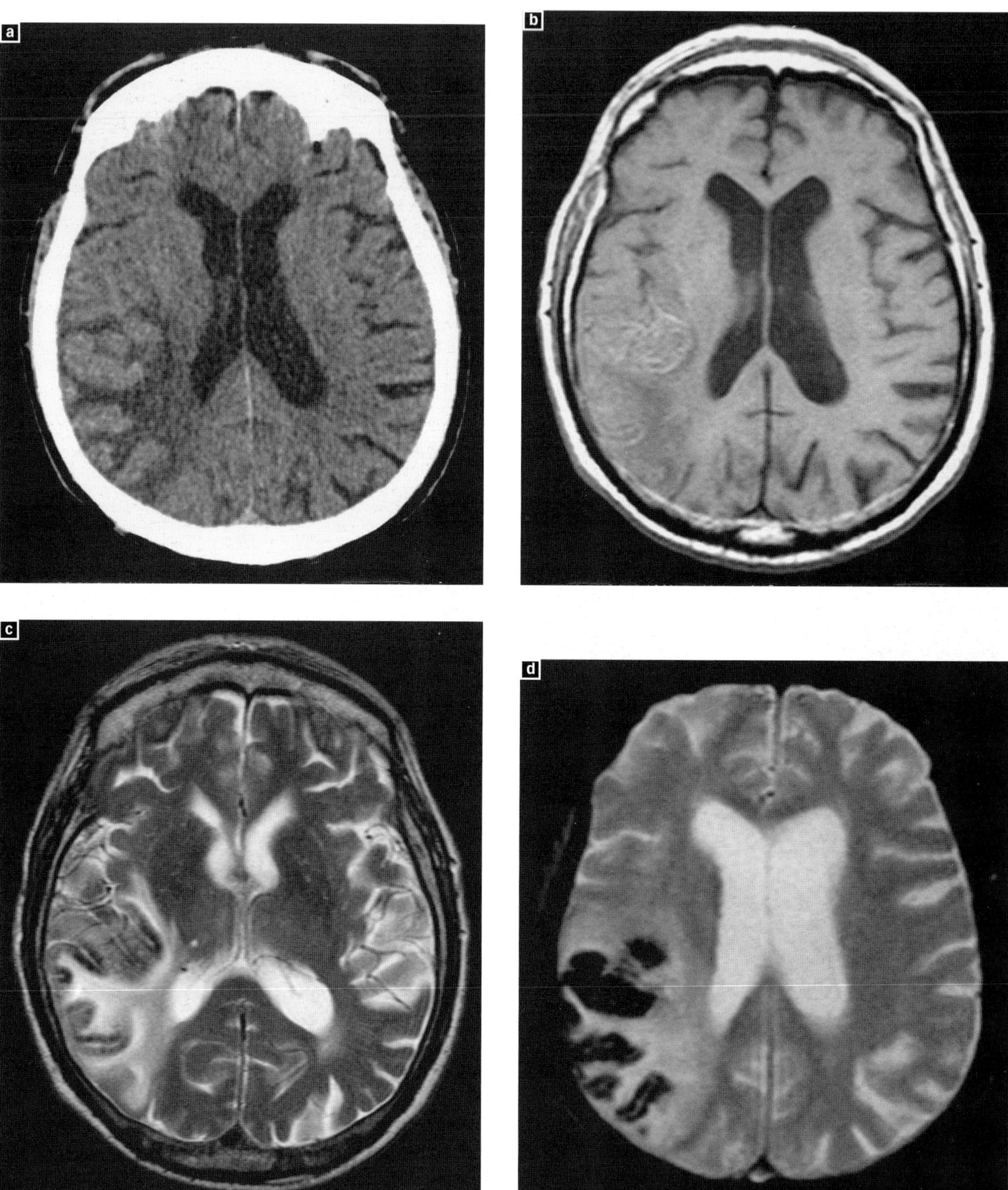

Fig. 8.35. **Subacute right MCA infarct. (a) CT shows swollen, minimally hyperdense gyri without frank hemorrhagic transformation. There is minimal (b) gyriform T1 hyperintensity and (c) T2 hypointensity suggesting minimal blood-breakdown products. (d) GRE imaging shows prominent hemorrhagic transformation in the infarct zone.**

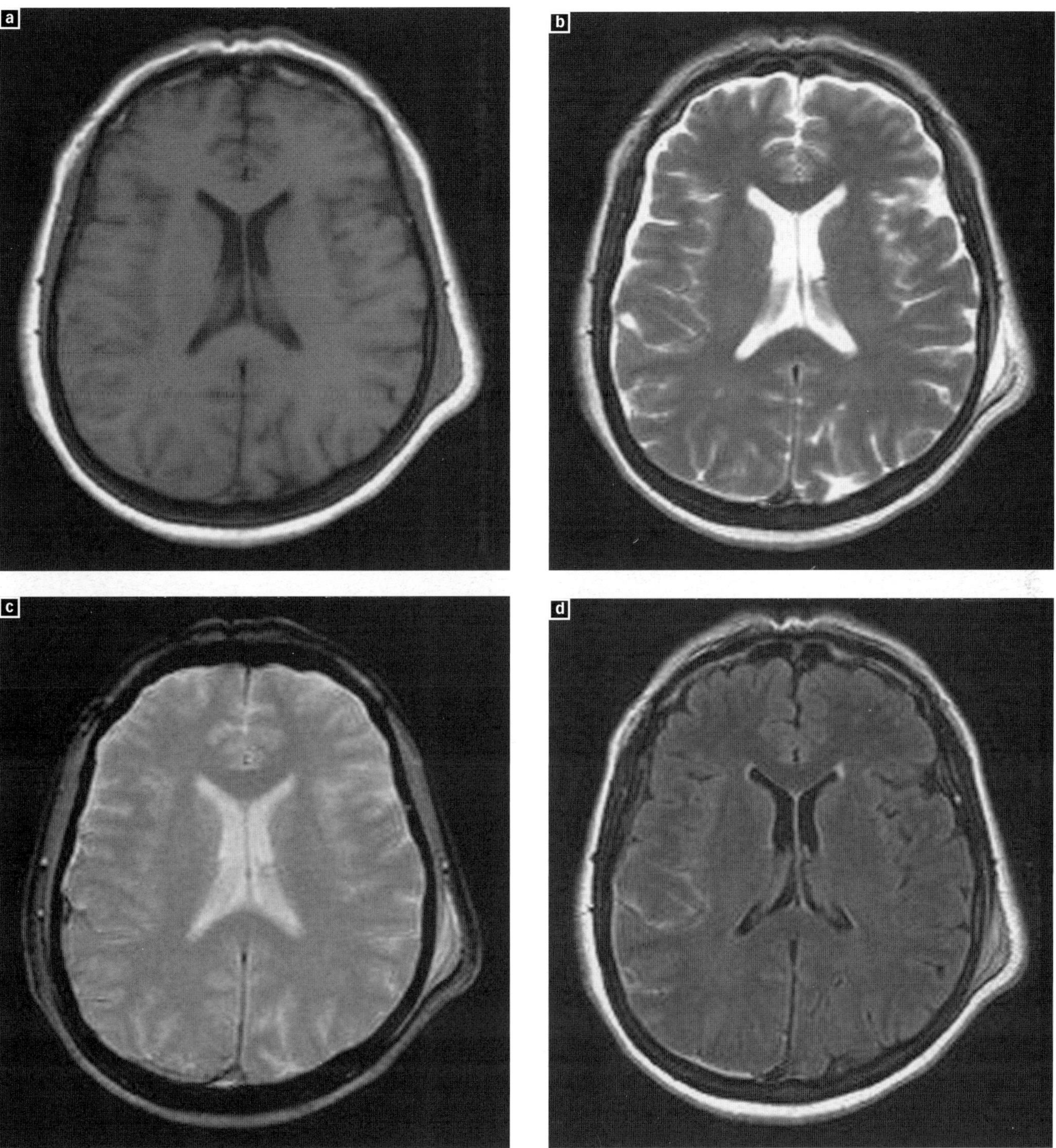

Fig. 8.36. **(a)** T1, **(b)** T2, **(c)** GRE T2, and **(d)** FLAIR images in a patient with an acute post-traumatic right temporo-parietal subarachnoid bleed (and a very small subdural bleed). Note that the subarachnoid hemorrhage is visible only on the FLAIR sequence, and is not detectable on GRE.

parenchymal hemorrhage and are superior to CT in detecting very early hemorrhagic transformation in an infarct (Fig. 8.35).

A study known as the HEME study was conducted at UCLA and the NIH Stroke Center at Suburban Hospital, evaluating whether GRE MRI could detect acute cerebral hemorrhage as well as CT. The conclusion of the study was positive, stating that, "MRI may be as accurate as CT for the detection of acute hemorrhage in patients presenting with acute focal stroke symptoms and is more sensitive than CT

for the detection of chromic intracerebral hemorrhage."
(Kidwell *et al.*, 2004). Another concurrent study supported
the use of MR as the sole imaging modality in the screening
of acute stroke patients (Fiebach *et al.*, 2004). This study
concluded: "Hyperacute ICH [intracranial hemorrhage] causes
a characteristic imaging pattern on stroke MRI and is
detectable with excellent accuracy … Stroke MRI alone
can rule out ICH and demonstrate the underlying pathology in hyperacute stroke."

One issue not sufficiently discussed in this vein, in the
author's opinion, is that of subarachnoid hemorrhage.
Contrary to popular belief, GRE MRI cannot rule out subarachnoid bleed (Fig. 8.36). This is a critical point often
misunderstood by residents. Subarachnoid blood is in the
oxyhemoglobin phase, and hence has no susceptibility
effects. FLAIR images show excellent sensitivity when the
subarachnoid bleed extends beyond the basal cisterns,
because the proteinaceous fluid replaces CSF in the cisterns
and sulci. However, FLAIR takes a long time to acquire, and is
sometimes not included in the acute stroke MRI protocol.

Another issue raised by MRI evaluation is that of the significance of microbleeds found on GRE MRI (Fig. 8.37). These
microbleed foci have been reported in 6 percent of healthy
adults and in 12 percent of patients presenting with stroke.
Are they a contra-indication for stroke thrombolysis? The
answer is currently unclear, and will require further
research. For further reading, refer to Kidwell *et al.*, 2002b.

(3) If the presence or absence of a PWI–DWI mismatch is to be
used as an inclusion–exclusion criterion for thrombolysis,
some decision needs to be made regarding which PWI
parameter will be used to assess the perfusion deficit.

Depending on the parameter, there can be significant differences in the degree of PWI–DWI mismatch. For example, using MTT or T_{max}, hypoperfusion regions are
significantly smaller than those obtained when using TTP.
Also, setting some sort of threshold value for hypoperfusion –
such as that the MTT or TTP needs to be at least 4 seconds

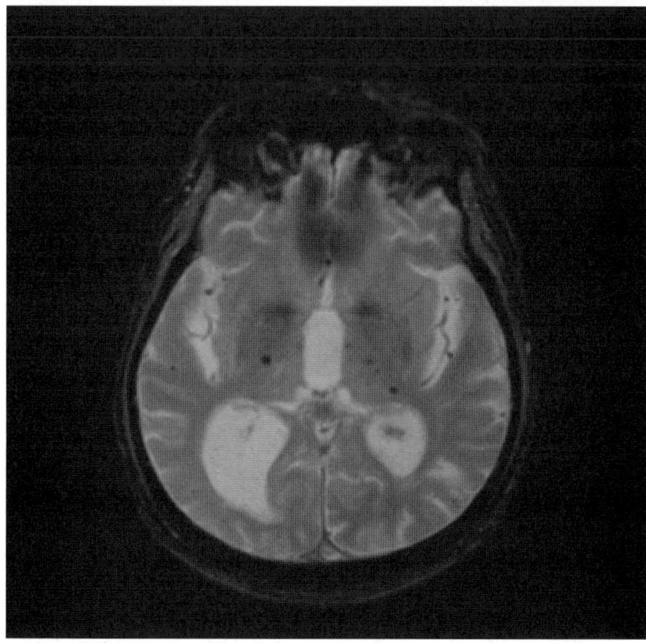

Fig. 8.37. **GRE axial images show multiple punctuate foci of hypointensity consistent with microbleeds.**

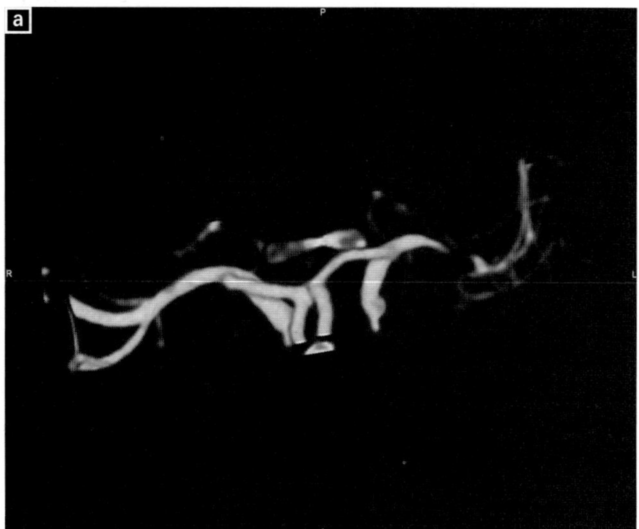

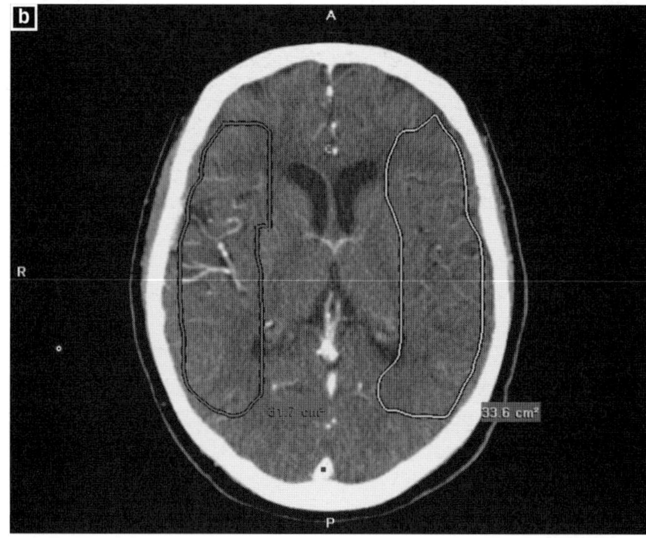

Fig. 8.38. **CT perfusion study in a patient with recurrent TIAs, but without acute infarct. (a) CT angiogram shows a high grade focal stenosis in the left horizontal MCA. (b) Raw CT perfusion data image shows less contrast enhancement in the left MCA territory. (c) MTT image shows a clearly prolonged MTT in the left MCA territory consistent with hypoperfusion. CT can also provide direct quantitation for specified regions of interest. (d) Quantitative MTT estimates show an MTT of 2.9 seconds on the right, and a markedly prolonged MTT of 6.5 seconds on the left. (e) Quantitative CBF mapping shows a normal CBF of 64 ml/100 g per min on the right, and a significant reduction to 29 ml/100 g per min on the left. (f) The quantitative CBV map shows a value of 2.1 ml/100 g on the right and 2.8 ml/100 g on the left, reflecting the known compensatory increase in CBV in the face of hypoperfusion. See plate section for color images.**

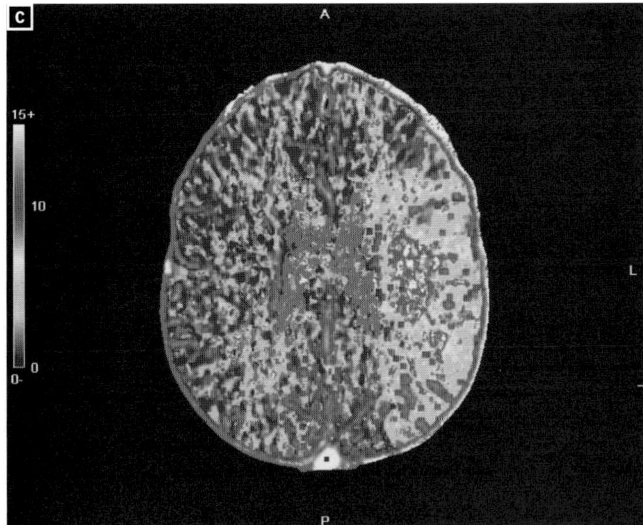
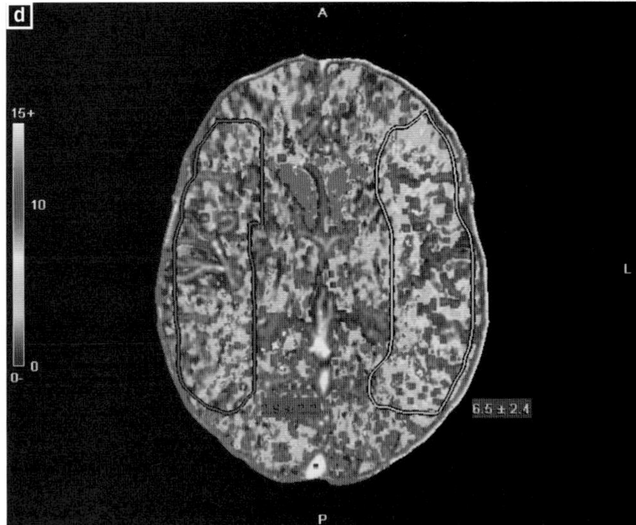
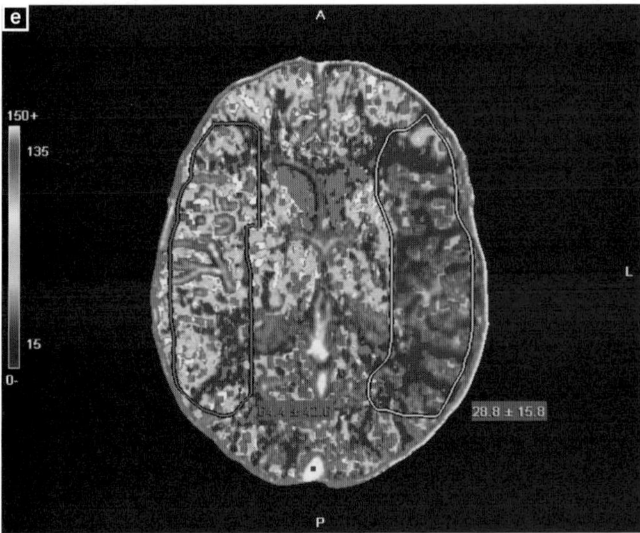
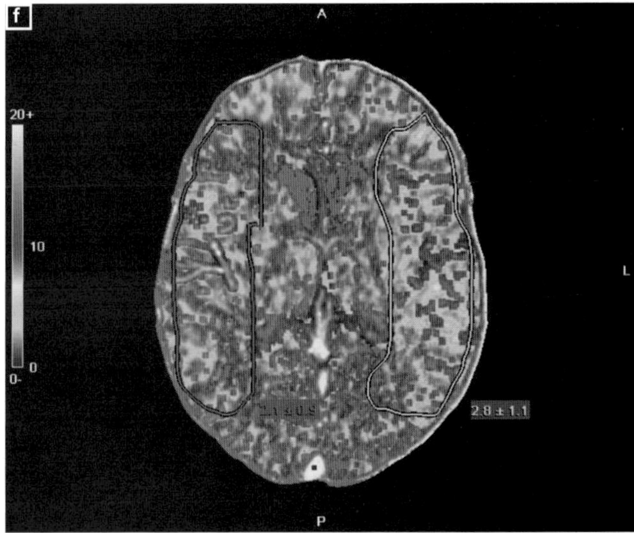

Fig. 8.38 **(cont.)**

longer than the contralateral side – significantly lessens the frequency of PWI–DWI mismatch (Butcher *et al.*, 2005). However, the precise definition here may not really be critical, as studies such as DIAS and DEDFAS have shown that an eyeball estimate of PWI–DWI mismatch may be sufficient. Such issues, though, will become more critical in threshold analysis.

(4) The role of advanced CT needs to be elucidated. We have spent most of the chapter on the role of advanced MRI. However, advanced CT, which includes perfusion imaging, also has the capacity to offer significant information about cerebral perfusion. Instead of PWI–DWI mismatches, investigators have looked at such things as CBV–CBF mismatches. CT has a definite advantage over MRI in that it can be more quantitative regarding the absolute levels of cerebral perfusion (Fig. 8.38).

Once these methodological issues are sorted out, we will hopefully be in a new and moe efficacious era of stroke thrombolysis.

Before ending this long journey through stroke diagnosis and treatment, we stress that a significant part of imaging, which we have not touched on, has to do with issues of stroke prevention. This is at least as important, and probably more fruitful, than stroke treatment ("an ounce of prevention…", etc.). We will try to remedy this deficit, as well as redeem the case-based structure of this book, by ending this chapter with the following clinical case.

Case 1

69-year-old male presents with 10 minutes of aphasia and right hemiparesis, which spontaneously resolved. On neurological examination, the patient showed no focal weakness, and no evidence of aphasia or dysarthria. There was an audible bruit over the left neck.

(1) *Where do you think the lesion is?*

The description is highly suggestive of a transient ischemic attack in the distribution of the left middle cerebral artery. This suggests possible carotid stenosis, or embolic disease from a cardiac source.

(2) *MRA, followed by conventional angiography, were performed (Fig. 8.39). What are the findings?*

(3) *Discuss the importance of detecting and accurately grading carotid stenosis.*

According to the North American Symptomatic Carotid Endarterectomy Trial (NASCET), symptomatic patients with severe carotid artery stenosis (70–99 percent) derive a clear benefit from elective endarterectomy, resulting in an overall decrease in stroke and mortality risk. Patients in this group have a 9 percent risk of stroke over 2 years after carotid endarterectomy, versus a 26 percent 2-year stroke risk when treated medically, representing a 17 percent absolute risk reduction (North American Symptomatic Carotid Endarterectomy Trial Collaborators, 1991). Recent updated results from the North American Symptomatic Carotid Endarterectomy Trial (NASCET) demonstrate a small but statistically significant improvement in outcome for endarterectomy in symptomatic patients with stenoses in the 50–69 percent range as well, although the guidelines for patient selection for surgery are less clear. In this group, there is overlapping of the confidence intervals of the stroke-free survival curves for the medical versus surgical arms, as well as a higher perioperative complication rate compared to the severe stenosis group. This is in contradistinction to the severe (greater than 70 percent) stenosis group, where there is clear benefit to surgery and no overlap in the confidence intervals of stroke-free survival curves (Barnett *et al.*, 2002). These considerations are profoundly reflected in the NNT numbers (number needed to treat to prevent one stroke): 19 for the moderate (50–69 percent) stenosis group versus 6 for the severe (greater than 70 percent) stenosis group. Meanwhile, the European Carotid Surgery Trial (ECST) study showed a 9.8 percent perioperative complication rate for patients with moderate stenoses, and an overall negative benefit for endarterectomy, and no calculable NNT in this group (Barnett *et al.*, 2002).

In asymptomatic patients, the Asymptomatic Carotid Atherosclerosis Study (ACAS) trial demonstrated a small stroke risk reduction in patients with a greater than 60 percent stenosis (Executive Committee for the Asymptomatic Carotid Atherosclerosis Study, 1995). However, these results are often viewed with significant skepticism, as the absolute average annual risk reduction in stroke was only 1 percent, yielding a two-year NNT of 83 (it is necessary to operate on 83 patients in order to prevent one additional stroke in 2 years) (Barnett *et al.*,2002). In light of this, our surgeons do not routinely consider asymptomatic endarterectomy until the stenosis approaches approximately 80 percent.

Given the small benefit for mid-range symptomatic stenoses (50–69 percent), as well as the lack of stratification of the ACAS data and the small overall benefit for asymptomatic patients, it is important to accurately delineate carotid stenosis. The gold standard for doing this has been direct carotid angiography.

(4) *Discuss the risks of angiography as well as available non-invasive imaging techniques for delineating the degree of carotid stenosis.*

The risks of carotid angiography are generally estimated to be in the 1 percent range. The ACAS angiographic stroke rate was 1.2 percent. Recent angiographic series report transient neurologic deficit rates of 0.55 to 2.2 percent, and persistent neurologic deficit rates of up to 0.5 percent. However, in atherosclerotic "high risk" patients, the rate of persistent deficit can be as high as 2 percent (Heiserman *et al.*, 1994).

It has been our clinical experience that for a large portion of patients, and depending on the institution, ultrasound alone, or a combination of ultrasound and MRA is regularly utilized in lieu of arteriography before endarterectomy is performed. The accuracy of these studies for surgical decision making is a subject of active debate. In one study (Johnston and Goldstein 2001), the misclassification rate in surgical decision-making was 28 percent for UTZ, 18 percent for MRA, and 7.9 percent for concordance of the two exams.

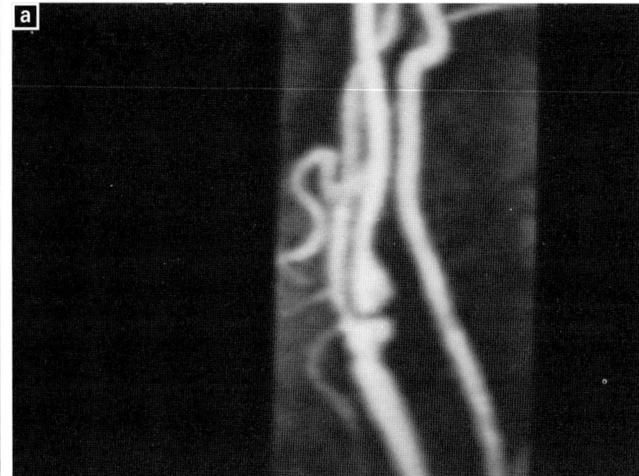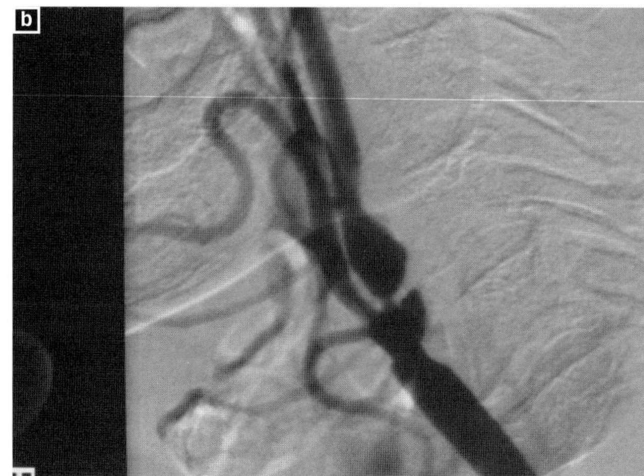

Fig. 8.39. **(b) The conventional angiogram displays a high grade stenosis in the proximal left internal carotid artery. (a) The MRA suggests the same findings, displaying a focal flow gap in the proximal left ICA, consistent with a high grade stenosis.**

An important consideration in analyzing such numbers, however, has to do with the methodology for deciding "misclassifications" by non-invasive tests. In the work of Johnston and Goldstein (2001), for example, the surgical population was defined as symptomatic patients with 50–99 percent stenoses, and asymptomatic patients with 60–99 percent stenoses. As stated earlier, the data on the efficacy of carotid endarterectomy in symptomatic patients with moderate stenoses and in asymptomatic patients in general raise serious concerns whether these are appropriate cutoff points.

CT angiography may be somewhat more accurate than MRA or ultrasound in the detection of surgically significant stenosis. A review of several recent reports showed sensitivities ranging from 82–100 percent, and specificities ranging from 94–100 percent in the detection of surgically relevant stenosis (70–99 percent) (Marks, 1996).

References

Abciximab in Ischemic Stroke Investigators. Abciximab in acute ischemic stroke: a randomized, double-blind, placebo-controlled, dose-escalation study. *Stroke* 2000; **31**: 601–609.

Adams, H. P., Jr, Brott, T. G., Furlan, A. J., *et al*. Guidelines for thrombolytic therapy for acute stroke: a supplement to the guidelines for the management of patients with acute ischemic stroke: a statement for healthcare professionals from a special writing group of the Stroke Council, American Heart Association. *Circulation* 1996; **94**: 1167–1174.

Albers, G. W. Expanding the window for thrombolytic therapy in acute stroke: the potential role of acute MRI in patient selection. *Stroke* 1999; **30**: 2230–2237.

Barber, P. A., Darby, D. G., Desmond, P. M. *et al*. Prediction of stroke outcome with echoplanar perfusion- and diffusion-weighted MRI. *Neurology* 1998; **51**(2): 418–426.

Barnett, H. J. M., Meldrum, H. E., and Eliasziw, M. The appropriate use of carotid endarterectomy. *Canadian Medical Association Journal* 2002; **166**(9): 1169–1179.

Becker, K. J., and Brott, T. G. Approval of the Merci clot retriever: a critical view. *Stroke* 2005; **36**: 400–403.

Buchan, A. M., Barber, P. A., Newcommon, N. *et al*. Effectiveness of t-PA in acute ischemic stroke: outcome relates to appropriateness. *Neurology* 2000; **54**: 679–684.

Butcher, K. S., Parsons, M., MacGregor, L. *et al*. Refining the diffusion-perfusion mismatch hypothesis. *Stroke* 2005; **36**: 1153–1159.

Chalela, J. A., Kand, D. W., Luby, M. *et al*. Early magnetic resonance imaging findings in patients receiving tissue plasminogen activator predict outcome: insights into the pathophysiology of acute stroke in the thrombolysis era. *Annals of Neurology* 2004; **55**(1): 105–112.

Demchuk, A. M., and Coutts, S. B. Alberta Stroke Program Early CT Score in Acute Stroke Triage. *Neuroimaging Clinics of North America* 2005a; **15**: 409–419.

Demchuk, A. M., Hill, M. D., Barber, P. A., *et al*. Importance of early ischemic computed tomography changes using ASPECTS in NINDS rtPA stroke study. *Stroke* 2005b; **36**: 2110.

Desmond, P. M., Lovell, A. C., Rawlinson, A. A., *et al*. The value of apparent diffusion coefficient maps in early cerebral ischemia. *American Journal of Neuroradiology* 2001; **22**: 1260–1267.

Executive Committee for the Asymptomatic Carotid Atherosclerosis Study. Endarterectomy for asymptomatic carotid artery stenosis. *Journal of the American Medical Association* 1995; **273**: 1421–1428.

Executive Committee of the ASITN; Intraarterial Thrombolysis: Ready for Prime Time? *American Journal of Neuroradiology* 2001a; **22**: 55–58.

Executive Committee of the ASITN; Intraarterial thrombolysis. *The American Journal of Neuroradiology AJNR* 2001b; **22**: S18-S21.

Fiebach, J. B., Schellinger, P. D., and Gass, A. Stroke magnetic resonance imaging is accurate in hyperacute intracerebral hemorrhage: a multicenter study on the validity of stroke imaging. *Stroke*, 2004; **35**(2): 502–506.

Fisher, M., Pessin, M. S., and Furian, A. J. ECASS: lessons for future thrombolytic stroke trials. European Cooperative Acute Stroke Study. *Journal of the American Medical Association* 1995; **274**(13): 1058–1059.

Furlan, A., Higashida, R., and Weschler, L. Intra-arterial prourokinase for acute ischemic stroke: The PROACT II Study: a randomized controlled trial. *Journal of the American Medical Association* 1999; **282**: 2003–2011.

Furlan, A. J., Eyding, D., Albers, G. W. *et al*. the DEDAS Investigators. Dose escalation of desmoteplase for acute ischemic stroke (DEDAS): evidence of safety and efficacy 3 to 9 hours after stroke onset. *Stroke* 2006; **37**(5): 1227–1231.

Garcia, J. H. Experimental ischemic stroke: a review. *Stroke* 1984; **15**: 5–14.

Gaskill-Shipley, M. F. Routine CT evaluation of acute stroke. *Neuroimaging Clinics of North America* 1999; **9**(3): 411–422.

Gonzalez, R. G., Schaefer, P. W., Buonanno, F. S. *et al*. Diffusion-weighted MR imaging: diagnostic accuracy in patients imaged within 6 hours of stroke symptom onset. *Radiology* 1999; 210: 155–162.

Grossman, R. I., and Yousem, D. M. *Neuroradiology: the Requisites*. Philadelphia, Pennsylvania: Mosby Publishers, 2003, 195.

Hacke, W., Kaste, M., Fieschi, C. *et al*. Intravenous thrombolysis with recombinant tissue plasminogen activator for acute hemispheric stroke. The European Cooperative Acute Stroke Study (ECASS). *Journal of the American Medical Association* 1995; **274**: 1017–1025.

Hacke, W., Kaste, M., Fieshchi, C. *et al*. Randomized double-blind, placebo-controlled trial of thrombolytic therapy with intravenous alteplase in acute ischemic stroke (ECASS II) *Lancet* 1998a; **352**: 1245–1251.

Hacke, W., Bluhmki, E., Steiner, T. *et al*. Dichotomized efficacy end points and global end-point analysis applied to the ECASS intention-to-treat data set: post hoc analysis of ECASS I. *Stroke* 1998b; **29**: 2073–2075.

Hacke, W., Donnan, G., Fieschi, C. *et al*., on behalf of the ATLANTIS Trials Investigators, ECASS Trials Investigators, NINDS rt-PA Study Group Investigators; Association of outcome with early stroke treatment: pooled analysis of ATLANTIS, ECASS, and NINDS rt-PA stroke trials. *Lancet* 2004; **363**: 768–774.

Hacke, W., Albers, G., Al-Rawi, Y. *et al*. DIAS Study Group; The Desmoteplase in acute ischemic stroke trial (DIAS): a phase II MRI-based 9-hour window acute stroke thrombolysis trial with intravenous desmoteplase. *Stroke* 2005; **36**(11): 66–73.

Heiserman, J. E., Dean, B. L., Hodak, J. A. *et al*. Neurologic complications of cerebral angiography. *American Journal of Neuroradiology* 1994; **15**: 1401.

Hjort, N., Butcher, K., Davis, S. M. *et al*. Magnetic resonance imaging criteria for thrombolysis in acute cerebral infarct. *Stroke* 2005; **36**: 388–410.

Johnston, D. C. and Goldstein, L. B. Clinical carotid endarterectomy decision-making: noninvasive vascular imaging versus angiography. *Neurology* 2001; **56**: 1009–1015.

Kidwell, C. S., Saver, J. L., Mattiello, J. *et al*. Thrombolytic reversal of acute human cerebral ischemic injury shown by diffusion/perfusion magnetic resonance imaging. *Annals of Neurology* 2000; **47**(4): 462–469.

Kidwell, C. S., Saver, J. L., Starkman, S. *et al*. Late secondary ischemic injury in patients receiving intra-arterial thrombolysis. *Annals of Neurology* 2002a; **52**: 698–705.

Kidwell, C. S., Saver, J. L., Villablanca, J. P. *et al*. Magnetic resonance imaging detection of microbleeds before thrombolysis: an emerging application. *Stroke* 2002b; **33**(1): 95–98.

Kidwell, C. S., Chalela, J. A., Saver, J. L. *et al*. Comparison of MRI and CT for detection of acute intracerebral hemorrhage. *Journal of the American Medical Association* 2004; **292**(15): 1823–1830.

Kim, J.-A., Chung, J. I., Yoon, P. H. *et al*. Transient MR signal changes in patients with generalized tonicoclonic seizure or status epilepticus: peri-ictal diffusion-weighted imaging. *American Journal of Neuroradiology* 2001; **22**: 1149–1160.

Kleindorfer, D., Kissela, B., Schneider, A. *et al*. Eligibility for recombinant tissue plasminogen activator in acute ischemic stroke: a population-based study. *Stroke* 2004; **35**(2):E27–E29.

Liebeskind, D. S., Kidwell, C. S. for the UCLA Thrombolysis Investigators. Advanced MR imaging of acute stroke: the University of California at Los Angeles endovascular therapy experience. *Neuroimaging Clinics of North America* 2005; **15**: 455–466.

Lewandowski, C., Frankel, M., Tomsick, T. *et al*. Combined intravenous and intra-arterial r-TPA versus intra-arterial therapy of acute ischemic stroke. Emergency management of stroke (EMS) bridging trial. *Stroke* 1999; **30**: 2598–2605.

Leys, D., Pruvo, J. P., Godefroy, O. *et al*. Prevalence and significance of hyperdense middle cerebral artery in acute stroke. *Stroke* 1992; **23**: 317–324.

Lyden, P. Early major ischemic changes on computed tomography should not preclude use of tissue plasminogen activator. *Stroke 2003*; **34**: 821–822.

Manelfe, C., Larrue, V., von Kummer, R. *et al*. Association of hyperdense middle cerebral artery sign with clinical outcome in patients treated with tissue plasminogen activator. *Stroke* 1999; **30**: 769–772.

Marks, M. P. Computed tomography angiography. *Neuroimaging Clinics of North America* 1996; **6**(4): 899.

Marler, J. R., Tilley, B. C., Lu, M. *et al*. Early stroke treatment associated with better outcome: the NINDS rt-PA stroke study. *Neurology* 2000; **55**(11): 1649–1655.

Meschia, J. F., Miller, D. A., and Brott, T. G. Thrombolytic treatment of acute ischemic stroke. *Mayo Clinic Proceedings* 2002; **77**: 542–551.

Mlynash, M., Eyngorn, I., Bammer, R. *et al*. Automated method for generating the arterial input function on perfusion-weighted M R imaging: validation in patients with stroke. *American Journal of Neuroradiology* 2005; **26**: 1479–1486.

Mullins, M. E., Schaefer, P. W., Sorensen, A. G. *et al*. CT and conventional and diffusion-weighted MR imaging in acute stroke: study in 691 patients at presentation to the emergency department. *Radiology* 2002; **224**: 353–360.

National Institute of Neurological Disorders and Stroke rt-PA Stroke Study Group; Tissue plasminogen activator for acute ischemic stroke. *New England Journal of Medicine*, 1995; **333**: 1581–1587.

NINDS t-PA Stroke Study Group. Intracerebral hemorrhage after intravenous t-PA therapy for ischemic stroke. *Stroke* 1997a Nov; **28**(11): 2109–2118.

NINDS t-PA Stroke Study Group. Generalized efficacy of t-PA for acute stroke: subgroup analysis of the NINDS t-PA stroke trial. *Stroke* 1997b; **28**: 2119–2125.

North American Symptomatic Carotid Endarterectomy Trial Collaborators. Beneficial effect of carotid endarterectomy in symptomatic patients with high-grade carotid stenosis. *New England Journal of Medicine* 1991; **325**: 445–453.

Oppenheim, C., Stanescu, R., Dormont, D. *et al*. False-negative diffusion-weighted MR findings in acute ischemic stroke. *American Journal of Neuroradiology* 2000; **21**: 1434–1440.

Oppenheim, C., Grandin, C., Samson, Y. *et al*. Is there an apparent diffusion coefficient threshold in predicting tissue viability in hyperacute stroke? *Stroke* 2001; **32**: 2486–2491.

Parsons, M. W., Barber, P. A., Chalk, J. *et al*. Diffusion- and perfusion-weighted MRI response to thrombolysis in stroke. *Annals of Neurology*, 2002; **51**(1): 28–37.

Patel, S. C., Levine, S. R., Tilley, B. C., *et al*. Lack of clinical significance of early ischemic changes on computed tomography in acute stroke. *Journal of the American Medical Association* 2001; **286**: 2830–2838.

Qureshi, A. I., Siddiqui, A. M., Suri, M. F. *et al*. Aggressive mechanical clot disruption and low-dose intra-arterial third-generation thrombolytic agent for ischemic stroke: a prospective study. *Neurosurgery* 2002; **51**: 1319–1329.

Qureshi, A. I., Siddiqui, A. M., and Kim, S. H. Reocclusion of recanalized arteries during intra-arterial thrombolysis for acute ischemic stroke. *American Journal of Neuroradiology* 2004; **25**(2): 322–328.

Qureshi, A. I., Suri, M. F., Nasar, A. *et al*. Thrombolysis for ischemic stroke in the United States: data from National Hospital Discharge Survey 1999–2001. *Neurosurgery* 2005; **57**(4): 647–654.

Qureshi, A. I., Ezzedine, M. A., Nasar, M. S. *et al*. Is IV tissue plasminogen activator beneficial in patients with hyperdense artery sign? *Neurology* 2006; **66**: 1171–1174.

Rohl, L., Ostergaard, L., Simonsen, C. Z., *et al*. Viability thresholds of of ischemic penumbra of hyperacute stroke defined by perfusion-weighted MRI and apparent diffusion coefficient. *Stroke* 2001; **32**: 1140–1146.

Romero, J. M., Ackerman, R. H., Dault, N. A. *et al*. Noninvasive evaluation of carotid atery stenosis: indications, strategies and accuracy. *Neuroimaging Clinics of North America* 2005; **15**: 351–365.

Schaefer, P. W., Ozsunar, Y., He, J. *et al*. Assessing tissue viability with MR diffusion and perfusion imaging. *American Journal of Neuroradiology* 2003; **24**: 436–443.

Schafer, P. W., Copen, W. A., Lev, M. H. *et al*. Diffusion-weighted imaging in acute stroke. *Neuroimaging Clinics of North America* 2005; **15**: 503–530.

Schellinger, P. D. The evolving role of advanced MR imaging as a management tool for adult ischemic stroke: a Western European perspective. *Neuroimaging Clinics of North America* 2005; **15**: 245–258.

Shih, L. C., Saver, J. L., Alger, J. R. *et al*. Perfusion-weighted magnetic resonance imaging thresholds identifying core, irreversibly infarcted tissue. *Stroke* 2003; **34**(6): 1425–1430.

Suarez, J., Sunshine, J., Tarr, R. *et al*. Predictors of clinical improvement, angiographic recanalization, and intracranial hemorrhage after intra-arterial thrombolysis for acute ischemic stroke. *Stroke* 1999; **30**: 2094–2100.

Sugg, R. M., Noser, E. A., Shaltoni, H. M. *et al*. Intra-arterial reteplase compared to urokinase for thrombolytic recanalization in acute ischemic stroke. *American Journal of Neuroradiology* 2006; **27**(4): 769–773.

Thijs, V. N., Somford, D. M., Bammer, R. *et al*. Influence of arterial input function on hypoperfusion volumes measured with perfusion-weighted imaging. *Stroke* 2004; **35**(1): 94–98.

Thomalla, G., Schwark, C., Sobesky, J. *et al*. Outcome and symptomatic bleeding complications of intravenous thrombolysis within 6 hours in MRI-selected stroke patients: comparison of a German multicenter study with the pooled data of ATLANTIS, ECASS, and NINDS tPA trials. *Stroke* 2006; **37**: 852–858.

Tomsick, T. A., Brott, T. G., Chambers, A. A., *et al*. Hyperdense middle cerebral artery sign on CT: Efficacy in detecting middle cerebral artery thrombosis. *American Journal of Neuroradiology* 1990; **11**: 473–477.

Tomsick, T., Brott, T., Barsan, W. *et al*. Prognostic value of the hyperdense middle cerebral artery sign and stroke scale score before ultraearly thrombolytic therapy. *American Journal of Neuroradiology* 1996; **17**(1): 79–85.

Unger, M., Littlefield, J., and Gado, M. Water content and water structures in CT and MR signal changes: possible influence in detection of early stroke. *American Journal of Neuroradiology* 1988; **9**: 687–691.

von Kummer, R., Allen, K. L., Holle, R. *et al*. Acute stroke: usefulness of early CT findings before thrombolytic therapy. *Radiology* 1997; **205**: 327–333.

von Kummer, R., Bourquain, H., Bastianello, S. *et al*. Early prediction of irreversible brain damage after ischemic stroke at CT. *Radiology* 2001; **219**: 95–100.

Wolpert, S. M., Bruckmann, H., and Greenlee, R., Neuroradiologic evaluation of patients with acute stroke treated with recombinant tissue plasminogen activator. *American Journal of Neuroradiology* 1993; **14**: 3–13.

Wu, O., Ostergaard, L., and Sorensen, A. G. Technical aspects of perfusion-weighted imaging. *Neuroimaging Clinics of North America* 2005; **15**: 623–637.

Xavier, A. R. and Farkas, J.; Catheter-based recanalization techniques for acute ischemic stroke. *Neuroimaging Clinics of North America* 2005; **15**: 441–453.

Index